Ultimate Review
for the
Neurology Boards

Second Edition

Ultimate Review
for the
Neurology Boards
Second Edition

Hubert H. Fernandez, MD
Associate Professor
Associate Chair of Academic Affairs
Program Director, Neurology Residency and Movement Disorders Fellowship Training
Co-Director, Movement Disorders Center
Director, Clinical Trials for Movement Disorders
Department of Neurology
University of Florida College of Medicine
Gainesville, Florida

Stephan Eisenschenk, MD
Clinical Associate Professor
Clinical Director, Adult Neurology Comprehensive Epilepsy Program
Evelyn F. and William L. McKnight Brain Institute
Department of Neurology
University of Florida College of Medicine
Gainesville, Florida

Michael S. Okun, MD
Adelaide Lackner Associate Professor
Co-Director, Movement Disorders Center
Departments of Neurology, Neurosurgery, and Psychiatry
University of Florida College of Medicine
Gainesville, Florida

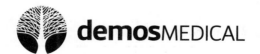

New York

Acquisitions Editor: Beth Barry
Cover Design: Steve Pisano
Compositor: Publication Services, Inc.
Printer: Hamilton Printing

Visit our website at www.demosmedpub.com

Medicine is an ever-changing science. Research and clinical experience are continually expanding our knowledge, in particular our understanding of proper treatment and drug therapy. The authors, editors, and publisher have made every effort to ensure that all information in this book is in accordance with the state of knowledge at the time of production of the book. Nevertheless, the authors, editors, and publisher are not responsible for errors or omissions or for any consequences from application of the information in this book and make no warranty, express or implied, with respect to the contents of the publication. Every reader should examine carefully the package inserts accompanying each drug and should carefully check whether the dosage schedules mentioned therein or the contraindications stated by the manufacturer differ from the statements made in this book. Such examination is particularly important with drugs that are either rarely used or have been newly released on the market.

Library of Congress Cataloging-in-Publication Data

Fernandez, Hubert H.

Ultimate review for the neurology boards / Hubert H. Fernandez, Stephan Eisenschenk, Michael S. Okun.—2nd ed.
     p. ; cm.
     Rev. ed. of: The ultimate review for the neurology boards / Hubert H. Fernandez . . . [et al.]. c2005.
     Includes bibliographical references and index.
     ISBN 978-1-933864-20-4
     1. Neurology—Outlines, syllabi, etc. 2. Neurology—Examinations—Study guides. I. Eisenschenk, Stephan. II. Okun, Michael S. III. Title.
     [DNLM: 1. Neurology—education—Outlines. 2. Internship and Residency—Outlines. 3. Licensure, Medical—Outlines. 4. Specialty Boards—Outlines. WL 18.2 F363u 2009]
    RC343.6.U48 2009
    616.80076—dc22   2009013097

Made in the United States of America
09 10 11 12   5 4 3 2 1

This book is dedicated to

Our beautiful children, Annella Marie, Austin Christian, Aiden Christian, and Jack Robert, for inspiring us daily and reminding us of the meaning of life

And to our wonderful and hardworking residents at the University of Florida, for whom this book was written.

Hubert H. Fernandez

Stephan Eisenschenk

Michael S. OKun

CONTENTS

Text Portion

CONTENTS

Pediatric Neurology

Subspecialties

Basic Neurosciences

Psychiatry, Neurobehavior, and Neuropsychology

CONTENTS

Web Portion

www.ultimateneurology.com
Enter registration code UltNeur2E

Case-Based Neuropathology and Neuroradiology Mini-Atlas

Tumors

Vascular/Stroke

Pediatrics/Congenital

Eye

Neurodegenerative

Other Imaging Sequences

Miscellaneous

Neurophysiology Case Review

EEG

EMG

Sleep Studies

High-Yield Information Flash Cards

Dementia

Neuromuscular

Epilepsy

Movement Disorders

Neurotoxicology and Nutritional Disorders

Sleep Disorders

Pediatric Neurology

Neuro-oncology

Neurogenetics

Medications Data Bank

PREFACE TO THE SECOND EDITION

We are overwhelmed by the reception and feedback we received from the first edition of *Ultimate Review for the Neurology Boards*! We are also flattered to note that since the release of our book, more review manuals have been published to help neurology students navigate their yearly in-service examination and especially for the actual neurology board examination. It is a testament to the growing need for a concise yet comprehensive book that will "put everything together" for the busy clinician, as the fund of knowledge required to competently practice neurology in the new millennium is rapidly and ever expanding.

As in the first edition, this book contains 24 detailed chapters on all subjects included on the neurology board examination (including the Psychiatry portion), as well as a web-based self-assessment and review tool (http://www.ultimateneurology.com) with hundreds of interactive flash cards and cases keyed to specific chapters in this text. For maximal retention with the shortest amount of time, we have kept the expanded outline format of this manual. The topics are arranged from the most familiar (i.e., clinical topics) to the least familiar (i.e., basic neuroscience topics) so that you will read the easiest-to-remember first and the most-likely-to-be-forgotten just before you take your board exams.

However, in this *expanded* second edition, we made even more enhancements:

- More diagrams and illustrations have been added, especially in Chapter 21 on neuroanatomy (such as the ascending and descending spinal tracts, thalamic nuclei and their connections, the complex vestibular and auditory systems, vascular territories, etc.) to help solidify concepts and simplify (and retain) dense information.
- We added a "Mini-Atlas" of high-yield EEG tracings at the end of Chapter 4 to supplement the text.
- We updated the contents in each chapter to stay current with the times. We included the pivotal trials in stroke prevention and treatment; new medications in Parkinson's disease and multiple sclerosis; antibiotics for CNS infections; AAN guidelines and various diagnostic criteria for headaches, multiple sclerosis, sports concussions, and stroke; recently reported gene mutations in various disorders, etc.
- We expanded and clearly marked the "N.B." items that are sprinkled throughout the text. These items are *high yield* information that are *frequently* asked in the Annual Residency In-Service Training Examination (RITE) and actual board examination.
- We added an "Additional Notes" section at the end of each chapter, where the reader can write any update to make this book a "living manual" for use throughout residency training, during board preparation, and beyond.
- We added more tables throughout the text to help organize key concepts and enhance learning and memorization.
- On the website, we have improved the utility of the flashcards, added new stroke and imaging cases, and created two new modules for neurophysiology case review and medications.

- And finally, we added a new section, "Are You *Really* Ready?," which includes practice questions with answers and explanations to help the reader gauge his or her preparedness for the RITE or actual neurology board examination.

We sincerely hope that the improvements made in this expanded second edition of the *Ultimate Review for the Neurology Boards* will make everyone's review effortless and fun.

PREFACE TO THE FIRST EDITION

As medical science continues to expand at an exponential rate, clinicians are forced to carry the burden of keeping abreast with the latest developments in the diagnosis and treatment of disorders in their specialty to ensure that every patient, at the minimum, receives the ever-changing current standard of care from his or her doctor. Neurology as a specialty is no exception. In fact, fueled by the discoveries during the "decade of the brain" in the 1990s, neurology is now at the forefront of cutting-edge research and innovation. Almost every day, there is a new drug for epilepsy, Parkinson's disease, or multiple sclerosis; a faster magnetic resonance imaging machine; a new imaging technique; a diet that delays Alzheimer's disease; a vitamin that prevents strokes; and so on.

As the bar is raised to improve the standard of care, so is the bar of required medical knowledge for today's clinicians. Unfortunately, the painful reality of competency testing is a necessary evil with good intentions. It is not, by any means, a perfect process, but it tries to ensure that neurologists certified by their own society have been carefully critiqued and deemed safe and competent to provide the ultimate privilege of improving the lives of others.

It is the aim of this book to ease the pain of this almost essential step in a clinician's maturation process. We hope to lessen the anxiety of needing to acquire and retain a huge volume of, at times, seemingly trivial medical information. We hope this book provides the framework needed for the candidate's successful completion of his or her certification examination.

Although this book is not meant to replace the more detailed classic texts of neurology, it does provide a concise review of the clinically important aspects of neurology that a neurologist in training might find useful for both day-to-day patient care and preparation for the yearly in-service examination (e.g., Residency In-Service Training Examination [RITE]).

The practicing clinician might also find this book useful when the date for board recertification approaches.

From those of us who have crossed the finish line, we say, "Good luck, Colleague!"

SPECIAL CONTRIBUTIONS

M. Cecilia Lansang, MD, MPH
Assistant Professor, Interim Chief, Division of Endocrinology
University of Florida College of Medicine
Neuroendocrinology

Ramon L. Rodriguez, MD

Clinical Assistant Professor
Director, Movement Disorders Clinic
University of Florida College of Medicine
Pediatric Neurology

Dylan P. Wint, MD

Assistant Professor
Department of Psychiatry
Emory University School of Medicine
Adult Psychiatry
Child Psychiatry
Neurobehavior and Neuropsychology

William Friedman, MD

Professor and Chairman
Department of Neurosurgery
University of Florida College of Medicine
Cases (Web-based Review)

Kelly D. Foote, MD

Co-Director, Movement Disorders Center
Department of Neurosurgery
University of Florida College of Medicine
Cases (Web-based Review)

David Peace

Medical Illustrator
Department of Neurosurgery
Anatomic Illustrations

Fabio J. Rodriguez, MD

Associate Professor
Department of Radiology
University of Florida College of Medicine
Cases (Web-based Review)

Ilona Schmalfuss, MD

Assistant Professor
Department of Radiology (Neuroradiology)
University of Florida College of Medicine
Cases (Web-based Review)

Anthony T. Yachnis, MD

Associate Director of Anatomic Pathology
Chief, Neuropathology Section
Department of Pathology, Immunology, and Laboratory Medicine
University of Florida College of Medicine
Cases (Web-based Review)

INTRODUCTION

Preparing for Your Boards

I. How to Use This Book and Web-Based Review

As you prepare for your neurology board examination, you will be faced with the dilemma of what books to read. Neurology covers a broad spectrum of disease processes. Moreover, your certification examination will also include psychiatry and other neurologic subspecialties such as neuro-ophthalmology, neuro-otology, and neuroendocrinology, to name a few. Unfortunately, there is not one convenient book that you can read that will contain everything you need to know to pass your boards. Although this book is entitled *Ultimate* **Review for the Neurology Boards**, it is not intended to be your single source of study material in preparing for your examination. Rather, it presumes that throughout your residency training, or at the very least, several months before your board examination date, you will have already read primary references and textbooks (and, therefore, carry a considerable fund of knowledge) on the specific broad categories of neurology. However, because you cannot possibly retain all the information you have assimilated, we offer this book and web review tool as a convenient way of tying it all together. It is best used 1–3 months before your examination date.

Ultimate **Review for the Neurology Boards** contains 24 detailed chapters on all subjects included on the neurology board examination, as well as a web-based self-assessment and review tool (http://www.ultimateneurology.com) with hundreds of interactive flash cards and cases keyed to specific chapters in the text.

For maximal retention with the shortest amount of time, we have used an expanded outline format in the *text portion* of this manual. The topics are arranged from the most familiar (i.e., clinical topics) to the least familiar (i.e., basic neuroscience topics) so that you will read the easiest-to-remember first and the most-likely-to-be-forgotten just before you take your boards.

The main headings and subtopics are in **bold**. A few phrases or a short paragraph is spent on subtopics that we think are of particular importance. Crucial or essential data within the outline are *italicized*. Thus, we present three levels of learning in each chapter. We suggest that you first read the entire chapter, including the brief sentences on each subtopic. After which, you should go back a second time, focusing only on the headings and subtopics in **bold** and the *italicized* words within the outline. If you need to go back a third time to test yourself, or, alternatively, if you feel you already have a solid fund of knowledge on a certain topic, you can just concentrate on the backbone outline in **bold** to make sure you have, indeed, retained everything.

Whenever appropriate, illustrations are liberally sprinkled throughout the text to tap into your "visual memory." Quick pearls (such as mnemonics to remember long lists and confusing terminology, tables to organize a complex body of information) and high-yield topics are preceded with this symbol "**NB:**" (for *nota bene*, Latin for "note well"), to make sure you do not miss them.

Some chapters overlap. For example, some diseases discussed in the Pediatric Neurology chapter and the Neurogenetics chapter can also be found in the individual chapters of the Clinical Neurology section. This is intended to maximize memory retention through repetition.

The *interactive web component* of this manual presents a case-based "mini-atlas" on gross and microscopic neuropathology and, whenever possible, their corresponding neuroradiologic picture. For this edition, we have also developed a totally new case module for neurophysiology review. All of the cases are designed to help you think through histories, imaging, and pathology and to prepare you for the "pictures" that will appear on the boards. We believe that pictures are most remembered when cases are tagged along with them. After all, your residency training was predominantly a case-based learning program, and recognizing these pictures correctly is only useful if you can apply or relate them to the daily cases you confront in your practice. The web component also contains several hundred terms in flash card format. The flash cards are a tool designed to help you master difficult-to-remember minutiae. Based on excellent comments from users of the first edition, we have improved the flashcards to be more intuitive. In addition, we added a dedicated section for reviewing medications.

The flash cards are divided into nine categories (based on the chapters in the textbook) of difficult-to-remember facts that often appear on board exams. Each flash card is paired as a term with a second flash card that contains its definition. The design of the flash cards is such that you will be able to quickly drill yourself on the computer until you have memorized all of the rare facts that may appear on the examination. Additionally, each flash card contains a reference to the chapter(s) in which you may review the details of the subject.

After reviewing the categories of questions, you may choose to look at either *each* category of flash cards in random order or *all* of the flash cards in random order. The randomized feature allows you to solidify your knowledge of difficult-to-remember facts.

As a suggested approach for using this book and web-based review, you might first review the relevant chapters in the book and then review the related category of flash cards so as to test your knowledge and understanding of the print material. Later, you can review the flash cards in a given category in random order to help maintain your currency and understanding of the material. Finally, after reading the entire book and reviewing the flash cards by section, both in order and randomly, you may wish to review all of the flash cards in random order to determine how well you have learned and retained the material in the review book.

The cases are divided into seven categories (tumor, vascular/stroke, pediatrics/congenital, eye, neurodegenerative, other imaging sequences, and miscellaneous). Cases include combinations of common and uncommon histories, imaging, and pathology. The cases are designed to allow you to think through the answer based on the information provided before proceeding to the next screen within the case. For example, many cases offer a history, then an image, then the imaging diagnosis, then the pathology, and then the pathologic diagnosis. It is in this way that we hope you will learn to think through cases and recognize common pictures. You may review the cases in order in each topic module, or you may select a random presentation of cases within any given module. We have also created a new section for neurophysiology review containing case examples of EEG, EMG, and sleep studies.

For the oral board preparation, this Introduction includes tips on how to prepare for your oral boards, how to lessen your anxiety, and how to improve your presentation skills.

Good luck and we hope you pass your boards in one attempt!

II. Preparing for Your Board Examination

Although most residents initially feel that after a busy residency training, it is better to "take a break" and postpone their certification examination, we believe that, in general, it is best to take your examination right after residency, when "active" and "passive" learning are at their peaks. There will never be "a perfect time" (or "enough time") to review for your boards. The board examination is a present-day reality that you will need to prepare for whether you are exhausted, in private practice, expecting your first child, renovating your newly purchased 80-year-old house, or burning candles in your research laboratory. You just need to squeeze in the time to study.

Here are a few pointers to help you prepare for the Board Examination. All or some of them may be applicable to you:

A. Board preparation starts from day 1 of your residency training. Although most residency programs are clinically oriented and have a case-based structure of learning, here are some suggestions as to how you can create an "active" learning process out of your clinical training, rather than just passively learning from your patients and being content with acquiring clinical skills.

1. Imagine you are on your sixth month of a boring ward rotation carrying eight patients on your service. Below is a table containing the diagnoses of your patients in the neurology ward and the reading initiative we recommend.

Patient	Diagnosis	Reading initiative
1	Thalamic lacunar stroke	Master the anatomy of the thalamus.
2	Embolic stroke	Become familiar with the literature on the use of heparin vs. aspirin.
3	Guillain-Barré syndrome	Master the differential diagnosis of axonal vs. demyelinating polyneuropathy.
4	Amyotrophic lateral sclerosis	Master the differential diagnosis of motor neuron diseases.
5	25-year-old with stroke, unclear etiology	Master the data on stroke risk factors.
6	Seizure breakthrough for overnight observation	Know all the mechanisms of action of antiepileptic agents.
7	Hemorrhagic stroke	Know and be able to differentiate the magnetic resonance imaging picture of a hyperacute, acute, subacute, chronic bleed.
8	Glioblastoma multiforme (a "dump" from neurosurgery)	Know the pathology of all glial tumors

2. Always carry a small notebook that fits in your coat pocket so you can write down all the questions and observations that may arise in the course of your day. If possible, do not sleep without answering those questions. Likewise, jot down all the new information you have learned. Read through these notes one more time before you call it a night.

3. Follow your grand rounds schedule. Read the topic(s) beforehand. This will help you in two ways: (1) the talk itself will serve as reinforcement because you already read about it; and (2) you can ask more intelligent questions that will, at the very least,

impress your colleagues and mentors, if not make you learn and appreciate neurology even more.

4. For the driven resident: have a monthly schedule of books or book chapters to read. Maximize your reading on your light or elective rotations. On the average, a "good" resident reads 25–50 pages per day (from journals, notes, books, etc.). If you read more than 50 pages per day, you are driven and will be rewarded with an almost effortless board review period. If you read less than 10 pages per day, or, even worse, are an occasional reader, you are relying on passive learning and will need to make up a lot of lost time (and knowledge) during your board review.

B. Take your RITE/in-service examination seriously. If possible, prepare for it weeks in advance. People who do well every year are the ones who pass their written board examination on the first attempt.

C. Know all board examination requirements several months before you finish your residency training. Know all the deadlines. Check the name on your identification and the name on your admission slip to make sure they are identical. Contact the American Board of Psychiatry and Neurology (ABPN) if they are not. Ideally, you should be distracted as little as possible when your examination date approaches.

D. Start your formal board review midway (that is January 2) of your senior year. Make a general, realistic schedule. Do not make it too ambitious or too detailed. Otherwise, you will find yourself frustrated and always catching up to your schedule. As we mentioned, there will never be a perfect time to study for your boards—you need to create your own time.

E. In general, start with topics you know the most about (and, therefore, are least likely to forget), such as clinical neurology, and end with topics you know the least about (and, thus, are more likely to forget in a short amount of time), such as neurogenetics, metabolic disorders, neuroanatomy, neurochemistry, etc. The flow of this book is arranged such that the clinical topics are first and the technical topics are last.

F. Use your book allowance wisely. Read and underline books during residency that fit your taste and that you are likely to use for your board review. Underlined books are less overwhelming, provide a sense of security that you have already been through the material (even if you have forgotten its contents), make review time more efficient, and significantly reinforce learning and retention.

G. End your formal review at least two weeks before the date of your written boards. Earmark one week for the psychiatry portion (do not forget to read on child psychiatry) and one week for recapping high-yield topics; questions and answers; looking at radiology and pathology pictures; and reading the answers to past RITE/in-service examinations (they do repeat!).

H. Arrive at your examination site city at least 24 hours before. You do not want to realize on the day of your examination that your hotel reservation was inadvertently misplaced or that your flight was canceled because of a snow storm. Print directions to your testing site on both *Yahoo* (http://www.yahoo.com) and *MapQuest* (http://www.mapquest.com). Make sure your cell phone is fully charged and you have your driver's license with you.

I. You might consider bringing ear plugs, an extra sweater, and a reliable watch. When one of us took our boards in the basement of a hospital, there was a general announcement through the public-address system every 30 minutes. We have heard different stories: the heater was not working, a dog convention was going on in the next room, etc. It is best to be prepared.

J. If this is the second or third time you are taking the Boards, consider the benefits of a small study group or having a study partner. You will be amazed that two or three people assigned the same topic to read will emphasize different items. It could very well be that you are underlining the wrong words and need someone to give you a different perspective. At the very least, a study group will keep you on pace with your schedule.

III. Preparing for the Oral Portion (for those who graduated residency on or before June 30, 2007)

Adult neurology candidates will take three examinations:

- One 1-hour examination in clinical adult neurology (with a live patient)
- One 1-hour examination in clinical adult neurology (case vignettes)
- One 1-hour examination in clinical child neurology (case vignettes)

Child neurology candidates will take three examinations:

- One 1-hour examination in clinical child neurology (with a live patient)
- One 1-hour examination in clinical child neurology (case vignettes)
- One 1-hour examination in clinical adult neurology (case vignettes)

NB: Distribution and number of adult and pediatric case vignettes may vary from year to year.

Here are some tips to help you prepare for your oral boards:

1. Right after you pass the written portion, start preparing the materials to read for your oral boards. You will need a good book for (1) differential diagnosis of adult neurologic disorders, (2) differential diagnosis for pediatric neurologic disorders, and (3) neurologic emergencies (pediatric and adult) and critical care neurology (pediatric and adult).
2. As you read and prepare, create a list of all the medications per disease and memorize the exact dose and frequency of each. Pay particular attention to the doses of all antiepileptic agents (especially in status epilepticus of both the adult and the child), drugs that lower intracranial pressure, plasmapheresis, intravenous immunoglobulin, interferons, etc.
3. Practice! Practice! Practice! This is the only way you can gain confidence in your delivery. Practice case vignettes with someone you are least comfortable with, someone in your department who has been an examiner several times, or someone who recently took (and preferably passed) the oral boards.
4. If your funds permit, consider taking oral board review courses given before the examination. Participating in it gives you more practice and makes you more confident, and watching others mess up their presentation allows you to learn from their mistakes. Remember, the oral portion is only a "fair" examination and a true test of your knowledge and competence as a clinician if your nervousness is not in the way.
5. Prepare your medical bag. Have all your instruments ready.

On the day itself . . .

1. Do not forget to wear a reliable watch. You may be going from one hospital to another for the three parts of your oral boards.
2. Go to the bathroom before you leave your hotel room.
3. Wear formal, conventional, neat yet comfortable attire. Make sure there are no holes or stains. Blue, black, and dark green are the best colors. Have a neat/conventional haircut. No earrings for men. Cut your nails. In other words, do not do or wear anything that will attract undue attention. Give the impression that you are a mature, balanced, intelligent, humble, and affable neurologist.

4. The first thing your examiners would like to make sure of is that you are a *safe* neurologist. Therefore try to stick with conventional treatment options (especially in the neurologic emergencies and critical care portions). If you are making a last ditch effort, and you have an unconventional plan for your patient, then say "at this point, I shall consider what some neurologists may classify as nonstandard . . ."

5. Do not place used safety pins back in your medical bag. Do not hurt the patient. Be nice to your patient and treat him/her with respect and dignity. Never show you are frustrated or getting impatient.

6. The next thing your examiners would like to make sure of is that you are an *organized* and *practical* thinker. When you begin your discussion, do not paraphrase the entire case. Choose a major problem (e.g., I am essentially faced with a 3-year-old boy with monoplegia. . .), then state and discuss your differential diagnosis pertinent to your case only, and end with your impression. You do not need to show off and give them a laundry list of differential diagnoses, especially if it is not pertinent to your case. It will only irritate your examiners.

7. The final thing they want to know is that you are *competent*. Make sure you know the basic diagnostic test and treatment for each of your differentials. They can interrupt you anytime to elaborate on a particular diagnosis. Do not forget to state the need to obtain vital signs, electrocardiogram, complete blood count, routine chemistry, urinalysis, blood culture, chest X-ray, etc., to rule out a general medical condition.

8. When given the choice, we recommend that you ask your examiners to read each case of the vignettes for you. This allows you to organize your thoughts while the case is being read.

9. Pretend that you have a panel of medical students and that you are teaching them. Answer your examiner's questions as if you are lecturing to students. They may not know the answers to their own questions and they are not necessarily more knowledgeable than you in a particular subject. The only clear difference is that they already passed the boards.

10. For the most part, your examiners are there to pass you, not to fail you. Be receptive to the clues they might be giving you to arrive at the correct diagnosis or answer.

11. For live pediatric cases, do not forget to check the head circumference (and if abnormal, check the parents' as well). Always do a funduscopy. Check for neurocutaneous lesions.

12. For live adult cases, do not forget to check for bruits, pulses, and blood pressure of both arms for stroke patients; check for tongue fasciculations for motor neuron disease patients; make patients with tremors write a sentence, perform a task, and draw concentric circles.

13. Always maximize the 30 minutes given to you to examine your live patient. Never finish early.

14. Take out all the instruments you will need to examine the patient and lay them out neatly on the table. Put them back in your medical bag one at a time after each use (except for the safety pin, which goes to the trash can). That way, at the end of your neurologic examination, you will be reminded if you missed a test because the instrument for that test would still be on the table. When your table is clean, you are confident that you performed a thorough neurologic examination.

15. Keep on talking. If you do not know the answer to a question, first tell them what you know about the topic or question before telling them that you do not know the answer to the particular question. But be honest. Do not bluff.

16. Be aware of the body language you send. Put your hands together or place them on your lap. Do not swivel your chair. Do not slouch. Do not cross your legs. Do not appear too relaxed or too tense. Show some calmness and sincerity.

Despite the horror stories on the oral portion that are passed on from generation to generation, it is actually, in some respects, a more balanced and fair assessment of your competence in your chosen field than the written portion of the boards. Just try to relax and show them that you are a safe, respectful, organized, practical, and competent clinician.

Clinical Neurology

CHAPTER 1

Stroke, Trauma, and Intensive Care (Including Brain Death)

I. Definitions

A. **Stroke:** sudden, nonconvulsive, focal neurologic deficit; apoplexy/shock/cerebrovascular accident (CVA); neurologic condition/deficit continues for >24 hours

B. **Transient ischemic attack (TIA):** focal neurologic deficit lasting *<24 hours; <20%* of strokes have prior TIA, but when present it *predates infarction rather than hemorrhage*

C. *Reversible ischemic neurologic deficit:* symptoms that exceed 24 hours and resolve within 3 weeks

D. *Cerebral infarction transient symptoms:* stroke based on brain imaging with fleeting symptoms

II. Epidemiology

A. **Stroke incidence:** the number of first cases of stroke over a defined time interval in a defined population; in the United States, *400,000–500,000 new cases* per year, with 175,000 deaths per year.

B. **Stroke prevalence:** measures the total number of cases, new and old, at a particular time in a defined population; in the United States, stroke *prevalence is 3,000,000.*

C. Stroke is the *third most common* cause of death in the United States; overall, accounts for 10% of all deaths in most industrialized countries.

D. With the decrease in coronary artery disease (CAD) and malignant hypertension, a 20% decrease in stroke incidence was noted between 1968 and 1976; but an increase was noted in incidence between 1980 and 1984, despite continued improvement in hypertension control, because of widespread use of computed axial tomography scan.

III. Frequency of Strokes

Type	Merritt's textbook of neurology	Mohr and Sacco
Ischemic	70–80%	
Thrombosis		15%
Embolism		25%
Lacunar		10%

Type	Merritt's textbook of neurology	Mohr and Sacco
Hemorrhage	10–30%	
Subarachnoid hemorrhage (SAH)	⅓–½	12%
Intracerebral hemorrhage (ICH)	⅔–½	13%
Others		
Arteritis/dissection	<5%	
Unknown		25%

IV. Pathophysiology
A. Cerebral blood flow (CBF)

Normal	*50 cc/100 g/min*
Change in electrophysiologic activity	20 cc/100 g/min
Irreversible ischemia	*10 cc/100 g/min*

B. Oxygen delivery equals the CBF multiplied by the blood oxygen content:

$$DO_2 = CBF \times Ca_{O_2}$$

C. When blood supply is interrupted for 30 seconds, brain metabolism is altered: *1 minute, neuronal function ceases; 5 minutes,* a chain of events that result in cerebral *infarction ensues;* evolution of an infarct: local vasodilatation → stasis of the blood column with segmentation of red cells; edema → necrosis of brain tissue
  1. *Coagulation necrosis:* the infarcted area is pale and swollen—blurred border between gray and white matter at *6–24 hours; "red neuron"* (neuronal shrinkage and eosinophilia); astrocytes and oligodendrocytes; microglial cells disintegrate and give rise to somewhat granular appearance of the background; polymorphonucleocytes surround vessels; red cell extravasation; edematous swelling (may occur in 3–4 days).
  2. *Liquefaction (or absorption):* represents removal of debris by macrophages *72–96 hours later;* glitter cells—lipid laden macrophages; sharpened demarcation between normal and infarcted tissue; tissue becomes mushy; there is hypertrophy (12–36 hours), then hyperplasia (48 hours to months) of astrocytes; macrophages clear debris at 1 cc/month.
  3. Atherosclerosis is the chief etiologic factor of CVA; it is rare for cerebral arteries to develop plaques beyond their first major branching; it is rare for cerebellar and ophthalmic arteries to show atheromatous involvement, except with hypertension; site of predilection.
    a. Bifurcation of common carotid artery into external carotid artery and internal carotid artery (ICA)—62%
    b. Origin of middle cerebral artery (MCA)—10%
    c. Origin of anterior cerebral artery (ACA)—1%
    d. Origin of vertebrobasilar artery—15%
    e. Others—11%
  4. Although atheromatous plaques narrow the lumen, complete occlusion is always the consequence of thrombosis; atherosclerotic thrombosis involves the deposition of fibrin and platelets.

V. Risk Factors
A. Nonmodifiable risk factors
  1. *Age: strongest determinant of stroke;* incidence rises exponentially with age >65 years

2. Sex: *men*
3. Race: in the United States, *blacks* (intracranial > extracranial disease) followed by *Hispanic = whites* (extracranial > intracranial disease); in Japan, hemorrhage is more common than atherothrombosis

B. **Modifiable risk factors**
1. *Hypertension: the most powerful risk factor after age;* risk rises proportionately with increased blood pressure (BP), especially among blacks; the risk for 10 mm Hg rise in BP is 1.9 for men and 1.7 for women, and, even in mild hypertension, the risk is approximately 1.5; elevated systolic BP or diastolic BP, or both, increases risk by accelerating the progression of atherosclerosis and predisposing to small vessel disease
2. *Cardiac disease:* atrial fibrillation; valvular heart disease; myocardial infarction (MI), CAD, left ventricular hypertrophy, and perhaps mitral valve prolapse
   a. *Chronic atrial fibrillation* affects >1,000,000 Americans with a *fivefold increase in stroke risk; stroke risk doubles in the presence of congestive heart failure.*
   b. *CAD* increases stroke risk by twofold.
   c. *Congestive heart failure* increases stroke risk by fourfold.
   d. *Left ventricular hypertrophy* carries a 2.3-fold increased stroke risk.
   e. Mitral annular calcification carries a 2.1-fold increased stroke risk.
3. *Diabetes: carries a 1.5–3.0 stroke risk,* depending on the type and severity; the effect is found in men and women, independent of age and hypertension (however, in the Framingham study, it was found independent only for older women)
4. *Blood lipids:* the degree of progression of atherosclerosis is directly related to cholesterol and low-density lipoprotein and inversely related to high-density lipoprotein; there is a quadratic or U-shaped relationship between serum total cholesterol and stroke; there is a dose-dependent, inverse relationship between high-density lipoprotein and TIA; others: lipoprotein A is associated with stroke risk; low-serum cholesterol may be associated with increased risk for intracranial hemorrhage (still needs confirmation)
5. *Cigarette smoking:* 1.7 (1.5–2.0) increased risk for stroke, greatest in heavy smokers and quickly reduced in those who quit; independent of carotid artery plaque thickness; stroke risk is greatest for SAH, intermediate for cerebral infarction, lowest for cerebral hemorrhage
6. *Alcohol:* the risk is controversial; in Framingham studies, a *J-shaped* relationship shows increased risk with moderate to heavy alcohol consumption (>14 oz of alcohol per month) and decreased risk with light drinking compared to nondrinkers; 2.2-fold increased risk in SAH for more than two drinks per day; not a risk factor for MI or CAD; mechanism is probably associated with hypertension
7. *TIA:* the annual stroke risk is 1–15%, with the 1st year after the TIA having the greatest stroke risk (>10× increased risk for stroke in the 1st year and 7× during the next 5 years); amaurosis fugax has a better outcome than hemiparetic TIA; TIA precedes cerebral infarction in <20% of cases
8. *Asymptomatic carotid artery disease:* >75% stenosis = annual stroke risk of 3.3%; <75% stenosis = annual stroke risk of 1.3%; Asymptomatic Carotid Atherosclerosis Study: prophylactic surgery was beneficial in >60% stenosis by angiography (provided the perioperative morbidity/mortality was low)

C. **Potential risk factors**
1. *Moderate physical activity:* reduced risk of stroke, whereas more vigorous activity did not provide further protection
2. *Oral contraceptives:* mostly in older users (>35 y/o); those who *smoke* and with other risk factors associated with thromboembolism; the risk is highest for SAH, especially for

older smokers; in a Framingham study, the stroke risk is 2.0 in women; however, the Nurses Health Study and National Health and Nutrition Examination Survey reported decreased risk with use of postmenopausal hormones

3. *Drug abuse:* includes opiates (e.g., heroin, amphetamines, cocaine, phencyclidine); mechanism is dramatic increase in BP/MI/intravenous (i.v.) drug abuse arteritis (e.g., amphetamine causes necrotizing angiitis of medium-sized arteries)/toxicity/vasospasm/hypersensitivity; cocaine causes infarction and hemorrhage in any mode of drug administration; seizures are the most common neurologic complication; mechanism for cocaine-induced stroke: vasculitis, vasospasm, MI, ventricular arrhythmia; it is prudent to perform an angiogram on any patient with stroke due to cocaine use to look for saccular aneurysm or arteriovenous malformation (AVM)

4. *Coagulopathy*
   a. Disorders predisposing to hemorrhage: classic *hemophilia, factor deficiencies* (9, von Willebrand, 6, 7, 12, 13)
   b. *Antithrombin III:* predisposes to *venous thrombosis* and pulmonary embolism; a few cases of arterial thrombosis have been described; can be inherited as autosomal dominant or acquired (in severe renal disease–nephrotic syndrome)
   c. *Protein S* deficiency: may cause stroke, but data unclear
   d. *Lupus anticoagulants:* can cause *venous or arterial* thrombosis; most have prolonged partial thromboplastin time (PTT); lab confirmation: false-positive VDRL, lupus anticoagulant antibodies, radioimmunoassay, or enzyme-linked immunosorbent assay for anticardiolipin antibodies; history of spontaneous abortions
   e. *Antiphospholipid antibodies* syndrome: *young female*; minority with systemic lupus erythematosus (SLE); history of thrombosis or CVA and history of *spontaneous abortion*; pathology: thrombotic occlusion without inflammation; labs: 50% have low titer antinuclear antibody, 33% have low platelets, 50% have prolonged PTT (lupus anticoagulant +); echocardiogram—may have mitral valve lesions; associated signs and symptoms: *migraine, amaurosis, chorea, livedo reticularis*; the incidence of antibodies in TIA or stroke patients is 6–8%

5. Others
   a. *Heredity*
   b. *Patent foramen ovale (PFO)*
   c. *Atrial septal defect*
   d. *Spontaneous echo contrast ("smoke" finding on transesophageal echocardiography)*
   e. *Aortic arch plaques (>4 mm) presumed hypercoagulable states*
   f. *Homocystinuria*
   g. *Migraine*
   h. *Snoring*
   i. *Other inflammatory disease associated with stroke: ulcerative colitis, Crohn's disease, Wegener's granulomatosis*
   j. *Sickle cell disease:* 10% of hemoglobin SS will develop stroke (75% being arterial thrombosis, 25% from ICH); sickle cell patients are at increased risk for stroke due to *cerebral infarction, SAH, ICH, venous sinus thrombosis*
   k. Risk for *sagittal sinus thrombosis: postpartum* female
   l. *Epidural hematoma* caused by laceration of *middle meningeal* arteries
   m. *Subdural hematoma* caused by laceration of *bridging veins*

VI. Clinical Stroke Syndromes

A. **Common carotid/ICA:** anatomy: the right common carotid artery arises from the brachiocephalic (innominate) artery, and the left common carotid directly from the aortic arch; the common carotids ascend to the C4 level (just below the angle of the jaw) then divides into external and internal branches; common carotid occlusion accounts for <1%, most are due to internal carotid; most variable of clinical syndromes, because ICA is not an end vessel, no part of the brain is completely dependent on it; presentations range from devastating major hemispheric infarction to small cortical lesions; also dependent on the state of anastomosis

1. *Two mechanisms:* embolus from and ICA thrombus goes to distal vessel *(artery-to-artery embolism)* or occlusion of carotid artery (thrombosis) leads to ischemia in the distal field *(watershed or borderzone, 17%);* the incidence of anterior vs. posterior borderzone infarcts is approximately equal

2. *MCA/posterior cerebral artery (PCA) borderzone:* affects temporo-occipital portion of distal MCA territory; produces quadrant/hemianopic field defect, transcortical aphasia, or hemi-inattention (depending on hemisphere)

3. *MCA/ACA borderzone:* affects superficial frontal and parietal parasagittal cortical area; produces *proximal >> distal sensory motor deficit* in the contralateral upper extremities; variable lower extremity involvement, sparing face and hand

4. ICA nourishes *optic nerve and retina: transient monocular blindness occurs in 25%* of symptomatic carotid occlusion; stenosis, ulcerations, dissections of ICA may be a source of fibrin platelet emboli or may cause reduction of blood flow

B. **MCA:** most frequent; *principal mechanism is embolism;* four segments: M1—main MCA trunk with deep penetrating vessels and lenticulostriate arteries, M2—in the Sylvian fissure where the two divisions arise, M3—all cortical branches, M4—over the cortical surface

1. *Territory* encompasses
   a. Cortex and white matter of the *inferior parts of frontal lobe,* including areas 4 and 6, centers for lateral gaze, Broca's area
   b. Cortex and white matter of *parietal lobe,* including sensory cortex and *angular and supramarginal*
   c. *Superior parts of the temporal lobe* and insula, including Wernicke's area
   d. Penetrating branches: *putamen, outer globus pallidus, posterior limb of internal capsule, body of caudate, corona radiata*

2. *Stem occlusion:* blocking deep penetrating and superficial cortical branches—*contralateral hemiplegia* (face, arm, and leg), *hemianesthesia, homonymous hemianopia,* deviation of head and eyes toward side of the lesion; left hemisphere lesions—*global aphasia;* right hemisphere—*anosognosia and amorphosynthesis;* stem occlusion is relatively infrequent (2–5% of MCA occlusion); most are embolic that drift into superficial branches

3. *Superior division:* supplying rolandic and prerolandic areas—dense sensorimotor of face and arm >> leg; ipsilateral deviation of head and eye; brachiofacial paralysis, no impairment of consciousness; left-sided lesions—initial global aphasia, then predominantly motor
   a. *Ascending frontal branch:* initial mutism and mild comprehension defect, then slightly dysfluent, agrammatic speech with normal comprehension
   b. *Rolandic branches:* sensorimotor paresis with severe dysarthria but little aphasia
   c. *Cortical-subcortical branch:* brachial monoplegia
   d. *Ascending parietal:* no sensorimotor defect, only a conduction aphasia

4. *Inferior division: less frequent* than superior; nearly always due to cardiogenic emboli; left sided—*Wernicke's* aphasia; right sided—*left visual neglect;* superior *quadrantanopia* or homonymous hemianopia; agitated confusional state from temporal lobe damage

5. Other cortical syndromes
   a. Dominant parietal lobe: *Gerstmann syndrome*—finger agnosia, acalculia, right-left confusion, alexia (supramarginal gyrus), alexia with agraphia (angular gyrus), and ideational apraxia

      b. Nondominant parietal lobe: anosognosia, autoprosopagnosia, neglect, constructional apraxia, dressing apraxia

      c. Bilateral anterior poles of the temporal lobes: *Klüver-Bucy* syndrome; docility, hyperoral, hypersexual, hypomobile, hypermetamorphosis, visual agnosia

NB: In addition to prosopagnosia (deficit in facial recognition), other *non-dominant* hemisphere deficits include: auditory agnosia (deficit in recognition of sounds), autotopagnosia (inability to localize stimuli on the affected side), phonagnosia (inability to recognize familiar voices). Pure word deafness (inability to recognize spoken language) is a *dominant* hemisphere deficit!

      d. Aphasias

Type	Comprehension	Fluency	Repetition	Naming
Broca	Normal	Impaired	Impaired	Impaired
Wernicke	Impaired	Normal	Impaired	Impaired
Conduction	Normal	Normal	Impaired	Normal/impaired
Transcortical motor	Normal	Impaired	Normal	Impaired
Transcortical sensory	Impaired	Normal	Normal	Impaired
Mixed transcortical	Impaired	Impaired	Normal	Impaired
Global	Impaired	Impaired	Impaired	Impaired

C. **ACA:** supplies anterior three-fourths of the medial surface of cerebral hemisphere, including medial-orbital surface of frontal lobe, strip of lateral surface of cerebrum along the superior border; anterior four-fifths of corpus callosum; deep branches supplying anterior limb of internal capsule, inferior part of caudate, anterior globus pallidus

    1. *Stem occlusion:* proximal to the anterior communicating artery, usually well tolerated; if both arteries arise from one ACA, paraplegia, abulia, motor aphasia, frontal lobe personality changes; distal to the anterior communicating artery—sensorimotor defect of contralateral foot >> shoulder and arm; motor in foot and leg >> thigh; sensory is more of discriminative modalities and is mild or absent; head and eyes deviated ipsilaterally, urinary incontinence, contralateral grasp reflex, paratonic rigidity (gegenhalten); left sided—may have alien hand

    2. *Branch occlusions:* fragments of the total syndrome (usually spastic weakness and cortical sensory loss of foot or leg); occlusion of Heubner's artery: may give rise to transcorticomotor aphasia

    3. *Penetrating branches:* transient hemiparesis, dysarthria, and abulia or agitation; left side—stuttering and language difficulty; right side—visuospatial neglect; bilateral caudate—syndrome of inattentiveness, abulia, forgetfulness, sometimes agitation and psychosis

D. **Anterior choroidal artery:** long narrow artery from ICA just above the posterior communicating artery; supplies: internal globus pallidus, posterior limb of internal capsule, contiguous structures like the optic tract; choroid plexus of lateral ventricles; clinical: contralateral hemiplegia, hemihypesthesia, and homonymous hemianopsia; cognitive function is spared; no uniform syndrome

E. **PCA:** in 70%, both PCAs originate from the bifurcation of the basilar artery; in 20–25%, one of the PCAs comes from the ICA; in the remainder, both PCAs from ICA

    1. *Anatomy*

      a. *Interpeduncular branches/mesencephalic artery:* supply red nucleus, substantia nigra, medial cerebral peduncles, medial longitudinal fasciculi and medial lemnisci

      b. *Thalamoperforate/paramedian thalamic arteries:* inferior, medial, and anterior thalamus

NB: Contralateral hemianesthesia and hemiparesis followed by spontaneous pain in the affected limbs is due to the involvement of the thalamoperforate branches of the PCA. Some of these branches also supply portions of the posterior limb of the internal capsule and may produce contralateral hemiparesis in addition to sensory changes and a thalamic pain syndrome.

    c. *Thalamogeniculate branches:* geniculate body, posterior thalamus
    d. *Medial branches:* lateral cerebral peduncles, lateral tegmentum, corpora quadrigemina, pineal gland
    e. *Posterior choroidal:* posterosuperior thalamus, choroid plexus, posterior hypothalamus, psalterium (decussation of fornices)
    f. *Cortical branches:* inferomedial temporal lobe, medial occipital, including lingula, cuneus, precuneus, and visual areas 17, 18, and 19

2. *Syndromes*
    a. Anterior and proximal syndromes, involves interpeduncular, thalamic perforant, thalamogeniculate branches
      i. *Thalamic syndrome of Dejerine and Roussy:* infarction of sensory relay nuclei (due to occlusion of thalamogeniculate)—deep and cutaneous sensory loss contralateral, with transient hemiparesis; after an interval, pain, paresthesia, hyperpathia of affected parts; distortion of taste, athetotic posturing of hand; depression
      ii. *Central midbrain and subthalamic syndromes:* due to occlusion of interpeduncular branches; oculomotor palsy with contralateral hemiplegia *(Weber syndrome)*, palsies of vertical gaze, stupor, coma, movement disorders (usually contralateral ataxic tremor)
      iii. *Anteromedial-inferior thalamic syndromes:* occlusion of thalamoperforate branches; hemiballismus, hemichoreoathetosis; deep sensory loss, hemiataxia, tremor; occlusion of dominant dorsomedial nucleus gives rise to *Korsakoff syndrome*
    b. *Cortical syndromes*
      i. Occlusion of branches to temporal and occipital lobes: homonymous hemianopsia; macular and central vision may be spared owing to collateralization of occipital pole from distal branches of MCA (or ACA); visual hallucination in blind parts *(Cogan)* or metamorphopsia, palinopsia
      ii. Dominant hemisphere: alexia, anomia (most severe for colors and visually presented material—may describe their function and use them but not name them), visual agnosia, occasional memory impairment
    c. Bilateral cortical syndromes: result of successive infarctions from embolus or thrombus of upper basilar artery
      i. *Cortical blindness:* bilateral homonymous hemianopia with unformed visual hallucinations; pupillary reflexes preserved, optic discs are normal; patient may be unaware *(Anton syndrome)*
      ii. If confined to occipital poles, may have homonymous central scotomas

NB: Hemiachromatopsia, disturbance with the recognition of color in one visual field, occurs only with inferior posterior occipital lesions.

      iii. *Balint's syndrome:* from bilateral occipital-parietal borderzones
        (A) Psychic paralysis of fixation of gaze
        (B) Optic ataxia (failure to grasp objects under visual guidance)
        (C) Visual inattention (affecting mainly periphery of visual field)

    iv. Bilateral inferomedial temporal lobes: *Korsakoff amnestic state*
    v. Bilateral mesial-temporal-occipital lesions: prosopagnosia

F. **Vertebral artery**
 1. *Anatomy:* chief arteries of the medulla; supplies lower three-fourths of pyramid, medial lemniscus, all or lateral medullary region, restiform body, posterior-inferior part of cerebellar hemisphere; long extracranial course and pass through transverse processes of C6-C1 before entering the cranial cavity—may be subject to trauma, spondylotic compression
 2. *Syndromes*
  a. *Lateral medullary syndrome/Wallenberg syndrome:* vestibular nuclei (nystagmus, oscillopsia, vertigo, nausea, vomiting); spinothalamic tract (contralateral impairment of pain and thermal sense over one-half the body); descending sympathetic tract (ipsilateral Horner's—ptosis, miosis, anhidrosis); cranial nerves (CNs) IX and X (hoarseness, dysphagia, ipsilateral paralysis of palate and vocal cord, diminished gag); otolithic nucleus (vertical diplopia and illusion of tilting of vision); olivocerebellar and/or spinocerebellar fibers/restiform body (ipsilateral ataxia of limbs, falling to ipsilateral side); nucleus and tractus solitarius (loss of taste); descending tract and nucleus of V (pain, burning, impaired sensation on ipsilateral one-half of face; rarely nucleus cuneatus and gracilis (ipsilateral numbness of limbs); most likely due to occlusion of vertebral artery (eight-tenths) or posterior-inferior cerebellar artery

NB: A lesion in the nucleus tractus solitarius may result in fluctuating hypertension, just like in pheochromocytoma.

  b. *Medial medullary syndrome:* involves medullary pyramid (contralateral paralysis of arm and leg); medial lemniscus (contralateral impaired tactile and proprioceptive sense over one-half the body); CN XII (ipsilateral paralysis and, later, hemiatrophy of the tongue)
  c. *Posterior medullary region:* ipsilateral cerebellar ataxia and, rarely, a hiccup
  d. *Avellis syndrome:* tegmentum of medulla: CN X, spinothalamic tract (paralysis of soft palate and vocal cord and contralateral hemianesthesia)
  e. *Jackson syndrome:* tegmentum of medulla: CN X, XII, corticospinal tract (Avellis syndrome plus ipsilateral tongue paralysis)

G. **Basilar artery**
 1. *Branches*
  a. Paramedian
  b. Short circumferential (supplying lateral two-thirds of pons and middle and superior cerebellar peduncles)
  c. Long circumferential (anterior-inferior cerebellar artery and superior cerebellar artery)
  d. Paramedian (interpeduncular) at the bifurcation of the basilar artery supplying subthalamic and high midbrain
 2. *Syndromes*
  a. *Basilar artery syndrome:* bilateral corticobulbar and corticospinal tracts (paralysis/weakness of all extremities plus all bulbar musculature); ocular nerves, medial longitudinal fasciculus, vestibular apparatus (diplopia, paralysis of conjugate gaze, internuclear ophthalmoplegia, horizontal and/or vertical nystagmus; visual cortex (blindness; visual field defects); cerebellar peduncles and hemispheres (bilateral cerebellar ataxia);

tegmentum of midbrain/thalami (coma); medial lemniscus-spinothalamic tracts (may be strikingly intact, syringomyelic, reverse, or involve all modalities)

b. *Medial inferior pontine syndrome* (occlusion of paramedian branch of basilar artery): paramedian pontine reticular formation (paralysis of conjugate gaze to the side of lesion but preservation of convergence); vestibular nuclei (nystagmus); middle cerebral peduncle (ipsilateral ataxia of limbs and gait); CN VI (ipsilateral diplopia on lateral gaze), corticobulbar and corticospinal tract (contralateral paresis of face, arm, and leg); medial lemniscus (contralateral tactile dysfunction and proprioceptive sense over one-half the body)

c. **NB:** *Lateral inferior pontine syndrome* (occlusion of anterior-inferior cerebellar artery): CN VIII (horizontal and vertical nystagmus, vertigo, nausea, oscillopsia, deafness, and tinnitus); CN VII (ipsilateral facial paralysis); paramedian pontine reticular formation (paralysis of conjugate gaze to side of lesion); middle cerebellar peduncles and cerebellar hemisphere (ipsilateral ataxia); main sensory nucleus and descending tract of V (ipsilateral impairment of sensation over face); spinothalamic tract (contralateral impairment of pain and thermal sense over one-half the body)

d. *Millard-Gubler syndrome* (base of pons): CN VI and VII and corticospinal tract (facial and abducens palsy plus contralateral hemiplegia)

e. *Medial midpontine syndrome* (paramedian branch of midbasilar artery): middle cerebellar peduncle (ipsilateral ataxia of limbs and gait); corticobulbar and corticospinal tracts (contralateral paralysis of face, arm, and leg; deviation of eyes); medial lemniscus (variable—usually pure motor)

f. *Lateral midpontine syndrome* (short circumferential artery): middle cerebellar peduncle (ipsilateral ataxia); motor nucleus of V (ipsilateral paralysis of masticatory muscles); sensory nucleus of V (ipsilateral sensory facial impairment)

g. *Medial superior pontine syndrome* (paramedian branches of upper basilar artery): superior and middle cerebellar peduncle (ipsilateral cerebellar ataxia); medial longitudinal fasciculus (ipsilateral internuclear ophthalmoplegia); central tegmental bundle (rhythmic myoclonus of palate, pharynx, vocal cords, etc.); corticobulbar and corticospinal tracts (contralateral paralysis of face, arm, and leg); medial lemniscus (rarely with sensory impairment)

h. *Lateral superior pontine syndrome (syndrome of superior cerebellar artery):* middle and superior cerebellar peduncles, dentate nucleus (ipsilateral ataxia, falling to side of lesion); vestibular nuclei (dizziness, nausea, horizontal nystagmus); descending sympathetic fibers (ipsilateral Horner's); spinothalamic tract (contralateral impairment of pain and temperature sense of face, limb, trunk); medial lemniscus—lateral portion (contralateral impaired touch, vibration, position sense of leg >> arm); other—ipsilateral paresis of conjugate gaze, skew deviation

i. Base of midbrain (*Weber syndrome*): CN III (ipsilateral oculomotor palsy) plus corticospinal tract (crossed hemiplegia)

j. Tegmentum of midbrain (*Claude syndrome*): CN III, red nucleus, and brachium conjunctivum (contralateral cerebellar ataxia and tremor)

k. *Benedikt syndrome:* CN III, red nucleus, plus corticospinal tract

l. *Nothnagel syndrome:* CN III (unilateral or bilateral); superior cerebellar peduncles (ocular palsies, paralysis of gaze, cerebellar ataxia); usually caused by a tumor

m. *Parinaud syndrome:* dorsal midbrain—supranuclear mechanism for upward gaze and other structures in periaqueductal gray (paralysis of upward gaze and accommodation, fixed pupils)

VII. TIA

A. **Mechanism:** a reduction of CBF below 20–30 mL/100 g/minute produces neurologic symptoms; mechanisms include angiospasms, embolism, hemodynamic factors (decreased BP); disturbance of intracranial vascular autoregulation, arterial thrombosis; when it precedes a stroke, almost always stamp the process as thrombotic

B. **Natural history:** one-third have CVA within 5 years (usually within the 1st month); one-third have continued TIAs, one-third cease to have symptoms; 50–80% of CVA victims never experience TIA; crescendo TIAs: two or more TIAs within 24 hours—a medical emergency; a single transient episode or multiple episodes of different pattern (may be due to embolus—especially if prolonged), as opposed to brief, repeated ones of uniform type (warning sign of impending vascular occlusion from thrombosis); 21% rate of MI; therefore, predictor of CVA and MI; two-thirds are men and/or hypertensive

C. **Symptomatology:** 90% anterior, 7% vertebrobasilar, and 3% difficult to fit; in the carotid artery system, tends to involve either (not both) cerebral hemisphere (contralateral sensorimotor) or eye (ipsilateral visual disturbance); early-onset transient monocular blindness is usually not associated with stroke (mechanism probably migraine or antiphospholipid antibody); vertebrobasilar insufficiency symptoms tend to be less stereotyped and more prolonged, also more likely to culminate in stroke

VIII. Lacunar Stroke: due to occlusion of small arteries, 50–200 μm in diameter; strong correlation of lacunar state with hypertension, atherosclerosis, and, to a lesser degree, diabetes

A. *Pathology: lipohyalin degeneration* and occlusion in smaller lacunes; atheroma, thrombosis, and embolus in larger lacunes

B. **Location** (in descending order): putamen, caudate, thalamus, basis pontis, internal capsule, convolutional white matter

C. *Syndromes*
   1. *Pure motor* hemiparesis: lacune in the territory of lenticostriate artery (internal capsule or adjacent corona radiata); face = arm = leg
   2. *Pure sensory* stroke: lacune in the lateral thalamus or parietal white matter
   3. *Clumsy hand-dysarthria:* in the basis pontis; may also be pure motor hemiplegia but sparing of the face and with ipsilateral paresis of conjugate gaze
   4. *Ataxia-hemiparesis:* lacunar infarction in the pons, midbrain, capsule, parietal white matter

IX. Embolic Infarction: *most frequently,* a fragment from a *cardiac thrombus* (75% of cardiogenic embolus lodge in the brain—atrial fibrillation is most common cause), less frequently, *intra-arterial;* rarely, due to *fat, tumor cells, fibrocartilage, or air;* usually arrested at the bifurcation or site of natural narrowing of lumen, ischemic infarction follows, which may be pale, hemorrhagic, or mixed (hemorrhagic infarction nearly always indicates embolism, although most embolic infarcts are pale); superior division of the MCA is most frequent; two hemispheres equally affected

A. *Etiology:* paroxysmal *atrial fibrillation* or flutter may be etiology; arteriosclerotic (5X) and rheumatic (17X) atrial fibrillation are more liable to stroke than age-matched normal rhythm; other sources: *cardiac catheterization* or surgery (especially valvuloplasty); *mitral and aortic valve prosthesis; atheromatous ulcerated plaque* from carotid or vertebral artery; *aortic dissections, fibromuscular disease; atheromatous plaques in ascending aorta/arch (plaques >4 mm); disseminated cholesterol emboli; paradoxic embolism from PFO; vegetations of acute and subacute bacterial endocarditis; marantic or nonbacterial endocarditis (from carcinomatosis or lupus); mitral valve prolapse; pulmonary veins—from pulmonary suppurative disease, Osler-Weber-Rendu disease; neck and thorax surgery; arteriography; cardiac myxomas and other tumors; fat embolism from bone trauma; air embolism from abortion, scuba diving, or cranial, cervical, or thoracic operations involving large venous sinuses; unknown in 30%*

B. **Clinical picture:** develops most rapidly; full blown picture within seconds; usually getting up to go to the bathroom

C. **Lab picture:** frequently the first sign of MI is embolism; therefore, electrocardiography should be obtained in all patients with stroke of unknown origin; Holter, carotid studies/magnetic resonance angiography looking for plaques, transesophageal echocardiography (important in evaluation of young patient with probable PFO, aortic plaque); 30% of cerebral embolism produces a hemorrhagic infarct, particularly if scan is repeated on 2nd or 3rd day; in embolism due to subacute bacterial endocarditis, cerebrospinal fluid (CSF) white blood cell count may reach 200; may have equal number of red blood cells and fair xanthochromia; protein elevated, glucose normal; no bacteria in culture; in contrast, CSF from acute bacterial endocarditis may be that of purulent meningitis; 10–20% of patients will have their second embolus within 10 days but seldom before the 3rd day

X. Intracranial Hemorrhage: third most frequent cause of stroke—due to (1) hypertensive/spontaneous hemorrhage, (2) ruptured saccular aneurysm, and (3) vascular malformation and bleeding disorders; *Duret hemorrhages* (small brain stem hemorrhages from temporal lobe herniation); hypertensive encephalopathy and brain purpura do not simulate a stroke

A. **Primary (hypertensive) ICH:** predominantly due to hypertension and degenerative changes of cerebral arteries; bleeding occurs within brain tissue, resulting in distortion and compression; size and location determine degree of upper brain stem compression; massive: several centimeters; small: 1–2 cm; slit: old collapsed hemorrhage or petechial; vessel involved is usually a penetrating artery

1. **CSF is bloody in >90%** but almost never ruptures through the cortex—blood reaches subarachnoid space through ventricular system; computed tomography (CT) shows edema and mass effect from extruded serum as hypodense; surrounding edema recedes after 2–3 weeks; totally reliable for ≥1 cm in diameter

2. Most common sites: *putamen and adjacent internal capsule (50%); lobar; thalamus; cerebellar hemisphere; pons*

3. Pathogenesis: effects of hypertension—lipohyalinosis and false aneurysm (microaneurysm) of Charcot-Bouchard; amyloidosis—associated with lobar sites, *familial forms in the Netherlands and Iceland, sporadic with apolipoprotein e-4*

4. Clinical picture: usually no warning, headaches and vomiting may be prominent; average age is lower than thrombotic stroke but no age predilection; higher in blacks, Japanese; onset while up and active; usually only one episode (if with recurrent bleeding—think of aneurysm or AVM); acute reactive hypertension, far exceeding patient's chronic hypertensive level, always suggests hemorrhage; other frequent findings—headache, nuchal rigidity, vomiting

   a. Seizures found in 10%—usually in the first few days

   b. Ocular signs: putaminal—eyes deviated to opposite side of paralysis; thalamic—downward deviation, unreactive pupils; pontine—eyeballs are fixed, pupils are tiny but reactive; cerebellar—eyes deviated to the opposite side of lesion with ocular bobbing

   c. Course and prognosis: for large- and medium-sized clots—30% die within 30 days; volume ≤30 mL has favorable outcome

B. Magnetic resonance imaging (MRI) findings of hemorrhage

	T1	T2
Acute (3 hrs–3 days)	Iso-/hypointense	Iso-/hypointense
Subacute (3–7 days)	Hyperintense	Hypointense
Subacute (>7 days)	Hyperintense	Hyperintense
Chronic		
Hemosiderin	Hypointense	Hypointense
Resorbed	Hypointense	Hyperintense

XI. Spontaneous Subarachnoid Hemorrhage *(ruptured saccular aneurysm):* fourth most frequent cerebrovascular disorder; called *berry* aneurysm—small, thin-walled blisters protruding from arteries of circle of Willis or its major branches, usually due to developmental *defect in media and elastica;* 90–95% on the anterior part of the circle of Willis

A. *Alternate theory:* hemodynamic forces at apices of bifurcation cause focal destruction of internal elastic membrane, causing the intima to bulge outward

B. Vary in size from 2 mm to 3 cm; average, 7.5 mm; those that rupture have >10 mm; site of rupture is usually at the dome of the aneurysm; rare in childhood; peak between *35 and 65 y/o;* increased incidence in congenital *polycystic kidneys, fibromuscular dysplasia, moyamoya, coarctation of the aorta, Ehlers-Danlos syndrome, Marfan's syndrome, pseudoxanthoma, 5% of AVM*—usually the main feeding artery of the aneurysm

C. **Hypertension:** more frequently present than in general population, but most are normotensive; no increased risk in pregnancy; atherosclerosis probably plays no part

D. **Several types other than saccular:** *mycotic* (caused by septic emboli that weakens the wall of the vessel); *fusiform, diffuse, and globular* (enlargement of the entire circumference of the involved vessels, usually carotid, vertebral or basilar, also called atherosclerotic aneurysms, may press or become occluded by thrombus but rarely ruptures)

E. **Clinical picture:** usually asymptomatic before rupture; rupture usually occurs during active hours, sexual intercourse, straining at stool, lifting heavy objects; because hemorrhage is confined to subarachnoid space, there are few or no lateralizing signs; convulsive seizure—usually brief and generalized, occur during bleeding or rebleeding; do not correlate with location, do not alter prognosis; fundi—reveals smooth-surfaced, sharply outlined collections of blood that cover retinal vessels, preretinal, or subhyaloid hemorrhages; in summary, the clinical sequence of sudden headache, collapse, relative preservation of consciousness with paucity of lateralizing signs, and neck stiffness is diagnostic of SAH due to a ruptured saccular aneurysm

F. *Complications*
   1. *Vasospasm:* causing delayed hemiplegia, occurs 3–12 days after rupture; most frequent in arteries surrounded by the largest collection of blood
   2. *Hydrocephalus:* acute—patient becomes confused or unconscious; subacute—may occur 2–4 weeks after
   3. Most feared complication is *rerupture*—may occur anytime from minutes to 2–3 weeks later; *rebleeding* rate 2.2% per year for the first decade

G. **Lab findings**
   1. CT confirms SAH in 95% of cases; lumbar puncture should be undertaken in all other cases when clinical features suggest an SAH; CSF is usually bloody; deep xanthochromia

after several hours; increased CSF pressure (differentiates traumatic tap); protein may be elevated, glucose may be low.

2. Carotid and vertebral angiography is the only certain means of demonstrating an aneurysm.

3. Electrocardiography changes: large peaked T waves, hyponatremia, albuminuria, glycosuria, water retention, natriuresis, and, rarely, diabetes insipidus; leukocytosis with normal erythrocyte sedimentation rate (ESR); outstanding characteristic: tendency to rebleed at the same site; no way of predicting; those that cannot be visualized angiographically have better prognosis.

H. *Perimesencephalic hemorrhage:* accounts for *10% of SAH* and 50% of SAH with negative angiograms; cisterns surrounding midbrain and upper pons are filled with blood; mild headache and vasospasm do not develop; good prognosis

I. **Surgery:** advised for unruptured aneurysms >7 mm

XII. Arteriovenous Malformations: tangle of dilated vessels that form an abnormal communication between the arterial and venous system; developmental abnormality representing persistence of an embryonic pattern of blood vessels; one-tenth as frequent as saccular aneurysms; male = female

A. **Natural history:** hemorrhage in 42%, seizures in 18%; most common between ages 10 and 30 years; first clinical manifestation is SAH (50%), seizures (30%), or headache (20%); SAH has a partly intracerebral portion causing hemiparesis, etc.; seizures are usually focal motor; headache may be chronic, recurrent; rate of hemorrhage in untreated cases is 4% per year

B. *Cavernous angioma:* composed mainly of *thin-walled vessels (veins) without arterial feeders; little or no intervening nervous tissue;* tendency to bleed is no less than that of AVMs, but hemorrhages are small and clinically silent; one-half are not visible on angiograms; diagnosis is based on clinical manifestations or MRI; one-half lie in the brain stem (may be misdiagnosed as multiple sclerosis); 10% multiple, 5% familial; treated by surgery or low-dose proton radiation

XIII. Other Causes of Intracranial Bleeding

A. *Anticoagulant therapy:* most common cause after hypertensive hemorrhage; treat with fresh frozen plasma and vitamin K

B. *Amyloid angiopathy:* major cause of lobar hemorrhages in the elderly, especially if in succession or multiple; associated with apolipoprotein e-4; accounts for up to 10% of intracranial hemorrhages

NB: The deposition of beta amyloid protein in the media and adventitia of small meningeal and cortical vessels result in lobar hemorrhages in amyloid angiopathy.

C. *Hematologic conditions:* for example, leukemia, aplastic anemia, thrombocytopenic purpura; less common: liver disease, uremia on dialysis, lymphoma; factors involved: reduced prothrombin and clotting elements, bone marrow suppression by antineoplastic drugs, disseminated intravascular coagulation

D. *Acute extradural and subdural hemorrhage*

E. *Primary intraventricular hemorrhage:* may be traced to an AVM or to neoplasm

F. **Hemorrhage into a primary** (glioblastoma and medulloblastoma, pituitary adenoma) **or secondary** (choriocarcinoma, melanoma, renal cell carcinoma, bronchogenic carcinoma) **brain tumor**

XIV. Inflammatory Disease of Brain Arteries

A. *Meningovascular syphilis, tuberculous meningitis, fungal meningitis, and subacute bacterial meningitis* may be accompanied by inflammatory changes and cause *occlusion of arteries or veins.*

1. *Typhus and other rickettsial diseases* cause capillary and arteriolar changes, and perivascular inflammatory cells are found in the brain.
2. *Mucormycosis* may *occlude ICA in diabetic* patients as part of the orbital and cavernous sinus infections; it is unclear how trichinosis causes cerebral symptoms, bland emboli from the heart.
3. *Cerebral malaria* blocks *capillaries and precapillaries* by parasitized red blood cells causing coma, convulsions, and focal symptoms.
4. *Schistosomiasis* may implicate cerebral and spinal arteries.

B. **Subdivided into giant cell arteritides:** temporal arteritis, granulomatous arteritis of the brain, aortic branch arteritis (e.g., Takayasu's); and inflammatory diseases of cranial arteries: polyarteritis nodosa, Churg-Strauss, Wegener's granulomatosis, SLE, Behcet's, post-zoster, acquired immunodeficiency syndrome arteritis; in most of the above diseases, there is an abnormal deposit of complement-fixing immune complex on the endothelium, leading to inflammation, occlusion, rupture.

1. *Temporal arteritis/giant cell arteritis/cranial arteritis:* usually elderly; *external carotid system*, particularly the temporal branches, are sites of subacute granulomatous inflammatory exudate consisting of lymphs, monos, neutrophils, and giant cells; affected parts of the artery become thrombosed; ESR is characteristically >80 mm/hour; few cases <50
   a. Headache and head pain are the chief complaints; may have aching, stiffness of proximal limb muscles; clinical picture overlaps with polymyalgia rheumatica; less frequent manifestations: fever, anorexia, weight loss, anemia, and mild leukocytosis; dementia; occlusion of branches of ophthalmic artery resulting in blindness in one or both eyes occurs in 25%
   b. Significant inflammatory involvement of intracranial arteries is uncommon, but strokes occur rarely with occlusion of ICA or vertebral arteries; suspect in the elderly with severe and persistent headache, with tender and thrombosed or thickened cranial artery; may need to biopsy both sides owing to the interrupted distribution of granulomatous lesions
   c. Treatment: prednisone, 50–75 mg/day; gradually diminishing for at least several months or longer—guided by symptoms and ESR
2. *Intracranial granulomatous arteritis: small-vessel, giant cell arteritis;* presenting as a low-grade, nonfebrile meningitis with sterile CSF, followed by infarction over one or several parts of the cerebrum or cerebellum
   a. May have severe headaches, focal cerebral or cerebellar signs, gradual evolution to confusion, memory loss; CSF pleocytosis, elevated protein, and papilledema from increased intracranial pressure (ICP); symptoms persist for several months
   b. Angiography demonstrates irregular narrowing and blunt ending of small cerebral arteries; CT/MRI show multiple irregular white matter changes and small cortical lesions; occasionally, white matter lesions become confluent and simulate Binswanger's disease or hypertensive encephalopathy; affected vessels are 100–500 μm, surrounded by lymphocytes, plasma cells, monocytes, and giant cells; meninges are infiltrated with inflammatory cells, and usually only a part of the brain is affected
   c. Differentiating it from sarcoid, lymphomatoid granulomatosis and Churg-Strauss are *sparing of lungs and other organs, no eosinophilia, normal ESR*
   d. Some have responded to steroid and cyclophosphamide
3. *Aortic branch disease (Takayasu's Disease, occlusive thromboaortopathy):* mainly *aorta and the large arteries* arising from the arch; similar to giant cell arteritis except its propensity to involve the proximal rather than distal branches of the aorta; young, Asian, female

a. Constitutional symptoms, elevated ESR, later occlusion of innominate, subclavian, carotid, and vertebral artery—*pulseless disease* (usually due to atherosclerosis); may involve coronary, renal, pulmonary artery; usual neurologic findings: blurred vision on activity, dizziness, hemiparetic, hemisensory syndromes

b. Pathology: *periarteritis with giant cells*

c. Death usually in 3–5 years; treatment: corticosteroids in acute inflammatory stage, reconstructive vascular surgery in later stages

4. *Polyarteritis (periarteritis) nodosa:* inflammatory necrosis of *arteries and arterioles through-out the body, but lungs are spared* (distinguishing from Churg-Strauss); vasa nervorum is frequently involved, causing *mononeuropathy multiplex, or axonal type of peripheral neuropathy;* central nervous system (CNS) involvement is unusual (<5%)—widespread microinfarcts: manifested by headache, confusion, fluctuating cognitive disorders, convulsions, hemiplegia, brain stem signs

5. *Wegener's granulomatosis:* rare, adults, male > female (2:1); subacutely evolving *necrotizing granulomas of upper and lower respiratory tracts,* followed by necrotizing glomerulonephritis and *systemic vasculitis (both small arteries and veins)*

a. Neurologic complications (50%) come later: peripheral neuropathy, mononeuropathy multiplex, or multiple cranial neuropathy (as a result of direct extension of nasal and sinus granuloma); orbits involved in 20% simulating lymphoma or pseudotumor

b. Elevated ESR, rheumatoid factor, antiglobulin factors, C-ANCA (antineutrophil cytoplasmic antibodies)—specific and sensitive for Wegener's (also in lymphomatoid granulomatosis)

c. Treatment: cyclophosphamide, 1–2 mg/kg/day; in acute cases: prednisolone, 50–75 mg/day with immunosuppressant

6. *SLE:* CNS is involved in 75% of cases; usually later stage; usual manifestations: disturbance in mentation, seizures, CN palsies; widespread microinfarcts in the cerebrum and brain stem due to destructive changes of arterioles and capillaries—do not represent vasculitis in the strict sense; other causes are hypertension, endocarditis (gives rise to cerebral embolism); thrombotic thrombocytopenic purpura (terminal phase) and corticosteroid use—muscle weakness, seizures, psychosis

7. Arteritis symptomatic of underlying systemic disease

a. *Acquired immunodeficiency syndrome and drug abuse* (mainly cocaine) are associated with vasculitis similar to polyarteritis nodosa

b. True cerebral and spinal cord vasculitis in *systemic lymphoma* (particularly Hodgkin's)—probably related to circulating immune complexes

c. Small vessel arteritis as a hypersensitivity phenomenon

8. *Behcet's disease:* chronic, recurrent vasculitis, involving small vessels with prominent neurologic manifestations (30%); most common in Turkey and Japan; male > female

a. Triad: *relapsing iridocyclitis, recurrent oral and genital ulcers;* other symptoms: erythema nodosum, thrombophlebitis, polyarthritis, ulcerative colitis; neurologic: encephalitis, meningitis, CN palsies (particularly abducens), cerebellar ataxia, and corticospinal tract signs—symptoms are abrupt, clear in a few weeks, then recur

b. Small perivascular and meningeal infiltration of lymphocytes, cerebral venous thrombosis

c. Pathergy test: formation of sterile pustule at site of needle prick

d. Treatment: corticosteroids

9. *Vasculitic workup: rheumatoid factor, antinuclear antibody, C-reactive protein, ESR, complement (C3, C4, CH50), P-ANCA, C-ANCA, Scl-70, anticentromere antibody, angiotensin-converting enzyme (ACE) level, immunoglobulins, cryoglobulins, Coombs' test, Schirmer tests, CSF*

XV. Less Common Causes of Occlusive Cerebrovascular Disease

A. **Fibromuscular dysplasia:** *segmental, nonatheromatous, noninflammatory arterial disease;* uncommon; first described affecting the renal artery; in the nervous system, ICA is most frequent, followed by vertebral and cerebral arteries; female > male; 75% >50 y/o

1. Radiology: irregular *string of beads* or a tubular narrowing; bilateral in 75%; usually only extracranial; 20% have intracranial saccular aneurysm; 12% with arterial dissections

2. Pathology: narrowed arterial segments show degeneration of elastic tissue and irregular arrays of fibrous and smooth muscle tissue in a mucous ground substance; dilatations are due to atrophy of coat of the vessel wall; some with atheroma, others with dissection, others marked stenosis

3. Treatment: excision of affected segments if symptoms are related, conservative if incidental finding; endovascular dilatations now possible; saccular aneurysms >4–5 mm should be surgically removed

B. **Dissection of ICA:** should be suspected in a young adult woman (late 30s to early 40s) as a spontaneous occurrence or in relation to direct trauma, whiplash injury, violent coughing; pregnancy and delivery; most have warning attacks of unilateral cranial or facial pain—nonthrobbing, around the eye, frontal, temporal area, angle of mandible, or high neck; followed by TIA or ICA hemispheric stroke; with unilateral Horner's

1. Magnetic resonance angiography/angiography: reveals elongated, irregular, narrow column of dye beginning 1.5–3.0 cm above carotid bifurcation extending to the base of the skull—string sign

2. Treatment: immediate anticoagulation to prevent embolism; warfarin may be discontinued in several months to 1 year if magnetic resonance angiography shows lumen patent and smooth-walled

3. Pathogenesis: cystic medial necrosis

C. **NB: Moyamoya disease and multiple progressive intracranial arterial occlusions:** *cloud of smoke;* network of small anastomotic vessels at the base of the brain around and distal to the circle of Willis, along with segmental stenosis or occlusion of terminal parts of both ICAs; mainly in infants, children, adolescents; male = female; usually, weakness of an arm or leg that tends to clear rapidly but recurs; occasional headache, convulsions, visual disturbance, nystagmus; in older patients, SAH was most common; more frequent in persons of Asian descent

1. Pathology: adventitia, media, internal elastic lamina were all normal; *only intima was thickened with fibrous tissue;* no inflammation; with *microaneurysm due to weakness of elastic lamina;* may be primary genetic or secondary to various conditions such as radiation therapy involving the circle of Willis, sickle cell disease, neurofibromatosis.

2. There is association with Down syndrome and HLA types—favoring hereditary basis; multiple progressive intracranial arterial occlusion: same age period but no cloud of anastomosis

D. **Binswanger's disease and familial subcortical infarction:** widespread degeneration of cerebral white matter having a vascular causation observed in the context of hypertension, atherosclerosis of small vessels, and multiple strokes; dementia, pseudobulbar state, gait disorder; *cerebral autosomal dominant arteriopathy with subcortical infarcts and leukoencephalopathy*—autosomal dominant, European families, *chromosome 19,* recurrent small strokes beginning in early adulthood, culminate in subcortical dementia

NB: CADASIL is a mutation in the Notch-3 gene. Diagnosis can be made by skin muscle biopsy demonstrating thickening of smooth arteriopathic muscle cells that eventually degenerate. Electron microscopy shows granular, osmophilic materials in the arterial smooth muscle.

XVI. Other Forms of Cerebrovascular Disease

A. **Thrombosis of cerebral veins and venous sinuses:** usually in relation to infections of the ear and paranasal sinuses or hypercoagulable states that may lead to increase in ICP (*pseudotumor cerebri*)

 1. Diagnosis is difficult except in known clinical settings, such as taking *birth control pills, postpartum, postoperative states characterized by thrombocytosis and hyperfibrinogenemia, hypercoagulable states in cancer, congenital heart disease, cachexia in infants, sickle cell disease, antiphospholipid antibody syndrome, protein S or C deficiency, antithrombin III deficiency, resistance to activated protein C (relative risk for venous thrombosis is 2.7 for patient with point mutation for gene encoding factor V resulting in resistance to activated protein C), primary or secondary polycythemia or thrombocytopenia, and paroxysmal nocturnal hemoglobinuria* (can also cause cerebral and SAH), following head injury

 2. Somewhat slower evolution of clinical syndrome; multiple lesions not in typical arterial territories; greater epileptogenic and hemorrhagic tendency

 a. *Anterior cavernous sinus thrombosis:* marked chemosis, proptosis, painful ophthalmoplegia, CN III, IV, VI and ophthalmic division of V palsy

 b. *Sagittal sinus and cerebral vein thrombosis:* seizures and hemiparesis, predominantly leg first on one side then the other; with severe headache

 c. *Posterior cavernous sinus thrombosis:* palsies of CN VI, IX, X, XI without ptosis; involvement of the superior petrosal sinus will be accompanied by CN V palsy

 d. In *superior sagittal sinus,* jugular vein and torcular thrombosis, there is increased ICP without ventricular dilatation

 3. Enhanced CT, arteriography, or magnetic resonance venography facilitate diagnosis

 4. Treatment: heparin for several days followed by warfarin, combined with antibiotics (if inflammatory); mortality remains high at 10–20%

B. **Marantic endocarditis and cerebral embolism:** *sterile vegetations,* terminal or *nonbacterial thrombotic endocarditis;* consists of fibrin and platelets and are loosely attached to the mitral valves and contiguous endocardium; one-half of cases are associated with malignant neoplasm; remainder in debilitated patients; no distinctive clinical features that permit differentiation from cerebral embolism; apoplectic nature distinguishes it from tumor metastasis; rheumatic arteritis: lesions of small cerebral arteries in rheumatic heart disease; probably secondary to diffuse embolism; anticoagulation is probably risky in debilitated patients

C. **Thromboangiitis obliterans of cerebral vessels (Winiwarter-Buerger disease):** little evidence that this is a recognizable entity; thin, thread-like white leptomeningeal arteries and borderzone infarction

D. **Stroke as a complication of hematologic disease**

 1. *Antiphospholipid antibodies:* suspect in migraine, *thrombocytopenia, TIAs or stroke in the young adult; related to SLE* in some cases; most frequent neurologic abnormality is a TIA (usually amaurosis fugax); stroke is more common in patients with migraine, hyperlipidemia, (+) antinuclear antibody, smokers, taking oral contraceptive pills; one-third had thrombocytopenia; 23% with false-positive VDRL; vascular lesions are mainly white matter

 2. *Sneddon syndrome:* deep blue-red lesions of *livedo reticularis and livedo racemosa in association with multiple strokes;* most but not all with high antiphospholipid antibody titers; 30–35 y/o; MRI lesions are small, deep, and multiple; tendency to recur; skin biopsy aids in diagnosis; international normalized ratio (INR) close to 3 for effective prevention of stroke; plasma exchange in fulminant cases; aspirin and heparin in patients with recurrent fetal loss

3. *Thrombotic thrombocytopenic purpura (Moschowitz syndrome):* uncommon but serious, mainly young adults; pathology: widespread occlusions of arterioles and capillaries of all organs; fever, anemia, symptoms of renal and hepatic disease, thrombocytopenia, confusion, delirium, seizures, and altered states of consciousness—sometimes remittent or fluctuating

4. *Thrombocytosis and thrombocytopenia:* platelets >800,000; generally a form of myeloproliferative disease, with enlarged spleen, polycythemia, chronic myelogenous leukemia, or myelosclerosis; present with recurrent thrombotic episodes, often minor; treatment: cytapheresis (to reduce platelets); antimitotic drugs (hydroxyurea) suppress megakaryocyte formation—relieve neurologic symptoms

5. **NB:** *Sickle cell disease:* presence of hemoglobin S in red blood cells; clinical abnormalities occur only with sickle cell disease, not trait; ischemic lesions of the brain occur in 25% of sickle cell disease, both large and small, are most common; cerebral, subarachnoid, and subdural hemorrhage occurs; *large artery stenosis and occlusion is common in children (80% occur before 15 years of age); in adults, high risk of both infarction and hemorrhage;* treatment: i.v. hydration *and transfusion* (for primary and secondary prevention) and use of narcotic analgesics for pain control; STOP trial (Stroke Prevention Trial in Sickle Cell Anemia): high-risk patients based on transcranial Doppler, had <1% per year stroke risk with transfusion compared to 10% per year without transfusion

NB: Hemoglobin S fraction must be kept below 30% for stroke prevention. Transcranial Doppler helps predict risk of stroke. Treat with chronic transfusion therapy.

6. *Polycythemia vera:* myeloproliferative disorder of unknown cause, marked increase of red cell mass (7–11 million/mL^3) and blood volume, often with increase in white blood cell count and platelets; secondary forms—white blood cell count and platelets remain normal; leads to thrombosis due to high blood viscosity and reduced rate of flow; majority have TIA and small strokes; essential thrombocythemia (limited to thrombocytosis), with splenomegaly, severe hemorrhage manifestations, thrombo-occlusive events, involving retina, brain, and distal arteries

7. *Disseminated intravascular coagulation:* perhaps the most common and most serious disorder of coagulation affecting the nervous system; release of thromboplastic substances resulting in activation of coagulation process and formation of fibrin, in the course of which, clotting factors and platelets are consumed; occurrence of widespread fibrin thrombi in small vessels resulting in numerous infarctions in various organs; also results in hemorrhage; decreased platelet counts with prolonged prothrombin time and PTT

8. *Hypercoagulable state workup: serum viscosity; fibrinogen; antithrombin III; protein C and S; bleeding time; serum protein electrophoresis; human immunodeficiency virus; factor V Leiden; factor VII, VIII, IX, X, XI, XII, XIII; thrombin time; fibrin degradation products; sickle prep; antiphospholipid antibodies*

XVII. Treatment
A. Atherothrombotic infarct and TIA
1. Patients should remain in a nearly horizontal position on the 1st day unless edema is prominent.
2. Reactive hypertension after ischemic stroke is prevalent and has a tendency to decline without medications during the first few hospital days; therefore, treatment of previously unappreciated hypertension is deferred until later when neurologic deficit is stabilized; avoid antihypertensive drugs in the first few days unless there is active MI or if BP is high enough to pose a risk to other organs (particularly the kidney).

3. *Thrombotic agents:* recombinant tissue-type plasminogen activator and streptokinase convert plasminogen to plasmin to hydrolyze fibrin, fibrinogen, and other clotting agents; incidence of cerebral hemorrhage is 20% through intra-arterial route; National Institute of Neurological and Communicative Disorders and Stroke and Stroke rt-PA Study Group: treatment within 3 hours of i.v. recombinant tissue-type plasminogen activator at 0.9 mg/kg (10% given as a bolus, followed by 1-hour infusion) led to a *30% increase in little or no neurologic deficit when re-examined 3 months later—for all types of stroke (including lacunes); 6% risk of cerebral hemorrhage.*

4. Acute surgical revascularization: if the common carotid artery or ICA has just become thrombosed, immediate removal of clot or the performance of a bypass procedure may restore function; if interval is longer than 12 hours, little value cerebral edema and increased ICP.

5. *Controlled ventilation* is a useful temporary procedure; *i.v. mannitol,* 1 g/kg, then 50 g every 2 or 3 hours, or *glycerol* by mouth, 30 mL every 4–6 hours, or i.v. of 50 g dissolved in 500 mL of 2.5% saline solution; corticosteroids of little value; *hemicraniectomy* combined with duraplasty—if patient is progressing from stuporous state to coma and imaging shows increasing mass effect (futile in long periods of coma, bilaterally enlarged pupils, or midbrain damage by MRI).

6. *Anticoagulant drugs:* the administration of anticoagulants is not of great value once the stroke is fully developed; it is uncertain whether it prevents recurrence; there is a possibility of hemorrhagic complication.
   a. Two situations in which anticoagulation may be useful: (1) fluctuating basilar artery thrombosis and impending carotid artery occlusion, and (2) cardioembolic cerebral infarction/*atrial fibrillation*
   b. Low-molecular-weight heparin (Nadoheparin [or antifactor Xa]) at 4000 U subcutaneously given within first 48 hours shows improved outcome when measured after 6 months, with no increased hemorrhagic frequency
   c. *Warfarin-Aspirin Recurrent Stroke Study Trial:* no difference between acetylsalicylic acid (ASA) vs. warfarin in patients with stroke not due to cardioembolic sources
   d. *Warfarin-Aspirin Symptomatic Intracranial Disease Study Trial:* early termination of the trial comparing warfarin vs. aspirin for symptomatic intracranial lesions owing to increased complications
   e. *PFO in Cryptogenic Stroke Study:* no difference in outcome with warfarin vs. ASA among patients with PFO; there was also no difference in the 2-year event rates in patients with no, small, or large PFOs

7. *Anti-platelet drugs*
   a. *ASA:* acetyl moiety combines with platelet membrane and *inhibits platelet cyclo-oxygenase,* preventing thromboxane A2 and prostacyclin
   b. *Ticlopidine,* 250 mg bid; inhibits platelet aggregation induced by adenosine Po_4; does not inhibit cyclo-oxygenase

NB: Leucopenia has been reported with ticlopidine.

   c. *Clopidogrel:* 8% nonsignificant relative risk reduction rate of stroke compared to ASA; *Management of Atherothrombosis with Clopidogrel in High-Risk Patients Study:* no significant difference in stroke risk reduction in clopidogrel vs. ASA/clopidogrel combination

NB: TTP has been reported with ticlopindine and clopidogrel.

   d. *ASA/extended release dipyridamole:* 23% relative risk reduction in stroke compared to 50 mg ASA; ESPRIT Trial: among 2,739 patients randomized to ASA/extended release dipyridamole vs. ASA alone, 13% of patients on ASA and dipyridamole and 16% of patients on ASA alone met primary outcome (death from vascular causes) (hazard ratio: 0.80; absolute risk reduction of 1% per year)

8. Cholesterol lowering treatments: in a meta analysis of 90,056 patients
   a. The risk of vascular events is directly proportional to and has a roughly linear relationship to the absolute reduction in LDL cholesterol.
   b. Every 40 mg/dl reduction in LDL cholesterol is associated with a 23% reduction in risk of vascular events (i.e., an 80 mg/dL reduction would likely reduce risk by 46%).
   c. The absolute risk reduction was approximately three times as high in patients with CAD than in those without.
   d. There was no increase in risk of cerebral hemorrhage (RR: 1.05; 99% CI 0.78-1.41).

9. Surgery
   a. *North American Carotid Endarterectomy Trial* and European Carotid Surgery Trial: carotid endarterectomy for symptomatic lesions >70% stenosis (relative risk reduction = 70%; absolute risk reduction = 9%); among patients with 50–69% stenosis, certain subgroups, primarily men without diabetes benefited most from surgery
   b. Superficial temporal-middle cerebral anastomosis for intracranial lesions: no benefit
   c. Asymptomatic carotid stenosis: *Asymptomatic Carotid Atherosclerosis Study:* strokes are reduced from 11% to 5% over 5 years by removing plaques in asymptomatic patients with stenosis >60% (surgical complication rate = 2.4%); European trial: asymptomatic carotid stenosis <70% carries only a 2% risk for stroke over a 3-year period, and in >70% stenosis only 5.7%; endarterectomy is not justified in asymptomatic cases

10. *Folate and vitamins*
   a. The *Swiss Heart study* looked at the effect of homocysteine-lowering therapy with folic acid, vitamin B_{12}, and vitamin B_6 on clinical outcome after percutaneous coronary intervention; randomized to placebo or folate, 1 mg, + B_{12}, 400 µg, + B_6, 10 mg, in patients undergoing angioplasty/stent for acute coronary events; found a dramatic and significant reduction in the rate of restenosis and a 30% reduction in cardiac events in the vitamin group; suggested that homocysteine might be causative of atherogenesis; another study showed decreased rate of coronary restenosis after lowering of plasma homocysteine levels
   b. The *Vitamin Intervention for Stroke Prevention:* a randomized controlled trial testing the efficacy of folate + B_{12} + B_6 for stroke prophylaxis (to prevent recurrent stroke, MI, and death); the study found *no vitamin effect*
   c. Third study out of Germany and the Netherlands, similar to the Swiss Heart Study, found that vitamin treatment was associated with *worse* outcome; the authors suggested that the difference might relate to the fact that in their study, all the patients were stented; in the Swiss Heart Study, only approximately one-half were stented, and the vitamin effects were mainly in the people who underwent angioplasty without stent

11. *Physical therapy* should be started early to prevent contracture and periarthritis; should be moved from bed to chair as soon as illness permits

B. **American Heart Association (AHA)/American Stroke Association (ASA)/American Academy of Neurology (AAN) Guidelines**

1. Recommendations for vascular risk factors

Risk Factor	Recommendation	Class/Level of Evidence
Hypertension	Antihypertensive treatment is recommended for prevention beyond the hyperacute period	Class I, Level A
	Should be considered for all ischemic strokes and TIAs	Class IIa, Level B
	Data support the use of diuretics and ACE inhibitors; choice should be individualized	Class I, Level A
Diabetes	More rigorous control of BP and lipids in patients with DM	Class IIa, Level B
	Most patients require >1 agent; ACE inhibitors, ARBs recommended as first choice in patients with DM	Class I, Level A
	Glucose control to near-normoglycemic levels to reduce microvascular complications	Class I, Level A
	Goal for Hgb A1c should be ≤7%	Class IIa, Level B
Cholesterol	Managed according to NCEP III guidelines, including lifestyle, diet modifications, medications	Class I, Level A
	Statins are recommended; goal should be LDL-C of <100 mg/dL; LDL-C of <70 for very high risk patients	Class I, Level A
	Patients with low HDL-C may be considered for treatment with niacin or gemfibrozil	Class IIb, Level B
Smoking	All patients should not smoke	Class I, Level A
Alcohol	Heavy drinkers should eliminate or reduce their consumption of alcohol	Class I, Level A
	Light to moderate levels of ≤2 drinks per day for men; 1 drink per day for nonpregnant women may be considered	Class IIb, Level C
Obesity	Weight reduction with a goal of a BMI of 18.5–24.9kg/m^2, waist circumference <35 in for women, <40 in for men	Class IIb, Level C
Physical activity	At least 30 minutes of moderate-intensity physical exercise on most days	Class IIb, Level C

2. Recommendations for interventional approaches to patients with CVA from large-artery atherosclerotic disease

Risk factor	Recommendation	Class/Level of Evidence
Extracranial carotid disease	Symptomatic 70–99% carotid stenosis: CEA by a surgeon with perioperative morbidity/mortality of <6%	Class I, Level A
	Symptomatic 50–69% carotid stenosis: CEA recommended depending on patient-specific factors (age, gender, co-morbidities)	Class I, Level A

Risk Factor	Recommendation	Class/Level of Evidence
	<50% stenosis: no indication for CEA	Class III, Level A
	When stenosis is difficult to access surgically, other risks, CAS is not inferior to CEA and may be considered	Class IIa, Level B
Extracranial vertebrobasilar disease	Endovascular treatment may be considered when patients are symptomatic despite medical treatment (antithrombotics, statins, etc.)	Class IIb, Level C
Intracranial arterial disease	Usefulness of endovascular therapy (angioplasty and/or stent placement) is uncertain; considered investigational	Class IIb, Level C

3. Recommendations for patients with cardioembolic stroke types

Risk factor	Recommendation	Class/Level of Evidence
AF	Persistent and paroxysmal AF, anticoagulation with target INR = 2.5 (range 2–3)	Class I, Level A
	For patients unable to take anticoagulants, ASA 325 mg/d	Class I, Level A
Acute MI and LV thrombus	Oral anticoagulation is reasonable, INR between 2–3 for 3 months to 1 year	Class IIa, Level B
	ASA in doses up to 162 should be used concurrently	Class IIa, Level A
Cardiomyopathy	Either warfarin or anti-platelet therapy may be considered	Class IIb, Level C
Rheumatic mitral valve disease	Warfarin is reasonable, INR target 2.5 (range 2–3)	Class IIa, Level C
	Anti-platelets should not be routinely added to warfarin	Class III, Level C
	Add ASA if with recurrent embolism while receiving warfarin	Class IIa, Level C
MVP	Long-term anti-platelet therapy is reasonable	Class IIa, Level C
MAC	For MAC not documented to be calcific, anti-platelet therapy may be considered	Class IIb, Level C
	If with mitral regurgitation from MAC, anti-platelet or warfarin may be considered	Class IIb, Level C
Aortic valve disease	Anti-platelets may be considered	Class IIa, Level C
Prosthetic heart valves	Oral anticoagulants are recommended, INR target of 3.0 (range 2.5–3.5)	Class I, Level B
	CVA despite warfarin, add ASA 75–100 mg/d	Class IIa, Level B

Risk factor	Recommendation	Class/Level of Evidence
	For bioprosthetic heart valves, warfarin with INR target between 2–3	Class IIb, Level C

4. Recommendations for stroke patients with other specific conditions

Risk Factor	Recommendation
Arterial dissection	Warfarin for 3–6 months or anti-platelet agents are reasonable
	Beyond 3–6 months, long-term antiplatelet therapy is reasonable; anticoagulant therapy if with recurrent events
	Definite recurrent events despite antithrombotic therapy, endovascular therapy may be considered
	Fail or not candidates of endovascular therapy, surgery is reasonable
Patent foramen ovale	Anti-platelet therapy is reasonable
	Warfarin for high risk (underlying hypercoagulable state, evidence of venous thrombosis)
	Insufficient evidence for PFO closure for first time stroke
Hyperhomocystenemia	Daily standard multivitamins to reduce homocysteine levels reasonable; but no evidence that reducing homocysteine levels will reduce CVA
Inherited thrombophilias	Should be evaluated for DVT (an indication for anticoagulant therapy)
	Anticoagulation or anti-platelet therapy are reasonable
	Long-term anticoagulation for recurrent thrombotic events
Antiphospholipid antibody (APA) syndrome	Anti-platelet therapy is reasonable
	APA with venous or arterial occlusive disease, miscarriages, livedo reticularis, oral anticoagulation with INR target 2–3
Sickle-cell disease	General treatment and use of anti-platelet agents
	Consider: regular blood transfusion to reduce Hb S to <30–50% of total Hb, hydroxyurea, or bypass surgery for advanced occlusive disease
Cerebral venous thrombosis	UFH or LMWH is reasonable even in the presence of hemorrhagic infarction
	Continue anticoagulation for 3–6 months, followed by anti-platelet therapy
Pregnancy	High risk: adjusted dose UFH throughout pregnancy; adjusted LMWH with factor Xa monitoring; UFH or LMWH until week 13, warfarin in the middle trimester, low dose ASA last trimester
	Low risk: UFH or LMWH for first trimester, low dose ASA for the remainder

C. *ICH:* general medical management is same as ischemic stroke
  1. For large hemorrhages, controlled *hyperventilation* to a P_{CO_2} of 25–30 mm Hg; ICP monitoring and tissue-dehydrating agents: *mannitol* (with osmolality kept between 295 and 305 mOsm/L and Na at 145–150 mEq), limitation of fluid intake to 1200 mL/day, given as i.v. normal saline.
  2. Virtually all patients are hypertensive immediately after the stroke, and natural trend is for BP to diminish over several days; rapid reduction is not recommended because it risks compromising cerebral perfusion in the setting of increased ICP from bleeding; however, mean BP >110 mm Hg may exaggerate cerebral edema—use β-blockers (esmolol or labetalol) or ACE inhibitors. Diuretics are helpful in combination; avoid calcium channel blockers and nitrates as they can increase ICP; *PROGRESS trial* (Perindopril Protection Against Recurrent Stroke Study) included patients with ICH, and these patients did well on combined ACE inhibitor and diuretic therapy.
  3. Consider *surgery* in deteriorating clinical state, hemorrhage >3 cm; most successful in lobar and putaminal hemorrhage; surgical evacuation of cerebellar hematoma is a more urgent matter because of proximity to brain stem and risk for abrupt onset of coma and respiratory failure; hematomas >3 or 4 cm pose the greatest risk and should be evacuated no matter what clinical state.
D. **SAH:** influenced by the general and neurologic state as well as location and morphology of aneurysm

Grade	Hunt and Hess classification
Grade I	Asymptomatic or with slight headache
Grade II	Moderate to severe headache, nuchal rigidity, no focal or lateralizing signs
Grade III	Drowsy, confusion, mild focal deficit
Grade IV	Persistent stupor, semicoma, early decerebrate rigidity
Grade V	Deep coma and decerebrate rigidity

  1. General medical management: bed rest, fluids above-normal circulating volume and venous pressure (due to volume contraction from bed rest, sodium loss from release of antinuclear factor), elastic stockings, stool softener, propranolol, i.v. nitroprusside to maintain systolic BP ≤150 mm Hg, pain relievers for headache generally avoid anticonvulsants unless a seizure has occurred; *nimodipine,* 60 mg orally every 4 hours, to reduce vasospasm; operate early (within 36 hours) for grades I and II; timing of surgery for grade III is controversial (may need to be aggressive if general medical condition allows); outcome for grade IV is dismal no matter what course is taken.
  2. *International Subarachnoid Aneurysm Trial:* comparing clipping vs. platinum coiling; relative risk reduction at 1 year for endovascular arm was 22.6% and absolute risk reduction of 6.9%; coiling has become standard for basilar tip aneurysms and is used in ICA and proximal circle of Willis.

XVIII. Coma and Brain Death
  A. Coma

1. *Glasgow Coma Scale*

Eye Opening	Spontaneous	4
	To voice	3
	To pain	2
	None	1
Best Motor Response	Obeys commands	6
	Localizes pain	5
	Withdraws to pain	4
	Flexor posturing	3
	Extensor posturing	2
	None	1
Best Verbal Response	Conversant and oriented	5
	Conversant and disoriented	4
	Inappropriate words	3
	Incomprehensible words	2
	None	1

2. Respiratory patterns associated with coma

Pattern	Description	Location
Cheyne-Stokes	Hyperapnea (in a crescendo-decrescendo pattern) followed by apnea	Bilateral diencephalon or cerebrum
Central neurogenic hyperventilation	Regular, rapid, deep hyperapnea	Brainstem tegmentum
Apneustic	Hyperapnea pauses at full inspiration	Pons
Ataxic	Irregular rate and depth of respiration	Medullary reticular formation

3. Pupillary clues in the comatose state

Description	Lesion
Small and reactive	Diencephalon
Ipsilateral pupillary constriction	Hypothalamus
Pinpoint but still reactive	Pons
Large and fixed	Tectum
Midposition and fixed	Midbrain
Dilated and fixed	Uncal herniation

B. Cause is *known and irreversible; no severe overlying medical condition* (electrolytes, acid/base disturbances, endocrine abnormalities); *no drug intoxication* or poisoning; core temperature is *at least 90°F (32°C)*
   1. *Cardinal features*
      a. *Unresponsive (no motor response to pain)*
      b. *No brain stem reflexes*
      c. No pupil response to light
      d. No oculocephalic reflex (doll's eyes maneuver)
      e. No caloric vestibular reflex: using 50 mL of cold water, allow 1 minute for each ear and 5 minutes between ears
      f. No corneal reflex; no grimacing to pain
      g. No gag reflex; no cough or bradycardia with suction
   2. *Apnea test*
      a. Temperature at least 97°F (36.5°C); systolic BP at least 90 mm Hg; no diabetes insipidus or positive fluid balance in the past 6 hours.
      b. Preoxygenate the patient to get P_{O_2} to at least 200 and P_{CO_2} to 40 or lower.
      c. Shut off vent for 8 minutes; stop test if you see respiratory movements, systolic PB <90 mm Hg, P_{O_2} significant desaturation, or cardiac arrhythmia.
      d. Draw arterial blood gas: test is *positive if P_{CO_2} is at least 60 or 20 mm Hg increase over baseline.*
C. **Confirmatory tests (optional)**
   1. *Angiography:* no filling at level of carotid bifurcation or circle of Willis
   2. *Electroencephalography:* electrocerebral silence
   3. *Transcranial Doppler ultrasound:* no signal
   4. *Technetium 99 hexamethylpropyleneamine oxime brain scan:* no uptake
   5. *Somatosensory evoke potentials:* no response of N20–P22
   6. *Repeat examination in 6 hours*

NB: Electroencephalography criteria: no electrical activity during at least 30 minutes, 2 mV, electrodes 10 cm apart, system check, qualified operator.

XIX. Craniocerebral Trauma: in persons up to 44 y/o, trauma is the leading cause of death, more than one-half due to head injuries; 80% of head injuries are seen first by a general physician in the emergency room; <20% ever require neurosurgical intervention
   A. **Definitions**
      1. *Concussion:* violent shaking or jarring of the brain and a resulting *transient functional impairment*
      2. *Contusion:* bruising of the brain without interruption of its architecture
         a. Coup injury: head is struck while immobilized; the focus of the injury is at the site of impact
         b. Contre-coup injury: the head is not immobilized (i.e., it is in motion, accelerating or decelerating)
   B. **Mechanisms of brain injury:** the majority of the injury is opposite the side of the head from impact
      1. Cranium distorted by forceps
      2. Gunshot wound to the head
      3. Falls
      4. Blows on the chin
      5. Injury to the skull by falling objects

C. **Fractures:** although not necessary in fatal head injuries, are a rough measure of force to which the brain was exposed; warns possibility of cerebral injury (20 times more frequent than without fractures), indicates site and possible severity, potential for ingress of bacteria or air or egress of CSF

1. *Basilar fractures*

   a. *Fracture of petrous pyramid:* deforms external auditory canal—*otorrhea, hemotympanum; 8th nerve damage*—deafness (sensorineural as compared to high-tone hearing loss in cochlear damage and conduction deafness due to bleeding); postural vertigo and nystagmus; facial palsy

   b. *Damage posteriorly (sigmoid sinus): Battle sign*—boggy and discolored mastoid process

   c. *Anterior skull: raccoon eyes or panda bear* appearance (blood leaking into periorbital tissues)

   d. Commonly, existence of *basilar fractures* are indicated by CN damage; *anosmia and loss of taste* (more of aromatic flavors and not elementary modalities) are frequent sequelae of displacement of brain and tearing of olfactory nerve filaments at the cribriform plate due to fall on back of the head

   e. *Fracture near the sella: tear pituitary stalk*—diabetes insipidus, impotence, reduced libido, amenorrhea

   f. *Fracture of sphenoid bone:* may *lacerate optic nerve* and cause blindness—pupil dilated and unreactive to light but intact consensual reflex; damage to 4th nerve is most common cause of diplopia

2. *Carotid-cavernous fistula:* may result from *fracture through the sphenoid bone, lacerating ICA;* within hours or days, disfiguring pulsating *exophthalmos* as arterial blood distends superior and inferior ophthalmic veins; orbit feels tight, painful, eye may become immobile; *6th nerve affected most often;* may have vision loss due to ischemia of optic nerve; 5–10% recover spontaneously, remainder by interventional radiology or surgery; etiology may be from trauma, ruptured saccular aneurysm, Ehlers-Danlos (may be unexplained)

3. *Pneumocephalus, aerocele, and rhinorrhea:* nasal discharge can be identified as CSF by *diabetic test tape (mucus has no glucose);* presence of fluorescein dye injected in lumbar subarachnoid space

   a. *Most rhinorrhea heal by themselves;* if persistent, with episodes of meningitis, repair is warranted.

   b. *Aerocele:* may be secondary to *fracture or prolonged neurosurgical procedure;* potential route of entry for bacteria; occasionally, may require needle aspiration if clinical signs are present.

   c. *Depressed fractures* are of significance only if underlying dura is lacerated or brain compressed—should be *repaired within 24–48 hours.*

4. *Cerebral concussion:* reversible traumatic paralysis is always immediate; effects are variable; optimal condition for production of concussion is a change in momentum of the head (either accelerative or decelerative)

   a. *Mechanism:* when the head is struck, movement of the partly tethered but suspended brain always lags (inertia), but when it eventually does move, it must rotate, for it occupies a round skull whose motions describe an arc; the shearing stress centered at point of tethering at the level of high midbrain and subthalamus disrupts upper reticular formation, explaining immediate loss of consciousness; also explains surface brain injuries: bony prominences of base of skull, injuries to corpus callosum as it is flung against the falx

     b. *Clinical:* loss of consciousness, suppression of reflexes, transient arrest of respiration, brief bradycardia, and hypotension are characteristic; time of recovery is variable; *duration of anterograde amnesia is the most reliable index of severity of injury*

     c. Pathologic changes of severe head injury: blow to the front of the head mainly produces *coup* lesions; back of the head—*contrecoup;* side of the head—either or both

D. ***Approach to the patient with head injury***

   1. *Minor head injury (patients who are conscious or rapidly regaining consciousness):* most frequently encountered; most cases, little need of neurologic consultation; *hospitalization is not required*, provided that a family member is able to report changes; *1 in 1000 chance* of developing *intracranial hemorrhage* if without fracture and mentally clear; 1 in 30 if with fracture; still unresolved whether to routinely obtain films of head and neck

     a. *Post-traumatic syndrome:* headaches, giddiness, fatigability, insomnia, and nervousness

     b. *Delayed fainting after head injury:* simply a vasodepressor syncopal attack, related to pain and emotional upset—must be distinguished from a "lucid interval of epidural bleed"

     c. *Transient traumatic paraplegia, blindness, and migrainous phenomena:* both legs become temporarily weak, with bilateral Babinski sign, occasional sphincteric incontinence; symptoms disappear after a few hours

     d. *Delayed hemiplegia or coma:* usually young adults after relatively minor athletic or road injury; massive hemiplegia, hemianesthesia, hemianopsia, aphasia—represents either *dissecting aneurysm of internal carotid, late evolving epidural or subdural hematoma, ICH, or preexisting AVM;* with fracture of large bones and pulmonary symptoms 24–72 hours later, traumatic fat embolism should be considered

   2. *Patients who have been comatose from the time of head injury*

     a. Pathology usually discloses *increased ICP, cerebral contusions, lacerations, SAH, zones of infarction, scattered ICHs; diffuse axonal injury.*

     b. Immediate arrest of respiration: bradyarrhythmia may be sufficient to damage brain; diagnosis of brain death should not be made immediately to not be confused with anoxia, drug or alcohol intoxication, and hypotension.

     c. *Traumatic delirium:* when stupor gives way to a confusional state, may last for weeks; associated with aggressive behavior or uncooperativeness.

     d. *Traumatic dementia:* once the patient improves, he or she is slow in thinking and unstable in emotion, with faulty judgment.

     e. Small groups are in *persistent vegetative state:* normal vital signs but do not speak and are capable only of primitive reflexes.

   3. *Concussion followed by a lucid interval and serious cerebral damage:* initial and temporary loss of consciousness is due to concussion but later deterioration because of *delayed expansion of subdural hematoma, worsening brain edema, or epidural clot*

     a. *Acute epidural hemorrhage:* due to *temporal or parietal fracture with laceration of the middle meningeal artery or vein;* less often a tear in dural venous sinus; visualization of the fracture line across the groove of the middle meningeal artery and knowledge of the site of trauma aid in diagnosis; meningeal vessels may be torn without a fracture; CT: *lens-shaped clot with a smooth inner margin;* treatment: burr holes, craniotomy or drainage (prognosis is poor if with bilateral Babinski sign, decerebrate posturing sets in before procedure)

     b. *Acute subdural hematoma:* may be unilateral or bilateral; may have a lucid interval; more often, patient is comatose from the time of injury and coma deepens progressively; frequently combined with epidural hematoma; CT detects in 90%; less acute hematomas may be isodense to the cortex and present only as a ventricular shift; treatment: craniotomy

c. *Chronic subdural hematoma:* traumatic injury may be trivial or forgotten; due to *tearing of bridging veins;* period of *weeks follow before onset* of headaches, giddiness, slowness of thinking, confusion, apathy, drowsiness, or seizures; focal sign is usually hemiparesis; usually not hemianopsia or hemiplegia; sign may be ipsilateral or contralateral (remember *Kernohan-Woltman false localizing sign*); dilatation of the ipsilateral pupil is more reliable than the side of hemiparesis; CSF may be clear, bloody, acellular to xanthochromic; *subdural hygroma* (collection of blood and CSF in subdural space) may form after an injury or after meningitis in the infant or young

d. *Cerebral contusion:* severe closed head injury is almost universally accompanied by cortical contusions and surrounding edema, which can cause shifts and increased ICP; on CT, appear as edematous areas of cortex and subcortical white matter admixed with areas of higher density (representing leaked blood); main concern is tendency of contused areas to swell or to develop hematomas, giving rise to delayed clinical deterioration; swelling may be precipitated by excessive administration of i.v. fluid

e. *Traumatic ICH:* may be immediate or delayed *(spatapoplexie);* clinical picture similar to hypertensive brain hemorrhage

E. **Penetrating wounds of the head**

1. *Missiles and fragments:* air is compressed in front of the bullet so that it has an explosive effect on entering tissue; if brain is penetrated at the lower brain stem level, death is instantaneous from respiratory or cardiac arrest; if vital centers are untouched, immediate problem is bleeding, increased ICP, swelling; *treatment: (1) rapid and radical debridement, (2) control ICP with mannitol or dexamethasone, (3) prevent systemic complications; epilepsy is the most troublesome sequelae* (more than one-half of patients)

F. **Sequelae of head injury**

1. *Post-traumatic epilepsy:* most common *delayed sequela* of craniocerebral trauma (5% in closed head injury, 50% in compound skull fracture); interval between head injury and epilepsy varies; interval is longer in children; either focal or generalized (not petit mal); tend to decrease in frequency as years pass; individuals with early attacks are more likely to have complete remission; etiology: abnormality of dendritic branching, providing the groundwork for the excitatory focus or deafferentation of residual cortical neurons

2. *Autonomic dysfunction syndrome in the vegetative state:* occurrence of episodic violent extensor posturing, profuse diaphoresis, hypertension, tachycardia, lasting minutes to an hour; precipitated by painful stimuli, distention of viscus, or spontaneously; result of decortication, allowing hypothalamus to function independently; narcotic and diazepines with slight benefit; bromocriptine with sedative or small doses of morphine is more effective

3. *Post-traumatic nervous instability (postconcussion syndrome): post-traumatic headache/ traumatic neurasthenia;* headache, generalized or localized variable quality, precipitated by straining, emotion, etc., relieved by rest, quiet room; dizziness is also prominent (more of lightheadedness or giddiness); patient is intolerant to noise, emotional excitement, crowds; also tense, restless, decreased concentration; tends to resist all varieties of treatment; eventually symptoms lessen; almost unknown to children

4. *Post-traumatic Parkinson syndrome: controversial* (most probably had Parkinson's disease [PD] or postencephalitic parkinsonism brought to light by head injury) *except in exboxers*

5. *Punch-drunk encephalopathy (dementia pugilistica):* dysarthric speech; forgetful, slow thinking; movements are slow, stiff, uncertain; legs with shuffling, wide-based gait;

often with parkinsonian syndrome and ataxia; pathologically: enlargement of lateral ventricles, thinning of corpus callosum, widened cavum septum pellucidum; fenestration of septal leaves; *diffuse plaques* and Alzheimer's changes; *no Lewy bodies*

6. *Post-traumatic hydrocephalus:* postmortem examinations reveal *adhesive basilar arachnoiditis;* shunt is treatment

7. *Post-traumatic cognitive and psychiatric disorders:* general rule: the lower score on Glasgow Coma Score, longer anterograde amnesia, and, more likely, permanent cognitive and personality changes

NB: Most common sequelae of traumatic brain injury is personality changes.

G. *Treatment*

1. *Patients with only transient unconsciousness:* antidepressants (amitriptyline, imipramine, or selective serotonin reuptake inhibitor); analgesics: aspirin, acetaminophen, or nonsteroidal anti-inflammatory drugs; litigations should be settled as soon as possible

2. *Severe head injury:* first step is to clear the airway and ensure adequate ventilation; careful search for other injuries; Glasgow Coma Score provides a means of evaluating state of consciousness; control factors that raise ICP, such as hypoxia, hypercarbia, hyperthermia, awkward head positions, and high mean airway pressure

   a. If ICP exceeds 15–20 mm Hg, induce hypocarbia by controlled ventilation; maintain P_{CO_2} at 28–33 mm Hg (good for 20–40 minutes—sometimes up to a few hours)

   b. *Hyperosmolar dehydration* (0.25–1.0 g of 20% mannitol every 3–6 hours or 0.75 mg/kg of furosemide) to maintain serum osmolality at 290–300 mOsm/L; sodium level should be between 136–141 mEq/L

   c. Fluids with free water (5% dextrose; 0.5% saline) should be avoided; last resort for increased ICP: *hypothermia and barbiturates;* unless BP is above 180/95, it can be disregarded; β-blockers and ACE inhibitors are drugs of choice in lowering BP; avoid agents that dilate cerebral vasculature, such as nitrates, hydralazine, calcium channel blockers

3. *General measures:* if coma persists >48 hours, oral gastric tube must be placed; cimetidine, 300 mg/day, or equivalent i.v. every 4 hours to keep acidity pH above 3.5; not in favor of prophylactic use of antiepileptic drug; diazepam for restlessness; avoid haloperidol in the acute stage; acetaminophen or cooling blanket for fever; early rehabilitation; age and duration of traumatic amnesia are good prognostic factors (good for the young and children, and amnesia lasting <1 hour up to 24 hours)

H. **Spinal injury:** may be classified as nonmissile and missile; if damaged vertebra are still capable of moving, the fracture/injury is called *unstable,* the rest of injuries are classified as *stable;* spinal cord dysfunction can be *transient, caused by impaired axonal conduction, edema, or compression by extradural or subdural blood*

1. *Traumatic hematomyelia:* collection of blood within the cord; often extending to some distance above and below the level of the central canal; reactive changes: hyperplasia of astrocytes, microglia and blood vessels; long term: *narrowing* of the spinal cord at the level of the injury, *wallerian degeneration, post-traumatic syringomyelia*

2. *Compression of the spinal cord:* effects depend on the rate of development of the compressive lesion; once large enough, it will interfere with blood supply

   a. Majority of compressing lesions arise in the *spinal extradural space* (metastatic carcinoma, lymphoma, myeloma, subacute pyogenic abscess from staphylococci or coliform bacteria, extension of a tuberculoma of the vertebral body, prolapsed intervertebral disc, vascular malformations, and tumors of mesenchymal origin

   b. *Intradural extramedullary lesions:* meningiomas and schwannomas

    c. *Intramedullary lesions:* tumors, vascular malformations and syringomyelias

    d. Treatment: standard treatments for spinal cord compression include corticosteroids, radiotherapy, and surgery; in 101 patients with spinal cord compression from metastatic cancer randomized to surgery + radiotherapy vs. radiotherapy alone, the 30 day mortality rate for surgery was 6% and for radiotherapy alone was 14%; with more patients in the combined treatment group able to recover ability to walk and for longer periods

  3. **Syringomyelia:** cavitation or syrinx that extend over metameric segments; most often *cervicothoracic segments;* most often *single but can be multiple;* occupies the center of the spinal cord, involving *the midline crossing fibers of pain and temperature* (giving cape-like distribution of sensory loss if affecting the cervical region); may fuse laterally with the entering sensory roots or affect the anterior horn cell, may traverse laterally; in majority, extends to the inferior portion of the brain stem but seldom involves the pons; in the medulla, has three types (lateral, midline, and anterior slit)

    a. *Dysraphic theory:* closure defect of the neural tube at the level of the posterior raphe

    b. *Hydrodynamic theory:* distribution of outflow of CSF—increased CSF pressure, causing dilatation of central canal

I. **Concussion in sports**

  1. *Grade I:* no loss of consciousness; transient confusion; symptoms resolve in less than 15 minutes

  2. *Grade II:* no loss of consciousness; transient confusion; symptoms last more than 15 minutes

  3. *Grade III:* any loss of consciousness, either brief (seconds) or prolonged (minutes)

  4. When to return to play after removal from a contest

Grade I concussion	May return to contest if symptoms resolve in <15 minutes
Multiple Grade I concussion	1 week
Grade II concussion	1 week
Multiple Grade II concussion	2 weeks
Grade III concussion—brief LOC	1 week
Grade III concussion—prolonged LOC	2 weeks
Multiple Grade III concussions	1 month or longer

ADDITIONAL NOTES

CHAPTER 2

Dementia

I. Delirium

A. *Definitions*

1. **Confusional state**: characterized by inability to think with proper speed and clarity, impaired immediate recall, and *diminution of attention and concentration*

2. **Delirium:** an *acute confusional state*, marked by *prominent alterations in perception and consciousness* and associated with vivid hallucinations, delusions, heightened alertness, and agitation; hyperactivity of psychomotor and autonomic functions; insomnia; etc.

3. **Dementia:** a syndrome characterized by deterioration of function in *memory, plus two other cognitive domains* (e.g., executive functioning, praxis, language, etc.); compared to previous baseline cognitive ability; *severe enough to interfere with usual social functioning and activities of daily life*

B. *Etiology of delirium*

Intoxication	*Drugs:* alcohol, anticholinergics, sedative hypnotics, opiates, digitalis derivatives, steroids, salicylates, antibiotics, anticonvulsants, antihypertensives, H_2 blockers, antineoplastics, lithium, antiparkinsonian agents, indomethacin, etc.
	Inhalants: gasoline, glue, ether, nitrous oxide, nitrates
	Toxins: carbon disulfide, organic solvents, bromide, heavy metals, organophosphates, carbon monoxide, plants and mushrooms, venom
Withdrawal syndromes	Alcohol
	Sedatives/hypnotics: barbiturates, benzodiazepines, glutethimide, meprobamate, etc.
	Amphetamines
Metabolic disorders	Hypoxia
	Hypoglycemia
	Hepatic, pulmonary, renal, pancreatic insufficiency
	Errors of metabolism: porphyria, carcinoid, Wilson's disease
Nutritional disorders	Vitamin deficiencies: B_{12}, nicotinic acid, thiamine, folate, pyridoxine
	Hypervitaminosis: vitamin A and D intoxication
	Fluid/electrolyte disorders: dehydration or water intoxication; alkalosis/acidosis; excesses or deficiencies of Na, Ca, Mg, etc.
Hormonal disorders	Hyper-/hypothyroidism
	Hyperinsulinism
	Hypopituitarism

	Addison's disease
	Cushing's syndrome
	Hypo-/hyperparathyroidism
Infection	Systemic (especially pneumonia and urinary tract infection)
	Intracranial: encephalitis, meningitis, herpes, rabies, etc.
Neoplasms	Metastases, meningeal carcinomatosis
	Paraneoplastic
	Primary tumors of the temporal lobe, parietal lobe, or brain stem
Inflammatory	Central nervous system vasculitis
Trauma	Subarachnoid hemorrhage
	Postconcussive delirium
	Cerebral contusions or lacerations
Miscellaneous	Postconvulsive
	Postoperative/intensive care unit
	Mixed
	Poststroke

II. Dementia
A. *Etiology of dementia*

Trauma	Dementia pugilistica
	Diffuse axonal injury
	Chronic subdural hematoma
	Postconcussion syndrome
Inflammatory/ infection	Chronic meningitis (tuberculosis, cryptococcus, cysticercosis)
	Syphilis *(general paresis of the insane, gumma, vasculitic)*
	Postherpes simplex encephalitis
	Focal cerebritis/abscess
	Human immunodeficiency virus dementia and opportunistic infections
	Progressive multifocal leukoencephalopathy
	Creutzfeldt-Jakob disease (CJD)
	Lyme disease
	Parenchymal or cerebral sarcoidosis
	Subacute sclerosing panencephalitis
	Whipple's disease of the brain
Neoplastic	Benign and malignant tumors
	Paraneoplastic limbic encephalitis
Metabolic	Hypothyroid

Vitamin B$_1$ deficiency *(Wernicke-Korsakoff)*

Vitamin B$_{12}$ deficiency

Vitamin E deficiency *(neuropathy, ataxia, encephalopathy in celiac disease)*

Nicotinic acid deficiency *(pellagra)*

Uremia/dialysis dementia

Chronic hepatic encephalopathy

Chronic hypoglycemic encephalopathy

Chronic hypercapnia/hyperviscosity/hypoxemia

Chronic hypercalcemia/electrolyte imbalance

Addison's/Cushing's diseases

Hartnup's disease

Vascular Multi-infarct dementia

Binswanger's encephalopathy

Amyloid dementia

Specific vascular syndromes (thalamic, inferotemporal, bifrontal)

Triple borderzone watershed infarction

Diffuse hypoxic/ischemic injury

Mitochondrial disorders (mitochondrial encephalomyopathy with lactic acidosis and stroke-like episodes)

Cerebral autosomal dominant arteriopathy with subcortical infarcts and leukoencephalopathy, migraine

Autoimmune Systemic lupus erythematosus

Polyarteritis nodosa

Temporal arteritis

Wegener's granulomatosis

Isolated angiitis of the central nervous system

Drugs/toxins Medications: β-blockers, neuroleptics, antidepressants, histamine receptor blockers, dopamine receptor blockers

Substances of abuse: alcohol, phencyclidine, mescaline, marijuana psychosis, etc.

Toxins: lead, mercury, arsenic

Demyelinating Multiple sclerosis, Schilder's disease, Baló concentric sclerosis

Electric injury-induced demyelination

Decompression sickness demyelination

Adrenoleukodystrophy

Metachromatic leukodystrophy

Other inflammatory/infectious processes

Obstructive Normal pressure hydrocephalus

Degenerative—adult	Obstructive hydrocephalus
	Alzheimer's disease (AD)
	Pick's disease
	Parkinson's disease (PD)
	Huntington's disease
	Frontotemporal dementia
	Progressive supranuclear palsy
	Dementia with Lewy bodies (DLB)
	Multiple systems atrophy
	Corticobasal ganglionic degeneration
	Hallervorden-Spatz disease
	Primary progressive aphasia
Degenerative—pediatric	Mitochondrial diseases (myoclonic epilepsy with ragged red fibers and mitochondrial encephalomyopathy with lactic acidosis and stroke-like episodes)
	Adrenoleukodystrophy
	Metachromatic leukodystrophy
	Kufs' disease *(neuronal ceroid lipofuscinoses)*
	GM_1 and GM_2 gangliosidoses
	Niemann-Pick II-C
	Krabbe's disease *(globoid cell leukodystrophy)*
	Alexander's disease
	Lafora's disease
	Cerebrotendinous xanthomatosis

B. *Diagnostic workup*

Basic	Complete blood cell count, erythrocyte sedimentation rate, creatinine, electrolytes, glucose, calcium, magnesium, liver function tests, thyroid-stimulating hormone, B_{12}, folate, VDRL, antinuclear antibodies, human immunodeficiency virus, chest x-ray, urinalysis, computed tomography of the head (with contrast if suspecting an enhancing lesion), electroencephalography, neuropsychologic testing, psychiatric consultation (if indicated), spinal tap (if indicated)
Expanded	Magnetic resonance imaging (MRI)with gadolinium
	Spinal tap—cells, protein, glucose, fungus, tuberculosis, virus, cytology, oligoclonal banding, immunoglobulin G, 14-3-3, glutamine, lactate
	Schilling test
	Arterial blood gas
	Toxic screen (drugs, poisons, metals)
	Hemoglobin A1c, insulin
	Vitamins B_1, B_6, E

Porphyrins

Vascular workup: lipid profile, anticardiolipin antibodies, carotid ultrasound, Holter monitor, echocardiogram

Quantitative plasma amino acids

Quantitative urine amino acids

Vasculitis workup: anti–double-stranded DNA, Ro, La, Sm, ribonucleoprotein, antineutrophil cytoplasmic antibodies, C3, C4, CH50

Tumor screen, paraneoplastic serum antibodies

If necessary — Positron emission tomography/single-photon emission computed tomography

Cerebral angiography for vasculitis

Biopsy: brain, meninges, nerve, muscle, skin, liver, kidney

C. *Suggested evaluations for dementia of undetermined cause*

Low-serum ceruloplasmin and copper, high-urine and liver copper	*Wilson's disease*
Plasma very-long-chain fatty acids	*Adrenoleukodystrophy*
White blood cell count arylsulfatase A	*Metachromatic leukodystrophy*
Serum hexosaminidase A and B	*Tay-Sachs disease*
	Sandhoff disease
Muscle biopsy (ragged red fibers on trichrome; polysaccharide nonmembrane bound structures)	*Mitochondrial encephalomyopathy with lactic acidosis and stroke-like episodes*
	Myoclonic epilepsy with ragged red fibers
	Lafora bodies
White blood cell count for galactocerebroside β-galactosidase	*Krabbe's disease*
Serum cholestanol or urine bile acids	*Cerebrotendinous xanthomatosis*
White blood cell count for β-galactosidase	*GM$_1$ gangliosidosis*
Skin biopsy for biochemical testing of fibroblasts	*Niemann-Pick II-C*
X-ray of hands for bone cysts, bone or skin biopsy for fat cells	*Polycystic lipomembranous osteodysplasia with sclerosing leukoencephalopathy*
Urine mucopolysaccharides elevated, serum α-N-acetyl glucosaminidase deficient	*Mucopolysaccharidoses*
Indications for biopsy	*Focal, relevant lesion(s) of undetermined etiology*
	Central nervous system vasculitis
	Subacute sclerosing panencephalitis, CJD, progressive multifocal leukoencephalopathy
	Krabbe's disease (periodic acid-Schiff–positive histiocytes)

Kufs' disease (intranuclear fingerprint pattern)

Neuronal intranuclear (eosinophilic) inclusion disease

D. **AD**: the *most common degenerative disease* of the brain; incidence increases sharply with age after 65; *age is the most important and common risk factor* (10% of patients >65 y/o, 50% of patients >85 y/o); *other risk factors: Down syndrome* (patient 30–45 y/o shows similar pathologic changes), *mother's age at birth, head injury, excess aluminum intake, apolipoprotein E genotype;* reported *protective factors: smoking, education, inheritance of apolipoprotein E2 allele*

NB: The Clinical Dementia Rating (CDR) Scale is a dementia staging instrument with an impairment range from none to maximal (0, 0.5, 1, 2, 3) in 6 domains: memory, orientation, judgment and problem solving, function in community, home and hobbies, and personal care.

1. *Clinical features:* common words, tasks, places, and events are forgotten; remote memory is also affected, difficulty remembering words, echolalia (repetition of spoken phrase), difficulty balancing checkbook; may progress to acalculia, difficulty parking car, putting arms in sleeves, lost on way to home; initially little change in behavior but later with paranoid delusions, anxiety, phobias, akinesia, mutism; day-night pattern changes; parkinsonian look; rigidity and fine tremor; myoclonus

NB: Early in the disease, AD patients are characterized by impaired word recall and normal digit span.

NB: *Mild cognitive impairment* refers to mild memory impairment or subtle changes in cognitive function that do not interfere with daily activities for which no underlying cause can be found.

2. *Pathology:* brain *volume is decreased* in advanced case up to 20% or more; ventricles enlarge proportionally; extreme *hippocampal atrophy;* atrophic process involves temporal, parietal, and frontal, but cases vary a lot; microscopically: *senile or neuritic plaques, neurofibrillary tangles, granulovacuolar degeneration* of neurons most prominent in pyramidal cell layer of hippocampus; *Hirano bodies*
   a. *Cholinergic neurons of the nucleus basalis of Meynert* (substantia innominata), *locus ceruleus, medial septal nuclei, and diagonal band of Broca are reduced;* with resulting deficiency of acetylcholine
   b. *Neurofibrillary tangles* are composed of clusters of abnormal tubules, and *senile plaques contain a core of amyloid;* tangles and plaques are found in all association cortex; *CA1 zone of the hippocampus* disproportionately affected

NB: Amyloid starts as an amyloid precursor protein, normally cleaved by a series of enzymes into a short version that can be easily excreted by the body. In AD, amyloid is incorrectly cleaved by beta-secretase and gamma-secretase (assisted by Presenilin-1). This abnormal cleaving results in amyloid aggregation that ultimately leads to plaque formation.

3. *Genetics: familial in 10%*
   a. A defective gene was identified on *chromosome 21* near the β-amyloid gene which codes for an errant *AAP (amyloid precursor protein) gene.*
   b. *Chromosome 14,* for the protein called *presenilin-1;* accounts for 80% of the familial cases.
   c. Gene mutation on *chromosome 1* for the protein *presenilin-2;* age of onset for all familial cases is earlier.
   d. *Apolipoprotein E4 on chromosome 19* is associated with tripling the *risk* of acquiring AD.

4. *Treatment*
   a. Cholinesterase inhibitors: pharmacologic characteristics

	Tacrine	Donepezil	Rivastigmine	Galantamine
Year available	1993	1996	2000	2001
Brain selectivity	No	Yes	Yes	Yes
Reversibility	Yes	Yes	Yes/slow	Yes
Chemical class	Acridine	Piperidine	Carbamate	Phenanthrene alkaloid
Enzymes inhibited				
Acetylcholinesterase	Yes	Yes	Yes	Yes
Butyrylcholinesterase	Yes	Negligible	Yes	Negligible
Nicotinic receptor modulation	No	No	No	Yes
Doses per day	4	1	2	2
Initial dose (mg/day)	40	5	3	8
Maximum dose (mg/day)	160	10	12	24
Given with food	No, unless nausea occurs	No	Yes	Yes
Plasma half-life (hrs)	2–4	~70	~1	~6
Elimination pathway	Liver	Liver	Kidney	50% Kidney 50% Liver
Metabolism by cytochrome P450	Yes	Yes	Minimal	Yes

   b. *Memantine:* a low to moderate affinity to *noncompetitive N-methyl-D-aspartate receptor antagonist* (N-methyl-D-aspartate receptors, by the excitatory amino acid glutamate, have been hypothesized to contribute to the symptomatology of AD); U.S. Food and Drug Administration (FDA)-approved for the treatment of moderate to severe dementia in AD; titrate doses up to 20 mg/day

NB: There is lack of definitive evidence that ginkgo biloba, estrogen, statins, or non-steroidal anti-inflammatory drugs can prevent or treat AD.

NB: Having Type II DM increases the risk of developing AD by 65%. Patients with DM and cognitive decline should be treated aggressively, including the use of insulin.

NB: At a severity of CDR 0.5, driving is mildly impaired and a referral for a driving performance evaluation should be considered. At a severity of CDR 1, driving is potentially dangerous and discontinuation of driving should be strongly considered.

E. **Frontotemporal dementia (FTD):** syndrome characterized by *prominent frontal lobe symptoms,* in contrast to the more pronounced amnestic symptoms in AD; reduced frontal cerebral blood flow; symmetric frontal and anterior temporal atrophy with frontal ventricular enlargement; striatum, amygdala, or hippocampus is usually spared

NB: Serotonergic deficit has been consistently reported in FTD such that some experts will treat with SSRIs even in the absence of depression. There is no evidence of significant cholinergic deficit in FTD.

1. *FTD of the frontal lobe degeneration type:* microscopically: microvacuolation and gliosis predominantly over the outer three laminae of cerebral frontal cortex; no Pick bodies, ballooned neurons, or Lewy bodies (LBs)
2. **NB:** *FTD of the Pick type:* more pronounced *frontal lobe atrophy and in addition to microvacuolation, gliosis, and neuronal loss have ballooned or inflated neurons and Pick bodies;* Pick bodies are most frequent in the medial parts of temporal lobes; clinically: gradual onset of confusion with personal neglect, apathy, focal disturbances (such as aphasia and apraxia), personality changes, abulia, frontal release signs, and sometimes Klüver-Bucy syndrome; incidence of depression is much less compared to PD, HD, or multiple sclerosis
3. *FTD of the motor neuron type:* previously described clinical and neuropathologic findings are *coupled with spinal motor neuron degeneration; motor neuron loss is most severe in the cervical and thoracic segments;* may be identical to amyotrophy-dementia complex

NB: *Semantic dementia* is a category of FTD characterized by insidiously progressive yet relatively focal disease until late in the course of their illness. They have fluent yet empty speech, with naming impairment and failure to understand the meaning of the words.

F. **DLB:** characterized by the clinical *triad of fluctuating cognitive impairment, recurrent visual hallucinations, and spontaneous motor features of parkinsonism;* in an attempt to define DLB as a distinct clinical syndrome, separate from AD and PD with dementia, a consensus workshop established a new set of diagnostic criteria

Mandatory	Presence of dementia, PLUS
	Core features (at least two out of three for probable DLB):
	Fluctuation of cognition, function, or alertness
	Visual hallucinations
	Parkinsonism
Supporting features	Repeated falls
	Syncope
	Transient loss of consciousness
	Neuroleptic sensitivity
	Systematized delusions
	Nonvisual hallucinations
	Depression
	Rapid eye movement sleep behavior disorder

1. *Clinical:* the degree to which an individual patient exhibits cognitive impairment, behavioral problems, and parkinsonian features is variable.
2. *Pathology:* the essential hallmark of DLB pathology is *the LB; these LBs are observed in the brain stem nuclei, subcortical regions, and cerebral cortices;* in the brain stem, pigmented neurons often present with the classic morphology of intracellular LBs, comprising an eosinophilic core with a peripheral halo; immunohistochemistry using antibodies

against ubiquitin or α-synuclein has been shown to be more sensitive and specific in the detection of cortical LB; the clinical overlap of AD, DLB, and PD with dementia similarly extends to their pathology—most cases of DLB have varying degrees of AD pathology, including deposits of β-amyloid protein and neurofibrillary tangles.

3. *Neurochemistry:* substantial *loss of cholinergic neurons* in the nucleus basalis of Meynert, suggesting a cholinergic mechanism of cognitive impairment in DLB, similar to that of AD; *deficits in acetylcholine, γ-aminobutyric acid, dopamine, and serotonin* neurotransmission have also been described in DLB; neocortical choline acetyltransferase, a synthetic enzyme for acetylcholine, is decreased significantly, similar to that seen in AD or PD with dementia; reduced dopamine and its metabolites have been shown in DLB brains, possibly accounting for its parkinsonian features.

4. *Treatment:* must be individualized.
   a. Although there are no officially approved drugs for DLB, limited experience from clinical trials, as well as past experience with treatment of AD and PD patients, provide some basis for making drug choices; the cholinergic deficit seen in DLB makes *cholinesterase inhibitor* drugs the mainstay of treatment for cognitive impairment; this class of drugs has also shown therapeutic benefit in reducing hallucinations and other neuropsychiatric symptoms of the disease.
   b. Patients with DLB are exquisitely sensitive to the extrapyramidal side effects of neuroleptic medications; thus, only *atypical antipsychotic agents,* such as quetiapine, should be considered as alternative treatment for psychosis.
   c. Anxiety and depression are best treated with *selective serotonin reuptake inhibitors,* whereas rapid eye movement sleep behavior disorder may be treated with low-dose *clonazepam.*
   d. Parkinsonism responds to dopaminergic agents; however, precipitation or aggravation of hallucinosis may occur; *levodopa* is preferred over dopamine agonists owing to its lower propensity to cause hallucinations and somnolence.

NB: DLB may present as parkinsonism with early-onset visual hallucinations and dementia; they are extremely sensitive to neuroleptics.

NB: The DLB Consortium has revised criteria for the diagnosis of DLB. REM sleep behavior disorder, severe neuroleptic sensitivity, and reduced striatal dopamine transporter activity on functional imaging are now given greater diagnostic weight as features suggestive of DLB. When any of these are present with one of the core features such as visual hallucinations, parkinsonism, or fluctuating attention, then the diagnosis of probably DLB is supported.

G. **Multi-infarct dementia:** history of one or more strokes is usually clear; deficit increases with strokes, and focality of deficits may indicate the type and location of strokes; multiple lacunar infarcts may also give rise to a pseudobulbar palsy with a history of stroke; **Binswanger's disease:** multi-infarct state of cerebral white matter associated with dementia; **cerebral autosomal dominant arteriopathy with subcortical infarcts and leukoencephalopathy** treatment: may respond to cholinesterase inhibitors.

H. *Other dementias*
   1. *Mesolimbocortical dementia of non-Alzheimer's type:* memory, initiative, and attention are affected more and early; histologically with cell loss and gliosis in hippocampi, caudate nuclei, thalami, and the ventral tegmental area of the mesencephalon
   2. *Thalamic dementia:* rapidly progressive (over few months) dementia associated with choreoathetosis; relatively pure degeneration of the thalamic neurons; myoclonus may be present; should be differentiated from CJD

3. *Hypoxic encephalopathy and acute inclusion body (herpes simplex) encephalitis:* these two conditions may cause injury to the inferomedial portion of both temporal lobes and may leave the patient with memory and learning difficulties
4. *Severe trauma:* especially in conditions when prolonged coma and stupor follow the injury, causes well-established cerebral deficits
5. *Primary progressive aphasia:* a linguistic syndrome of *progressive aphasia without initial dementia;* may exhibit neuropathologic features identical to FTD of the frontal lobe degeneration type, except that speech areas are more heavily involved; progressive aphasia has also been described in the context of AD, CJD, corticobasal ganglionic degeneration, and classic Pick's disease
6. *Prion disorders: CJD, Gerstmann-Straussler-Scheinker*
7. *Hydrocephalic dementia:* normal pressure hydrocephalus—dementia, gait disturbance (magnetic gait), and urinary incontinence
8. *Dementia pugilistica (punch drunk):* long recognized sequelae of multiple head injuries in boxing; pathology: demonstrate β-*amyloid protein-containing plaques and neurofibrillary tangles*

ADDITIONAL NOTES

CHAPTER 3

Neuromuscular Disorders

I. General Evaluation

  A. **History**

    1. Chief complaint

      a. Weakness vs. sensory

      b. Acute vs. subacute vs. chronic

      c. Symmetric vs. asymmetric

    2. Contributing history

      a. Family history

      b. Medications, toxins

      c. Trauma

      d. Infections

      e. Vaccinations

      f. Diet

      g. Concurrent medical conditions (i.e., autoimmune, rheumatologic, endocrinopathies, cardiovascular)

    3. Neurophysiologic studies (see Chapter 10: Clinical Neurophysiology)

  B. *Types of muscle fibers*

	Type 1	Type 2a	Type 2b
Axon innervating	Smaller	Larger	Larger
Type	Tonic	Phasic	Phasic
Color	Dark	Dark	Pale
Fiber diameter	Small	Larger	Largest
Twitch speed	Slow	Fast	Fast
Fatigability	Low	Low	High

  C. *Electromyography (EMG) of neuropathic, neuromuscular, and myopathic processes*

	SPMUPs	Frequency recruitment	Recruitment/force
Myopathy	+	Normal	Increased
Neuromuscular junction	+	Normal	Increased
Denervation	+	Normal or decreased	Increased
Reinnervation	+	Decreased	Possible decrease or no change

SPMUPs, short-duration, polyphasic motor unit potentials; +, present.

D. *Pathologic differentiation between myopathic and neurogenic processes*

Myopathic	Neurogenic
Marked irregularity of fiber size	Nests of atrophic fibers
Rounded fibers	Angular fibers
Real increase in number of muscle nuclei	Pseudo-increase of nuclei due to cytoplasmic atrophy
Centralized nuclei	Not present
Necrotic and basophilic fibers	Not present
Cytoplasmic alterations	Target fibers
Copious interstitial fibrosis	Minimal
Inflammatory cellular infiltrate	Not present

II. Peripheral Neuropathic Syndromes

A. *Classification and degrees of peripheral nerve injury*
   1. **Segmental demyelination**
      a. Conduction block
      b. Normal distal compound muscle action potential (CMAP) and sensory nerve action potential (SNAP)
   2. **Neurapraxia** and **axonotmesis:** both can lead to decreased motor unit recruitment
   3. *Wallerian degeneration: complete in 7–11 days*

	1st Degree	2nd Degree	3rd Degree	4th Degree	5th Degree
Pathology	Segmental demyelination; neurapraxia	Loss of axons with intact supporting structures; axonotmesis	Loss of axons with disrupted endoneurium; neurotmesis	Loss of axons with disrupted endoneurium and perineurium	Loss of axons with disruption of all supporting structures (discontinuous)
Prognosis	Excellent; usually complete recovery in 2–3 mos	Slow recovery dependent on sprouting and reinnervation	Protracted, and recovery may fail because of misdirected axonal sprouts	Recovery unlikely without surgical repair	Recovery not possible without surgical repair

B. **Mononeuropathies**
   1. **Sciatic mononeuropathy**
      a. *Common causes*
         i. Hip replacement/fracture/dislocation
         ii. Femur fracture
         iii. Acute compression (coma, drug overdose, intensive care unit [ICU], prolonged sitting)
         iv. Gunshot or knife wound
         v. Infarction (vasculitis, iliac artery occlusion, arterial bypass surgery)

      vi. Gluteal contusion or compartmental syndrome (during anticoagulation)

      vii. Gluteal injection

      viii. Endometriosis (catamenial sciatica)

NB: The sciatic nerve is composed of a peroneal division and tibial division. The only muscle above the knee supplied by the peroneal division is the short head of the biceps femoris.

  2. **Footdrop**

    a. *Common causes*

      i. Deep peroneal mononeuropathy

      ii. Common peroneal mononeuropathy

      iii. Sciatic mononeuropathy

      iv. Lumbosacral plexopathy (especially of the lumbosacral trunk)

      v. Lumbar radiculopathy (L5 or, less commonly, L4)

      vi. Motor neuron disease

      vii. Parasagittal cortical or subcortical cerebral lesion

NB: To differentiate a peroneal nerve lesion from an L5 lesion in a patient with a footdrop, test the foot invertors. Peroneal nerve lesions should not involve the foot invertors. Foot evertors will be involved with damage to the superficial peroneal nerve. The majority of the peroneal palsies occur at the level of the fibular head.

Clinical Assessment of Footdrop

	Peroneal neuropathy	L5 radiculopathy	Lumbar plexopathy	Sciatic neuropathy
Common causes	Compression/trauma	Disk herniation, spinal stenosis	Pelvic surgery, hematoma, prolonged labor	Hip surgery, injection injury
Ankle inversion	Normal	Weak	Weak	Normal or mildly weak
Plantar flexion	Normal	Normal	Normal	Normal or mildly weak
Ankle jerk	Normal	Normal	Normal	Normal or depressed
Sensory loss	Peroneal only	Poorly demarcated except big toe	L5 dermatome	Peroneal and lateral cutaneous of calf

  3. **Piriformis syndrome**

    a. Clinically: *buttock and leg pain worse during sitting without low back pain;* exacerbated by internal rotation or abduction and external rotation of the hip; local tenderness in the buttock; soft or no neurologic signs

    b. EMG/nerve conduction velocity (NCV): *denervation seen in branches after the piriformis muscle, but normal if branches before the piriformis muscle*

  4. **Femoral mononeuropathy**

    a. Clinically: *acute thigh and knee extension weakness; numbness of anterior thigh;* absent knee jerk; normal thigh adduction

    b. Common causes

      i. *Compression in the pelvis:* retractor blade during pelvic surgery (iatrogenic), abdominal hysterectomy, radical prostatectomy, renal transplantation, and so forth; iliacus or psoas retroperitoneal; hematoma; pelvic mass

      ii. *Compression in the inguinal region:* inguinal ligament during lithotomy position (vaginal delivery, laparoscopy, vaginal hysterectomy, urologic procedures); inguinal hematoma; during total hip replacement; inguinal mass

      iii. *Stretch injury* (hyperextension)

      iv. Others: radiation; laceration; injection

  5. **Tarsal tunnel syndrome:** compression of the tibial nerve or any of its three branches under the flexor retinaculum

    a. *Clinically:* sensory impairment in the sole of the foot; Tinel's sign; muscle atrophy of the sole of the foot; rarely weak (long toe flexors are intact); ankle reflexes normal; sensation of the dorsum of the foot normal; note: not associated with footdrop

NB: Nocturnal pain is common, such as in carpal tunnel syndrome (CTS). There is an anterior tarsal tunnel syndrome caused by compression of the deep peroneal nerve at the ankle that results in paresis of the extensor digitorum brevis alone.

    b. Differential diagnosis

      i. Plantar fasciitis

      ii. Stress fracture

      iii. Arthritis

      iv. Bursitis

      v. Reflex sympathetic dystrophy

      vi. High tibial or sciatic mononeuropathy

      vii. Sacral radiculopathy

      viii. Bilateral peripheral neuropathy

  6. **Meralgia paresthetica**

    a. *Anatomy*

      i. Entrapment of the *lateral femoral cutaneous nerve,* which is a pure sensory branch via L2 and L3 nerve roots

      ii. Enters through the opening between the inguinal ligament and its attachment to the anterior superior iliac spine

    b. Etiologies

      i. Obesity

      ii. Wearing tight belt or girdle

      iii. Pregnancy

      iv. Prolonged sitting

      v. More common in diabetics

      vi. Abdominal or pelvic mass

      vii. Metabolic neuropathies

    c. Clinical: *burning dysesthesias in the lateral aspect of the upper thigh just above the knee;* may be exacerbated by clothing; may improve with massage; bilateral in 20% of cases

    d. Differential diagnosis

      i. Femoral neuropathy

      ii. L2 or L3 radiculopathy

      iii. Nerve compression by abdominal or pelvic tumor

    e. Treatment: usually spontaneous improvement; nonsteroidal anti-inflammatory drugs for 7–10 days for pain; avoid tight pants/belts; use suspenders, if able

  7. **Ulnar nerve mononeuropathy**

    a. Localization of ulnar neuropathy

      i. Guyon's canal (wrist) entrapment: sensory loss of the palmar and dorsal surfaces of the little and ring fingers and the ulnar side of the hand

    ii. Sensory loss of medial half of the ring finger that spares the lateral half (pathognomonic of ulnar nerve lesion; not seen in lower trunk or C8 root lesion)

    iii. *If flexor carpi ulnaris and flexor digitorum profundus are both abnormal with axonal loss, the lesions are localized proximal to the elbow.*

    iv. *Purely axonal lesions with normal flexor carpi ulnaris and flexor digitorum profundus suggest lesions around the wrist.*

    v. Ulnar entrapment syndromes at the elbow

      (A) *Cubital tunnel syndrome:* proximal edge of the flexor carpi ulnaris aponeurosis (arcuate ligament)

      (B) Subluxation of the ulnar nerve at the ulnar groove: often caused by repetitive trauma

      (C) *Tardy ulnar palsy:* may occur years after a distal humeral fracture in association with a valgus deformity

      (D) Idiopathic ulnar neuropathy at the elbow

      (E) Other causes of compressive ulnar neuropathy at the elbow: pressure; bony deformities; cubital tunnel syndrome; chronic subluxation

    vi. *Martin-Gruber anastomosis: patients with apparent conduction block of the ulnar motor fibers at the elbow should undergo further investigation to rule out the presence of anomalous nerves (Martin-Gruber anastomosis), which occur in 20–25% of the normal population*

  b. Clinical signs of ulnar neuropathy: Tinel's sign at the elbow; sensory exam may be normal despite symptoms; ulnar claw hand (caused by weakness or by flexion of the interphalangeal joints of the 3rd and 4th lumbricals); *Froment's sign;* fascicular phenomenon (variable weakness and numbness distally due to propensity for partial focal lesions to affect fascicles differentially within that nerve)

NB: Ulnar nerve lesions do not cause sensory symptoms proximal to the wrist. If such symptoms are present, think about a proximal lesion (e.g., root).

Lesion site	Nerve affected	Clinical
Guyon's canal	Main trunk of ulnar nerve	Ulnar palmar sensory loss and weakness of all ulnar intrinsic hand muscles
	Ulnar cutaneous branch	Ulnar palmar sensory loss only
Pisohamate hiatus	Deep palmar branch (distal to branch to the abductor digiti minimi)	Weakness of ulnar intrinsic hand muscles with sparing of the hypothenar muscles and without sensory loss
NB: Pure motor lesion!		
Midpalm (rare)	Deep palmar branch (distal to hypothenars)	Weakness of adductor pollicis, the 1st, 2nd, and possibly the 3rd interossei only, sparing the 4th interossei and hypothenar muscles, without sensory loss

8. **Radial nerve mononeuropathy**
  a. Anatomy
    i. Arises from *posterior divisions* of three trunks of the brachial plexus
    ii. Receives contribution from C5 to C8
    iii. Winds laterally along spiral groove of the humerus

      iv. Distinguished from brachial plexus posterior cord injury by sparing deltoid (axillary nerve) and latissimus dorsi (thoracodorsal nerve)

  b. Etiologies and localization

      i. *Spiral groove* (most common)

      ii. *Saturday night palsy:* acute compression at the spiral groove

     iii. Humeral fracture

     iv. Strenuous muscular effort

      v. Injection injury

     vi. Trauma

  c. Clinical

      i. *Axillary compression:* less common than compression in the upper arm; etiologies: secondary to misuse of crutches or during drunken sleep; clinical: weakness of triceps and more distal muscles innervated by radial nerve

      ii. *Mid–upper-arm compression:* site of compression: spiral groove, intermuscular septum, or just distal to this site; etiologies: Saturday night palsy, under general anesthesia; clinical: weakness of wrist extensors (wristdrop) and finger extensors; triceps are normal

     iii. *Forearm compression:* Radial nerve enters anterior compartment of the arm above the elbow and gives branches to brachialis, brachioradialis, and extensor carpi radialis longus before dividing into posterior interosseous nerve and the superficial radial nerve; the posterior interosseous nerve goes through the supinator muscle through fibers known as arcade of Frohse.

NB: The posterior interosseous nerve is purely motor. A lesion results in fingerdrop. The superficial radial nerve is mainly sensory.

      (A) *Posterior interosseous neuropathy*

        (1) Etiologies: lipomas, ganglia, fibromas, rheumatoid disease

        (2) Clinical: extensor weakness of thumb and fingers (fingerdrop)—distinguished from radial nerve palsy by less to no wrist extensor weakness; no sensory loss

NB: Posterior interosseous syndrome spares the supinator, which receives innervation proximal to the site of compression.

      (B) *Radial tunnel syndrome (supinator tunnel syndrome)*

        (1) Contains radial nerve and its two main branches including posterior interosseous nerve and superficial radial nerve

        (2) Etiologies: fourth supination or pronation or inflammation of supinator muscle (tennis elbow)

        (3) Clinical: pain in the region of common extensor origin at the lateral epicondyle; tingling in distribution of superficial radial nerve; usually no weakness

NB: Cheiralgia paresthetica is a pure sensory syndrome by lesion of the superficial cutaneous branch of the radial nerve in the forearm. It causes paresthesias and sensory loss in the radial part of the dorsum of the hands and the dorsal aspect of the first 3½ fingers.

  9. **Median nerve entrapment**

    a. The two most common sites of entrapment of the median nerve: transverse carpal ligament at the wrist *(CTS);* and upper forearm by pronator teres muscle *(pronator teres syndrome)*

b. Anatomy
  i. Contribution from C5 to T1.
  ii. In the upper forearm, it passes through the pronator teres, supplying this muscle, and then branches to form the purely motor anterior interosseous nerve, which supplies all the muscles of finger and wrist flexion; it emerges from the lateral edge of the flexor digitorum superficialis and later passes under the transverse carpal ligament.
  iii. The transverse carpal ligament attaches medially to the pisiform and hamate.
  iv. The palmar cutaneous branch arises from the radial aspect of the nerve proximal to the transverse carpal ligament and crosses over the ligament to provide sensory innervation to the base of the thenar eminence.

c. **Carpal Tunnel Syndrome (CTS)**
  i. Etiologies
    (A) *Trauma:* repetitive movement; repetitive forceful grasping or pinching; awkward positioning of hand or wrist; direct pressure over carpal tunnel; use of vibrating tools
    (B) *Systemic conditions:* obesity; local trauma; transient development during pregnancy; mucopolysaccharidosis V; tuberculous tenosynovitis
    (C) Other: dialysis shunts
  ii. Differential diagnosis
    (A) Cervical radiculopathy, especially C6/C7
    (B) Neurogenic thoracic outlet syndrome: sensory manifestations are in C8/T1 distribution
    (C) Peripheral polyneuropathy: manifestations in legs; hyporeflexia/areflexia
    (D) *High median mononeuropathy: e.g., pronator syndrome, compression at the ligament of Struthers in the distal arm; both have weakness in the long finger flexors*
    (E) Cervical myelopathy
  iii. Clinical
    (A) Dysesthesias with numb hand that may awaken patient at night: palm side of lateral 3½ fingers, including thumb, index, middle, and lateral half of ring finger; dorsal side of the same fingers distal to the proximal interphalangeal joint; radial half of palm
    (B) Weakness of hand: particularly grip strength
    (C) *Phalen's test:* 30–60 seconds of complete wrist flexion reproduces pain in 80% of cases
    (D) *Tinel's sign:* paresthesia or pain in median nerve distribution produced by tapping carpal tunnel in 60% of cases
  iv. *EMG/NCV*
    (A) The electrophysiologic hallmark of CTS is *focal slowing of conduction at the wrist.*
    (B) Normal in 15% of cases of CTS.
    (C) *Sensory latencies are more sensitive than motor latencies.*
    (D) Normal median nerve should be at least 4 milliseconds faster than ulnar nerve.

Degree	Sensory NCV latency (msecs)	Motor NCV latency (msecs)
Normal	<3.7	<4.5
Mild	3.7–4.0	4.5–6.9
Moderate	4.1–5.0	7.0–9.9
Severe	>5.0 or no response	>10.0

      v. Lab testing
        (A) Diabetes: fasting glucose
        (B) Thyroid disease (myxedema)
        (C) Multiple myeloma: complete blood count
      vi. Treatment
        (A) Nonsurgical: rest; nonsteroidal anti-inflammatory drugs; neutral position splint; local steroid injection
        (B) Surgical: carpal tunnel release
  d. **Pronator teres syndrome**
      i. *Etiologies:* direct trauma; repeated pronation with tight handgrip
      ii. Nerve entrapment between two heads of pronator teres
      iii. Clinical: vague aching and fatigue of forearm with weak grip; not exacerbated during sleep; pain in palm distinguishes this from CTS because median palmar cutaneous branch transverses over the transverse carpal ligament
C. **Radiculopathies**
  1. Clinical
    a. **Lumbosacral radiculopathy**
      i. *L5 radiculopathy:* most common radiculopathy

Clinical Presentations in Lumbosacral Radiculopathy

	S1	L5	L4	L2/L3
Pain radiation	Buttock	Buttock	Hip	Groin
	Posterior thigh and leg	Posterior thigh and leg	Anterior thigh	Anteromedial thigh
			Knee	
	Lateral foot	Dorsal foot	Medial leg	
Sensory impairment	Posterior thigh	Lateral leg	Anterior thigh	Groin
		Dorsal foot	Medial leg	Medial thigh
	Lateral foot	Big toe		
	Little toe			
Weakness	Plantar flexion	Toe dorsiflexion	Knee extension	Hip flexion and knee extension
	Toe flexion	Ankle dorsiflexion	Ankle dorsiflexion	
		Inversion		
		Eversion		
Diminished reflexes	Ankle jerk	None	Knee jerk	Knee jerk

    b. *Cervical radiculopathies*

Clinical Presentations in Cervical Radiculopathy

	C5	C6	C7	C8
Pain	Parascapular area shoulder	Shoulder	Posterior arm forearm	Medial arm
		Arm		
	Upper arm	Forearm	Index/middle fingers	Forearm

Clinical Presentations in Cervical Radiculopathy

	C5	C6	C7	C8
Sensory impairment	Upper arm	Thumb/index finger Lateral arm Forearm Thumb/index finger	Index/middle fingers	Little/ring fingers Medial arm Forearm Little finger
Weakness	Scapular fixators Shoulder abduction Elbow flexion	Shoulder abduction Elbow flexion Forearm pronation	Elbow extension Wrist and finger extension	Hand intrinsics and long flexors and extensors of finger
Diminished reflexes	Biceps brachioradialis	Biceps brachioradialis	Triceps	None

2. Differential diagnosis of radiculopathies
   a. Congenital
      i. Meningeal cyst
      ii. Conjoined nerve root
   b. Acquired
      i. Spinal stenosis
      ii. Spondylosis
      iii. Spondylolisthesis
      iv. Ganglion cyst of facet joint
   c. Infectious
      i. Diskitis
      ii. Lyme disease
   d. Neoplastic
   e. Vascular
   f. Referred pain syndromes
      i. Kidney infection
      ii. Kidney stone
      iii. Gallstones
      iv. Appendicitis
      v. Endometriosis
      vi. Pyriformis syndrome
3. Electrophysiologic studies in radiculopathies
   a. *Needle EMG: the most sensitive electrodiagnostic test for diagnosis of radiculopathy in general.*
   b. The goals of EMG in radiculopathy: exclude more distal lesion; confirm root compression; localize the compression to either a single root or multiple roots.
   c. Differential diagnosis of lumbosacral plexopathy and lumbosacral radiculopathy depends on: *EMG in paraspinal muscles → abnormal in radiculopathy; SNAP__ abnormal in plexopathy*

NB: Lesions proximal to the dorsal root ganglion will manifest clinically with sensory loss, but sensory NCVs will be normal.

     d. *Two criteria for diagnosing radiculopathy: denervation in a segmental myotomal distribution, and normal SNAP*

     e. SNAP-correlated levels

         i. L4: saphenous

         ii. S1: sural

         iii. L5: superficial peroneal

D. **Plexopathies**

   1. **Brachial plexopathy**

     a. Etiologies

         i. Tumor (Pancoast's syndrome): usually lower plexus

         ii. Idiopathic peripheral plexitis: usually upper plexus or diffuse; antecedent or concurrent upper respiratory tract infection occurred in 25% of cases; one-third have bilateral involvement; predominant symptom is acute onset of intense pain with sudden weakness, typically within 2 weeks

         iii. Viral

         iv. After radiation treatment

         v. Diabetes

         vi. Vasculitis

         vii. Hereditary

         viii. Traumatic

     b. Clinical: more common in young women; weakness of the hand with wasting of the thenar; greater than hypothenar eminence; variable pain and paresthesia in the medial aspect of the upper extremity; exacerbated by upper extremity activity; minimal involvement of the radially innervated muscles; after 1 year, 60% of upper plexus lesions are functionally normal, whereas lower plexus lesions have persistent symptomatology

         i. **Erb-Duchenne palsy** *(upper radicular syndrome): upper roots (C4, C5, and C6) or upper trunk of the brachial plexus;* blow to neck or birth injury; clinical: *Waiter's/bellhop's tip; weak arm abduction/elbow flexion, supination, and lateral arm rotation*

         ii. **Klumpke's palsy** (lower radicular syndrome): *C8 and T1 lesion* (clinically, as if combined median and ulnar damage); sudden arm pull or during delivery; clinical: paralyzed thenar muscles and flexors; flattened simian hand

         iii. **Middle radicular syndrome:** *C7 or middle trunk lesion; crutch injury;* clinical: loss of radially innervated muscles (except brachioradialis and part of triceps); *EMG/NCV:* usually takes up to 3 weeks for electrophysiologic findings; chronic denervation (large motor unit potentials [MUPs]) in needle electromyographs; low or absent SNAP in the ulnar nerve with normal SNAP of median nerve

NB: In a patient with breast cancer and history of radiation, the plexus may be affected by carcinomatous invasion of the plexus vs. radiation-induced plexopathy. Carcinomatous invasion is usually painful, whereas radiation-induced plexopathy is usually painless and may present myokymic discharges in EMG.

   2. **Lumbosacral plexopathy**

     a. *Etiologies*

i. *Pelvic masses:* malignant neoplasms (lymphoma; ovarian, colorectal, and uterine cancer); retroperitoneal lymphadenopathy; abscess

ii. *Pelvic hemorrhage:* iliacus hematoma (only femoral nerve); psoas hematoma; extensive retroperitoneal hematoma

iii. *Intrapartum*

iv. Pelvic fracture

v. Radiation injury

vi. Diabetes

vii. Idiopathic lumbosacral plexitis

b. *Anatomy and clinical findings*

  i. Lumbar plexus

    (A) From ventral rami of L1, L2, L3, and most of L4 roots, which divide into dorsal (femoral nerve without L1) and ventral (obturator nerve without L1) branches

    (B) Plexus also posteriorly gives rise directly to iliacus, psoas muscles, and three other nerves

  ii. *Lumbosacral trunk (lumbosacral cord)*

    (A) Primarily L5 root

    (B) Travels adjacent to the sacroiliac joint while being covered by psoas muscle, except the terminal portion at the pelvic rim where the S1 nerve root joins

    (C) *Lesion will cause weakness of inversion and eversion in addition to footdrop; may have variable hamstring and gluteal muscle weakness*

  iii. *Sacral plexus*

    (A) Fusion of lumbosacral trunk and ventral rami of S1, S2, S3, and S4 roots

    (B) Gives rise to sciatic nerve and superior and inferior gluteal nerves

    (C) *Lesion will cause sciatica-like symptom with gluteal muscle involvement*

E. **Cauda equina syndrome and conus medullaris syndrome**

	Conus medullaris syndrome	Cauda equina syndrome
Onset	Sudden	Gradual
Localization	Bilateral	Unilateral
Spontaneous pain	Symmetric in perineum or thighs	Prominent asymmetric severe radicular-type pain
Sensory deficit	Bilateral symmetric sensory dissociation	Saddle anesthesia but no dissociation
Motor loss	Symmetric ± fasciculations	—
Autonomic symptoms	Prominent early	Late
Reflexes	Ankle jerk absent	Ankle jerk absent
	Knee jerk preserved	Knee jerk absent
Other	—	Urinary retention (90%)
	—	Diminished anal tone

F. **Diabetic neuropathies**
   1. *Pathophysiology:* most common cause of neuropathy; 50% of patients with diabetes and neuropathic symptoms or abnormal NCV on electrophysiologic testing; up to 25% of diabetic patients have signs and symptoms of neuropathy; most common after age 50 years
      a. *Pathology: loss of myelinated fibers is the predominant finding; segmental demyelination-remyelination; may have axonal degeneration*
      b. *EMG/NCV:* both demyelinating and axonal findings may be present; decreased amplitude; peroneal nerve is best predictor
   2. *Classification of diabetic neuropathy*
      a. **Distal symmetric polyneuropathy**
         i. Mixed sensory-motor-autonomic
         ii. Predominantly sensory
            (A) Types: small fiber (including autonomic); large fiber; mixed
            (B) Signs/symptoms: symmetric; lower extremities affected > upper extremities; presents with pain, paresthesia, and dysesthesia; chronic and slowly progressive; accelerated loss of distal vibratory sensation
      b. **Asymmetric polyradiculoneuropathy:** proximal asymmetric motor neuropathy (amyotrophy); thoracic radiculopathy
      c. **Cranial mononeuropathy:** typically pupil, sparing cranial nerve III lesion; cranial nerves VI and VII may also be involved; spontaneous recovery in 2–3 months
      d. **Entrapment mononeuropathy:** median mononeuropathy at the wrist (CTS); ulnar mononeuropathy; peroneal mononeuropathy
      e. **Diabetic amyotrophy** (subacute diabetic proximal neuropathy)
         i. Usually older than 50 years with mild type 2 diabetes.
         ii. Two-thirds have associated predominantly sensory polyneuropathy but minimal sensory loss in distribution.
         iii. Recovery usually occurs in less than 3–4 months but may take up to 3 years.
         iv. Recurrent episodes may occur in up to 20%.
         v. Abrupt onset of asymmetric pain in hip, anterior thigh, knee, and sometimes calf.
         vi. Weakness of quadriceps, iliopsoas, and occasionally thigh adductors.
         vii. Loss of knee jerk.
         viii. Weakness is usually preceded by weight loss.
         ix. EMG shows involvement of paraspinals but no evidence of myopathy.
      f. **Autonomic neuropathy**
         i. Often superimposed on sensorimotor polyneuropathy
         ii. Symptoms: involves bladder, bowel, circulatory reflexes; orthostatic hypotension; impotence; diarrhea; constipation
         iii. Pathology: degeneration of neurons in sympathetic ganglia; loss of myelinated fibers in splanchnic and vagal nerves; loss of neurons and intermediolateral cell column
         iv. Treatment of orthostatic hypotension: elevate head of bed; sodium diet; elastic stockings; fludrocortisone, 0.1 mg/day, up to 0.5 mg bid; indomethacin, 25–50 mg tid; ihydroergotamine; caffeine

NB: Midodrine may also be used for the treatment of orthostatic hypotension without the mineralocorticoid effects.

G. **Mononeuritis multiplex**
   1. *Diabetic neuropathies (see section II.F)*
   2. *Vasculitis*

  a. Multiple systemic symptoms, including weight loss, fever, malaise with potential multiple organ involvement

  b. Elevated sedimentation rate

  c. Prominent prolonged sensory NCV

  d. Diagnosis made by sural nerve biopsy

  e. Treatment with immunosuppressive agents

  f. Etiologies

   i. Polyarteritis nodosa

   ii. Rheumatoid arthritis

   iii. Systemic lupus erythematosus

   iv. Wegener's granulomatosis

   v. Progressive systemic sclerosis

   vi. Sjogren's syndrome

   vii. Churg-Strauss syndrome (allergic granulomatosis and angiitis)

   viii. Temporal arteritis

   ix. Behcet's disease

   x. Hypersensitivity vasculitis

   xi. Lymphomatoid granulomatosis

3. *Multifocal motor neuropathy*

  a. *Subacute to chronic progression typically involving upper extremities*

  b. *Pure motor involvement in 50% of cases, but mild sensory symptoms and signs can be present*

  c. Tendon reflexes are usually reduced or absent

  d. Controversy over whether this is a variant of chronic inflammatory demyelinating polyradiculoneuropathy (CIDP)

  e. Males > females

  f. *Asymmetric distal upper extremity weakness, particularly in three-fourths of cases*

  g. Progresses slowly

  h. Mimics motor neuron syndromes

  i. *Elevated anti-GM1 antibody (Ab) titers in 40–60% of cases; the importance of GM1 Ab in the diagnosis and treatment of multifocal motor neuropathy is not compelling*

  j. Presence of conduction block appears to correlate with pathologic alteration in sural and motor nerves and is a better guide to management

  k. NCV: demyelinating neuropathy with multifocal conduction block in motor nerves but relatively normal sensory conduction

  l. *Pathology: demyelination with remyelination ± inflammation*

  m. *Treatment: intravenous immunoglobulin (IVIg); plasma exchange (PE); cyclophosphamide; prednisone relatively ineffective*

NB: The characteristics of a demyelinating polyneuropathy are decreased in conduction velocity and temporal dispersion of the CMAP.

4. *Sarcoidosis*

  a. *5% have nervous system involvement*

  b. *3% have central nervous system (CNS) findings without systemic manifestations*

  c. Organs commonly involved include lungs, skin, lymph nodes, bones, eyes, muscle, and parotid gland; hypothalamic involvement may produce diabetes insipidus

  d. Pathology: primarily involves leptomeninges, but parenchymal invasion may occur; noncaseating granulomas with lymphocytic infiltrate

  e. Predilection for posterior fossa

    f. May produce basilar meningitis

    g. Clinical

       i. *Mononeuritis multiplex:* most common; usually large and irregular areas of sensory loss can be distinguishing feature

       ii. *Cranial neuropathies* (particularly facial palsies)

NB: In a patient with bilateral facial nerve palsies, think of Lyme disease and sarcoidosis.

       iii. *Polyneuropathy*

       iv. *Mononeuropathy* (usually early on course)

    h. Serum testing: angiotensin-converting enzyme elevated in 80% with active pulmonary sarcoidosis but only in 11% with inactive disease

    i. Cerebrospinal fluid (CSF): subacute meningitis with elevated pressure, mild pleocytosis (10–200 cells) that are mainly lymphocytes, elevated protein, and reduced glucose; CSF angiotensin-converting enzyme level elevated in 50% of neurosarcoidosis

    j. NCV: axonal involvement

    k. Treatment: steroids or other immunosuppressants if steroids ineffective

  5. *Lyme disease*

    a. Pathophysiology: *caused by* Borrelia burgdorferi; v*ector: via* Ixodes immitis *tick;* early summer most common

    b. Clinical: acute form: more severe signs and symptoms and often with cranial nerve palsy (facial palsy most common); presentations: erythema chronicum migrans; headache; myalgias; meningismus; cranial neuropathy (cranial nerve VII most common); radiculopathy; mononeuritis multiplex; peripheral neuropathy (one-third have neuropathies)

    c. Diagnosis: *sural biopsy demonstrates perivascular inflammation and axonal degeneration*

    d. Treatment

       i. *Facial palsy: doxycycline, 100 mg bid for 3 weeks*

       ii. *CNS involvement: 3rd-generation intravenous cephalosporin (eg. ceftriaxone, 2 mg intravenously q12h); penicillin, 3.3 million units intravenously q4h; treatment for 2–3 weeks*

  6. *Leprosy*

  7. *Human immunodeficiency virus (HIV)*

H. **Multiple cranial nerve palsies**

  1. Differential diagnosis

    a. Congenital (e.g., *Möbius' syndrome):* facial diplegia; affects cranial nerve VI in 70%; external ophthalmoplegia in 20%; ptosis in 10%; voice paralysis in 15–20%

    b. Infectious: chronic meningitis (e.g., spirochete, fungal, mycoplasma, viral, including HIV, tuberculous [cranial nerve VI most frequent])

    c. Lyme disease

    d. Neurosyphilis

    e. Acute fungal infection (cryptococcus, aspergillosis, mucormycosis)

    f. Traumatic (particularly skull base fracture)

    g. Tumor: for example, meningioma, adenocarcinoma, glomus jugular tumors, carcinomatous meningitis, primary CNS lymphoma

    h. Wegener's granulomatosis

    i. Sarcoidosis

    j. Inflammatory

    k. Acute inflammatory demyelinating polyneuropathy (IDP)

    l. Entrapment syndromes: eg. Paget's disease, fibrous dysplasia

I. *Chronic sensorimotor polyneuropathy*
   1. Diabetic neuropathy (see section II.F)
   2. CIDP (see section III.B)
   3. Nutritional
      a. Mechanism of production of the nutritional neuropathies
         i. Chronic alcoholism
         ii. Food/nutritional dietary fads
         iii. Malabsorption
         iv. Drugs
      b. *Neuropathic beriberi*
         i. *Disease of the heart and peripheral nerves*
         ii. Clinical features: slow onset and evolution of a generalized peripheral neuropathy with weakness and wasting affecting the lower extremities distally, followed by involvement of the upper extremities distally; similar distribution of sensory loss involving all methods of sensation; reflexes are absent or reduced; vagal involvement; cranial neuropathies (rare); subacute loss of vision (rare)
         iii. Pathology: axonal degeneration affecting the distal segments of lower > upper extremities; vagus and phrenic nerves often affected (late); chromatolytic changes occur in the dorsal root ganglion and alpha motor neuron cell bodies; secondary degeneration of dorsal columns may occur; accumulation of membrane-bound sacs and depletion of neurotubules and neurofilaments of the distal ends of motor and sensory axons.
      c. *Strachan's syndrome:* amblyopia; painful neuropathy; orogenital dermatitis; caused by deficiency of the B vitamins
      d. *Burning feet syndrome:* subacute onset of a neuropathy characterized by severe burning pain in the extremities with hyperhidrosis of the feet: may be associated with deficiencies of the B vitamins, including pantothenic acid, thiamine, nicotinic acid, and riboflavin
      e. *Vitamin B_{12} deficiency*
         i. Pathogenesis: pernicious anemia with absence or marked reduction of intrinsic factor; posterior column involvement more significant than peripheral neuropathy
         ii. *Clinical:* slowly progressive; numbness and paresthesias of the feet followed by ataxia, weakness, and wasting of distal lower extremities (upper extremities become involved in severe); *loss of vibration and position sense is prominent early, followed by a distal loss of pain and temperature perception*
         iii. Lab testing: reduced vitamin B_{12} levels; if uncertain, *Schilling test* or test for intrinsic factor blocking Ab should be done
         iv. Treatment: *vitamin B_{12}, 1,000 g intramuscularly daily for 4 days, followed by the same dosage monthly*

NB: Vitamin B_{12} deficiency may involve the dorsal columns as well as pyramidal tracts, causing subacute combined degeneration.

      f. *Vitamin E deficiency:* chronic axonal sensory neuropathy; clinical: increased creatine phosphokinase (CPK); ataxia; ophthalmoplegia
      g. *Alcoholic polyneuropathy*
         i. Pathogenesis: likely secondary to dietary deficiency and alcoholic gastritis; significant weight loss may also be contributory; thiamine deficiency has a major role and may cause axonal degeneration in experimental models

      ii. Clinical: chronic slowly progressive neuropathy; distal weakness and wasting affecting mainly the lower extremities; mild pansensory impairment distally; ankle jerks usually absent; *peripheral neuropathy occurs in 80% of patients with Wernicke-Korsakoff syndrome;* NCV of motor and sensory nerves are mildly reduced

      iii. Pathology: axonal degeneration

      iv. Treatment: balanced high-calorie diet; supplemental B vitamins daily (thiamine 25 mg, niacin, 100 mg, riboflavin 10 mg, pantothenic acid 10 mg, pyridoxine 5 mg)

4. Connective tissue disease
5. Paraneoplastic (see section II.J)
6. *Multiple myeloma*
   a. *Uncontrolled proliferation of plasma cells that infiltrate in bone and soft tissues*
   b. May be a hyperviscosity state due to paraproteinemia, renal failure, hypercalcemia, and amyloidosis, all of which affect nerve excitation and conduction or fiber degeneration
   c. Clinical
      i. Neuropathy due to direct effect of neoplastic tissue: root compression due to deposits or from vertebral collapse produces radicular pain, which is the most common neurologic symptom in multiple myeloma; cauda equina syndrome; sensorimotor polyneuropathy
      ii. Neuropathy due to compression with amyloid deposits
      iii. Amyloid generalized neuropathy
      iv. Neuropathy due to remote effect of multiple myeloma
      v. Osteosclerotic myeloma with polyneuropathy
7. *Monoclonal gammopathy of undetermined significance*
   a. *50% of neuropathies associated with M-protein*
   b. *Anti-MAG Ab in 50% of cases*
   c. Typically men > 50 y/o
   d. Slow progressive ascending demyelinating sensory neuropathy with weakness
   e. May be associated with Raynaud's phenomenon, ataxia, and intentional tremor
   f. Treatment with immunosuppressive agents: PE; IVIg: steroids
8. *Waldenström's macroglobulinemia*
   a. *Usually affecting elderly with fatigue, weight loss, lymphadenopathy, hepatosplenomegaly, visual disturbances, and bleeding diathesis, and, hematologically, by a great excess of 19S IgM macroglobulin in the blood.*
   b. May occur in association with chronic lymphocytic leukemia, lymphosarcoma, carcinoma, cirrhosis of the liver, collagen vascular diseases, and in hemolytic anemia of the cold Ab type; in these conditions, symptoms are caused by involvement of nerve, CNS, and systemic manifestations.
   c. IgM M-protein class is usually κ light chain.
   d. Slowly progressive neuropathy.
      i. Early stage may be asymmetric.
      ii. In later stages, there is a typical sensorimotor neuropathy.
      iii. Sensory symptoms consisting of paresthesia, pain, and objective sensory loss, and there may also be marked weakness and wasting extremities.
      iv. Myopathy can also occur because of IgM binding to decorin.
   e. Treatment with immunosuppression: PE, chemotherapy
9. *Cryoglobulinemia*

a. *Characterized by the presence in the serum of a cryoglobulin that precipitates on cooling and redissolves on rewarming to 37°C*
b. Types of cryoglobulinemia
    i. *Idiopathic: monoclonal gammopathy such as myeloma, macroglobulinemia, and lymphomas: M component is cryoprotein*
    ii. *Secondary: collagen vascular disorders, chronic infections (hepatitis C), mesothelioma, and the polyclonal gammopathies*
c. Neuropathy occurs in 7%
d. Usually, gradually progressive axonal neuropathy
e. Patients present with Raynaud's phenomenon, cold sensitivity, purpuric skin eruptions, and ulceration of the lower limbs
f. Over years, eventually develop asymmetric sensorimotor neuropathy (lower > upper extremities) accompanied by pain and paresthesia
g. Necessary to work up for a collagen vascular disorder, hematologic causes of an M protein, and for hepatitis C (50% of patients with chronic hepatitis C have cryoglobulinemia)
h. Treatment: avoidance of cold, plasmapheresis, cytotoxic agents, corticosteroids; in hepatitis C, neuropathy may respond to interferon-α

10. *Uremic polyneuropathy*
  a. *Two-thirds of dialysis patients*
  b. *May begin with burning dysesthesias*
  c. Painful distal sensory loss followed by weakness (lower > upper extremities)
  d. Uremia is also associated with CTS and ischemic monomelic neuropathy
  e. Treatment: hemodialysis improves signs/symptoms; renal transplant: complete recovery in 6–12 months

11. *Leprosy*
  a. *Most common cause of neuropathy globally but rare in the United States*
  b. *Laminin-2 has been identified on the Schwann cell-axon unit as an initial neural target for the invasion of* Mycobacterium leprae
  c. *Trophic ulcers, Charcot joints, and mutilated fingers are common due to anesthesia*
  d. *Tuberculoid leprosy:* causes mononeuritis multiplex; skin lesions consist of asymmetric hypesthetic macules; superficial nerve fibers are always affected and may be palpable as skin; sensory loss is earliest for pain and temperature; ulnar, median, peroneal, and facial nerves are especially prone; superficial cutaneous radial, digital, posterior auricular, and sural are the commonly affected sensory nerves
  e. *Lepromatous leprosy:* hematogenous spread to skin, ciliary bodies, testes, nodes, and peripheral nerves; lesions tend to occur on other cooler parts of the body: the dorsal surface of hands, dorsomedial surface of forearm, dorsal surface of feet, and anterolateral aspects of legs with loss of pain and temperature
  f. Pathology: segmental demyelination
  g. Treatment: combination of dapsone, 100 mg daily, and rifampin, 600 mg monthly, for 6 months

12. *Critical illness polyneuropathy*
  a. *50% of critically ill ICU patients (length of stay > 1 week), particularly if patient has concurrent sepsis and multiorgan failure*
  b. *Primarily axonal degeneration (motor > sensory)*

NB: There is also a critical care myopathy known as myosin-losing myopathy.

13. *HIV neuropathy*
   a. Clinical
      i. *IDP*
         (A) Acute inflammatory demyelinating polyradiculoneuropathy (AIDP) and CIDP have been associated with HIV-1 infection.
         (B) Main features that distinguish HIV-1–infected individuals from HIV-1–seronegative patients with IDP.
            (1) HIV-1–infected patients with IDP frequently have a lymphocytic CSF pleocytosis of 20–50 cells.
            (2) HIV-1 infected individuals have polyclonal elevations of serum immunoglobulins.
         (C) Electrophysiologic features of IDP in HIV-1–seropositive individuals are not different.
      ii. *Mononeuritis multiplex:* with and without necrotizing vasculitis
      iii. *Distal predominantly sensory polyneuropathy:* several factors involved, including age, immunosuppression, nutritional status, and chronic disease
      iv. *Distal symmetric polyneuropathy associated with neurotoxic drugs:* dose-dependent neuropathy (e.g., zalcitabine, didanosine, stavudine, lamivudine
      v. *Autonomic neuropathy:* more frequently in the late stage
      vi. *Polyradiculoneuropathy associated with cytomegalovirus:* patients have low CD4 lymphocyte counts; clinical: stereotypic development of a rapidly progressive cauda equina syndrome; upper extremities are usually spared until late in the course; rapidly fatal if untreated
J. *Carcinomatous/paraneoplastic neuropathy*
   1. Syndromes
      a. *Antineuronal nuclear Ab type 1 (ANNA-1)*
         i. *Aka anti-Hu Ab syndrome*
         ii. Panneuronal Ab binding to both nucleus and cytoplasm of neurons of both the peripheral nervous system and CNS
         iii. Associated with *small-cell lung carcinoma* and more recently found to be associated with the gastroenterologic neuropathy typically presenting as a pseudo-obstruction syndrome; may also be associated with prostate and breast cancer
         iv. Two-thirds are female
         v. Tumor may not be discovered for up to 3 years after onset of signs/symptoms or not until autopsy
         vi. Antigen reactive with ANNA-1 has been identified in homogenized small-cell lung carcinoma tissue
         vii. Clinical: subacute sensory neuropathy (most common); motor neuron disease; limbic encephalopathy; cerebellar dysfunction; brainstem dysfunction; autonomic dysfunction
      b. *ANNA-2*
         i. *Aka anti-Ri and anti-Nova Ab syndrome*
         ii. Associated with carcinoma of the breast
         iii. Antigens are 55- and 80-kDa CNS proteins
         iv. Clinical: cerebellar ataxia; opsoclonus; myelopathy; brain stem dysfunction
      c. *Anti-Purkinje cytoplasmic Ab type 1 (PCAb1)*
         i. *Aka anti-Yo Ab syndrome*
         ii. Ab reacts with the cytoplasm of cerebellar Purkinje cells, particularly rough endoplasmic reticulum, and also cytoplasm of cerebellar molecular neurons and Schwann cells

iii. PCAb1 is a serologic marker for *ovarian carcinoma and, less often, breast carcinoma*
iv. Clinical: subacute cerebellar syndrome (most common); neuropathy (rare)

Ab	Structure	Cancer	Neurologic syndrome
ANNA-1 (anti-Hu)	Panneuronal	Small-cell lung cancer	Sensory neuronopathy
			Pseudo-obstruction syndrome
ANNA-2 (anti-Ri or -Nova)	Neuronal nucleus	Breast cancer	Cerebellar myelopathy
PCAb1 (anti-Yo)	Purkinje cytoplasmic	Ovarian and breast cancer	Subacute cerebellar dysfunction

2. *Clinical patterns of neuropathies associated with cancer*
   a. *Sensory neuronopathy*
      i. Approximately 20% of the paraneoplastic neuropathies.
      ii. Underlying malignancy is almost always a lung carcinoma and usually oat cell; other causes include esophageal and cecal carcinoma.
      iii. Females > males.
      iv. Mean age of onset is 59 years.
      v. Neuropathy usually precedes diagnosis of the tumor by approximately 6 months to 3 years.
      vi. Subacute onset and slow progression.
      vii. Sensory symptoms predominate, including numbness and paresthesia of the extremities, aching limb pains, and a sensory ataxia.
      viii. Motor weakness and wasting are minimal until more advanced.
      ix. Pseudoathetosis may develop due to sensory dysfunction.
      x. Removal of the underlying tumor does not usually alter course.
      xi. Mean duration from onset of neuropathy to death is approximately 14 months.
      xii. Pathology: dorsal root ganglia cells degenerate and are replaced by clusters of round cells *(residual nodules of Nageotte);* dorsal root fibers and the dorsal columns are degenerated; perivascular lymphocytic infiltration affecting the dorsal root ganglia and also the hippocampus, amygdaloid nucleus, brain stem, and spinal cord.
   b. *Mild terminal sensorimotor neuropathy:* little disability; malignant disease was known to have been present for 6 months or longer in 70% of patients and for 2 years in 40%; mean interval from onset of the neuropathy to death was 11 months
   c. *Acute and subacute sensorimotor neuropathy*
   d. *Remitting and relapsing neuropathy*
   e. *Pandysautonomia:* sympathetic and parasympathetic dysfunction resulting in orthostatic hypotension and anhidrosis
K. **Neuropathy associated with lymphoma, lymphoproliferative, and Hodgkin's disease**
   1. Cranial neuropathies by local compression, leptomeningeal involvement, or direct invasion; *cranial nerves III, IV, VI, and VII are the most commonly affected.*
   2. Root compression occurs from extension of vertebral deposits or from vertebrae collapse; may present as cauda equina syndrome.
   3. Other presentations: plexopathy; lumbosacral > cervical; mononeuropathies.
L. **Neuropathy associated with myeloma**
   1. *Multiple myeloma*
      a. Uncontrolled proliferation of plasma cells that infiltrate in bone and soft tissues

b. May be a hyperviscosity state due to paraproteinemia, renal failure, hypercalcemia, and amyloidosis, all of which affect nerve excitation and conduction or fiber degeneration

c. Clinical

   i. Neuropathy due to direct effect of neoplastic tissue: root compression due to deposits or from vertebral collapse produces radicular pain, which is the most common neurologic symptom in multiple myeloma; cauda equina syndrome; sensorimotor polyneuropathy

   ii. Neuropathy due to compression with amyloid deposits

   iii. Amyloid generalized neuropathy

   iv. Neuropathy due to remote effect of multiple myeloma

   v. Osteosclerotic myeloma with polyneuropathy

M. *Medication-induced neuropathies*

1. *Amiodarone:* 5–10% of patients have symptomatic peripheral neuropathy invariably associated with a static or intention tremor and possible ataxia (possible cerebellar dysfunction); demyelinating; slowly progressive symmetric distal sensory loss and motor neuropathy with areflexia.

2. *Amitriptyline:* chronic axonal sensorimotor neuropathy.

3. *Cisplatin:* predominantly sensory neuropathy often occurs when dose exceeds a total of 400 mg/m^2; axonal; Lhermitte's phenomenon; distal paresthesia in lower and upper extremities followed by progressive sensory ataxia; loss of all sensory methods in glove and stocking distribution but more prominent loss of vibration and joint position sense; areflexia; differential diagnosis is paraneoplastic sensory neuropathy.

4. *Colchicine:* binds tubulin and interferes with mitotic spindle formation and axonal transport; chronic axonal sensorimotor neuropathy; association with an acute myopathy that superficially resembles acute polymyositis (PM).

5. *Dapsone:* chronic distal axonal motor neuropathy; sparing of sensory function.

6. *Disulfiram (Antabuse®):* chronic distal axonal sensorimotor neuropathy; begins with distal paresthesia and pain and progresses to distal sensory loss and weakness; more common in patients taking 250–500 mg/day of disulfiram; treatment: discontinuing disulfiram or lowering it to <125 mg/day typically results in gradual but complete recovery.

7. *Isoniazid:* chronic distal axonal sensory > motor neuropathy; begins with symmetric distal paresthesia in the feet and hands; progressing to include painful distal sensory loss; relative preservation of proprioception; treatment: pyridoxine (15–50 mg/day) appears to prevent the neuropathic side effects of isoniazid.

8. *Lithium:* chronic axonal sensorimotor neuropathy.

9. *Metronidazole:* chronic axonal sensory neuropathy.

10. *Nitrofurantoin:* chronic axonal sensorimotor neuropathy.

11. *Phenytoin:* chronic axonal sensory neuropathy.

12. *Pyridoxine:* chronic axonal sensory neuropathy: usually taking megadoses (1–5 g/day), but minimum dose of pyridoxine that has been associated with neuropathic symptoms is 200 mg/day; neuropathic symptoms may begin with ataxia in combination with Lhermitte's phenomenon (may be misdiagnosed as multiple sclerosis); motor or autonomic involvement is rare; treatment: limit pyridoxine to 50–100 mg/day.

13. *Statins:* distal painful polyneuropathy; axonal neuropathy.

14. *Vincristine:* chronic axonal motor neuropathy.

N. *Heavy metal-induced neuropathies*

1. *Arsenic*

  a. Clinical

    i. Acute axonal sensory neuropathy begins 5–10 days after ingestion.

      ii. Most typical history is that of an acute gastrointestinal illness followed by burning painful paresthesia in the hands and feet with progressive distal muscle weakness.

     iii. CNS symptoms may develop rapidly in acute poisoning, with drowsiness and confusion progressing to stupor or psychosis and delirium.

     iv. Hyperkeratosis and sloughing of the skin on the palms and soles may occur several weeks after ingestion and be followed by a more chronic state of redness and swelling of the hands and feet.

      v. Nail changes (*Mees' lines*).

     vi. With chronic poisoning, may have aplastic anemia.

  b. Diagnosis

      i. Acute intoxication: renal excretion >0.1 mg arsenic in 24 hours

     ii. Chronic intoxication: hair concentrations >0.1 mg/100 g of hair; slow-growing hair, such as pubic hair, may be elevated as long as 8 months after exposure

  c. Treatment: acute oral ingestion—gastric lavage with 2–3 L of water followed by instillation of milk or 1% sodium thiosulfate; British anti-Lewisite (BAL) is given parenterally in a 10% solution

  d. Prognosis: mortality in severe arsenic encephalitis: >50–75%; once neuropathy occurs, treatment is usually ineffective

2. *Gold*

  a. Pathophysiology: used in the treatment of arthritis, lupus erythematosus, and other inflammatory conditions; ingestion of jewelry

  b. Clinical: chronic distal axonal sensory > motor neuropathy; painful, producing burning or itching in the palms of the hands or soles of the feet; myokymia; brachial plexopathy; AIDP

  c. Pathology: loss of myelin as well as active axonal degeneration

  d. Treatment: chelation therapy with BAL has been used but is usually unnecessary

3. *Mercury*

  a. Clinical

      i. Acute: inflammation of the mouth, salivation, and severe gastrointestinal disturbances followed by hallucinations and delirium

     ii. Chronic

        (A) Chronic axonal sensory neuropathy

        (B) Constriction of visual fields, ataxia, dysarthria, decreased hearing, tremor, and dementia

        (C) Parkinsonism

        (D) In children: *acrodynia*

  b. Treatment: chelating agents (eg. D-Penicillamine, BAL, ethylenediaminetetraacetic acid)

4. *Thallium*

  a. Clinical

      i. Hallmark: *alopecia*

     ii. Acute

        (A) Gastrointestinal symptoms develop within hours of ingestion.

        (B) Large doses (>2 g) produce cardiovascular shock, coma, and death within 24 hours.

        (C) Moderate doses produce neuropathic symptoms within 24–48 hours, consisting of limb pain and distal paresthesia with increasing distal-to-proximal limb sensory loss accompanied by distal limb weakness.

        (D) May produce AIDP-like syndrome.

     iii. Chronic: chronic axonal sensorimotor neuropathy

    c. Treatment: chelating agents such as Prussian blue (potassium ferric hexacyanoferrate, BAL, dithizone, diethyldithiocarbamate; if acute, can also perform gastric lavage

5. *Lead*
    a. Pathophysiology
       i. Passes placental barriers.
      ii. Diminishes cerebral glucose supplies.
     iii. Brain is also unusually sensitive to the effects of triethyl lead.
     iv. Triethyl lead chloride intoxication decreases the incorporation of labeled sulfate into sulfatides, resulting in inhibition of myelin synthesis and demyelination.
      v. Adults: use of exterior paints and gasoline; more likely to present with neuropathy.
     vi. Children: pica and eating lead-based paints; more likely to present with encephalopathy.
    b. Clinical
       i. Neuropathy
         (A) Chronic axonal motor neuropathy
         (B) Classic neurologic presentation: wristdrop
         (C) Typical clinical triad: abdominal pain and constipation; anemia; neuropathy
      ii. CNS toxicity
         (A) Adult: prodrome: progressive weakness and weight loss; ashen color of the face; mild persistent headache; fine tremor of the muscles of the eyes, tongue, and face; progression into encephalopathic state; may have focal motor weakness.
         (B) Children: prodrome usually nonspecific, evolving into encephalopathic state (50%); if large amounts of lead are ingested, prodrome symptoms may be present.
    c. Treatment: chelating agents such as BAL, ethylenediaminetetraacetic acid, penicillamine
    d. Prognosis
       i. Mild intoxication: usually complete recovery
      ii. Severe encephalopathy: mortality high but lessened by the use of combined chelating agent therapy
     iii. Residual neurologic sequelae: blindness or partial visual disturbances, persistent convulsions, personality changes, and mental retardation
     iv. Prognosis worse in children than in adults

O. ***Hereditary polyneuropathy***
  1. *Inherited axonal neuropathies*
    a. *Predominantly motor axonal neuropathies*
       i. *Hereditary motor and sensory neuropathy type 2 (Charcot-Marie-Tooth type 2)*
         (A) Pathophysiology: autosomal dominant (AD): three types: types 2a, 2b, 2c, with some linkage to chromosome 1p
         (B) Clinical: symptoms start in early adulthood; stork leg appearance (peroneal muscular atrophy); rarely totally incapacitated; mildly slowed conduction velocity with decreased CMAP and SNAPs
      ii. *Acute intermittent porphyria*
         (A) Pathophysiology: actually an inborn error of metabolism; AD
         (B) Clinical: 90% never have symptoms; symptoms begin at puberty; *Motor neuropathy develops in proximal distribution (arms > legs); 50% of patients with neuropathy can have mild sensory involvement in the same distribution.*

b. *Predominantly sensory axonal neuropathies*
   i. *Hereditary sensory and autonomic neuropathies*

	Type 1	Type 2	Type 3 (Riley-Day syndrome, familial dysautonomia)	Type 4
Inheritance	AD	AR	AR (Ashkenazi)	AR
Age of onset	2nd decade	Infancy or at birth	At birth	Infancy
Clinical	Pain in feet and legs with ulcers of the feet	Hypotonia Affects hands, feet,	Present at birth with hypotonia Diagnosis by	Congenital insensitivity to pain, anhidrosis,
	Sensory loss in feet is a constant feature but is variable in the hands	trunk, and forehead Diffuse loss of pain perception	pilocarpine or histamine test	and mental retardation Usually present with symptoms related to
	Dissociative sensory loss (pain	Decreased sweating		anhidrosis in infancy
	and temperature first)	Absent SNAPs with normal CMAP and motor CV		Fungiform papillae of the tongue No sensory evoked potentials, SNAPs, no response on histamine testing, and absent sweat glands on skin biopsy

AR, autosomal recessive; CV, conduction velocity.

c. *Sensorimotor axonal neuropathies*
   i. *Giant axonal neuropathy*
      (A) Pathophysiology: rare; AR; affects both central and peripheral axons
      (B) Clinical; usually presents by age 3 years with gait problems, distal leg atrophy, and severely impaired vibration and proprioception; diagnosis: *sural nerve biopsy with enlarged axons with disrupted neurofilaments that are surrounded by a thin or fragmented myelin sheath (secondary demyelination)*
   ii. *Familial amyloid neuropathy*
      (A) Pathophysiology: *AD; chromosome 18; associated with gene for prealbumin*
      (B) Clinical: involves sensation, then autonomic function, and then motor late in course; have marked autonomic dysfunction: impotence, incontinence, anhidrosis, and cardiac involvement; death within 15 years; Portuguese heritage: young adulthood and predominantly involves the legs; Swiss heritage: less severe form affecting predominantly the arms; nerve conduction studies

(NCSs) show axonal sensory motor polyneuropathy; diagnosis: amyloid on sural biopsy

   iii. **Friedreich's ataxia:** *AR;* primarily affects the *corticospinal tracts, dorsal columns, and spinocerebellar tracts;* late in the disease course, can affect peripheral nerves; EMG/NCV: absent SNAPs and normal motor conduction studies

  2. *Inherited demyelinating neuropathies*

Patients with inherited demyelinating neuropathies have uniform slowing of the conduction velocities of all nerves without signs of conduction block, whereas acquired demyelinating neuropathies will tend to have multifocal slowing.

   a. **Charcot-Marie-Tooth type 1 (hereditary motor and sensory neuropathy type 1)**
     i. Pathophysiology
       (A) Most common
       (B) *AD mostly but can also be AR or X-linked*
       (C) *Genetically heterogeneous group*
       (D) *Three gene products have been identified as abnormal*
         (1) *Peripheral myelin protein 22 (PMP22)*
         (2) *Myelin protein zero (MPZ)*
         (3) *Connexin 32*
       (E) *Men affected more severely and commonly*
       (F) *Segmental demyelination and onion bulb formation*
     ii. Clinical: symptoms begin in 2nd decade; clubfoot and high arches followed with atrophy of the peroneal musculature; atrophy later involves upper leg and upper extremities; characteristic gait abnormality results from bilateral footdrop; have palpable nerves and loss of vibration and proprioception, then ankle jerks, and then diffuse reflex loss; NCV: slow with limited temporal dispersion.

NB: In CMT Type 1A, there is *duplication* of the PMP 22 gene; in Hereditary neuropathy with liability to pressure palsies (HNPP), there is *deletion* of PMP 22 gene. CMT 2 is the *axonal* phenotype!

   b. **Dejerine-Sottas (hereditary motor and sensory neuropathy type 3)**
     i. Pathophysiology: *AR; defect: PMP22 and point mutation of MPZ; onion bulb formation with segmental demyelination*
     ii. Clinical: delayed motor milestones in infancy; pes cavus; muscle cramps; palsies of the 6th and 7th cranial nerves; adults have severe truncal ataxia; NCV: severe slowing

   c. **Hereditary neuropathy with pressure palsies (tomaculous neuropathy)**
     i. Pathophysiology: *AD, chromosome 17; deletion of PMP22*
     ii. Clinical: asymmetric; associated with minor nerve compression or trauma; NCV: conduction block in areas not associated with entrapment; Biopsy: reveals tomacula

   d. **Congenital hypomyelinating neuropathy**
     i. Pathophysiology: *AR; MPZ point mutation; severe hypomyelination or complete lack of myelination of peripheral nerves*
     ii. Clinical: Biopsy: lack onion bulbs; hypotonia; severe distal weakness; difficulty with respiration and feeding; may be associated with arthrogryposis congenital; NCV: extremely slow

  3. **Multiple endocrine neoplasia type 2B**
   a. Pathophysiology: rare; *AD; gene linked to chromosome 10q11.2*
   b. *Clinical: medullary carcinoma of the thyroid (can metastasize); pheochromocytoma; ganglioneuromatosis; abnormalities of bony and connective tissue elements, peroneal muscular*

atrophy and pes cavus foot deformity with or without hammer toes, multiple endocrine disturbances develop

III. Acute and Chronic IDP
A. AIDP
1. Epidemiology: aka Guillain-Barré syndrome; 1–2 cases per 100,000 in North America; progressive increase with age, reaching 8.6/100,000 in individuals 70–79 y/o; male > female; antecedent respiratory and enteric infections in one-half to two-thirds of cases
2. Clinical
   a. Core features: acute onset; *ascending predominantly motor polyradiculoneuropathy typically beginning in the lower limbs;* CSF changes of elevated protein with normal cell count; areflexia
   b. Onset within 1–3 weeks after a benign upper respiratory or gastrointestinal illness
   c. Associated with AIDP
      i. Antecedent viral infection: cytomegalovirus, Epstein-Barr virus, HIV, Smallpox-vaccinia viruses, Hepatitis B
      ii. Antecedent bacterial infections: *Campylobacter jejuni: 20% of AIDP cases, Mycoplasma pneumoniae, Borrelia burgdorferi* (Lyme disease)
      iii. Vaccines: Rabies vaccine, Tetanus toxoid vaccine, Polio vaccine
      iv. Drugs
      v. Surgery
      vi. Pregnancy
      vii. Lymphoma
   d. Maximal weakness over the course of a few days to 6 weeks
   e. Facial weakness to some degree occurs in >50%
   f. May also have development of sensory loss
   g. Dysautonomia, mainly cardiovascular, manifested as tachycardia and orthostatic hypotension and associated with increased mortality.
   h. CSF: increase in protein associated with a cell count <10
   i. *Electrophysiologic findings: conduction slowing/block; prolonged distal latency; prolonged F-wave latencies; may be delayed for several weeks (usually 10–14 days, depending on severity of clinical symptoms)*

NB: The F-wave may be the first abnormal finding in NCV in acute stage of Guillain-Barré syndrome.

NB: There is an axonal form of the disease, which has a poor prognosis.

   j. Clinical variants
      i. *Autonomic variant:* core features: acute or subacute onset; widespread sympathetic and parasympathetic failure; relative or complete sparing of somatic fibers; sympathetic: orthostatic hypotension; anhidrosis; parasympathetic: dry eyes; dry mouth; bowel and bladder dysfunction; Schirmer test confirms reduced tear secretion.
      ii. *Miller-Fisher variant:* triad: *ophthalmoplegia; ataxia; areflexia;* 5% of AIDP cases; many cases are associated with motor involvement; associated with a particular serotype of *C. jejuni* (GQ1b epitope); CSF protein increased; EMG/NCV: demyelinating neuropathy; patients may respond to plasmapheresis better than IVIg.
3. Differential diagnosis
   a. Periodic paralysis
   b. Neuromuscular transmission (myasthenia gravis [MG], botulism, tick paralysis)
   c. Peripheral nerve axon (porphyria, toxins)

    d. Cell body (poliomyelitis)

    e. Acute myelopathy

    f. Drugs/toxins

       i. Acute hexacarbon neuropathy from volatile solvents (paint lacquer vapors, glue sniffing)

       ii. Nitrofurantoin

       iii. Dapsone

       iv. Organophosphates

       v. Saxitoxin

    g. Infection

       i. Cytomegalovirus

       ii. Diphtheria

       iii. Lyme disease

       iv. HIV: AIDP develops as patients seroconvert or have acquired immunodeficiency syndrome-related complex; usually have CSF pleocytosis (>40 cells)

4. Mechanisms

    a. Demonstration of IgM Abs that bind to carbohydrate residues of peripheral nerve in 90% of patients with AIDP at the onset of the disease.

    b. Abs may induce demyelination by binding to C1q and activating the complement cascade or potentially bind to the Fc receptor on macrophages.

    c. Therapeutic IVIg is capable of neutralizing neuromuscular blocking Abs in AIDP by an Ab-mediated mechanism.

5. Prognosis

    a. Monophasic, but 3–5% of cases may relapse; onset to peak in excess of 4 weeks may have a greater risk of relapse

    b. 75% have full functional recovery, and 10% have significant functional deficit

    c. Factors indicating good prognosis

       i. Young age

       ii. Mild disease

       iii. Acute (onset to peak at 1–3 weeks) but not hyperacute (onset to respirator support at 1–3 days) evolution

       iv. Improvement within 1 week of peak severity

    d. Factors indicating poor prognosis

       i. Old age

       ii. Hyperacute onset

       iii. Severe illness

       iv. Marked reduction in CMAP >80%

       v. Delayed onset of recovery

    e. Mortality rate: 5–8%; most commonly resulted from ventilator-associated pneumonia

6. Treatment

    a. Supportive care

       i. Forced vital capacity (FVC), respiration, and pulse rate q1h

       ii. ICU setting due to potential for rapid evolution

       iii. Ventilator support if FVC <1 L or if PO_2 <70 mm Hg on room air

    b. Interventional treatment

       i. PE

         (A) Patient who is deteriorating or has severe disease

(B) Mechanism of action of PE is not known but may be due to the removal of Ab, complement components, immune complexes, lymphokines, and acute-phase reactants

(C) Regimen: six PEs over 2 weeks with 3.0–3.5 L exchanged per treatment

(D) Adverse effects: transient hypotension, paresthesia, hypersensitivity reactions, nypocalcemia

  ii. IVIg

    (A) 0.4 g/kg per treatment

    (B) Five treatments over 3 or 6 days

    (C) Adverse effects: 5% of patients; congestive heart failure, hypotension, deep vein thrombosis, acute renal failure, anaphylaxis, aseptic meningitis, cerebral infarction, encephalopathy

  iii. Oral corticosteroids are not recommended.

 c. Rehabilitation

  i. 40% must go to rehab

  ii. More likely to require rehab

    (A) Ventilator support

    (B) Dysautonomia

    (C) Increased acute and total length of hospital stay

    (D) Cranial nerve dysfunction

B. **CIDP**

1. Pathophysiology and epidemiology; inflammatory (macrophage-dependent) demyelination of nerve roots and peripheral nerves; immune-mediated disease possibly triggered by an influenza-like infection or other viral infections; prevalence 1–2 per 100,000 (6–7 per 100,000 in those >70 y/o); male > female; 30–50% have relapsing-remitting course

2. Clinical

 a. Two courses

  i. Monophasic course: slow, stepwise, or steady dysfunction

  ii. Relapsing course

 b. *Symmetric, affecting both motor and sensory fibers with muscle weakness and sensory loss*

 c. Weakness of both proximal and distal muscles ± atrophy

 d. Sensory symptoms include numbness and paresthesias

 e. Decreased or absent deep tendon reflexes (DTRs)

 f. Cranial nerve involvement far less common than in AIDP

 g. CSF: *protein elevated between 60 and 200 mg*; CSF pleocytosis uncommon and should exclude other conditions (HIV-1, Lyme disease, and lymphoproliferative disorders)

 h. NCV/EMG: multifocal demyelination; motor conduction velocities <80% of normal; temporal dispersion of the CMAP; variable degree of conduction block; EMG: chronic denervation

3. Prognosis

 a. 10% die due to complications.

 b. 5% recover completely.

 c. 60% work with residual deficits.

 d. 10% confined to a wheelchair.

 e. Patients with significant denervation and loss of nerve fibers do worse.

4. Treatment

 a. Prednisone: both progressive and relapsing course improved

b. PE: be wary of long-term costs and difficulty maintaining venous access.

c. IVIg: 0.4 g/kg per treatment; 3–5 treatments over 7–14 days

Comparison of AIDP and CIDP

	AIDP	CIDP
Viral infection	Common	Uncommon
Onset to peak	<6 wks	>6 wks
Relapses	Uncommon (<5–7%)	More common
Facial weakness	>50%	<50%
Respiratory failure	Common	Uncommon
Sensory loss	Minimal	Moderate
Abnormal electrophys-iologic studies	Patchy May be normal for initial 2 wks	Diffuse
Treatment	PE IVIg	Prednisone PE IVIg
Prognosis	Good	Variable

Comparison of Chronic Acquired Immune-Mediated Demyelinating Polyneuropathies

Disorder	CIDP	Distal acquired demyelinating symmetric neuropathy	Multifocal acquired demyelinating sensory and motor neuropathy	Multifocal motor neuropathy
Clinical features				
Distribution of weakness	Symmetric; proximal and distal	Symmetric; predominantly distal; sometimes no weakness	Asymmetric; distal > proximal; upper > lower limbs	Asymmetric; distal > proximal; upper > lower limbs
Reflexes	Symmetrically reduced	Symmetrically reduced	Reduced (multifocal or diffuse)	Reduced (multifocal or diffuse)
Sensory deficits	Symmetric	Symmetric	Multifocal	None
Lab findings				
CSF protein	Usually elevated	Usually elevated	Usually elevated	Usually normal
Monoclonal protein	Occasionally present; IgG or IgA	IgM-κ present in the majority; 50–70% are positive for myelin-associated glycoprotein	Rare	Rare

Disorder	CIDP	Distal acquired demyelinating symmetric neuropathy	Multifocal acquired demyelinating sensory and motor neuropathy	Multifocal motor neuropathy
Anti-GM1 Abs	Rare	Absent	Rare	Present 50% of the time
Neurophysiology				
Abnormal CMAPs (demyelinat-	Usually symmetric	Usually symmetric; prolonged distal	Asymmetric; multifocal	Asymmetric; multifocal
ing features)		latencies		
Conduction block	Frequent	Rare	Frequent	Frequent
Abnormal SNAPs	Usually symmetric	Usually symmetric	Asymmetric; multifocal	Normal SNAPs
Treatment				
PE	Good	Poor[a] or Good	Unclear	Poor
Prednisone	Good	Poor[a] or Good	Good	Poor
Cyclophospha-mide	Good	Poor[a] or Good	Unclear	Good
IVIg	Good	Poor[a] or Good	Good	Good

[a]Treatment response when associated with IgM-monoclonal gammopathy of undetermined significance.

IV. Neuromuscular Junction Disorders
A. **MG**
  1. Pathophysiology
      a. Abnormal production of *acetylcholine (ACh) receptor Abs in thymus gland*
      b. Thymus gland *with lymphoid hyperplasia in >65–75% of MG cases and 15% with thymomas;* thymus gland in patients with MG contains an increased number of B cells, and thymic lymphocytes in tissue culture secrete ACh receptor Abs
      c. ACh receptor Abs interfere with ACh binding and decrease the number of ACh receptors
      d. 2–10 per 100,000
      e. Bimodal distribution
          i. In those <40 y/o, 3× more women than men
          ii. In those >50 y/o, men > women and more frequently have thymomas
      f. Passive transfer of MG from humans to mice using patient IgG
      g. Normal number of quanta of ACh released from the presynaptic membrane of the terminal axon at the neuromuscular junction in response to a nerve action potential, and each quantum contains a normal number of ACh molecules; miniature end-plate potential frequency in MG is normal, whereas amplitude is decreased (approximately 80%), related to the decreased number of available ACh receptors
      h. *Normal-amplitude CMAP (Note: small CMAP seen in the Lambert-Eaton syndrome and in botulism)*

2. Clinical
    a. Three cardinal signs/symptoms
        i. Fluctuating weakness: worse with increased activity
        ii. Distribution of weakness: ocular and facial weakness in 40% at presentation and 85% at some point
        iii. Response to cholinergic agents
    b. Initial symptoms/signs of MG
        i. Extraocular muscles (ptosis, diplopia): 50%
        ii. Leg weakness: 10%
        iii. Generalized fatigue: 9%
        iv. Dysphagia: 6%
        v. Slurred/nasal speech: 5%
        vi. Difficulty chewing: 5%
        vii. Weakness of the face: 3%
        viii. Weakness of neck: 3%
        ix. Weakness of arms: 3%
    c. *Transient neonatal myasthenia*
        i. *12% of infants born to mothers with MG*
        ii. *At birth, hypotonia with respiration and feeding dysfunction*
        iii. *Symptoms usually begin during the first 24 hours after birth and may last for several weeks*
        iv. May have fluctuating ptosis
        v. Arthrogryposis multiplex congenita as a result of lack of fetal movement in utero
        vi. Difficulty in feeding, generalized weakness, respiratory difficulties, weak cry, and facial weakness
        vii. Some improvement with edrophonium
        viii. EMG: repetitive stimulation abnormal in weak muscles; repetitive stimulation abnormal after sustained activity for 5 minutes in strong muscles; increased jitter
    d. *Slow channel syndrome: AD;* weakness in facial and limb musculature; muscle can be atrophic; usually after infancy in childhood, but onset may delay to adulthood; EMG: decreased repetitive stimulation but not in all muscle
    e. *Congenital acetylcholinesterase (AChE) deficiency*
        i. Clinical: neonatal generalized weakness; sluggish pupillary reactivity; develop postural problems and fixed spinal column deformities; no response to AChE inhibitors
        ii. EMG: repetitive stimulation at 2 Hz; demonstrates decrement in all muscles; single stimuli elicit repetitive CMAPs; for 6–10 milliseconds after the initial response; these fade quickly during repetitive stimulation, even at rates as low as 0.2 Hz

NB: Congenital myasthenic syndromes such as slow channel syndrome, congenital AChE deficiency, end-plate deficiency of AChE are *not* related to an immune process but are caused by genetic defects affecting the neuromuscular junction (NMJ).

    f. *Limb-girdle syndrome:* clinical onset during adolescence; progressive weakness responds to AChE inhibitors
    g. *Exacerbation of MG*
        i. Etiologies
            (A) Medications
                (1) D-Penicillamine
                (2) Aminoglycosides
                (3) Quinidine
                (4) Procainamide

       (5) β-Blockers
       (6) Synthroid
       (7) Lithium
       (8) Chlorpromazine
     (B) Infection
   ii. Myasthenic crisis
     (A) ICU setting to monitor FVC
     (B) Intubation if FVC <1 L
     (C) Often provoked by medications or infection
   iii. Cholinergic crisis
     (A) Overmedication resulting in miosis, increased salivation, diarrhea, cramps, and fasciculations
     (B) Treatment: withdrawal of medications under close observation
   iv. If unsure if myasthenic crisis vs. cholinergic crisis, use Tensilon® (edrophonium chloride) test challenge
  h. Differential diagnosis of MG
    i. Psychogenic neurasthenia
   ii. Progressive external ophthalmoplegia
   iii. Oculopharyngeal dystrophy
   iv. Amyotrophic lateral sclerosis (ALS)
    v. Progressive bulbar palsy
   vi. Lambert-Eaton syndrome
   vii. Botulism
   viii. Intracranial mass lesions compressing cranial nerves
   ix. Intranuclear ophthalmoplegia of multiple sclerosis
3. Diagnosis
  a. History
  b. PE: ptosis with prolonged upgaze or decremental weakness after repetitive activity (particularly proximal muscles)
  c. Tensilon® test
    i. Short-acting AChE inhibitor
   ii. Procedure
     (A) Determine weak muscles (i.e., ptosis).
     (B) *Edrophonium chloride, 10 mg intravenously, and normal saline (maintain atropine, 1 mg, at bedside for side effects such as bradycardia, hypotension, or arrhythmias).*
     (C) Inject 2 mg edrophonium chloride and observe.
     (D) Inject 2 mg normal saline and observe (for assessment of functional patients).
     (E) If no response, inject 4–8 mg edrophonium chloride and observe.
  d. *Cooling test*
    i. Place ice on muscles affected and observe.
   ii. Cooling muscles (particularly eyelid muscles) will produce weakness.
  e. *Repetitive nerve stimulation testing (Jolly test):* slow repetitive nerve stimulation at 2–3 Hz produces a decremental response of the CMAP that is maximal with the 3rd or 4th stimulus.
  f. *ACh receptor Ab test: generalized MG: 80–90% positive; ocular MG: 30–40% positive; does not correlate to severity of MG*

NB: Anti-MuSK antibody is now found to be positive in some patients considered "seronegative."

  g. *Antistriated muscle Ab: positive in 85% of patients with thymomas*

    h. Single fiber EMG: *increased jitter and blocking;* should only be performed by experienced electromyographers; 90% of MG positive; may be positive for other conditions (see Chapter 10: Clinical Neurophysiology)

NB: Single fiber EMG of the frontalis muscle has been reported as the most sensitive test for the diagnosis of MG.

    i. Other testing for differential diagnosis
        i. Autoimmune battery (antinuclear Ab, erythrocyte sedimentation rate, rheumatoid factor, double-stranded DNA)
        ii. Thyroid function test
        iii. B_{12} level
        iv. Chest x-ray ± chest computed tomography (CT)
        v. Purified protein derivative of tuberculin (before initiating immunosuppressant treatment)
        vi. Pulmonary function tests/FVC
  4. Treatment
    a. General
        i. Pace activities
        ii. Get plenty of rest
        iii. High-potassium diet
        iv. Avoid exacerbants of weakness caused by infections, fever, heat, cold, pain, overexertion, emotional stress, and medications that can exacerbate MG
    b. Continued scheduled treatment
        i. AChE inhibitors
        (A) *Pyridostigmine (Mestinon®)*
           (1) Onset: 30 minutes
           (2) Peak: 2 hours
           (3) Duration: 4–6 hours ± 1 hour
           (4) Side effects: diarrhea, nausea/vomiting, sweating, increased salivation, miosis, bradycardia, hypotension (glycopyrrolate 1–2 mg q8h to reduce diarrhea and salivation; also can use to decrease salivation in ALS)
           (5) May induce cholinergic crisis if too much is taken by patient
        ii. Immunosuppression
        (A) *Prednisone*
           (1) Must hospitalize due to risk of acute exacerbation of MG induced by steroids
           (2) 1–1.5 mg/kg (60–100 mg) per day until clinical stabilization followed by slow outpatient taper
           (3) If minimal symptoms, outpatient prednisone, 10–20 mg, followed by 5-mg dose increase every 3–5 days until clinical stabilization or max of 60 mg/day (riskier due to risk of exacerbation)
           (4) Side effects: insomnia, hyperglycemia, peripheral edema due to fluid retention, peptic ulcer disease, osteoporosis, psychosis, aseptic necrosis
        (B) *Azathioprine (Imuran®):* use when steroids are contraindicated; begin 50 mg/day for 1 week and titrate up to 2–3 mg/kg/day if complete blood count stable; may take 6–12 months for benefit; side effects: *leukopenia, bone marrow suppression, macrocytic anemia, elevated liver function tests, pancreatitis*

(C) *Cyclosporine:* second-line immunosuppressive agent; 5 mg/kg/day divided into twice-per-day dosing with meals (100–200 mg bid); more rapid onset than azathioprine; side effects: kidney and liver toxicity, leukopenia, gingival hyperplasia, hypertension, tremor, hirsutism

iii. Immune modulation

(A) *PE*

(B) *IVIg, 0.4 g/kg/day*

iv. *Thymectomy:* in patients with or without the presence of thymoma; between ages 8 and 55 years, thymectomy is currently recommended; maximal response 1–4 years after thymectomy

c. Myasthenic exacerbation

i. Supportive care

(A) *FVC q4h (intubate if FVC <1 L; arterial blood gas may be misleading)*

(B) Neurologic checks q2–4h (if increased bulbar signs/symptoms, consider intubation)

ii. PE should be used because faster rate of effect compared to IVIg

d. *Cholinergic crisis*

i. Overmedication resulting in miosis, increased salivation, diarrhea, cramps, fasciculations

ii. Treatment: withdrawal of medications under close observation

B. **Lambert-Eaton syndrome**

1. Pathophysiology

a. Autoimmune response with *autoantibodies directed against voltage-gated calcium channels on the presynaptic nerve terminal* of the neuromuscular junction and autonomic synapses resulting in decreased presynaptic ACh release

b. Two types

i. Paraneoplastic condition: 50–66% have cancer, particularly small-cell (oat) lung carcinoma; *onset of Lambert-Eaton precedes diagnosis of cancer by 9–12 months*

ii. Primary autoimmune form: associated with various autoimmune disorders, including pernicious anemia, hypothyroidism, hyperthyroidism, Sjšgren's syndrome, rheumatoid arthritis, systemic lupus erythematosus, vitiligo, celiac disease, psoriasis, ulcerative colitis, juvenile diabetes mellitus, and MG

2. Clinical

a. Symmetric proximal weakness without atrophy

b. Decreased or absent reflexes

c. Oculo-orophrayngeal symptoms far less common than in MG

d. Increased strength with repetitive effort

e. Dysfunction of the autonomic nervous system

i. Dry mouth (most common)

ii. Impotence, decreased lacrimation and sweating, orthostatism, and abnormal pupillary light reflexes also present

f. EMG/NCV/single fiber EMG: small CMAP (as low as 10% of normal); decreased response to 3–5 Hz stimulation of muscle; facilitation after activation or during repetitive stimulation rates >20 Hz; EMG demonstrates markedly unstable motor unit action potentials (typical); NCV is typically normal but may be abnormal if associated with underlying malignancy; single fiber EMG: jitter with frequent blocking

g. Differential diagnosis

i. MG

ii. AIDP

     iii. PM
     iv. Peripheral neuropathy
     v. Plexopathy
     vi. Multiple radiculopathies
  3. Treatment
    a. Poor response to AChE inhibitors
    b. Increased response to neuromuscular blockers
    c. Improve with treatment of tumor
    d. First-line treatment: prednisone, 60–80 mg qod, with azathioprine, 2–3 mg/kg/day
    e. Other treatment
      i. Guanidine HCl: raise the intracellular calcium concentration, resulting in an increase in ACh
      ii. 3,4-diaminopyridine: inhibits the neuronal voltage-gated K^+ ion conductance, which prolongs action potential, allowing increased Ca^{2+} and increased neurotransmitter
      iii. Immunomodulation
        (A) PE
        (B) IVIg
C. **Toxin-induced: botulism**
  1. Pathophysiology
    a. Caused primarily by *Clostridium botulinum, which is gram-positive anaerobe*
    b. Three forms
      i. Food-borne botulism: 1,000 cases per year worldwide; usually *home-canned vegetables; most associated with type A spores*
      ii. Wound botulism: injection drug use with black tar heroin; post-traumatic
      iii. *Infant botulism:* most common in children *aged 1 week to 11 months:* usually neurotoxins types A and B; death in <2% of cases in the United States but higher worldwide

NB: Sluggish and fatiguable pupils are a characteristic finding in botulism (when accompanied by acute or subacute onset descending paralysis involving the cranial nerves, neck, and shoulder girdle).

    c. The most common form now is wound botulism and then subcutaneous heroin
    d. Neurotoxins types A, B, and E are usual cause, but, rarely, types F and G can also be symptomatic
    e. Irreversible binding to the presynaptic membrane of peripheral cholinergic nerves blocking ACh release at the neuromuscular junction
      i. Three-step process
        (A) Toxin binds to receptors on the nerve ending.
        (B) Toxin molecule I then internalized.
        (C) Within the nerve cell, the toxin interferes with the release of ACh.
      ii. *Cleavage of one of the SNARE (soluble N-ethylmaleimide–sensitive factor attachment protein receptor) proteins by botulinum neurotoxin inhibits the exocytosis of ACh from the synaptic terminal*
  2. Clinical
    a. Blurred vision, dysphagia, dysarthria, pupillary response to light, dry mouth, constipation, and urinary retention

NB: Blurred vision is secondary to paresis of accommodation.

      b. Tensilon® test: positive in 30% of cases

      c. Infant botulism: constipation, lethargy, poor sucking, weak cry

      d. Electrophysiologic criteria for botulism

         i. ↓CMAP amplitude in at least two muscles

         ii. ≥20% facilitation of CMAP amplitude with repetitive stimulation

         iii. Persistent facilitation for ≥2 minutes after activation

         iv. No postactivation exhaustion

         v. Single fiber EMG: ↑jitter and blocking

      e. Prognosis: most patients recover completely in 6 months

  3. Treatment

      a. Supportive care

      b. Antibiotics

         i. Wound botulism: penicillin G or metronidazole

         ii. Antibiotics are not recommended for infant botulism because cell death and lysis may result in the release of more toxin

      c. Horse serum antitoxin

         i. Types A, B, and E

         ii. Side effects of serum sickness and anaphylaxis

D. Differential diagnosis of neuromuscular junction disorders

  1. ALS

  2. Syringomyelia

  3. Polio

  4. Polyneuropathy

  5. Myopathies

  6. Oculocraniosomatic myopathy

      a. Like ocular MG clinically, but slowly progressive

      b. Tensilon® test negative

      c. Single fiber EMG: ↑jitter in facial muscles; EMG reveals myopathic findings in muscle in shoulders

      d. Biopsy: ragged red fibers

  7. Hypermagnesemia

      a. Interferes with action of calcium in the release of ACh

      b. Seen in renal disorders patients who receive laxatives, and preeclampsia

      c. Treated with magnesium

      d. Severe weakness occurs with levels of Mg >10 mEq/L

      e. Clinically resembles Lambert-Eaton syndrome

      f. Tensilon® test positive

      g. Neurophysiologic testing resembles botulism

  8. Organophosphates

      a. Pathophysiology: *irreversible ACh inhibitors;* organophosphates are found in *insecticides (e.g., parathion, malathion), pesticides, and chemical warfare agents (e.g., tabun, sarin, soman);* highly lipid soluble; may be absorbed through the skin, mucous membranes, gastrointestinal tract, and lungs

      b. Clinical

         i. Symptoms occur within a few hours of exposure

         ii. Neuromuscular blockade; autonomic and CNS dysfunction, including headache, miosis, muscle fasciculations, and diffuse muscle cramping; weakness; excessive secretions; nausea; vomiting; and diarrhea; excessive exposure may lead to seizures and coma

      iii. May cause a delayed neuropathy or myelopathy beginning 1–3 weeks after acute exposure

      iv. Electrophysiology: resembles slow channel syndrome and congenital AChE deficiency: increased spontaneous firing rate and amplitude of the miniature end-plate potential; depolarization block

  c. Treatment
      i. Remove clothing and clean exposed skin
      ii. Gastric lavage
      iii. Supportive care
      iv. Atropine, 1–2 mg: antagonizes excessive ACh at muscarinic receptor sites, autonomic ganglia, and CNS synapses, but not at the neuromuscular junction
      v. Pralidoxime, 1 g intravenously: cholinesterase reactivator

9. Envenomation by snakes (see Chapter 8: Neurotoxicology and Nutritional Disorders)

V. Motor Neuron Diseases

A. **ALS**

1. Epidemiology: aka Lou Gehrig disease; male to female ratio is 2:1; onset is usually after 6th decade; *5% of ALS is familial; approximately 20% is due to a defect in the superoxide dismutase gene on chromosome 21*

2. Pathology: *degeneration of the anterior horn cells and corticospinal tracts; Bunina bodies:* intracytoplasmic, eosinophilic inclusions in anterior horn cells; muscle biopsy: fascicular atrophy, neurogenic atrophy (small angulated fibers)

3. Clinical features
  a. Weakness, atrophy, fasciculations (lower motor neuron signs)
  b. Increased reflexes, spasticity, upgoing toes (upper motor neuron signs)
  c. Hands are often affected first, usually asymmetrically, and then the disease generalizes to involve the legs and bulbar muscles (dysphagia, dysarthria, sialorrhea)
  d. Muscle cramps due to hypersensitivity of denervated muscle
  e. Weight loss
  f. Sensation, extraocular muscles, and sphincter function are spared
  g. Death within 3–5 years
  h. *Variants: hemiplegic (Mills) variant—starts with weakness on one side of the body; bulbar ALS—starts with bulbar weakness*
  i. Emotional lability/pseudobulbar effect has been described in many ALS patients.

4. *Electrophysiologic findings:* NCSs are usually normal; EMG shows widespread denervation on at least three limbs, with giant MUPs, polyphasic MUPs, and fasciculations

5. Treatment
  a. *Riluzole,* a glutamate presynaptic inhibitor, has a slight effect of prolonging survival of ALS patients by approximately 2–3 months. Recently, a study on Irish ALS population over a 5-year period showed that riluzole reduced mortality rate by 23% and 15% at 6 and 12 months, respectively, and prolonged survival by 4 months. Survival benefit was more marked in the bulbar-onset disease.
  b. A double-blind, placebo-controlled, randomized study *of vitamin E* plus riluzole vs. riluzole alone showed no effect on survival after 12 months of treatment, but patients given vitamin E were less likely to progress from the milder to the more severe state.
  c. *Anti-epileptic drugs with mild glutamate inhibitory properties* (such as gabapentin and topiramate) have been ineffective in well-designed trials.
  d. Results of *creatine* trials on improving strength in ALS patients are mixed.

e. *Noninvasive positive pressure ventilation* improves survival among ALS patients who can tolerate its use.

f. Placement of percutaneous endoscopic gastrostomy tube may improve survival and quality of life.

B. **Progressive spinal muscular atrophy (SMA)**

1. General description: spinal muscular atrophies, types 1–3, are *all AR and linked to chromosome 5 (mutation in the SMN gene);* pure lower motor neuron syndrome

2. Pathology: *degeneration of the anterior horn cells; in Fazio-Londe syndrome, there is loss of motor neurons in the hypoglossal, ambiguus, facial, and trigeminal motor nuclei*

3. Clinical

   a. *Werdnig-Hoffmann syndrome (SMA type 1)*

      i. Symptoms are evident at birth or before 6 months of age

      ii. A common etiology for floppy infant syndrome

      iii. Proximal muscles are first affect, but flaccid quadriplegia eventually ensues

      iv. Tongue fasciculations

      v. Absent reflexes

      vi. Extraocular muscles are spared

      vii. 85% die by age 2 years

   b. *SMA type 2*

      i. Onset is from age 6 months to 1 year.

      ii. Patients may survive past age 2 years.

      iii. Otherwise, clinical features are similar to SMA type 1.

   c. *Kugelberg-Welander disease (SMA type 3)*

      i. Onset in late childhood or adolescence

      ii. Slowly progressive gait disorder

      iii. Proximal arm weakness/wasting

      iv. Absent reflexes

      v. Fasciculations of the tongue and limb muscles

      vi. More benign course and may have a normal life span

      vii. Sensation, bulbar muscles, and intellect are generally spared

   d. *Fazio-Londe syndrome (childhood bulbar muscular atrophy)*

      i. Onset is late childhood to adolescence

      ii. Selective dysarthria, dysphagia, and facial diplegia

      iii. Tongue wasting with fasciculations

      iv. Weakness of the arms and legs can develop later, but symptoms may also remain restricted for years

   e. *Kennedy's disease (adult bulbar muscular atrophy)*

      i. *X-linked recessive and trinucleotide repeat disease.*

      ii. Symptoms generally begin after age 40 years.

      iii. Dysarthria and dysphagia appear first, followed by limb weakness; tongue fasciculations are present along with absent reflexes.

      iv. *Gynecomastia* is present in most cases.

4. Denervation is seen on NCS/EMG and muscle biopsy; creatine kinase is usually elevated

5. Treatment: a placebo-controlled trial of gabapentin in adults with SMA showed no benefit in slowing down the progression of weakness using quantitative strength testing; riluzole is currently being tested in SMA type 1

C. **Primary lateral sclerosis**

1. Epidemiology: rare and accounts for <5% of all motor neuron disorders.

2. Pathology: degeneration is confined to the corticospinal tracts; magnetic resonance imaging (MRI) is usually normal.
3. Clinical features: age of onset is usually after 40 years; usually starts as a slowly progressive spastic gait that later stabilizes; patients rarely lose the ability to walk with a cane or some other assistance; sphincter is usually preserved, but spastic bladder can occur rarely.
4. Differential diagnosis
   a. Multiple sclerosis (MS)
   b. ALS
   c. Cervical cord compression
   d. Adrenoleukodystrophy
   e. Tropical spastic paraparesis
   f. HIV-associated myelopathy
   g. Vitamin B_{12} deficiency
   h. Paraneoplastic myelopathy
D. **Postpolio syndrome:** patients often complain of fatigue, as well as a decline in functional abilities decades after the initial poliovirus infection; pyridostigmine has been previously studied with mixed results
E. **West Nile poliomyelitis**
   1. First recognized in the United States in 1999; the infection is caused by a *flavivirus that is transmitted from birds to humans through the bite of mosquitos.*
   2. In addition to meningoencephalitis, West Nile virus is associated with a lower motor neuron paralytic syndrome.
   3. Clinically and pathologically appears to be a form of poliomyelitis.
   4. Most of the cases had fever, meningitis, or encephalitis, and one-half had flaccid weakness that progressed over 3–8 days; the weakness tended to be proximal and asymmetric.
   5. CSF typically showed pleocytosis and elevated protein—positive for West Nile virus–specific IgM Abs.
   6. Pathology: anterior horn cell loss and perivascular inflammation.

VI. Myopathy
A. **Degenerative muscular dystrophy (MD)**
   1. General
      a. MD has five essential characteristics
         i. Myopathy by clinical, EMG, and pathologic processes; no evidence of denervation or sensory loss.
         ii. All symptoms are effects of limb or cranial muscle weakness.
         iii. Symptoms become progressively worse.
         iv. Histology implies degeneration and regeneration but no evidence of abnormal storage products.
         v. Heritable (even if no other evidence in other family members).
      b. Features of the most common MDs

	Duchenne's	Facioscapulohumeral	Myotonic
Age of onset	Childhood	Adolescence (rarely childhood)	Adolescence or later
Sex	Male	Either	Either
Pseudohypertrophy	Common	Never	Never

	Duchenne's	Facioscapulohumeral	Myotonic
Location of onset	Pelvic	Shoulder	Distal limbs
Weakness of face	Rare and mild	Always	Common
Rate of progression	Relatively rapid	Slow	Slow (variable)
Contracture deformities	Common	Rare	Rare
Cardiac disorders	Usually late	Rare	Common (conduction)
Inheritance	X-linked	Dominant	Dominant
Expressivity	Full	Variable	Variable
Genetic heterogeneity	Duchenne's/Becker's	None	Proximal limb weakness

2. **X-linked MD**
   a. *Duchenne's MD*
      i. Pathophysiology: *deletion or duplication at Xp21 in 60–70% of cases; abnormality of dystrophin (a cytoskeletal protein located in or near the plasma membrane and seems to be associated with membrane glycoproteins that link it to laminin on the external surface of the muscle fiber; when dystrophin is absent, the sarcolemma becomes unstable with subsequent excessive influx of calcium due to damage, which causes muscle necrosis)*
      ii. Clinical
          (A) *X-linked recessive trait* with females as carriers
          (B) Some carriers have mild manifestations
          (C) Begins with difficulties walking and running followed by difficulty climbing and rising from chairs *(Gowers' sign)*
          (D) Calf hypertrophy
          (E) Often have exaggerated lordosis to maintain upright posture
          (F) As disease progresses, arms and hands affected with slight facial weakness (but speech, swallowing, and ocular muscles are spared)
          (G) Iliotibial and heel cord contractures
          (H) By age 12 years, usually wheelchair bound
          (I) By age 20 years, usually respirator dependent
          (J) Heart spared, but abnormal electrocardiogram (ECG) (change in RS amplitude in V1 and deep narrow Q waves in left precordial leads)
          (K) Developmental delay in one-third of cases
   b. *Becker's MD:* essentially the same as Duchenne's MD except for two aspects—later age of onset (usually after 12 years), and lower rate of progression (still walking at age 20 years)
3. Facioscapulohumeral MD (Landouzy-Dejerine syndrome)
   a. Pathophysiology: *AD; chromosome 4q35-qter (but no gene product identified)*
   b. Clinical
      i. Associated disorders in childhood include deafness, oropharyngeal disorders, and, possibly, mental retardation; may have tortuous retinal vessels and Coats' disease (exudative telangiectasia of retina).
      ii. Initially involves the muscles of the face and trapezius, pectoralis, biceps, and triceps; muscles of the lower extremities are affected much later.

      iii. EMG: may show low-amplitude, short-duration, polyphasic MUPs recruited out of proportion to the degree of muscle force; presence of spontaneous discharges suggests the neuropathic form of this syndrome.

4. *Limb-girdle MD*
   a. Pathophysiology: *AR; several variants; men and women affected equally*
   b. Clinical
      i. Diagnosis of exclusion
      ii. Lower extremities usually affected first, followed by the upper extremities
      iii. Cranial nerves usually spared
      iv. Typically begins in the 2nd to 3rd decade with pelvic involvement and soon spreads to involve shoulders (face spared)
      v. Pseudohypertrophy may or may not occur in calves or deltoids
      vi. Slightly increased CPKs
      vii. Usually normal lifespan
      viii. Subdivided into myopathic and neurogenic forms
      ix. Conditions that simulate limb-girdle MD
         (A) Inflammatory (PM, dermatomyositis [DM], inclusion body myositis, sarcoid)
         (B) Toxic myopathies (chloroquine, steroid, vincristine, lovastatin, ethanol, phenytoin)
         (C) Endocrinopathies (hyper- and hypothyroid, hyperadrenocorticism, hyperparathyroidism, hyperaldosteronism)
         (D) Vitamin deficiency (vitamins D and E)
         (E) Paraneoplastic (Lambert-Eaton, carcinomatous myopathy)
         (F) MG
         (G) Metabolic disorders (late-onset acid maltase deficiency or carnitine deficiency)
         (H) SMA

5. *Myotonic dystrophy (aka Steinert's disease)*
   a. Pathophysiology: *most common of all MDs (incidence = 13.5/100,000); AD with almost 100% penetrance; chromosome 19q13.2 (CTG repeat >40); gene product—myotonin*
   b. Clinical
      i. Unlike any other form of major MD, it affects cranial muscles in addition to those of the face (ptosis, occasionally extraocular muscles are involved, dysphagia, dysarthria, temporalis muscle wasting)
      ii. Pathognomonic: *thin, narrow (hatchet) face; ptosis; thin/weak sternocleidomastoid; and frontal balding*
      iii. Other signs and symptoms
         (A) Weak voice due to involvement of laryngeal muscles.
         (B) Affects distal > proximal muscles (with prominent finger flexor weakness and footdrop with steppage gait)
         (C) Mental retardation
         (D) Cataracts are almost universal
         (E) Hypogonadism with testicular atrophy (endocrinopathy)
         (F) Cardiac arrhythmia or conduction abnormalities (first-degree heart block or bundle branch block)
         (G) Respiratory muscles may be affected even before limb muscles
         (H) Myotonia (impaired relaxation of muscle contraction) causing difficulty with shaking hands because letting go is difficult; may be able to elicit percussion myotonia

      iv. Congenital myotonic dystrophy
         (A) Affected parent is almost always mother
         (B) Ptosis
         (C) *Carp mouth—tented upper lip and open jaw—is diagnostic in infant*
         (D) Also note oropharyngeal difficulties
         (E) Developmental delay and, often, mental retardation
         (F) Arthrogryposis
         (G) Myotonia
      v. EMG/NCV: myopathic changes and waxing and waning after discharge of myotonia
      vi. CPK normal to moderately elevated (not to extent seen in Duchenne's MD)
   c. Pathology: atrophy of type 1 muscle fibers/long rows of central sarcolemmal nuclei and sarcoplasmic masses

NB: Defect is in chloride conductance.

   6. *Oculopharyngeal dystrophy*
     a. Pathophysiology: rare form of progressive ophthalmoplegia; *AD inheritance in French-Canadian families*
     b. Clinical
       i. Progressive ptosis and dysphagia develop late in life, with or without extraocular muscle weakness.
       ii. EMG: Polyphasic MUPs are recruited early in proximal muscles of the upper extremities.
       iii. NCVs are normal except low CMAPs.
       iv. Differential diagnosis: MG (difficult to differentiate clinically)—differentiated with ACh receptor Ab and Tensilon® test.
     c. Pathology: muscle biopsy: variation of fiber size, occasional, internal nuclei, small angulated fibers, and an intermyofibrillary network with moth-eaten appearance when stained with oxidative enzymes
   7. *Hereditary distal myopathy*
     a. Rare AD disorder
     b. Clinical
       i. Adult onset.
       ii. Unlike most dystrophies, predominantly affects distal muscles of upper extremities and lower extremities.
       iii. Weakness typically begins in intrinsic hand muscles, followed by dorsiflexors of the wrist and foot.
       iv. Typically spares proximal muscles.
       v. EMG: low-amplitude, short-duration MUPs during mild voluntary contraction.
     c. Pathology: muscle biopsy: vacuolar changes
   8. *Emery-Dreifuss syndrome*
     a. Pathophysiology: most have *X-linked inheritance* (but rare families have autosomal dominance)
     b. Clinical: weakness develops in humeroperoneal muscles; early contractures with marked restriction of neck and elbow flexion; also cardiac abnormalities causing atrial fibrillation (fib) and a slow ventricular rate
     c. Pathology: mixed pattern of myopathic and neurogenic change; absent emerin
B. **Infectious forms of myopathy**
   1. *Trichinosis* (only one that occurs relatively frequently)

  a. Infection due to undercooked pork containing encysted larvae of *Trichinella spiralis.*

  b. Post-initial gastroenteritis may have invasion of skeletal muscles, but weakness is mainly limited to muscles innervated by cranial nerves (tongue, masseters, extraocular muscles, oropharynx, and so on).

  c. Rarely, may have cerebral symptoms in acute phase due to emboli from trichinella myocarditis.

  d. Labs: eosinophilia, bentonite flocculation assay, and muscle biopsy.

  e. Treatment: symptoms usually subside spontaneously; if severe, thiabendazole, 25 mg/kg bid, plus prednisone, 40–60 mg/day.

 2. *Other infectious causes*

  a. *Toxoplasmosis*

  b. *Cysticercosis*

  c. *Trypanosomiasis*

  d. Mycoplasma pneumoniae

  e. *Coxsackie group B (pleurodynia or Bornholm disease)*

  f. *Influenza*

  g. *Epstein-Barr virus*

  h. *Schistosomiasis*

  i. *Chagas disease*

  j. *Legionnaire's disease*

  k. *Candidiasis*

  l. *Acquired immunodeficiency syndrome*

  m. *Influenza*

  n. *Rubella*

  o. *Hepatitis B*

  p. *Behcet's*

  q. *Kawasaki*

  r. *Echovirus*

C. *Endocrine processes*

 1. Thyroid disease

  a. *Hyperthyroid myopathy*

   i. In frequency of causative factor: hyper- (thyrotoxic myopathy) > hypothyroid.

   ii. Myopathy affects men more frequently than women (although thyrotoxicosis affects women more than men in general).

   iii. Clinical: some proximal weakness; typical weakness involves muscles of shoulder girdle more than pelvic girdle; usually normal DTRs but can be hyperactive; spontaneous muscle twitching and myokymia may develop.

   iv. EMG: myopathic features; quantitative EMG reveals low-amplitude, short-duration MUPs.

   v. Other neurologic conditions associated with thyrotoxicosis include exophthalmic ophthalmoplegia, MG, hypokalemic periodic paralysis.

  b. *Hypothyroid myopathy*

   i. Clinical: proximal muscle weakness, painful muscle spasm, and muscle hypertrophy; features of myxedema include Hoffman's sign (delayed muscle contraction), best demonstrated on eliciting an ankle reflex (brisk reflex with slow return to original position)

NB: Tapping the muscle causes a ridge of muscle contraction (aka myoedema). This may elevate creatine kinases and produce painful cramps.

    ii. EMG: increased insertional activity with some complex repetitive discharges (CRDs) (but no myotonia)

2. *Adrenal and pituitary disease*

    a. Similar weakness occurs with steroids/adrenocorticotropic hormone because steroids reduce the intracellular concentration of potassium.

    b. Dysfunction of the retinaculum or mitochondria may also contribute to the pathogenesis.

    c. Preferential weakness of pelvic girdle and thigh muscles (difficulty arising from a chair or climbing stairs).

    d. Muscle biopsy reveals type 2 atrophy, but neither necrosis nor inflammatory changes.

    e. *Cushing's disease:* hyperadrenalism with associated myopathic symptoms.

    f. *Acromegaly:* elevated growth hormone levels, increasing hand and foot size, thickened heel pad, frontal bossing, prognathism, macroglossia, hypertension, soft tissue swelling, headache, peripheral nerve entrapment syndrome, sweating.

3. Parathyroid disease

    a. *Hypoparathyroidism causes hypocalcemia, which results in tetany*

        i. Normally, influx of calcium into the axon terminal facilitates the release of ACh at the neuromuscular junction, resulting in excitation-contraction coupling; a reduction of calcium results in increased conductance for Na^+ and K^+, which causes instability and hyperexcitability of the cell membrane.

        ii. *EMG of tetany: doublets or triplets of MUPs; low-amplitude, short-duration MUPs recruit early in weak muscles; no spontaneous activity.*

        iii. NCV studies reveal reduced amplitude of CMAP but normal sensory and motor NCVs.

    b. *Hyperparathyroidism*

        i. Less frequently, neuromuscular symptoms in hypercalcemia may result from osteolytic metastatic disease, multiple myeloma, or chronic renal disease.

        ii. Varying proximal muscle weakness occurs in hyperparathyroidism (usually affecting the pelvic girdle more than the shoulder) with brisk DTRs, occasional Babinski, and axial muscle wasting.

D. **Becker's MD**

E. **Limb-girdle dystrophy**

F. **Fascioscapulohumeral MD**

G. **Emory-Dreifuss MD**

H. **Ocular pharyngeal dystrophy**

I. *Myotonic dystrophy*

1. Pathophysiology: characterized by muscle wasting and weakness associated with myotonia and a number of other systemic abnormalities; AD; incidence: 1:8,000; prevalence: 3–5 per 100,000; sodium conductance is altered as a result of abnormal opening of the channels at potentials that have no effect in normal muscle; this results in increased intracellular sodium concentrations

2. Genetic diagnosis

    i. *Chromosome 19q13.3*

    ii. *Amplified CTG repeat located in the 3′ untranslated region of the gene that encodes myotonin protein kinase*

    iii. Amplification in successive generations yields increasing severity

	Normal	Borderline	"Carriers"	Full mutation
Number of CTG repeats	5–37	38–49	50–99	>100
Clinical phenotype	Normal	Normal	Mild or no symptoms	Symptomatic

3. Clinical features
   a. Primary form
      i. Myotonia—delayed muscle relaxation after contraction
      ii. Weakness and wasting affecting facial muscles and distal limb muscles
      iii. Long face with wasting of the masseter and temporal muscles
      iv. Thin neck with wasting of the sternocleidomastoids
      v. Frontal balding in males
      vi. Cataracts
      vii. Cardiomyopathy with conduction defects
      viii. Gastrointestinal motility disturbances—cholecystitis, dysphagia, constipation, urinary tract symptoms
      ix. *Multiple endocrinopathies*
         (A) Hyperinsulinism, rarely diabetes
         (B) Adrenal atrophy
         (C) Infertility in women
         (D) Testicular atrophy: growth hormone secretion disturbances
      x. Low intelligence or dementia
      xi. Excessive daytime sleepiness
   b. Congenital form
      i. Children born to mothers with myotonic dystrophy
      ii. Significant hypotonia
      iii. Facial diplegia
      iv. Feeding and respiratory difficulties
      v. Skeletal deformities (e.g., clubfeet)
      vi. Delayed developmental progression during childhood
   c. EMG/NCV: myotonic discharges: bursts of repetitive potentials that wax and wane in both amplitude and frequency ("dive bomber" potentials)
   d. *Muscle biopsy: random variability in the size of fibers and fibrosis; multiple nuclei throughout the interior of the fibers and type 1 fiber atrophy; ring fibers*
   e. Treatment: rarely required unless symptoms are severe; phenytoin: membrane-stabilizing effect
J. **Congenital disorders of the muscle**
   1. *Myotonia congenita (Thomsen's disease)*
      a. Pathophysiology: *chromosome 7q35; almost always AD inheritance; dysfunctional chloride channel with decreased Cl⁻ conductance*
      b. Clinical
         i. Symptoms are only caused by myotonia or consequences thereof.
         ii. Differs from myotonic dystrophy because there is no muscle weakness or wasting, and also systemic manifestations, such as no cataracts; ECG abnormal, endocrinopathies, and so on, but the myotonia tends to be more severe.
         iii. Due to isometric contractions of myotonia, muscles tend to hypertrophy and make the patient look athletic (*mini-Hercules appearance*).

    iv. Myotonia may affect

      (A) Limbs: difficulty with grip; may often predominate in the lower extremities causing difficulty with ambulation

      (B) Oropharyngeal muscles (dysphagia)

      (C) Orbicularis oculi

      (D) Does not affect respiratory muscles

    v. Myotonia worse on initiation of activity, but decreases with gradually increasing exercise ("warming up" phenomenon) in the individual limb.

    vi. Movements begin slowly and with difficulty, especially after prolonged rest.

    vii. Diagnosis

      (A) Depends on signs and symptoms (including percussion myotonia) and positive family history.

      (B) In equivocal cases, exposure to cold can be a provocative test.

      (C) EMG helpful in that progressive nerve stimulation may cause progressive decline in successive evoked CMAPs due to increased muscle refractoriness (this may occur in any type of myotonic disorder).

    viii. Muscle biopsy: reveals absence of type 2B fibers and presence of internal nuclei.

  c. Treatment

    i. *Myotonia relieved with phenytoin or quinine sulfate (200–1,200 mg/day).*

    ii. *Acetazolamide occasionally effective.*

    iii. *Procainamide may ameliorate myotonia but may induce lupus.*

2. *Paramyotonia congenita of Eulenburg*

  a. AD; male = female

  b. Clinical

    i. Begins at birth or early childhood without improvement with age.

    ii. Paradoxically, the myotonia intensifies (instead of remits) with exercise.

    iii. *In cold, patient may have stiffness of tongue, eyelids, face, and limb muscles.*

    iv. EMG: discharges disappear with cooling despite increased muscle stiffness.

    v. Clinically similar to hyper-K^+ periodic paralysis in that there may be episodes of flaccid weakness.

    vi. May have elevated levels of serum K^+.

NB: Substantial decrease in the amplitude of the CMAP occurs with exposure to cold.

3. *Congenital myopathy*

  a. **Nemaline rod myopathy**

    i. *AD inheritance*

    ii. Clinical

      (A) Nonprogressive hypotonia that begins in early childhood

      (B) May be benign if onset is in childhood or adulthood, but fatal in newborn/ neonate

      (C) Diffuse weakness

      (D) Dysmorphism with reduced muscle bulk and slender muscles resulting in elongated face, high-arched palate, high-arched feet, kyphoscoliosis, and occasional scapuloperoneal distribution of weakness

      (E) Slightly elevated CPK

      (F) Muscle biopsy: patients and carriers have type 1 fiber predominance; *Gomori's trichrome stain shows typical rod-shaped bodies near sarcolemma staining bright red (not noted with other stains) that contain material identical to Z-bands of muscle fibers, involving either type 1 or 2, or both;* rods may be found in other disorders as nonspecific finding

(G) EMG: low-amplitude, short-duration MUPs with early recruitment, or, conversely, fibs and decreased number of high-amplitude, long-duration MUPs

NB: Most common presentation is congenital hypotonia.

b. **Centronuclear (or myotubular) myopathy**
   i. Pathophysiology: linked *to chromosome Xq28; inheritance varies (X-linked recessive, infantile-juvenile AR, and milder AD);* fetal myotubules persist into adult life; histology: the nuclei are positioned centrally instead of the normal sarcolemmal distribution and are surrounded by a pale halo.
   ii. Clinical: most have hypotonia, ptosis, facial weakness, and extraocular movement palsy at birth; may also affect proximal and distal muscles; course varies from death in infancy/childhood to mild progression with survival into adulthood.
      (A) *Muscle biopsy*
         (1) *Type 1 fiber atrophy and central nuclei (considered characteristic of fetal muscle).*
         (2) *The central part of the fiber is devoid of myofibrils and myofibrillar adenosine triphosphate (ATP) and, therefore, stains poorly with ATPase.*
         (3) *Oxidative enzymes may show decreased or increased activity in central region.*
      (B) EMG/NCV: excessive number of polyphasic, low-amplitude MUPs, fibs, positive sharp waves, and CRDs

NB: Centronuclear myopathy is the only congenital myopathy associated with spontaneous activity.

c. **Central core disease**
   i. Pathophysiology: histology: an amorphous area in the middle of the fiber stains blue with Gomori trichrome and contrasts with the peripheral fibrils that stain red; the cores are devoid of enzyme activity; *on electron microscopy, there are no mitochondria; AD—chromosome 19q13.1.*
   ii. Clinical
      (A) Hypotonia shortly after birth, developmental delay, and occasional hip dislocations.
      (B) Proximal muscle weakness but no distinct muscle atrophy.
      (C) May have skeletal deformities (lordosis, kyphoscoliosis, foot abnormalities).
      (D) Malignant hyperthermia has been reported in association with central core disease.
      (E) *Muscle biopsy: marked type 1 fiber predominance; central region of muscle fiber contains compact myofibrils devoid of oxidative and phosphorylase enzymes because of virtual absence of mitochondria (these central areas are referred to as* cores*); common in type 1 and less common in type 2 fibers; resemble target fibers, which indicate denervation and reinnervation, suggesting that central core disease may be a neurogenic process.*
      (F) EMG/NCV: suggest mixed myopathic–neurogenic process; usually insertional activity is normal with no spontaneous discharges, small MUPs with recruitment.
d. **Cytoplasmic body myopathy**
   i. Histology: accumulation of desmin
   ii. Clinical
      (A) Weakness characteristically involves the face, neck, and proximal limb muscles, as well as respiratory, spinal, and cardiac muscles; may have scoliosis; elevated CPK; abnormal ECG

      (B) Muscle biopsy: central nuclei, necrosis, fibrosis, and cytoplasmic bodies

      (C) EMG: myopathic findings

K. *Inflammatory myopathy*

If other connective tissue disease is concurrent, then designation is PM (or DM) with systemic lupus erythematosus, rheumatoid arthritis, and so on.

1. **Polymyositis (PM)**

    a. Pathogenesis: presumed to be cell mediated (unlike presumed humoral mediation in DM)

    b. Clinical

       i. Primarily affects adults with underlying connective tissue disease or malignancy.

         (A) Male—bowel, stomach, or lung cancer

         (B) Female—ovary or breast cancer

       ii. Usually no pain, fever, or initiating event; usually general systemic manifestations.

       iii. Proximal weakness (lower > upper extremities) with head lolling due to neck flexor (anterior compartment) weakness.

       iv. Affected muscles are nontender.

       v. No significant decrease in DTRs and no significant muscle atrophy.

    c. EMG: *"Myopathic changes" with small-amplitude, short-duration potentials and full recruitment; signs of muscle irritability may be noted with fibs and positive waves but no fasciculations; CRDs may be present*

    d. Pathology: *infiltration around normal muscle by CD8⁺ T lymphocytes; muscle necrosis and regeneration may be present (but differs from DM in that, with PM, there are no vascular lesions or perifascicular atrophy and differs from inclusion body by lack of vacuoles or inclusions)*

2. **Dermatomyositis (DM)**

    a. Pathogenesis

       i. Believed to be autoimmune but no direct evidence; most likely humorally mediated due to evidence of presence of more B cells than T cells in infiltrated muscle and a vasculopathy that deposits immune complexes in intramuscular blood vessels.

       ii. Tends to be associated with Raynaud's phenomenon, systemic lupus erythematosus, polyarteritis nodosa, Sjögren's syndrome, or pneumonitis.

    b. Clinical

       i. Usually begins with nonspecific systemic manifestations, including malaise, fever, anorexia, weight loss, and features of respiratory infection.

       ii. Skin lesions may precede, accompany, or follow myopathic process and vary from scaly eczematoid dermatitis to diffuse exfoliative dermatitis or scleroderma; characteristic heliotropic "lupus-like" facial distribution and on extensor surfaces of the extremities.

       iii. Also may have mild perioral and periorbital edema.

       iv. Usually proximal limb weakness, but cranial nerve musculature may also be involved with dysphagia in one-third of cases.

       v. Occurs in all decades of life, with peak before puberty and around age 40 years.

       vi. Females > males.

       vii. Higher incidence of associated connective tissue diseases and occurs in conjunction with tumors with approximately 10% of cases of women >40 y/o having an associated malignancy (lung, colon, breast, etc.).

    c. Pathology: *perifascicular atrophy (not seen in PM); inflammatory cells are found in the perimysium rather than within the muscle fiber itself*

    d. Childhood variant: in conjunction with DM, may have pain, fever, melena, hematemesis, and possible gastrointestinal perforation

    e. Treatment

       i. Prednisone, 60 mg/day (higher doses may be necessary in children)

       ii. Immunosuppressant medications

       iii. IVIg

       iv. Plasmapheresis ineffective

  3. **Inclusion body myositis**

    a. Pathogenesis: idiopathic, but viral origin suggested; like PM, low association with malignancy

    b. Clinical: more common in males, especially those >50 y/o; disproportionate affliction of distal limbs in conjunction with proximal limb involvement; weakness of hands may be early symptom and is one of only a few myopathies that affect the long finger flexors; dysphagia is rare; only slight increase in CPK

    c. Pathology: *muscle biopsy (distinctive): intranuclear and intracytoplasmic inclusions composed of masses of filaments and sarcolemmal whorls of membranes, combined with fiber necrosis, cellular infiltrates, and regeneration; also may have rimmed vacuoles*

    d. Treatment: poor response to treatment such as steroids

L. *Familial periodic paralysis*

	Hypokalemic periodic paralysis	Hyperkalemic periodic paralysis	Paramyotonia congenita
Age of onset	1st–2nd decade	1st decade	1st decade
Sex	Predominantly male	Equal	Equal
Incidence of paralysis	Interval of weeks to months	Interval of hours to days	May not be present
Degree of paralysis	Usually severe	Usually mild (occasionally severe)	Usually mild (occasionally severe)
Duration	Hours to days	Minutes to hours	Hours
Effect of cold	May induce attack	May induce attack	Usually induces attack
Effect of glucose	May induce attack	Relieves attack	Relieves attack
Effect of activity	Triggered by rest	Triggered by rest	Triggered by exercise
Serum potassium	Low	High	Normal but may be high
Oral potassium	Prevents attack	Precipitates an attack	Precipitates an attack
Myotonia	None	Occasional	Prominent
Genetics	AD	AD: Chromosome 17q13.1	AD
Channel	Calcium	Sodium	Possibly sodium

1. **Hypokalemic periodic paralysis**
   a. Pathophysiology: K$^+$ <3.0 mg/dL (often accompanied by high Na$^+$ levels); may be induced by injections of insulin, epinephrine, fluorohydrocortisone, or glucose; may follow high-carbohydrate diet; very rare; 3 males:1 female
   b. Clinical
       i. Attack usually begins after resting (commonly present at night or on awakening).
      ii. Weakness varies from mild to complete paralysis of all muscles of limbs and trunk (oropharyngeal and respiratory muscles are usually spared even in severe attacks).
     iii. Duration varies from few hours to 48 hours.
      iv. Some patients have improved strength with activity.
       v. Weakness especially likely on morning after ingesting high-carbohydrate meal.
      vi. Rarely, it is associated with peroneal muscle atrophy.
     vii. DTRs and EMG/NCVs are reduced proportionally to the severity of the attack (sensory NCVs are normal).
    viii. Not associated with any general medical problems.
      ix. Frequency of attacks tends to decrease as patient gets older and may cease after age 40–50 years.
       x. Fatalities are rare but may occur due to respiratory depression.
      xi. Diagnosis made during attack: *low K$^+$ and high Na$^+$; induction during glucose (100 g) or insulin (20 units) infusion*
     xii. Correlation with hyperthyroidism (especially in those of Asian decent).
    xiii. EMG: reduced recruitment of MUPs and decreased muscle excitability.
     xiv. Repetitive stimulation may result in incremental response.
   c. Pathology: light microscopy reveals few abnormalities; electron microscopy: vacuoles arising from local dilation of the transverse tubules and sarcoplasmic reticulum

NB: Vacuole formation in muscle fibers is the most common change in hypokalemic periodic paralysis. They are most prominent during the attacks.

   d. Treatment
       i. Acute attack: 20–100 mEq of KCl
      ii. Prophylactic therapy: *Carbonic anhydrase inhibitors (acetazolamide, 250–1,000 mg/day) helps prevent attacks in 90% of patients; if acetazolamide ineffective, may be treated with triamterene or spironolactone*

2. **Hyperkalemic periodic paralysis**
   a. Pathophysiology: *autosomal dominance with almost complete penetrance*; cellularly, extracellular Na$^+$ influx causes K$^+$ efflux from the cell
   b. Clinical
       i. Early age of onset (usually <10 years).
      ii. Attacks usually occur during the day and are shorter and less severe.
     iii. Myotonia demonstrable on EMG but usually not clinically relevant.
      iv. Myotonic lid-lag and lingual myotonia may be the only traits noted.
       v. *Elevated serum K$^+$ (may be due to leak from muscles).*
      vi. *Precipitated by hunger, rest, or cold and by KCl ingestion.*
   c. Treatment
       i. Acute attack: may be terminated by *calcium gluconate, glucose, or insulin*
      ii. Prophylactic: *acetazolamide, 250–1,000 mg/day, and thiazides or fludrocortisone*

3. **Paramyotonia congenita (Eulenburg's disease):** differs from ordinary myotonia in two ways
   a. Induced by cold
   b. Exacerbated by exercise

M. **Necrotizing polymyopathy (rhabdomyolysis) with myoglobinuria**
   1. Crush/infarction
   2. PM or DM with necrosis
   3. Toxic (alcohol, resins, poisoned fish [Haff disease])
   4. Hereditary disorders of glycolysis
      a. Myophosphorylase deficiency (McArdle's disease)
      b. Phosphofructokinase deficiency (Tarui's disease)
      c. Lipid storage myopathy
      d. Carnitine palmityltransferase deficiency
      e. Phosphoglycerate deficiency
   5. Excessive exercise
   6. Familial paroxysmal myoglobinuria
   7. *Malignant hyperthermia*
      a. Pathogenesis: *AD (rare); defect of phosphodiesterase; reduced reuptake of Ca^+ by the sarcoplasmic reticulum; highly susceptible to anesthetics including halothane and succinylcholine; the hyperthermia is thought to be secondary to abnormal depolarization of skeletal muscle by halothane.*
      b. Clinical
         i. After anesthetic induction, the patient develops fasciculations and increased muscle tone, followed by an explosive increase in temperature coinciding with muscle rigidity and necrosis.
         ii. If untreated, patient will die of hyperthermia (up to 42°C), acidosis, and recurrent convulsions, and, possibly, circulatory collapse.
      c. Treatment: stop anesthetic; cool the patient; intravenous dantrolene

N. *Medications associated with myopathy*
   1. Alcohol
   2. Colchicine
   3. Lovastatin
   4. Diazacholesterol
   5. Clofibrate
   6. Steroids
   7. Rifampin
   8. Kaliuretics
   9. Zidovudine (AZT)
   10. Chloroquine

NB: AZT inhibits mitochondrial DNA polymerase, producing mitochondrial DNA depletion. Muscle biopsy shows ragged red fibers, reflecting mitochondrial proliferation.

NB: Statin myopathy is a necrotizing myopathy due to the effects of the drug in inhibiting the synthesis of mevalonic acid, a precursor of several essential metabolites, including CoQ10.

NB: Chronic steroid myopathy may develop in cushing disease or during chronic steroid treatment. There is moderate to severe atrophy of type 2 fibers.

O. **Inherited metabolic disorders**
 1. *Glycogen storage diseases*
  a. **Acid maltase deficiency (type 2 glycogenosis, Pompe's disease)**
   i. *AR*
   ii. *Acid maltase deficiency leads to accumulation of glycogen in tissue lysosomes*
   iii. Clinical
    (A) Infantile (Pompe's disease): children develop severe hypotonia after birth and die within the first year of cardiac or respiratory failure.
    (B) Childhood: in less severe childhood and adult forms, symptoms mimic those of limb-girdle MD or PM with onset in childhood; results in proximal limb and trunk muscle weakness with variable progression; may die of respiratory failure by end of 2nd decade; increased net muscle protein catabolism has a part because this condition improves with a high-protein diet.
    (C) Adulthood: begin with insidious limb-girdle weakness during 2nd to 3rd decade followed by respiratory difficulty.
    (D) Elevated CPKs.
    (E) EMG: Infantile form = increased insertional activity, fibrillatory potentials, positive sharp waves, CRDs (due to anterior horn cells involvement).
   iv. Pathology
    (A) Histologically, anterior horn cells contain deposits of glycogen particles (as do other organs, including the heart, liver, and tongue [an enlarged tongue and cardiac abnormalities differentiate Pompe's from Werdnig-Hoffman disease])
    (B) Muscle biopsy: vacuolar myopathy affecting type 1 > type 2 fibers
  b. **Debrancher enzyme deficiency (type 3 glycogenosis)**
   i. Pathogenesis: *AR; absence of debrancher enzyme prevents breakdown of glycogen beyond the outer straight glucosyl chains;* consequently, glycogen with short-branched outer chains (aka phosphorylase-limit-dextrin) accumulates in the liver and striated and cardiac muscle; despite the generalized enzymatic defect, skeletal muscles may show little weakness.
   ii. Clinical
    (A) Child with hypotonia and proximal weakness with failure to thrive.
    (B) Accumulation of glycogen within the liver causes *hepatomegaly, episodic hypoglycemia, and elevated CPK.*
    (C) Clinical features of myopathy may develop after hepatic symptoms have abated.
    (D) Patients may improve in adolescence but may later develop distal limb weakness and atrophy (similar to motor neuron disease).
    (E) EMG: fibs, CRDs, and short-duration, small MUPs.
   iii. Pathology: muscle biopsy: subsarcolemmal periodic acid-Schiff–positive vacuoles in type 2 fibers without histologic signs of denervation
  c. **Myophosphorylase deficiency (McArdle's disease; type 5 glycogenosis)**
   i. Pathogenesis: 4 males:1 female; *usually AR (rarely AD);* myophosphorylase deficiency blocks the conversion of muscle glycogen to glucose during heavy exercise under ischemic conditions; abnormality is confined to skeletal muscle.
   ii. Clinical
    (A) Usually begins in childhood/adolescence; initially only causes muscle fatigability and weakness, but exercise intolerance develops by adolescence.

(B) Repetitive contraction causes cramping (which may improve if patient slows down and performs nonstrenuous activity due to mobilization of free fatty acids as an alternative energy source = *2nd-wind phenomenon*).

(C) Associated breakdown of muscle causes myoglobinuria.

(D) Neurologic exam between bouts demonstrates only mild proximal muscle weakness.

(E) Differential diagnosis
  (1) Phosphofructokinase deficiency: recurrent myoglobinuria and persistent weakness
  (2) Brody's disease: caused by deficiency of calcium ATPase in sarcoplasmic reticulum

(F) Confirmation study: ischemic exercise test (causing severe cramping); no rise in serum lactate with exercise.

d. **Phosphofructokinase deficiency (type 7 glycogenosis, Tarui's disease)**
  i. Pathogenesis: due to *defect of muscle phosphofructokinase, which is necessary for the conversion of F-6-phosphate to 1-6 diphosphate*
  ii. Clinical
    (A) Painful muscle contracture and myoglobinuria (similar to McArdle's) usually in infancy.
    (B) Infant usually has limb weakness, seizures, cortical blindness, and corneal opacities.
    (C) Differentiated from McArdle's by evaluation of phosphofructokinase activity in muscle.

NB: Myophosphorylase deficiency and phosphofructokinase deficiency do not have a normal rise in serum lactate with the ischemic exercise test.

2. *Lipid storage disease*
  a. *Carnitine deficiency*
    i. Pathogenesis
      (A) Whereas glycogen serves as the main energy source of muscle during rapid strenuous activity, circulating lipid in the form of free fatty acids maintains the energy supply at rest and during prolonged low intensity activity.
      (B) Carnitine palmitoyltransferase catalyzes the reversible binding of carnitine to plasma fatty acids; once carnitine is bound to the fatty acids, it can then transport the fatty acids across the mitochondrial membrane for oxidation.
      (C) AR (probable).
      (D) Two types
        (1) Restricted type: develops lipid storage predominantly in muscle, causing a lipid storage myopathy; probably develops due to decreased ability of muscle to uptake carnitine (despite normal serum carnitine levels).
        (2) Systemic type: insufficient synthesis lowers carnitine levels in liver, serum, and muscle.
    ii. Clinical
      (A) A congenital and slowly progressive myopathy of limb-girdle type and episodic hepatic insufficiency.
      (B) Severe defect may cause bulbar and respiratory defects with early death.
      (C) EMG/NCV: low-amplitude, short-duration, polyphasic MUPs.

       iii. Pathology: muscle biopsy: excess lipid droplets, mainly in type 1 fibers (which depend on the oxidation of long-chain fatty acids to a greater extent than type 2 fibers)

  b. *Carnitine palmitoyltransferase deficiency*

      i. Pathogenesis: *AR*; oxidation of lipid substrates is impaired because long-chain fatty acids (not coupled to carnitine) cannot move across the inner mitochondrial membrane.

      ii. Clinical

         (A) Painful muscle cramps; on prolonged exercise or fasting, recurrent myoglobinuria (first episode of myoglobinuria is usually in adolescence).

         (B) Muscle is strong between attacks, but cramping is elicited with exercise.

         (C) EMG/NCV: normal.

      iii. Pathology: muscle biopsy: no abnormalities, or only slight increase in intrafiber lipid droplets next to the mitochondria in type 1 fibers

3. *Mitochondrial encephalomyopathy*

  a. **Kearns-Sayre ophthalmoplegia** *(aka oculocraniosomatic neuromuscular disease)*

      i. Pathogenesis: most common type of mitochondrial myopathy; occurs sporadically (almost never familial)—believed to be due to a mutation in the ovum or somatic cells

      ii. Clinical

         (A) Triad

            (1) Age of onset <20 years

            (2) Progressive external ophthalmoplegia

            (3) Pigmentary retinopathy

         (B) Plus at least one of the following

            (1) Heart block

            (2) Cerebellar dysfunction

            (3) CSF protein >100 mg/dL

            (4) MRI/CT = leukoencephalopathy or basal ganglia calcification

         (C) May also commonly have lactic acidosis and dementia

         (D) Typical presentation: ptosis and extraocular muscle palsies appearing during childhood and adolescence; progressive weakness of extraocular muscles, cardiac abnormalities, and somatic complaints; progressive weakness and fatigue occur with a wide variety of neurologic deficits (including pigmentary degeneration of the retina, sensorineural deafness, cerebellar degeneration, endocrine abnormalities, sensorimotor neuropathy, and demyelinating polyradiculopathy)

         (E) Labs

            (1) Increased serum levels of lactate and pyruvate

            (2) Increased CSF pressure >100

      iii. Pathology: muscle biopsy: ragged red fibers

  b. **MERRF (myoclonic epilepsy with ragged red fibers)**

      i. Pathogenesis: *point mutation of nucleotide pair 8344 (nt-8344, or nt-8356): both are found in mitochondrial DNA gene for transfer RNA for lysine*

      ii. Clinical

         (A) Essential features

            (1) Myoclonic epilepsy

            (2) Cerebellar dysfunction

            (3) Myoclonus

   (B) Other features
    (1) Short stature
    (2) Ataxia
    (3) Dementia
    (4) Lactic acidosis
    (5) Weakness
   (C) MRI/CT: leukoencephalopathy and cerebellar atrophy
  iii. Pathology: muscle biopsy: ragged red fibers
 c. **MELAS (mitochondrial encephalopathy, lactic acidosis, and stroke-like episodes)**
  i. Pathogenesis: *point mutation at locus nt-3243 (the affected gene is the transfer RNA for leucine)*
  ii. Clinical
   (A) Age of onset <40 years
   (B) Short stature
   (C) Seizures
   (D) Dementia
   (E) Lactic acidosis
   (F) Recurrent headache
   (G) Stroke-like episodes
   (H) CT/MRI: Lesions do not conform to normal vascular distributions
  iii. Pathology: muscle biopsy: *ragged red fibers*
 d. *Respiratory chain defects (complex I, III; complex IV [cytochrome-c oxidase])*
 e. **Leigh's disease (subacute necrotizing encephalomyelopathy)**
  i. Pathogenesis: *cytochrome oxidase and pyruvate dehydrogenase deficiency*
  ii. Clinical
   (A) Age of onset usually <2 years
   (B) Developmental delay
   (C) Ataxia
   (D) Failure to thrive
   (E) Ophthalmoplegia
   (F) Hypotonia
   (G) Irregular respiration
   (H) Weakness
   (I) MRI: abnormality of brain stem and basal ganglia nuclei
   (J) Labs: increased serum pyruvate and lactate (which may also be increased in CSF)

P. **Muscle cramps and stiffness**
 1. *Myotonia*
  a. Once muscle membrane is activated, it tends to fire repetitively, inducing delayed muscle relaxation.
  b. Causes no pain, unlike cramping or spasm.
  c. During movement, myotonia may worsen initially but improve with warm-up period.
  d. Percussion myotonia elicited after muscle tap.
  e. Cold exacerbates both postactivation and percussion myotonia.
  f. Myotonic discharges with or without clinical myotonia occur with
   i. Hyperkalemic periodic paralysis.
   ii. Acid maltase deficiency.
   iii. Hyperthyroidism.
   iv. Familial granulovacuolar lobular myopathy.

      v. Malignant hyperthermia.

     vi. Diazacholesterol.

  g. Underlying process unknown but may be associated with sarcolemmal membrane; K^+ ions accumulate in the transverse tubules, resulting in negative afterpotentials; may also be associated with low chloride conductance.

2. **Neuromyotonia (Isaacs' syndrome)**

  a. Typically occurs sporadically

  b. Clinical

      i. Affects any age group

     ii. Begins insidiously and slowly progresses

    iii. *Spontaneous continuous muscle activity—myokymia*

    iv. Due to myokymia, may have abnormal postures of limbs

     v. Also have pseudomyotonia (caused by relapsing and remitting of myotonic bursts—not seen on EMG) and no percussion myotonia

    vi. Liability to cramps (failure to relax) with hyperhidrosis

    vii. Reduced/absent DTRs

   viii. Stiffness and myokymia are present at rest and persist in sleep and anesthesia

    ix. EMG

       (A) *Prolonged, irregular discharges of action potentials that are variable in amplitude and configuration (and some may resemble fibs).*

       (B) *Voluntary contraction produces more intense discharges that persist on relaxation.*

       (C) *A marked decrement of successive amplitude results from inability of the motor unit to follow rapidly recurring nerve stimuli.*

     x. Occasionally associated with paraneoplastic process

    xi. May have an increased level of γ-aminobutyric acid (GABA) in CSF

  c. Treatment: carbamazepine or phenytoin often controls symptomatology

3. **Tetany**

  a. Pathophysiology

      i. *Caused by hypocalcemia and alkalosis.*

     ii. *Decreased extracellular calcium increases sodium conductance, which leads to membrane depolarization and repetitive nerve firing.*

    iii. *Hypo-Mg^{2+} and hyper-K^+ also induce carpopedal spasm.*

    iv. *Tetanic contraction stops with infusion of curare (but not with peripheral nerve block); therefore, spontaneous discharges tend to occur at some point along the length of the nerve, which can be demonstrated with Chvostek's sign by tapping the facial nerve and Trousseau's sign by inducing ischemia.*

  b. Clinical

      i. Characterized by seizures, paresthesias, prolonged contraction of limb muscles, or laryngospasm.

     ii. Is accompanied by signs of excitability of peripheral nerves.

    iii. Occurs in hypo-Ca^{2+} (which, if latent, may produce tetany after hyperventilation), hypo-Mg^{2+}, or alkalosis; typical carpopedal spasms.

    iv. If spasm is severe, it may proceed to involve proximal limbs and axial muscles.

     v. In tetany, nerves are hyperexcitable as manifested by ischemia (Trousseau's sign) or percussion (Chvostek's sign).

    vi. Spasms are due to spontaneous firings of peripheral nerves (starting in the proximal portions of the longest nerves).

    vii. EMG: individual motor units discharging independently at a rate of 5–25 Hz (each discharge consists of a group of two or more identical potentials).

    c. Treatment: correcting metabolic disorder

4. **NB: Stiff-person syndrome (Moersch-Woltman syndrome)**
    a. Pathophysiology
        i. *Unknown but postulated that α and γ motor neurons are hyperactive by excitatory influences descending from the brain stem.*
        ii. May involve autoimmunity with Abs to glutamate decarboxylase found in serum and CSF.
        iii. *Abs have been demonstrated against glutamic acid decarboxylase, which is the rate-limiting enzyme for the synthesis of the inhibitory GABA.*
        iv. Occasionally paraneoplastic.
    b. Clinical
        i. Progressive muscular rigidity and painful spasms.
        ii. Slow progressive course over months to years.
        iii. Aching mainly in axial and proximal limb muscles.
        iv. Stiffness decreases in sleep and under general anesthesia.
        v. Later, painful reflex spasm occurs in response to movement, sensory stimulation, startle, or emotion.
        vi. Cocontraction of agonist and antagonist muscles may immobilize extremity in unnatural position.
        vii. Spasms may lead to joint deformities and may be powerful enough to tear muscle or cause fractures.
        viii. Passive muscle stretch produces an exaggerated reflex contraction that lasts several seconds.
        ix. Normal sensory and motor findings otherwise; seizures sometimes occur
        x. Continuous muscle activity relieved by benzodiazepines
        xi. Aka *stiff-man syndrome,* but changed because 80% are female.
        xii. EMG: continuous discharges of MUPs similar to voluntary contraction.
        xiii. Differentiated clinically from Isaacs' by the fact that Isaacs' affects mainly distal upper extremities and lower extremities and stiff-person affects the trunk.
    c. Treatment
        i. GABAergic drugs
            (A) Diazepam
            (B) Clonazepam
            (C) Baclofen
            (D) Vigabatrin
            (E) Tiagabine
        ii. Immunomodulation: IVIg: most successful immunomodulation

5. *Myokymia*
    a. *Consecutive repetitive contractions of adjacent muscle bands 1–2 cm in width.*
    b. *Due to lesion of peripheral branches of motor nerve causing continuous activity of motor units.*
    c. *Rest and sleep do not change myokymia.*
    d. Lidocaine (Xylocaine®) infusion of peripheral nerve trunk will block myokymic discharges.
    e. EMG: caused by brief tetanic contractions of repetitively discharging single or multiple motor units; typically occur alone without fibs or positive sharp waves.
    f. Facial myokymia.
        i. Usually suggests multiple sclerosis or pontine glioma, but also occurs in Bell's palsy, polyradiculoneuropathy, cardiopulmonary arrest, and, occasionally, metastatic tumor that interrupts the supranuclear pathway to the facial nerve

ii. Two EMG discharges characterize facial myokymia
   (A) Continuous type—rhythmic single or paired discharges of one or a few motor units recur at regular intervals of 100–200 milliseconds; tends to be more commonly associated with MS
   (B) Discontinuous type—bursts of single motor unit activity at 30–40 impulses per second last for 100–900 milliseconds and repeat regularly; more commonly associated with brain stem glioma
g. Treatment: carbamazepine

Q. **Miscellaneous**
   1. **Channels associated with neuromuscular disorders**

Disorder	Channel
Hypokalemic periodic paralysis	Calcium
Hyperkalemic periodic paralysis	Sodium
Paramyotonia congenita	Possible sodium
Myotonia congenita	Chloride
Malignant hyperthermia	Calcium
Central core disease	Calcium
Episodic ataxia and myokymia	Potassium
Barium-induced periodic paralysis	Barium blocks potassium channels

ADDITIONAL NOTES

CHAPTER 4

Epilepsy and Related Disorders

I. Miscellaneous

A. *Definitions*

1. *Seizure: reflects a sudden, sustained, and simultaneous discharge of very large numbers of neurons, either within a region of the brain or throughout the brain*

   a. *Partial:* focal cortical onset of epileptiform activity

      i. *Simple:* no definitive loss of awareness

      ii. *Complex:* loss of awareness at some level

   b. *Generalized:* diffuse cortical epileptiform activity

      i. *Primary:* immediate onset of diffuse cortical epileptiform activity

      ii. *Secondary:* spread of focal discharges throughout cortex

2. *Epilepsy: a tendency toward recurrent seizures unprovoked by systemic or neurologic insults*

B. *Incidence and prevalence*

1. Seizure: incidence: approximately 80/100,000 per year; *lifetime prevalence: 9% (one-third are benign febrile convulsions)*

2. Epilepsy

   a. Incidence: approximately 45/100,000 per year

   b. Point prevalence: 0.5–1.0% (2.5 million)

      i. ≤14 y/o: 13%

      ii. 15–64 y/o: 63%

      iii. ≥65 y/o: 24%

   c. Cumulative risk of epilepsy: 1.3–3.1%

C. **Impact of epilepsy in the United States**

1. Economic: the total cost to the nation for seizures and epilepsy is approximately $12.5 billion; direct costs: $1.7 billion (medical costs); indirect costs: $10.8 billion (productivity)

2. Psychosocial: self-esteem and behavior issues; depression and anxiety disorder; *sudden unexplained death in epilepsy (annual risk: 1/200–1/500;* cause unknown but suspected to be cardiopulmonary arrest)

D. **Experimental protocols to induce epilepsy in animal models**

1. Aluminum gel

2. Freezing

3. Penicillamine

4. Cobalt

5. Stimulation

6. Kainic acid

E. *Etiologies*

1. Metabolic

   a. Inborn erros: eg., gangliosidoses, glycogen storage diseases

   b. Acquired: hyponatremia, hypocalcemia, hypomagnesemia, hypophosphatemia, hypoglycemia or hyperglycemia, hyperthyroidism/thyrotoxicosis, uremia, hyperammonemia

   2. Toxic
      a. Alcohol toxicity or withdrawal
      b. Barbiturate toxicity or withdrawal
      c. Benzodiazepine toxicity or withdrawal
      d. Cocaine
      e. Phencyclidine
      f. Amphetamines
      g. Common medications that cause seizures
         i. Antidepressants (tricyclic antidepressants, bupropion)
        ii. Antipsychotics (chlorpromazine, thioridazine, trifluoperazine, perphenazine, haloperidol)
       iii. Analgesics (fentanyl, meperidine, pentazocine, propoxyphene, tramadol [Ultram®])
        iv. Local anesthetics (lidocaine, procaine)
         v. Sympathomimetics (terbutaline, ephedrine, phenylpropanolamine)
        vi. Antibiotics (penicillin, ampicillin, cephalosporins, metronidazole, isoniazid, pyrimethamine)
       vii. Antineoplastic agents (vincristine, chlorambucil, methotrexate, bischloroethylni-trosourea, cytosine arabinoside)
      viii. Bronchodilators (aminophylline, theophylline)
        ix. Immunosuppressants: cyclosporine, ornithine-ketoacid transaminase 3
         x. Others (insulin, antihistamines, atenolol, baclofen, cyclosporine)
   3. Neoplasm (metastasis, primary)
   4. Infection
      a. Meningitis
      b. Encephalitis
         i. Herpes simplex virus 1: most commonly causes temporal lobe seizures
        ii. Herpes simplex virus 2: infection acquired in birth canal
       iii. Human immunodeficiency virus
      c. Brain abscess
   5. Vascular: stroke (ischemia, hemorrhage), subarachnoid hemorrhage, arteriovenous malformation, cavernous malformation, venous sinus thrombosis, amyloid angiopathy
   6. Trauma: closed-head injury: subdural hematoma, contusion nonlesional; open-head injury
   7. Eclampsia
   8. Idiopathic: mesial-temporal sclerosis
   9. Congenital
  10. Perinatal insults
  11. Phakomatoses: tuberous sclerosis, Sturge-Weber syndrome
  12. Neuronal migration disorders
  13. Autoimmune: systemic lupus erythematosus; central nervous system (CNS) vasculitis
F. **Febrile seizures**
   1. *Uncommon before age 6 months and after age 6 years*
   2. *13% incidence of epilepsy if at least two factors*
      a. *Family history of nonfebrile seizures*
      b. *Abnormal neurologic examination or development*
      c. *Prolonged febrile seizure*
      d. *Focal febrile seizure with Todd's paralysis*

G. *Genetic basis for idiopathic epilepsies*

	Linkage
Benign familial neonatal convulsions	8q; 20q
Benign familial infantile convulsions	19q
Autosomal dominant nocturnal frontal lobe epilepsy (FLE)	20q
Partial epilepsy with auditory features	10q
Juvenile myoclonic epilepsy (JME)	6p
Generalized epilepsy with febrile seizures plus	19q; 2q
Febrile seizures	19p; 8q

H. **Differential diagnosis of seizures**
   1. Hypoglycemia
   2. Syncope
   3. Asterixis
   4. Tremor
   5. Cerebrovascular accident/transient ischemic attack
   6. Myoclonus
   7. Dystonia
   8. Narcolepsy
   9. Panic attack/anxiety
   10. Migraine
   11. Psychogenic seizures
   12. Malingering
   13. Breath-holding spells

NB: Breath-holding spells occur in up to 5% of infants, often triggered by frustration or sudden pain. Consciousness is lost prior to (occasional) brief clonic jerking

I. **Emergent evaluation of a patient with seizures**
   1. Airway, breathing, and circulation: protect airway by turning patient on side to reduce risk of aspiration
   2. Examination

Examination	Assess for focal deficits that may indicate a lesion (i.e., tumor, infections, stroke)
	Short-term memory deficits suggestive of temporal lobe epilepsy
	Frontal lobe executive dysfunction suggestive of FLE
History	History of seizures (type, duration, frequency)
	Intake of antiepileptic drugs (AEDs) and other medications that may cause seizures
	Family history of seizures
	History of head trauma with loss of consciousness >30 mins or penetrating head injury
	History of febrile seizures
	History of CNS infections
	History of substance abuse (especially ethyl alcohol [EtOH] and barbiturate; either intoxication or withdrawal)

3. Basic labs
   a. Electrolytes:↓Na^+, Ca^{2+}, Mg^{2+}
   b. ↑ or ↓ glucose
   c. Platelets (thrombotic thrombocytopenic purpura, disseminated intravascular coagulopathy)
   d. Toxicology screen (especially EtOH and barbiturate intoxication or withdrawal)
   e. AED levels
   f. Erythrocyte sedimentation rate (if vasculitis suspected)
   g. Infection: urinalysis, chest X-ray, ± Lumbar puncture (LP) (perform if recent fever, atypical mental status changes)
4. Diagnostic tests
   a. Radiographic: magnetic resonance imaging (MRI) > computed tomography (CT) (either should be acquired with or without contrast); evaluate for tumor, stroke, and/or infectious process; if patient stable, MRI preferred; if focal deficit, CT emergently followed by MRI
   b. LP: if there is any suggestion of fever, meningeal signs (nuchal rigidity), elderly, or behavioral signs → perform LP; once LP is performed, treat appropriately if any suggestion of infection clinically even before results are known; if LP cannot be performed and infection suspected, always treat patient and do not await availability of LP or results; may want to treat empirically with acyclovir, 10 mg/kg q8h, and third-generation cephalosporin
   c. Electroencephalography (EEG): obtain within 24–48 hours (increased epileptiform potentials are noted postictally within 24–48 hours); if persistent mental status changes, stat EEG to rule out nonconvulsive status epilepticus (SE)
5. *Treatment*
   a. Single seizure
      i. None (unless SE)
      ii. *Recurrence risk after a first unprovoked seizure*
         (A) *Year 1: 14%*
         (B) *Year 2: 29%*
         (C) *Year 3: 34%*
      iii. AEDs have no effect on risk or disease course
   b. Recurrent seizure or abnormality on evaluation
      i. Recommend, in most cases, to load with fosphenytoin, which provides rapid therapeutic effect (unless phenytoin [PHT] or rapid loading dose is contraindicated; may then convert patient to another AED of choice once patient is stabilized)
      ii. If recurrent self-limited seizures in emergency room, 1–2 mg of lorazepam (Ativan®) intravenously to max of 10 mg (or respiratory compromise significantly increases)
   c. If there is any history of EtOH abuse, administer thiamine, 100 mg intravenously, before glucose administration
   d. *If AED level is low, use volume of distribution to calculate bolus dose*

   Bolus dose (in mg) = V_d × (desired concentration – current concentration)

   V_d is in L/kg × body weight in kg

   Concentration is in mg/L

   V_d: *PHT = 0.6 L/kg*   *Phenobarbital (PB) = 0.6 L/kg*

                 Valproic acid (VA) = 0.1–0.3 L/kg   *Carbamazepine (CBZ) = 1–2 L/kg*

II. Classifications

A. *International classification of epileptic seizures*
1. *Partial*
    a. *Simple partial*
        i. With motor signs
        ii. With somatosensory or special sensory symptoms
        iii. With autonomic symptoms or signs
        iv. With psychic symptoms
    b. *Complex partial seizures (CPS)*
        i. Simple partial onset
        ii. With impairment of consciousness at onset
    c. *Partial seizures evolving to secondary generalized seizures*
        i. Simple partial seizures evolving to generalized seizures
        ii. CPS evolving to generalized seizures
        iii. Simple partial seizures evolving to CPS evolving to generalized seizures
2. *Generalized seizures*
    a. Absence seizures
        i. Typical absence
        ii. Atypical absence
    b. Myoclonic seizures
    c. Clonic seizures
    d. Tonic seizures
    e. Tonic-clonic seizures
    f. Atonic seizures
3. *Unclassified seizures*
B. *Revised international classification of epilepsies, epileptic syndromes, and related seizure disorder*
1. *Localization related*
    a. *Idiopathic (primary)*
        i. Benign childhood epilepsy with centrotemporal spikes
        ii. Childhood epilepsy with occipital paroxysm
        iii. Primary reading epilepsy
    b. *Symptomatic (secondary)*
        i. Temporal lobe epilepsies
        ii. Frontal lobe epilepsies
        iii. Parietal lobe epilepsies
        iv. Occipital lobe epilepsies
        v. Chronic progressive epilepsia partialis continua of childhood
        vi. Reflex epilepsies
    c. *Cryptogenic*
2. *Generalized*
    a. *Primary*
        i. Benign neonatal familial convulsions
        ii. Benign neonatal convulsions
        iii. Benign myoclonic epilepsy in infancy
        iv. Childhood absence epilepsy
        v. Juvenile absence epilepsy
        vi. JME
        vii. Epilepsy with generalized tonic-clonic (GTC) convulsions on awakening

      b. *Cryptogenic or symptomatic*
         i. West's syndrome
         ii. Lennox-Gastaut syndrome
         iii. Epilepsy with myoclonic astatic seizures
         iv. Epilepsy with myoclonic absences
      c. *Symptomatic*
         i. Nonspecific etiology
           (A) Early myoclonic encephalopathy
           (B) Early infantile epileptic encephalopathy with suppression burst
         ii. Specific syndromes
   3. *Epilepsies undetermined whether focal or generalized*
      a. With both focal and generalized seizures
         i. Neonatal seizures
         ii. Severe myoclonic epilepsy in infancy
         iii. Epilepsy with continuous spike waves during slow-wave sleep
         iv. Acquired epileptic aphasia (Landau-Kleffner syndrome)
      b. Special syndromes
      c. Situation-related seizure
      d. Febrile convulsions
      e. Isolated seizures or isolated SE
      f. Metabolic or toxic events
C. ***Primary generalized epilepsy***
   1. *Absence*
      a. *Typical*
         i. No aura or warning
         ii. Motionless with blank stare
         iii. Short duration (usually <10 seconds)
         iv. If seizure prolonged, eyelid fluttering or other automatisms may occur
         v. Little or no postictal confusion
         vi. 70% of cases can be precipitated by hyperventilation
         vii. EEG: 3-Hz spike and wave
      b. *Atypical*
         i. Similar to simple absence with motor activity or autonomic features
         ii. May have clonic, atonic, and tonic seizures
         iii. Longer duration
         iv. More irregular spike-wave with 2.5–4.5-Hz spike and wave, and polyspike discharges
   2. *Tonic*
   3. *Atonic*
      a. Typical in children with symptomatic or cryptogenic epilepsy syndromes, such as Lennox-Gastaut
      b. Duration: tonic mean, 10 seconds; atonic, usually 1–2 seconds
   4. *Tonic-clonic*
   5. *Myoclonic seizures*
      a. Brief, shock-like muscle contractions of head or extremities
      b. Usually bilaterally symmetric but may be focal, regional, or generalized
      c. Consciousness preserved unless progression into tonic-clonic seizure
      d. Precipitated by sleep transition and photic stimulation
      e. May be associated with a progressive neurologic deterioration

f. EEG: generalized polyspike-wave, spike-wave complexes

g. Subtypes of myoclonic epilepsy

    i. **NB: JME**

        (A) Onset is often *late adolescence (12–16 y/o) with myoclonic events followed by tonic-clonic seizures; within a few years, myoclonic events are more common in morning shortly after awakening*

        (B) *Genetically localized to chromosome 6p*

        (C) *Most common seizure induced by photic stimulation; also precipitated by alcohol intake and sleep deprivation*

        (D) May have severe seizures if missed AEDs

NB: Treatment of choice for JME is valproate (VPA), recurrence is likely if treatment is stopped.

    ii. *Progressive myoclonic epilepsy*

        (A) **Unverricht-Lundborg disease (Baltic myoclonus)**

            (1) Pathophysiology

                (a) *Mediterranean ancestry*

                (b) *Autosomal recessive (AR)*

                (c) *Genetic localization to chromosome 21q22.3, but may also occur sporadically*

                (d) Mutation is a dodecamer-repeat rather than a triplet-repeat disorder

                (e) Gene for cystatin B is the responsible gene

                (f) Two to 17 repeats is normal, but >30 repeats is positive for this disease

            (2) Clinical

                (a) *Relatively severe myoclonic-like events*

                (b) *Typically begin between 6 and 16 y/o*

                (c) *Progressive ataxia and dementia*

                (d) *EEG: diffuse background slowing in the θ frequency with a 3–5-Hz polyspike and wave discharge; may also have sporadic focal spike and wave discharges*

                (e) *Diagnosis is made by skin biopsy with a notation in sweat glands of vacuoles in one small series; pathology also demonstrates neuronal loss and gliosis of cerebellum, medial thalamus, and spinal cord*

                (f) Athena Diagnostics also has a lab test that is approximately 85% sensitive for genetic profile

        (B) **Lafora's body disease**

            (1) Pathophysiology: *AR; localized to chromosome 6q24*

            (2) Clinical

                (a) Significant myoclonus

                (b) Age of onset *is adolescence (10–18 y/o)*

                (c) *Tend not to have severe ataxia or myoclonus but do have relatively severe dementia*

                (d) Death by early- to mid-20s

                (e) *EEG demonstrates occipital spikes and seizures in approximately 50% of cases*

                (f) Abnormal somatosensory-evoked potentials

                (g) Diagnosis: *skin biopsy reveals Lafora bodies (polyglucosan neuronal inclusions in neurons and in cells of eccrine sweat gland ducts)*

                (h) Prognosis is poor

         (C) **Neuronal ceroid lipofuscinosis**

            Pathophysiology: *AR; defined by histology—by light microscope, neurons are engorged with periodic acid-Schiff–positive and autofluorescent material, and electron microscopy demonstrates that ceroid and lipofuscin are noted in abnormal cytosomes, such as curvilinear and fingerprint bodies that are diffusely distributed throughout the body* (although only have CNS manifestations)

(1) *Infantile (Santavuori's disease)*
   (a) *AR; association with genomic marker HY-TM1, located on short arm of chromosome 1*
   (b) Begins at approximately 8 months with progressive vision loss, loss of developmental milestones, severe myoclonic jerks, and microcephaly
   (c) Also have optic atrophy and macular degeneration with no response on electroretinogram

(2) *Late infantile (Bielschowsky-Jansky disease)*
   (a) Onset between ages 2 and 7 years
   (b) *AR; localized to chromosome 15q21-q23*
   (c) Progressive vision deterioration with abolished electroretinogram and retinal deterioration
   (d) Myoclonus, ataxia, and dementia are relatively severe, with rapid progression to vegetative state; death usually by 5–7 years

(3) *Juvenile (Spielmeyer-Vogt-Sjšgren disease)*
   (a) *AR*
   (b) *Localized to chromosome 16p12.1*
   (c) Most common neurodegenerative disorder of childhood
   (d) Storage material contains large amounts of adenosine triphosphate synthase subunit C protein
   (e) Variable onset usually between ages 4 and 12 years begins with progressive vision loss between ages 5 and 10 years due to pigmentary degeneration of the retina
   (f) Variable progression of myoclonus, ataxia, and dementia but death usually by 2nd decade
   (g) Diagnosis: skin biopsy reveals curvilinear inclusions noted

(4) *Adult (Kufs' disease)*
   (a) Onset typically between ages 11 and 34 years
   (b) *Autosomal dominant and recessive forms*
   (c) *More slowly progressive myoclonus, ataxia, and dementia but usually severe by 10 years after initial diagnosis*
   (d) No retinal degeneration and, therefore, no visual impairment
   (e) Diagnosis: *fingerprint profiles noted on skin biopsy*

(D) *Mitochondrial disorders*
   (1) **Myoclonic epilepsy with ragged red fibers**
      (a) *Point mutation of nucleotide pair 8344 (nt-8344 or nt-8356): both are found in mitochondrial deoxyribonucleic acid gene for transfer ribonucleic acid for lysine*
      (b) *Clinical:* age of onset: 3–65 years; essential features: myoclonic epilepsy, cerebellar dysfunction, myoclonus; other features: short stature, ataxia, dementia, lactic acidosis, weakness, and sensory deficits
      (c) MRI/CT: leukoencephalopathy and cerebellar atrophy
      (d) Diagnosis: muscle biopsy—ragged red fibers; genetic testing via Athena Diagnostics
   (2) **Leigh disease (subacute necrotizing encephalomyelopathy)**
      (a) Incidence: 1/40,000
      (b) *Inheritance: autosomal and X-linked recessive*

      (c) *Metabolic defect: pyruvate dehydrogenase complex, electron transport chain complexes*

      (d) Clinical pattern: usually appears in early infancy or childhood; characterized by a myriad of neurologic manifestations that may include lethargy or coma, swallowing and feeding difficulty, hypotonia, ataxia and intention tremor, involuntary movements, peripheral neuropathy, external ophthalmoplegia, ophthalmoplegia, optic atrophy and vision loss, impaired hearing, vascular-type headaches, and seizures

(E) **Sialidosis type 1**

    (1) *AR; chromosome 20*

    (2) *Decrease in α-neuraminidase; measured most reliably in cultured skin fibroblasts*

    (3) Pathology: *diffuse cortical atrophy with neuronal storage as well as vacuolar inclusions in liver*

    (4) Onset in adolescence

    (5) Severe myoclonus, visual impairment with disproportionate night blindness or loss of color vision, ataxia, cherry-red spots; death within 2–30 years

    (6) Myoclonus is generalized and may be stimulus-sensitive or increased by stress, excitement, smoking, or menses; GTC seizures are noted with disease progression; EEG shows progressive slowing of background activity and appearance of bilateral, fast-spike and wave activity, which is photosensitive

(F) **Schindler disease**

    (1) Incidence: very rare, with <10 described; *AR*

    (2) *Pathology: axonal spheroids are present in axons of cerebral cortex and myenteric plexus; α-β-Acetylgalactosaminidase deficiency*

    (3) Clinical

      (a) Acute form: onset in infancy, severe psychomotor deterioration; chronic form: adult onset, mild cognitive impairment

      (b) Psychomotor deterioration rapid, leading to marked spasticity, cortical blindness, and myoclonic epilepsy; exaggerated startle response noted at onset

(G) **Biotinidase deficiency disease**

    (1) Usually appearing in infancy *between 3 and 6 months of age*

    (2) Features include *hypotonia, GTC and myoclonic seizures, skin rash (seborrheic or atopic dermatitis), and alopecia*

    (3) *EEG shows multifocal spikes and slow waves*

    (4) *Treatment: oral biotin (5–20 mg/day); skin and neurologic features improve, whereas hearing and vision problems are more resistant*

(H) **GM$_2$ gangliosidosis**

	Type I Tay-Sachs	Type II Sandhoff
Inheritance	AR	AR
Onset	4–12 mos	4–12 mos
Enzyme defect	Hexosaminidase A	Hexosaminidase A and B
Clinical	Developmental delay, cherry-red spot maculae; startle seizures	Developmental delay, cherry-red spot maculae; startle seizures

(I) **Treatment of myoclonic epilepsies**
    (1) Clonazepam: may also improve ataxia
    (2) VPA
    (3) Topiramate
    (4) Zonisamide: anecdotal reports reveal zonisamide may slow the deterioration of progressive myoclonic epilepsies

(J) **Differential diagnosis of myoclonus**
    (1) Hypneic jerks
    (2) Exercise-induced (benign)
    (3) Benign infantile myoclonus
    (4) Photosensitive myoclonus
    (5) Infantile spasms
    (6) Lennox-Gastaut syndrome
    (7) Aicardi's infantile myoclonic epilepsy
    (8) JME
    (9) Progressive myoclonic epilepsy
    (10) Friedreich's ataxia
    (11) Ataxia telangiectasia
    (12) Wilson's disease
    (13) Hallervorden-Spatz disease
    (14) Huntington's disease
    (15) Mitochondrial encephalopathies
    (16) Sialidosis
    (17) Lipidoses
    (18) Alzheimer's disease
    (19) Multiple system atrophy
    (20) Progressive supranuclear palsy
    (21) Drugs: selective serotonin reuptake inhibitors, tricyclic antidepressants, lithium, levodopa, VA, CBZ, PHT
    (22) Metabolic: hepatic failure, renal failure, hypoglycemia, hyponatremia, dialysis, nonketotic hyperglycemia
    (23) Toxins: bismuth, heavy metals, methyl bromide, dichlorodiphenyl-trichloroethane
    (24) Posthypoxic
    (25) Post-traumatic
    (26) Electric shock
    (27) Focal CNS lesions affecting the cortex, thalamus, brain stem (palatal myoclonus), or spinal cord (segmental or spinal myoclonus)
    (28) Infectious: viral, subacute sclerosing panencephalitis, Creutzfeldt-Jakob disease, postinfections
    (29) Psychogenic

6. **West's syndrome**
    a. Onset: *age 3 months to 3 years*
    b. Prenatal causes are most common, including tuberous sclerosis (most common) and chromosomal abnormalities
    c. Truncal flexion, mental retardation, myoclonus
    d. *EEG: hypsarrhythmia*
    e. *Treatment: adrenocorticotropic hormone*

7. **Aicardi's syndrome**
    a. *X-linked dominant*

b. Onset at birth with infantile spasms, hemiconvulsions, coloboma, chorioretinal lacunae, agenesis of corpus callosum, and vertebral anomalies

c. *EEG: bursts of synchronous slow waves, spike waves, and sharp waves alternating with burst suppression*

d. *Treatment: adrenocorticotropic hormone*

8. **Lennox-Gastaut syndrome**

   a. Onset: *age 1–10 years*

   b. *Multiple seizure types, particularly atonic seizures, developmental delay*

   c. *EEG: slow spike-wave complex at 1.0–2.5 Hz (usually approximately 2 Hz), multifocal spikes and sharp waves, generalized paroxysmal fast activity*

   d. *Treatment: lamotrigine, VPA, vagal nerve stimulation*

D. *Partial seizures*

1. Simple partial seizures: no loss of awareness

2. CPS

   a. Impaired consciousness/level of awareness (staring)

   b. Clinical manifestations vary with origin and degree of spread

   c. Presence and nature of aura

   d. Automatisms (manual, oral)

   e. Dystonic motor activity

   f. Duration (typically 30 seconds to 3 minutes)

   g. Amnesia for event

3. Localization of partial seizures

   a. *Temporal* (Figure 4-1)

      i. *Approximately 70% of partial seizures*

      ii. Aura of déjà vu, epigastric sensation (rising), fear/anxiety, or olfactory sensation

      iii. Stare and nonresponsive

      iv. Oral and manual automatisms

      v. Usually 60–90 seconds

      vi. Contralateral, early dystonic upper extremity posturing has lateralizing value

      vii. Postictal language disturbance when seizures originate in dominant hemisphere

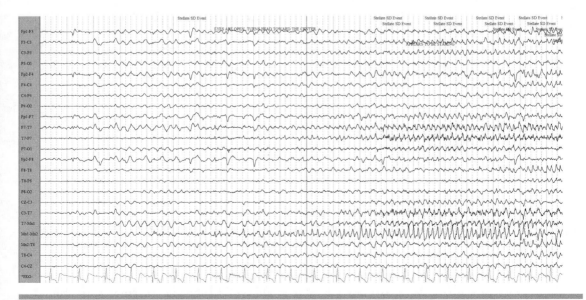

Figure 4-1. Temporal lobe complex partial seizure.

    b. *Frontal*
       i. *Approximately 20% of partial seizures*
      ii. Unilateral or bilateral (asymmetric) tonic posturing (bicycling and fencing posture)
     iii. Short duration (20–30 seconds) with minimal postictal confusion
     iv. Awareness and memory may be retained unless temporal spread present
      v. Localization: usually posterior-mesial-frontal gyrus/supplementary motor area (SMA).
     vi. Dorsolateral and orbitofrontal partial seizures may appear more similar to temporal lobe seizures with staring, nonresponsiveness, and automatisms
    vii. Posterior frontal may have focal clonic movements but no loss of awareness (consistent with simple partial seizures); SMA seizures are typically very brief (1–20 seconds) with dystonic posturing, fencing posture, or bicycling movements
       (A) Diagnostic features *of SMA seizures*
         (1) *Short duration <30 seconds)*
         (2) *Stereotypical events*
         (3) *Tendency to occur predominantly during sleep*
         (4) *Tonic contraction of arms in adduction*
         (5) *Note: scalp recordings of SMA seizures are frequently unremarkable*
    viii. Prominent nocturnal pattern—often 5–10 or more seizures in one night
    c. *Parietal and occipital*
       i. Approximately 10% of partial seizures
      ii. Parietal: aura consists of sensory manifestations
       (A) Anterior parietal: somatosensory sensation
       (B) Inferior posterior temporal parietal: formed hallucinations
     iii. Occipital: aura: nonspecific bright or colored objects
     iv. Spread often to ipsilateral > contralateral temporal lobes with resultant loss of awareness
  4. *Secondary generalized seizures*
    a. Assumed or observed to begin as simple and/or CPS
    b. Variable symmetry, intensity, and duration of tonic (stiffening) and clonic (jerking) phases
    c. Usual duration: 30–120 seconds; tonic phase: 15–60 seconds; clonic phase: 60–120 seconds
    d. If seizure duration >5 minutes, risk for continued development into SE is 40–70%
    e. Postictal confusion, somnolence, with or without transient focal deficit (Todd's paralysis)
E. *Psychogenic nonepileptic paroxysmal events*
  1. Represent genuine psychiatric disease
  2. 10–45% of refractory epilepsy at tertiary referral centers
  3. Females > males
  4. Psychiatric mechanism
    a. Dissociation
    b. Conversion
    c. Unconscious (unlike malingering)
  5. Association with physical, verbal, or sexual abuse in approximately 50–60% of cases
  6. Epileptic seizures and nonepileptic seizures may coexist in 10–20% of patients with pseudoseizures
  7. Video-EEG monitoring required to clarify the diagnosis
  8. Once recognized, approximately 50% respond well to specific psychiatric treatment

F. *Other:* *Hereditary hyperekplexia: linked to long arm of chromosome 5; point mutation of gene encoding the α-1 subunit of the glycine receptor*

III. Pediatric and Neonatal Seizures

A. *Neonatal seizures*
 1. Etiology
  a. Hypoxic-ischemic encephalopathy (50–60%); usually occur within first 24–48 hours
  b. Intracranial hemorrhage (10%)
   i. Subarachnoid hemorrhage: healthy baby; seizures after 24–48 hours
   ii. Subdural hemorrhage: focal seizures; within first 24–48 hours of birth
   iii. Germinal matrix hemorrhage: premature infants, particularly <27 weeks gestational age; seizures begin after 48–72 hours
  c. Metabolic: hypoglycemia; hypocalcemia; hypomagnesemia
  d. Infection (meningitis, encephalitis)
  e. Toxic (drug withdrawal of intoxication)
  f. Developmental

B. *Pediatric seizures*
 1. Etiology
  a. Idiopathic or genetic: 76%
  b. Development-related epilepsy: 13%
  c. Infection: 5%
  d. Head trauma: 3%
  e. Other causes: 2%
 2. **NB: Benign rolandic epilepsy**
  a. Onset between ages 18 months and 13 years; typically spontaneously ends by age 16 years
  b. *40% have family history of epilepsy or febrile seizures*
  c. Accounts for 10% of all childhood epilepsies
  d. Clinical: nocturnal seizures with somatosensory onset involving the tongue, lips, and gums followed by unilateral jerking that involves the face, tongue, pharynx, and larynx, causing speech arrest and drooling; no loss of awareness unless evolves into a secondary GTC seizure
  e. EEG: *centrotemporal spikes*
  f. Treatment: AEDs are typically unnecessary owing to isolated occurrence of seizures and overall cognitive effects of AEDs but may be necessary if recurrent GTC seizures; *CBZ is the treatment of choice, if necessary*

C. **Rasmussen's encephalitis**
 1. Rare, progressive neurologic disorder, characterized by frequent and severe seizures, loss of motor skills and speech, hemiparesis (paralysis on one side of the body), encephalitis (inflammation of the brain), dementia, and mental deterioration
 2. Affects a single brain hemisphere; generally occurs in children <10 y/o
 3. Treatment
  a. AEDs usually not effective in controlling the seizures
  b. When seizures have not spontaneously remitted by the time hemiplegia and aphasia are complete, *the standard treatment for Rasmussen's encephalitis is hemispherectomy*
  c. Alternative treatments may include plasmapheresis, intravenous (i.v.) immunoglobulin, ketogenic diet, and steroids

D. **Treatment of pediatric epilepsy**
 1. Greater degree of pharmacokinetic variability and unpredictability in pediatric patients.

2. Average clearance of antiepileptic medications during childhood is 2–4× adult; adult levels are reached between ages 10 and 15 years.
3. *PB in children may cause paradoxical excitation and agitation.*
4. *Levetiracetam has a significantly higher risk for hallucinations in children.*
5. *VPA has a markedly increased risk of hepatotoxicity in children <5 y/o, particularly on multiple AEDs.*
6. *Ketogenic diet*
   a. Predominantly used in children between age 2 years and adolescence.
   b. Purpose of the diet is to establish and maintain ketosis and acidosis along with partial dehydration.
   c. Often initiated in the hospital with starvation until ketosis occurs and then food is introduced.
   d. *Efficacy greatest for atonic, myoclonic, and atypical absence seizures; other seizure types (infantile spasms, tonic-clonic, secondarily GTC) and syndromes (Lennox-Gastaut syndrome) also respond.*
   e. Adverse effects
      i. During initiation, dehydration with metabolic acidosis may develop, requiring intervention
      ii. Renal stones (5–8%)
      iii. Long-term impact of hypercholesterolemia is unknown
      iv. Cardiac abnormalities and death (rare)

IV. Women and Epilepsy
A. **NB:** *AEDs that reduce oral contraceptive (OC) levels:* CBZ, PHT, PB, topiramate (doses >200 mg/day), oxcarbazepine, and lomotrigine; however, levetiracetam, gabapentin, tiagabine, vigabatrin, zonisamide, and topiramate have no effect on OC concentration.
B. 0.4% of pregnancies involve epileptic women.
C. Birth rates are reduced 30–60% by psychosocial and endocrine factors; optimizing management must be done preconceptually.
D. The percentage of women with epilepsy with children is lower than the average for the general population.

NB: Valproic acid and CBZ (and epilepsy itself) have been associated with an increased frequency of polycystic ovary syndrome.

1. Psychosocial factors
2. Difficulties with conception
3. Higher risk for spontaneous miscarriage
4. Birth defects
E. Risk for congenital malformations is 2–3× normal risk; but continuing AEDs during pregnancy is recommended as the risk of seizures off medication is higher.
   1. Valproate: higher incidence of congenital malformation (6–17%) compared with other AEDs (3–6%); third trimester exposure may result in lower IQ
   2. Carbamazepine: 5% rate of major malformations
   3. Lamotrigine: has most data among newer AEDs; 3% rate of malformation; 25-fold higher rate of cleft palate
   4. Levetiracetam: 2–4% rate of malformation
F. Seizure frequency may increase during pregnancy.
G. *Advise patient about risks and strategies to minimize risk factors.*
   1. *Appropriate anticonvulsant drug therapy*
   2. *Monotherapy*

3. *Lowest acceptable dose*
4. *Follow anticonvulsant levels every 4–6 weeks*
5. *Initiate folic acid, 4 mg/day, preconceptually*

H. *Breast-feeding is not contraindicated, with the exception of sedation to the infant.*

V. Treatment

A. *AEDs*

   1. **PHT (Dilantin®)**

Pharmacokinetics	
Mechanism	Sodium channel blocker
Range of daily maintenance dose	5–15 mg/kg/day
Minimum dose	Adult: once daily
	Child: bid
Time to peak serum concentration	4–12 hrs (oral)
Percent protein bound	90
Volume of distribution	0.45 L/kg
Half-life	9–140 hrs (average, 22 hrs); saturation kinetics
Time to steady state (SS)	7–21 days
Metabolism	Hepatic
Serum levels	10–20 µg/mL
Major metabolites	5-(p-hydroxy phenyl)-5-phenylhydantoin (inactive)
Absorption	Acid form poorly soluble in water but sodium salt is more so; do not give intramuscularly, owing to crystallization of drug and possibility of necrosis (Purple Glove syndrome); use fosphenytoin if i.v. access is questionable
Metabolism	Metabolized extensively by hepatic hydroxylase enzymes; <5% excreted unchanged in the urine; African descent may metabolize PHT slower; zero-order kinetics—the liver cannot increase rate of metabolism of PHT, and, therefore, only a fixed amount of drug can be removed regardless of the serum concentration
Half-life	Effective terminal half-life gradually increased as steady-state concentration rises as a result of the saturable nature of metabolism (zero-order kinetics)
Drug interaction	Effect of PHT on other drugs
	Potent inducer of hepatic enzymes: decrease coumadin, OCs, CBZ, benzodiazepine, other drugs
	Effect of other drugs on PHT
	Inhibition of PHT metabolism: increase PHT: VA
	Induction of PHT metabolism: decrease PHT: CBZ/chronic EtOH

Pharmacokinetics

	VA: results in increased free PHT but decreased total PHT
Adverse effects	Dose-dependent
	Neurologic: ataxia, nystagmus, diplopia, vertigo, tremor, dysarthria, headache, dyskinesias, peripheral neuropathy
	Hepatic: toxicity rare and usually within first 6 wks and accompanied by rash, fever, and lymphadenopathy and eosinophilia, suggestive of a hypersensitivity reaction
	Endocrine: accelerate cortisol metabolism; decrease free thyroid hormones and increase conversion of T_4 to T_3; long-term treatment may cause hypocalcemia and affect vitamin D metabolism, resulting in osteoporosis
	Hematologic: megaloblastic anemia, aplastic anemia, leukopenia, and lymphadenopathy
	Pregnancy: must give mother vitamin K at end of pregnancy and infant vitamin K at birth owing to increased risk of hemorrhage
	Dental: gingival hyperplasia
	Skin: hirsutism
	Teratogenicity: 2–3× normal level; cleft lip and palate; congenital heart defect; fetal hydantoin syndrome has been disputed; genetic defect in arene oxide detoxification may increase susceptibility to PHT birth defects
Pathophysiology	Reduces post-tetanic potentiation
Indications	CPS
	GTC
	Ineffective in absence seizure

2. **Sodium VPA (Depakote®)**

Pharmacokinetics

Mechanism	Sodium channel blocker
Range of daily maintenance dose	Adult: 20–40 mg/kg/day
	Child: 10–40 mg/kg/day
Serum concentration	50–150 µg/mL
Time to peak serum level	1–4 hrs (plain tabs)
	2–8 hrs (enteric coated)
Oral absorption	>95%

Pharmacokinetics

Percent bound to plasma protein	Approximately 90
Volume of distribution	0.1–0.4 L/kg
Elimination half-life	9–21 hrs
Time to SS after initiation	4 days
Major metabolites	w, w-1 oxidation products
Dose frequency	Depakote®: once daily to three times daily (tid)
	Depakote ER®: once daily
Distribution	Binding is reduced by free fatty acids, liver disease, hypoalbuminemia, and renal disease
Metabolism	Almost completely metabolized (97–99%) before excretion
	Major elimination path via conjugation with glucuronic acid (20–70%), with remainder via oxidative paths
	2-en metabolite of VA has antiepileptic activity, approximately 10% with parent compound having approximately 90% therapeutic effect
Half-life	Between 2 and 21 hrs with mean 12–13 hrs but may be shortened by other AEDs that induce oxidation of VA
	Half-life in neonate between 20 and 66 hrs but falls rapidly in first few months of life
Drug interaction	Effect of VA on other AEDs
	PB: VA increases PB levels (possibly owing to inhibition of metabolism of PB)
	PHT: VA displaces PHT from plasma protein and inhibits PHT metabolism; results in either increased free PHT or unchanged total levels
	Effect of other AEDs on VA
	PHT, CBZ, or PB decrease VA serum concentration owing to enzyme induction
	Salicylates possibly displace VA from plasma protein
Adverse effects	Gastrointestinal: anorexia, nausea/vomiting, dyspepsia, diarrhea, constipation
	Weight gain
	Skin: rash (rare)
	Reversible hair loss
	Hematologic: thrombocytopenia and bruising; reports of abnormal platelet function
	Neurologic: tremor (benign essential tremor and reversible)

Pharmacokinetics

	Hepatotoxicity: severe with occasional fatal outcome as idiosyncratic reaction that usually occurs within first 6 mos of treatment and most often in kids—1/50,000 risk overall (Black Box Warning)
	Hyperammonemia: rare; may cause encephalopathy
	Teratogenicity: spina bifida in approximately 1% of infants of mothers on VA due to depletion of folate; therefore, supplement with folic acid

NB: Polycystic ovary syndrome and fatal hemorrhagic pancreatitis may also occur with VA.

Indications	Absence seizures (up to 100% efficacy)
	Photosensitive epilepsy: drug of choice
	GTC
	Myoclonic epilepsy
	CPS (less effective for GTC but probably as efficacious as PHT/CBZ)
	Migraine headache (U.S. Food and Drug Administration [FDA] approved)
Other	Passes through placenta and via breast milk (0.17–5.40% of maternal concentration)

3. **CBZ (Tegretol®/Tegretol XR®/Carbatrol®)**

Pharmacokinetics

Mechanism	Sodium channel blocker
Range of daily maintenance	Adult: 15–40 mg/kg/day
	Child: 10–30 mg/kg/day
Serum concentration	4–12 µg/mL
Peak serum level	4–8 hrs
Percent protein bound	CBZ: 75
	Epoxide metabolite: 50
Volume of distribution	1.2 L/kg
Half-life	Single dose: 20–55 hrs
	Chronic
	Adult 10–30 hrs
	Child: 8–20 hrs
Time to SS after initiation	Up to 10 days (may increase with autoinduction)
Metabolism	Hepatic

Pharmacokinetics

Major metabolite	10,11-epoxide
Dose frequency	
Generic CBZ/standard Tegretol®	tid
Tegretol XR® and Carbatrol®	bid
Absorption	Slow and erratic; enhanced by taking with food
Bioavailability	75–85%
Distribution/binding	Highly lipid soluble; binding not influenced by other AEDs; brain concentration similar to serum
Metabolism	Mainly metabolized to 10,11-epoxide; 3–4 wks for maximal autoinduction of hepatic microsomal enzymes
Special situations	Transplacental transfer causes induction of fetal enzymes
Drug interaction	Effect of CBZ on other drugs
	Induce metabolism of other drugs, including VA, ethosuximide, PHT, clonazepam, OCs, coumadin
	Effect of other drugs on CBZ
	PHT/PB/myasthenia syndrome: decrease CBZ levels (but may increase epoxide levels)
	Enzyme-inhibiting drugs (cimetidine, propoxyphene, verapamil): increase CBZ levels
Adverse effects	Neurologic: nystagmus with blurred vision, dizziness, and diplopia and/or ataxia
	Hematologic: rare; bone marrow suppression with leukopenia, anemia, and/or thrombocytopenia; more rarely proliferative effects, such as eosinophilia and leukocytosis; incidence of aplastic anemia is 0.5/100,000/yr; 10% of patients have transient leukopenia usually within 1st mo
	Gastrointestinal: anorexia, nausea, and vomiting
	Hepatic toxicity: very rare
	Skin: rash in 3–5%; alopecia rarely occurs
	Endocrine: hyponatremia and decreased plasma osmolality; induces hepatic enzymes, resulting in increased risk of OC failure
	Teratogenicity: increased risk for spina bifida
Pathophysiology	CBZ suppresses seizures by limiting sustained repetitive firing of neurons
Indications	CPS
	GTC

4. Phenobarbital

Pharmacokinetics

Mechanism	γ-Aminobutyric acid-receptor agonist
Maintenance	Adult: 2–6 mg/kg/day
	Child: 3–8 mg/kg/day
Minimum dose frequency	Once daily
Time to peak serum level	1–6 hrs
Percent protein bound	45
Volume of distribution	0.5 L/kg
Half-life	Adult: 50–160 hrs
	Child: 30–70 hrs
Time to SS	Up to 30 days
Metabolism	Hepatic
Major metabolite	Para-hydroxy phenobarbitone
Therapeutic serum level	10–40 µg/mL
Distribution	Absorption rapid, but penetration of the brain is slow; PB sensitive to changes in the plasma pH because it has a pKa (7.3) close to physiologic pH; acidosis causes a shift of PB from plasma to tissues, and alkalosis results in higher plasma concentrations
Protein binding	45% bound (less susceptible to changes in plasma proteins)
Metabolism	11–55% excreted unchanged and remainder hydroxylated in the para position to para-hydroxy phenobarbitone; child metabolizes PB faster than adult and requires higher doses
Drug interactions	Potent inducer of hepatic mixed function oxidase enzymes but is also highly unpredictable in regard to the magnitude; VPA reduces PB metabolism: increases PB levels
Adverse effects	Neuropsychiatric (decreased cognition/sedation/paradoxical effect in children; may cause insomnia and hyperactivity in elderly); dependence occurs with withdrawal symptoms
	Hematologic: megaloblastic anemia and macrocytosis
	Endocrine: vitamin K–dependent coagulopathy; osteomalacia
Indications	CPS
	GTC

5. Primidone (Mysoline®)

Pharmacokinetics

Mechanism	γ-Aminobutyric acid-receptor agonist
Daily maintenance	Adult: 250–1,500 mg/day
	Child: 15–30 mg/kg/day
Minimum dose frequency	bid
Time to peak serum level	2–5 hrs
Percent protein bound	<20
Metabolism	Hepatic
Volume of distribution	0.6 L/kg
Major active metabolites	PB and phenylethylmalonamide
Elimination half-life	Primidone: 4–12 hrs
	Derived PB: 50–160 hrs
	Phenylethylmalonamide: 29–36 hrs
Time to SS after initiation	Up to 30 days for derived PB
Indications	CPS
	GTC

6. Ethosuximide (Zarontin®)

Pharmacokinetics

Mechanism	T-type calcium channel blocker
Daily maintenance	Adult: 500–1,500 mg/day
	Child: 10–15 mg/kg/day
Minimum dose frequency	Once daily
Time to peak concentration	1–4 hrs (faster with liquid)
Percent protein bound	Negligible
Volume of distribution	0.7 L/kg
Major metabolites (inactive)	Methyl succinimide derivatives
Half-life	Adult: 40–70 hrs
	Child: 20–40 hrs
Time to SS after initiation	Adult: up to 14 days
	Child: up to 7 days
Distribution	Rapidly crosses placenta, and 94% of serum level crosses into breast milk
Metabolism	Excreted as glucuronidase, with only 10–20% excreted unchanged
Indications	Typical absence seizures only

7. Oxcarbazepine (Trileptal®)

Pharmacokinetics

Daily maintenance	600–2,400 mg/day
Minimum dose frequency	bid
Time to peak concentration	3–8 hrs
Percent protein bound	50
Half-life	10–13 hrs
Time to SS after initiation	3 days
Major metabolites	Advantage is that it does not metabolize to the epoxide metabolite, which subsequently reduces side effects
Adverse effects	Side effects are milder than for CBZ and no definitive levels to follow, but may cause significant hyponatremia (free water restriction and increased use of salt may be helpful; worsened by sodium depleters, e.g., diuretics, selective serotonin reuptake inhibitors, etc.)
Drug interactions	OCs only
Indications	CPS
	GTC seizures

8. Lamotrigine (Lamictal®)

Pharmacokinetics

Mechanism	Voltage-gated sodium channel blocker
Daily maintenance	50–400 mg/day
Dose frequency	bid to tid
Time to peak concentration	2–3 hrs
Serum levels	2–12 µg/mL
Percent protein bound	55
Volume of distribution	1.1 L/kg
Half-life	Monotherapy: 10–13 hrs
	Concurrent with inducer: 8–33 hrs
	Concurrent with VPA: 30–90 hrs
Time to SS after initiation	3–15 days
Major metabolites	Glucuronide (inactive)
Adverse effects	If rash develops, must stop (Black Box Warning) because cannot tell if rash will be minor or evolve into Stevens-Johnson syndrome or toxic epidermal necrolysis; may also rarely have systemic organ failure
Indications	CPS

Pharmacokinetics

	Lennox-Gastaut
	Primary generalized (moderately effective but may worsen myoclonic seizures)

9. Gabapentin (Neurontin®)

Pharmacokinetics

Mechanism	Unknown
Daily maintenance	600–4,800 mg/day
Minimum dose frequency	tid to qid
Time to peak concentration	2–3 hrs
Percent protein bound	0
Volume of distribution	0.7 L/kg
Metabolism	Renal excretion
Half-life	5–7 hrs
Time to SS after initiation	2 days
Major metabolites	None
Dosing	Gastrointestinal absorption markedly reduced at single doses >1,200 mg
Drug interactions	None
Indications	CPS
	Neuropathic pain (FDA approved)

10. Zonisamide (Zonegran®)

Pharmacokinetics

Daily maintenance	100–400 mg/day (adults)
Minimum dose frequency	bid or once daily
Time to peak concentration	2.5–6.0 hrs
Percent protein bound	40–50
Half-life	50–70 hrs
Time to SS after initiation	5–12 days
Major metabolites	Many (probably inactive)
Adverse effects	Kidney stones (1.5% annual risk; increase fluid intake)
Metabolism	>90% hepatic (CYP3A4)
Indications	CPS
	GTC
	Progressive myoclonic epilepsy (anecdotal reports of slowing progression)

11. **Levetiracetam (Keppra®)**

Pharmacokinetics

Mechanism	Unknown
Daily maintenance	1,000–3,000 mg/day
Minimum dose frequency	bid
Percent protein bound	<10
Half-life	6–8 hrs (effective concentration longer in brain)
Metabolism	65% is renally excreted unchanged, 10% is metabolized by P450 system, and 25% is hydrolyzed by undetermined liver mechanisms
Drug interactions	None
Indications	CPS
	GTC
Adverse effects	Hallucinations in kids
	Moodiness and irritability in children and adults

12. **Topiramate (Topamax®)**

Pharmacokinetics

Mechanism	Unknown; possible sodium channel blocker
Daily maintenance	100–200 mg/day
Minimum dose frequency	bid
Percent protein bound	15
Half-life	18–23 hrs
Metabolism	55–65% renal excretion
Drug interactions	None at low dose; OCs at >200 mg/day
Indications	CPC
	GTC
	Primary generalized seizures except absence seizure
Adverse effects	Kidney stones (1.5% annual risk); paresthesias; naming and other cognitive dysfunction; elevated bicarbonate (likely clinically insignificant); *weight loss;*
	NB: can cause hypohydrosis and hyperthermia, esp. in children who exercise in hot weather

American Academy of Neurology Guidelines for Use of AEDs for Newly Diagnosed Epilepsy

AED	Newly diagnosed monotherapy partial/mixed	Newly diagnosed absence
Gabapentin	Yes[a]	No
Lamotrigine	Yes[a]	Yes[a]
Topiramate	Yes[a]	No
Tiagabine	No	No
Oxcarbazepine	Yes	No
Levetiracetam	No	No
Zonisamide	No	No

[a]Not FDA approved for this indication.

American Academy of Neurology Guidelines for Use of AEDs for Refractory Epilepsy

AED	Partial adjunctive-adult	Partial monotherapy	Primary generalized	Symptomatic generalized	Pediatric partial
Gabapentin	Yes	No	No	No	Yes
Lamotrigine	Yes	Yes	Yes[a] (only absence)	Yes	Yes
Levetiracetam	Yes	No	No	No	No
Oxcarbazepine	Yes	Yes	No	No	Yes
Tiagabine	Yes	No	No	No	No
Topiramate	Yes	Yes[a]	Yes	Yes	Yes
Zonisamide	Yes	No	No	No	No

[a]Not FDA approved for this indication.

Adjunctive Use of AEDs for Comorbid Conditions

Mood stabilization	Headache	Neuropathic pain	Obesity	PLMS	Tremor	Insomnia
Oxcarbazepine	Topiramate[a]	Gabapentin[a]	Topiramate	Clonazepam	PB	Tiagabine
VPA	VPA[a]	Oxcarbazepine	Zonisamide	Gabapentin	Primidone	
Lamotrigine	Zonisamide	CBZ		Topiramate	Clonazepam	
Topiramate	Oxcarbazepine	Topiramate		Zonisamide	Levetiracetam	
CBZ					Topiramate	

PLMS, periodic limb movements of sleep.
[a]FDA approved for this indication.

Summary of Serious and Nonserious Adverse Events of the Newer AEDs

AED	Serious adverse events	Nonserious adverse events
Gabapentin	None	Weight gain, peripheral edema, behavioral changes
Lamotrigine	Rash, including Stevens-Johnson and toxic epidermal necrolysis (increased risk for children, also more common with concomitant VPA use and reduced with slow titration); hypersensitivity reactions, including risk of hepatic and renal failure, diffuse intravascular coagulation, and arthritis	Tics and insomnia
Levetiracetam	None	Irritability/behavior change
Oxcarbazepine	Hyponatremia (more common in elderly), rash	None
Tiagabine	Stupor or spike-wave stupor	Weakness
Topiramate	Nephrolithiasis, open-angle glaucoma, hypohidrosis (predominantly children)	Metabolic acidosis, weight loss, language dysfunction
Zonisamide	Rash, renal calculi, hypohidrosis (predominantly children)	Irritability, photosensitivity, weight loss

Major Drug-Drug Interactions of the Anticonvulsants

Medication	Anticonvulsant	Resultant serum effect
Analgesics		
Aspirin	PHT	Transient increase of PHT level
	VPA	Transient increase in VPA level
Propoxyphene	CBZ	Increased CBZ level
Antibiotics		
Erythromycin	CBZ	Increased CBZ level
Sulfa drugs	PHT	Increased PHT level
Isoniazid	CBZ	Increased CBZ level
Gastrointestinal		
Cimetidine	CBZ, PHT	Increased PHT > CBZ level
Antacids	PHT, VPA	Unpredictable effects
Bronchial agents		
Theophylline	CBZ, PHT	Decreased theophylline level
Cardiovascular		
Digoxin	PHT	Decreased digoxin level
Diltiazem	CBZ	Increased CBZ level

Medication	Anticonvulsant	Resultant serum effect
Verapamil	CBZ	Increased CBZ level
Warfarin	CBZ	Decreased effect of warfarin
	PHT	Increased effect of warfarin
Immunosuppressants		
Cyclosporine	PHT, CBZ	Decreased cyclosporine level
	VPA	No significant effect on cyclosporine level
Contraceptives	PHT, CBZ	Decreased contraceptive level
Psychotropics		
Chlorpromazine	PHT, VPA	Increased PHT and VPA level
Haloperidol	CBZ, PHT	Decreased haloperidol level
	VPA	No effect
Imipramine	PHT	Increased PHT levels
Anticonvulsants		
PHT	CBZ	Decreased CBZ level
	VPA	Decreased PHT level
CBZ	PHT	Decreased PHT level
	VPA	Decreased VPA level
VA	PHT	Decreased PHT level
	CBZ	Increased CBZ level
Gabapentin	PHT, CBZ, VPA	No effect
Lamotrigine	VPA	Increased lamotrigine level
	PHT, CBZ	Decreased lamotrigine level
Tiagabine	PHT, CBZ, PB	Decreased tiagabine level

B. **Epilepsy surgery**
   1. Types
      a. Proven efficacy
         i. Resective
         ii. Multiple subpial transection
         iii. Vagal nerve stimulator
      b. Experimental
         i. Deep brain (thalamic) stimulator
         ii. Stereotactic radiosurgery
C. **Other treatments of refractory epilepsy**
   1. Ketogenic diet (see sec. III.D.6)

VI. Status epilepticus (SE)
   A. **Clinical**
      1. Definition: continuous seizure activity or recurrent seizures without regaining awareness that persist for >20 minutes.

2. Most generalized seizures are self-limited to 2–3 minutes. If seizure activity extends beyond 4–5 minutes, begin treatment for status, because a majority of these patients, if left untreated, will reach the criteria for the clinical diagnosis of SE.

3. Mean duration of SE without neurologic sequelae is 1.5 hours (i.e., must institute barbiturate coma by approximately 1 hour of onset).

4. SE is relatively common; 50,000–200,000 cases per year; approximately 10% of patients with epilepsy go into SE at some point in their lives; SE most common among children <5 y/o (~74% of cases), and next most common is elderly; approximately 30–50% of cases of SE are the patients' first seizures.

5. Etiologies
   a. Idiopathic: one-third of cases of SE
   b. Most common cause: AED noncompliance most common in adults
   c. In children: febrile seizures and meningitis (especially *Haemophilus influenzae* and *Streptococcus pneumoniae*) are common
   d. Electrolyte imbalance (especially hyponatremia)
   e. Drug intoxication (especially cocaine) or drug withdrawal
   f. Systemic effects of convulsive SE
      i. Cyanotic appearance may be due to tonic contraction, desaturation of hemoglobin, or impedance of venous return due to increased intrathoracic pressure
      ii. Cardiovascular system: stressed by repeated tonic contractions of skeletal muscles; tachycardia is invariable; bradycardia may occur owing to vagal tone modulation by the CNS; hyperkalemia may cause arrhythmia
      iii. Endocrine: may have elevation of prolactin, glucagon, growth hormone, and corticotropin; serum glucose may initially increase to 200–250 mg/dL, but, if seizure activity is persistent, hypoglycemia may develop
      iv. Rhabdomyolysis: due to tonic-clonic activity; may lead to renal damage; important to maintain hydration
      v. Metabolic-biochemical complications: respiratory and metabolic acidosis, hypokalemia, and hyponatremia
      vi. Autonomic disturbance due to activation of sympathetic and parasympathetic systems, including excessive sweating, hyperpyrexia, and salivary and tracheobronchial hypersecretion
      vii. Cerebrospinal fluid may demonstrate pleocytosis

6. *Classification* (Figure 4.2)

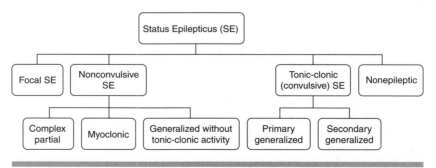

Figure 4-2. Classification of status epilepticus.

7. *Typical features of SE*

	Clinical manifestations	EEG pattern	Typical setting	Prognosis
Complex partial	Recurrent or continuous changes in mental status	Focal	History of seizures or focal brain lesion	Good
Myoclonic	Nonresponsive with myoclonic jerks	Generalized or burst suppression; EEG corresponds to myoclonus	Severe diffuse brain insult	Poor
Subtle generalized	Coma with subtle or no motor manifestations	Generalized	Severe diffuse brain insult	Variable, depending on underlying etiology
Absence	Recurrent or continuous changes in mental status	Generalized spike and wave pattern	History of seizures	Good
Focal (SE partialis)	Focal motor	Focal	Focal brain lesion	Variable, depending on underlying etiology but usually poor
Generalized convulsive	Bilateral tonic-clonic motor activity	Generalized or burst suppression; EEG corresponds to clonic movements	History of seizures with AED noncompliance, meningitis, encephalitis, electrolyte imbalance, or toxicity	Poor

B. **Morbidity and mortality**
   1. Related to three factors: CNS damage due to underlying insult, CNS damage from repetitive electric discharges, systemic and metabolic effects of repeated GTC seizures
   2. Increased duration of SE correlates to increased morbidity and mortality
   3. Convulsive SE
      a. Mortality: 8–12% acutely; up to 40–50% within 3 years (with large number due to underlying factors causing SE)
         i. Pediatric: 2.5%
         ii. Adult: 14%
         iii. Elderly: 38%
      b. In animal studies, neuronal death occurs after 60 minutes of seizure activity (despite paralyzing the animal to eliminate metabolic variables)
      c. In nonparalyzed primates in areas three, five, and six, cerebellum, hippocampus, amygdala, and certain thalamic nuclei; in paralyzed primates to minimize systemic

effects, mainly the hippocampus is damaged with only partial involvement of other areas (this supports theory that nonconvulsive SE may produce hippocampal neuronal damage); mechanism of neuronal damage is uncertain but may involve decreased inhibition by γ-aminobutyric acid system, enhanced glutaminergic excitatory activity with increased intracellular concentration of calcium and sodium, and calcium-mediated cell damage

C. **EEG:** initially EEG shows discrete seizures with interictal slowing; as SE continues, the seizures wax and wane, eventually evolving into continuous ictal discharges; if seizures persist, ictal discharges are interrupted by flat periods; in the final stage, paroxysmal bursts of epileptiform discharges arise from a flat background

D. **Motor systems:** initially, motor activity correlates to epileptiform discharges, but if seizures persist for >1 hour, then motor activity may diminish, although EEG activity continues; in final stages, may have electromechanical dissociation with no motor activity and periodic epileptiform discharges

E. **Systemic and metabolic effects**
   1. Phase one: ↑blood pressure/↑serum lactate and glucose/↓pH (indicative of acidosis)
   2. Phase two: blood pressure normalizes or hypotension develops; blood pressure no longer increases with each seizure

F. **Treatment of SE**

Time (mins)	Basic life support	Pharmacologic treatment
0–3	ABCs (airway, breathing, and circulation); evaluate respiration and give 2–4 L oxygen per nasal cannula (intubate if needed)	—
	i.v. access: thiamine, 100 mg intravenously followed by 50 cc 50% dextrose in water intravenously and continue normal saline or 5% dextrose in water; attain 2nd line for administration of treatment; ± naloxone (Narcan®), 0.4 mg intravenously	
	Draw blood for electrolytes, metabolic profile, complete blood cell count, toxicology, arterial blood gas, and AED levels	
	Obtain urinalysis and chest X-ray	
5	—	Lorazepam, 4–10 mg (0.1 mg/kg) bolus, or diazepam, 10 mg (0.2 mg/kg) bolus at 1–2 mg/min
8–10	Pyridoxine, 100–200 mg intravenously, in children <18 mos if seizures persist	Fosphenytoin (20 PE/kg) intravenously infused at a rate of no more than 0.75 mg/min/kg (max of 50 mg/min in adults)[a]
	Monitor electrocardiography and blood pressure during PHT administration	

Time (mins)	Basic life support	Pharmacologic treatment
10–15	Start continuous EEG monitoring	Benzodiazepine may be repeated up to max doses
45	CT scan LP	PB (20 mg/kg) infused at a rate of no more than 0.75 mg/min/kg of body weight (max of 50 mg/min in adults)
60–90		Pentobarbital: load with 3–5 mg/kg given over 3–5 mins followed by continuous infusion at 1 mg/kg/hr and increase continuous infusion at 1 mg/kg/hr with additional smaller loading doses until EEG shows burst-suppression
		or
		Midazolam (versed): 0.1–0.3 mg/kg bolus followed by continuous infusion at 0.05 mg/kg/hr and increasing by 0.05 mg/kg/hr q15mins up to 1 mg/kg/hr; if SE not controlled within 1 hr, start pentobarbital
		or
		Diazepam: 0.1 mg/kg i.v. bolus (if benzodiazepine not previously given) followed by 0.2 mg/mL at 0.5 mg/kg/hr up to 40 mg/hr to get a level of 0.2–0.8 mg/L; wean slowly over 8–12 hrs
		Note: Go to pentobarbital or another treatment if SE not controlled within 30–45 mins
		or
		Propofol drip: 1–2 mg/kg bolus followed by continuous infusion of 2–10 mg/kg/hr
		Note: Go to pentobarbital or another treatment if SE not controlled within 30–45 mins

PE = PHT equivalents.

[a]PHT (20 mg/kg) diluted in 300–500 cc saline can be substituted if fosphenytoin not available; i.v. PHT has risk of extravasation and tissue necrosis.

1. Fosphenytoin: should be substituted for i.v. PHT (Dilantin®); administration should not exceed 150 mg/minute because fosphenytoin can cause cardiac arrhythmias, prolongation of the QT interval, and hypotension; if i.v. access not available, may be given intramuscularly
2. Approximately 80% of prolonged seizures are brought under control with the combination of a benzodiazepine and PHT; if the seizure persists for >30 minutes, the patient should be transferred to an intensive care unit for probable intubation (likely secondary to decreased respiratory rate associated with barbiturate administration)
3. Comparison of commonly used AEDs in SE

Time	Diazepam	Lorazepam	PHT	PB
To reach brain	10 secs	2 mins	1 min	20 mins
To peak brain concentration	<5 mins	30 mins	15–30 mins	30 mins
To stop SE	1 min	<5 mins	15–30 mins	20 mins
Half-life	15 mins	6 hrs	>22 hrs	50 hrs

4. If on PHT, VA, or PB, give appropriate i.v. dose to achieve high or supratherapeutic serum level

$$\text{Bolus dose} = [(V_d)(\text{body weight})(\text{desired serum concentration} - \text{current serum concentration})]$$

Bolus dose (mg)
V_d: PHT = 0.6 L/kg   PB = 0.6 L/kg   VPA = 0.1–0.3 L/kg
Body weight (kg)
Serum concentration (mg/L)

VII. Sleep and Epilepsy
A. Mechanisms
1. Interictal discharges and seizures occur exclusively or primarily in nonrapid eye movement (NREM) sleep.
2. Neuronal synchronization with thalamocortical networks during NREM sleep results in enhanced neuronal excitability, facilitating seizures and interictal epileptiform discharges in partial epilepsy.
B. Timing of seizures in the sleep-wake cycle
1. Peak times for seizures
   a. Wake—three peaks
      i. 1–2 hours after awakening (7–8 a.m.)
      ii. Afternoon (3 p.m.)
      iii. Early evening (6–8 p.m.)
   b. Nocturnal—two peaks
      i. Early sleep (~10–11 p.m.)
      ii. 1–2 hours before awakening (~4–5 a.m.)
   c. Awakening seizures
      i. Associated with arousal (including awakening from daytime naps)
      ii. Typically are primary generalized seizures, including primary GTC, myoclonic, and absence seizures disorders
C. *Epileptiform activity during sleep*
1. *More frequent in NREM than in wake and REM sleep*

2. In generalized seizures, epileptiform discharges are sometimes facilitated by K complexes
3. NREM also facilitates focal spikes in partial seizures
4. In benign rolandic epilepsy, may have 20–60 spikes per minute in stages 1 and 2 sleep
D. **Effect of sleep deprivation:** increased interictal epileptiform discharges and ictal events
E. *Epileptic syndromes associated with sleep*

Epilepsy syndromes	Age of onset
Temporal lobe epilepsy	Late childhood to early adulthood
FLE	Late childhood to early adulthood
Benign rolandic epilepsy	3–13 yrs (peak 9–10)
Epilepsy with GTC seizures on awakening	6–25 yrs (peak 11–15)
JME	12–18 yrs (peak 14)
Absence seizures	3–12 yrs (peak 6–7)
Lennox-Gastaut syndrome	1–8 yrs (peak 3–5)
Electrical status of sleep	8 mos to 11.5 yrs

F. **Partial seizures ± secondary GTC seizures**
   1. 30% of partial epilepsies have both day and nocturnal seizures
   2. 40% of partial seizures with secondary GTC seizures have exclusively sleep epilepsy
   3. 15–40% of partial seizures without secondary GTC seizures have exclusively sleep epilepsy
   4. *FLE:* may occur primarily or predominantly during sleep; may be autosomal dominant with clustering of nocturnal motor seizures
   5. *Benign epilepsy of childhood with centrotemporal spikes (aka benign rolandic epilepsy)*
      a. Common childhood epilepsy accounting for 15–20% of childhood epilepsy
      b. Peak onset between ages 4 and 13 years; 60% males to 40% females; significant hereditary predisposition
      c. Neurologic examination normal
      d. 75% of seizures occur during sleep (most often in NREM sleep)
      e. Clinical ictal features: oropharyngeal signs, including hypersalivation and guttural sounds are common features; focal clonic activity also is prominent with facial contractions or hemiconvulsions; consciousness is preserved in most cases (unless there is secondary generalization)
      f. EEG: frequent focal rolandic/midtemporal spikes (5–10 per minute) remaining focal in wake and sleep
G. *Primary generalized seizures*
   1. *Primary GTC seizures on awakening*
      a. Clinical: >90% of GTC seizures occur at or immediately after awakening (sleep or nap) or in the evening when relaxing; myoclonic and absence seizures may coexist in 40–50%, suggesting that the same gene in JME may also be involved
      b. Photosensitivity and sleep deprivation are common precipitators
      c. Account for 2–4% of adult epilepsy
      d. EEG: generalized spike and wave discharges at 3–4 Hz and polyspike-wave complexes, which may be associated with K complexes
   2. *Absence epilepsy*

      a. Drowsiness and sleep activate spike and wave discharges that are most marked during the first cycle, max in NREM, and rare/absent in REM

      b. Morphology also affected in NREM with irregular polyspike and wave discharges predominating

   3. *Lennox-Gastaut syndrome:* NREM sleep is associated with increased 2.0–2.5-Hz spike- and slow-wave complexes and rhythmic 10-Hz spikes that may be accompanied by tonic seizures

   4. *JME*

      a. Begin in 2nd–3rd decade with myoclonic and generalized seizures

      b. 15–20% also have absence seizures

      c. Genetic basis: isolated to chromosome 6p (concordance rate of 70% in monozygotic twins, and 50% of first-degree relatives have primary generalized seizures)

      d. EEG: generalized 4–6-Hz polyspike wave discharge most prominent on awakening and at sleep onset; may be frequent in REM and deeper stages of NREM

H. *Other epilepsies associated with sleep*

   1. *Electrical SE of sleep*

      a. Almost continuous spike and wave complexes during NREM sleep (2.0–2.5-Hz generalized spike and wave discharges occurring in >85% of NREM sleep in REM and wakefulness → spike and wave complexes are less continuous and more focal

      b. Occurs in 0.5% of kids with epilepsy

      c. Average age onset: 8–9 years (range: 4–14 years) with spontaneous remission in 10 years

      d. Some have Landau-Kleffner syndrome: acquired aphasia with seizures, progressive language loss, and inattention to auditory stimuli

   I. **Differential diagnosis**

   1. Epileptic seizures

      a. FLE

      b. Temporal lobe epilepsy

      c. Generalized

      d. Benign rolandic epilepsy

   2. Nocturnal paroxysmal dystonia

   3. Sleep disorders

      a. Confusional arousals: body movement, automatic behaviors, mental confusion, fragmentary recall of dreams

      b. Night terrors

      c. Somnambulism

      d. REM sleep behavior disorder

      e. Periodic leg movements of sleep

      f. Sleep-onset myoclonus (hypnic jerk)

      g. Bruxism

      h. Rhythmic movement disorder

   4. Psychiatric disorders

      a. Nocturnal panic disorder

      b. Post-traumatic stress disorder

      c. Psychogenic seizures: patient is noted to be awake or drowsing on video-EEG

VIII. EEG "Mini-Atlas"

A. **Normal EEG**

   1. Normal background

a. Normal adult awake EEG

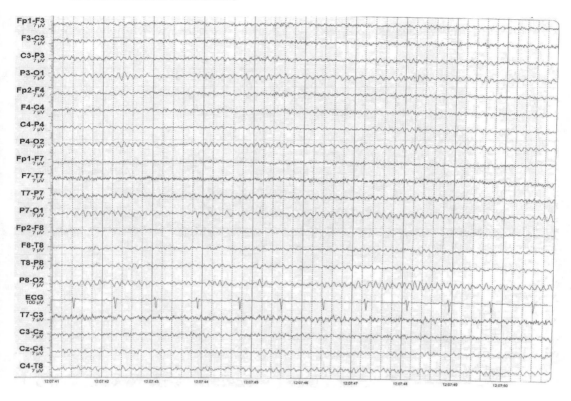

b. Normal light sleep (vertex wave)

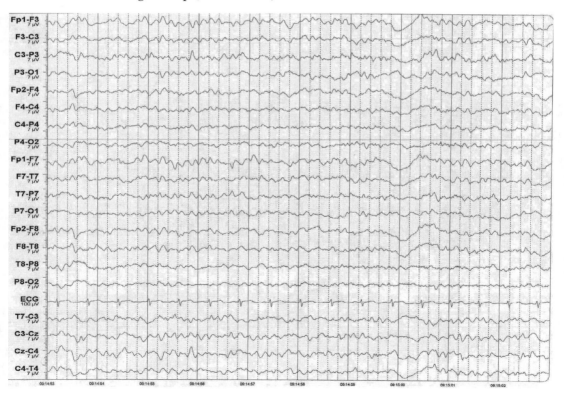

c. Normal light sleep (K complex): note that tech sneezed which may precipitate K complex

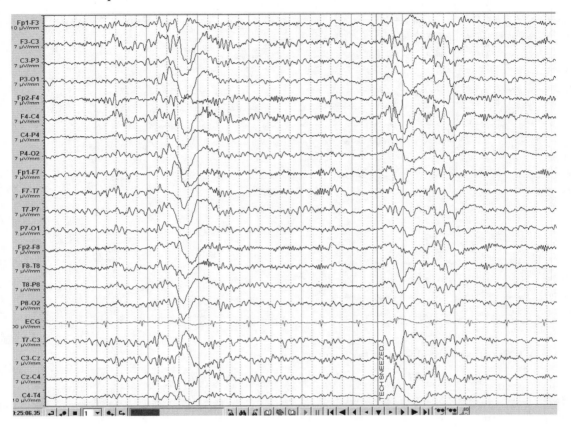

d. Normal deep sleep

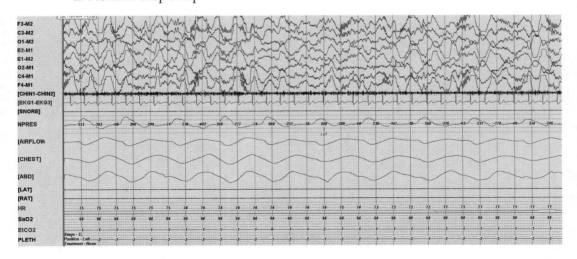

e. Normal REM sleep

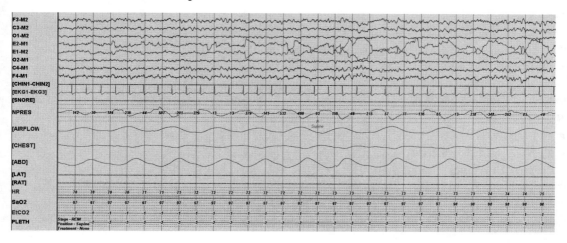

2. Normal variants
   a. Benign epileptiform transients of sleep (BETS): benign transients during sleep that occur typically between 30 to 60 years old and in children younger than 10 y/o

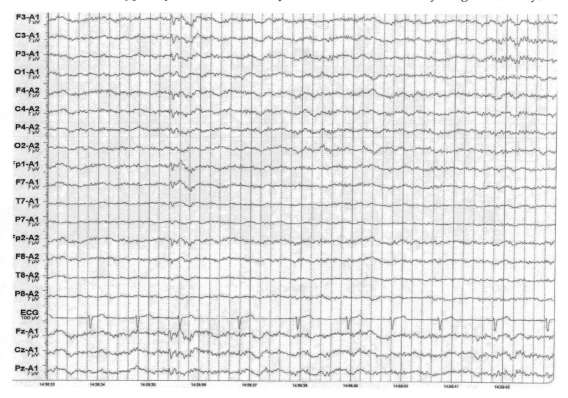

B. **Abnormalities**
   1. Diffuse slowing after anoxic brain injury

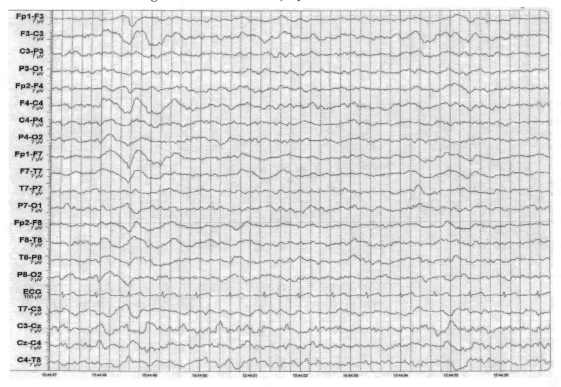

   2. Alpha coma: seen in comatose patients; in anoxic encephalopathy, signifies poor prognosis

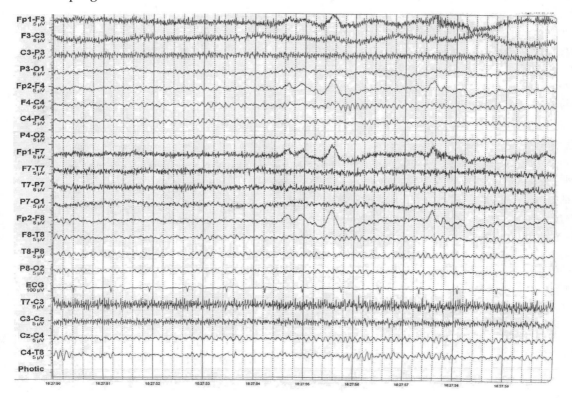

3. Breech: 35-year old following right anterior temporal lobectomy; due to craniotomy, cortical activity will have higher amplitude

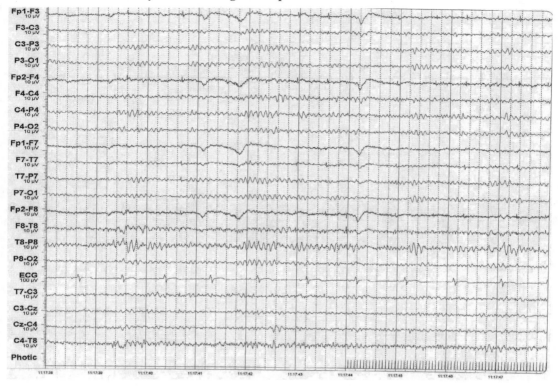

4. Burst suppression: 55-year old with uncontrolled seizures placed in burst-suppression with pentobarbital to control seizures; suppression of seizure activity is to control epileptiform activity that may damage neurons

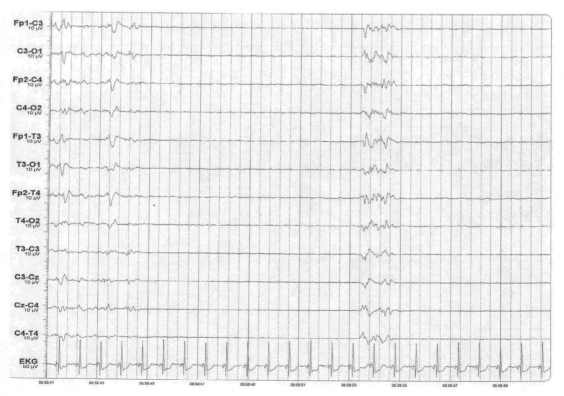

5. Focal slowing associated with left central parietal tumor

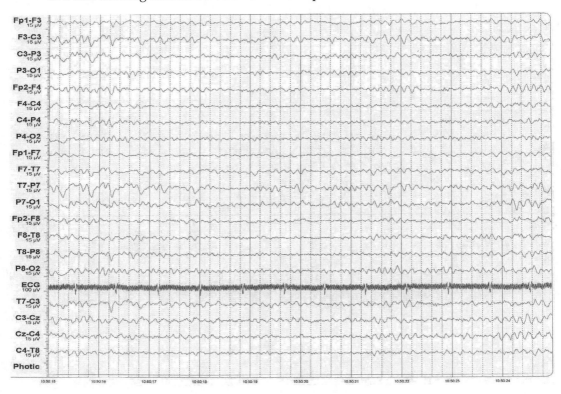

6. Periodic lateralized epileptiform discharges in patient with old stroke 6 months prior and no clinical symptoms

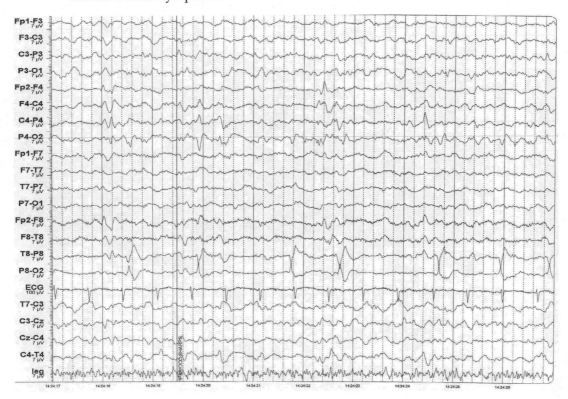

7. Frontal intermittent rhythmical delta activity (FIRDA): seen in multiple encephalopathies including mild anoxic brain injury, metabolic dysfunction; and normal variants

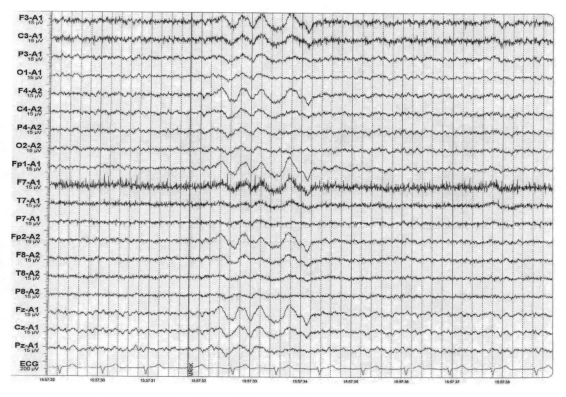

8. Triphasic waves in patient with renal failure

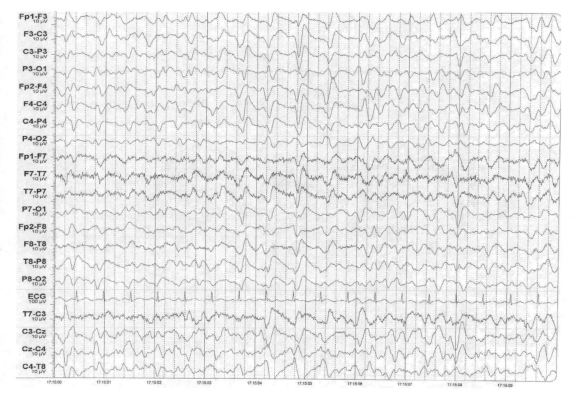

9. Seizure activity

a. Temporal lobe interictal seizure activity

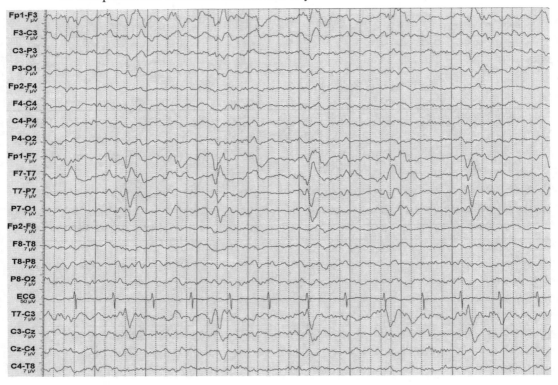

b. Polyspike wave generalized seizure activity

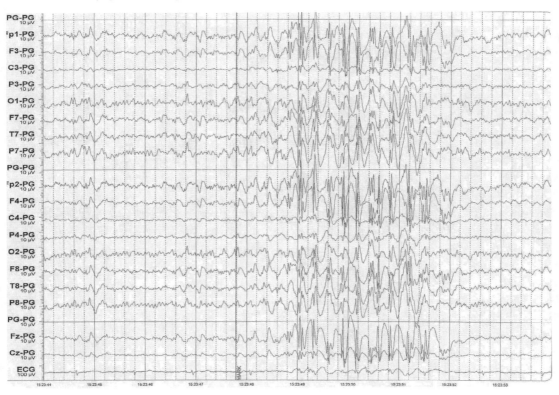

c. Temporal lobe ictal seizure activity and nonconvulsive status epilepticus due to herpes simplex encephalitis

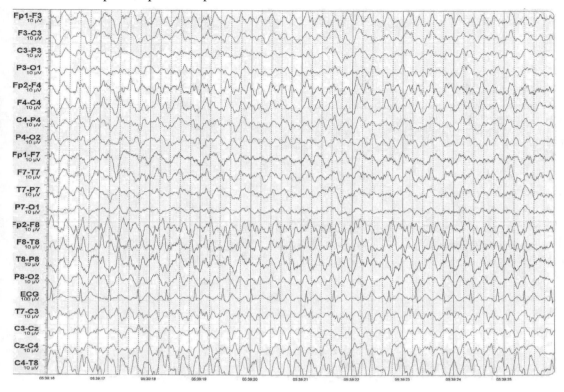

d. Frontal lobe ictal seizure

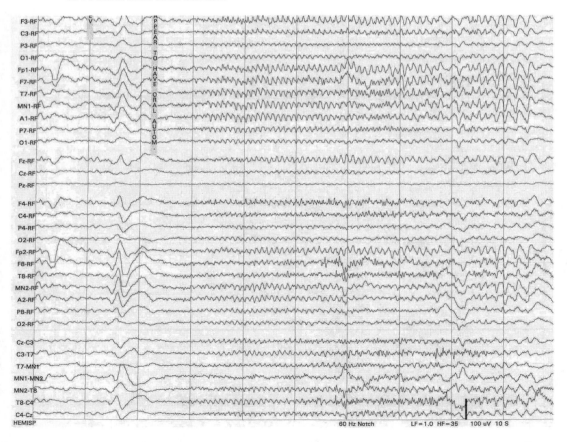

e. Absence seizure activity

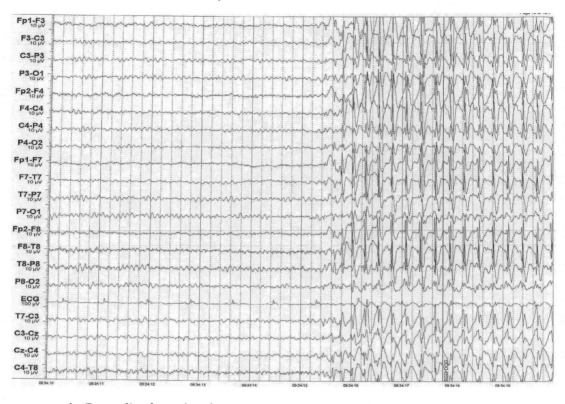

f. Generalized atonic seizure

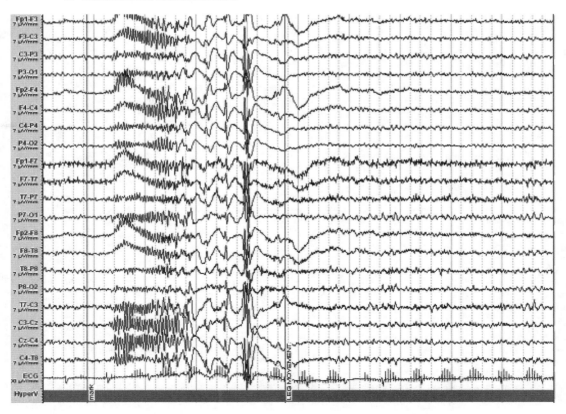

g. Generalized tonic-clonic seizure activity

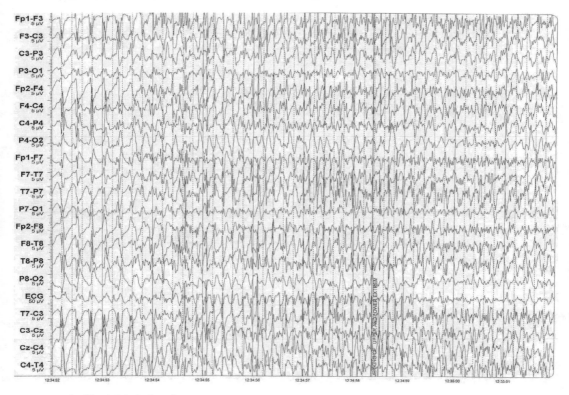

h. Post-ictal slowing

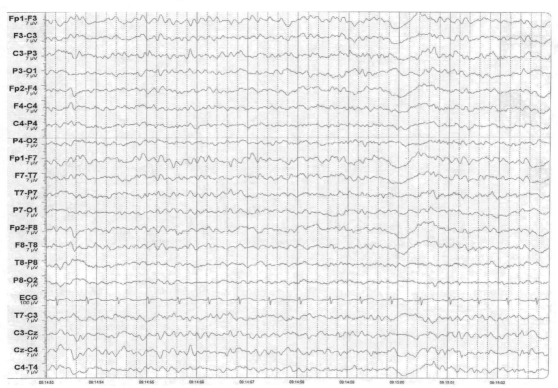

10. Artifact
   a. Electrode pop (four point star) due to poor impedance and EKG artifact (arrows)

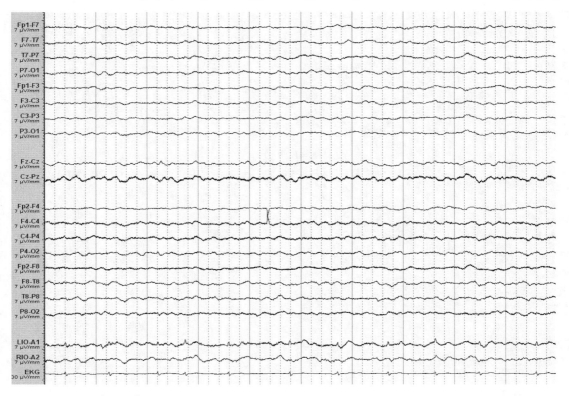

Muscle artifact

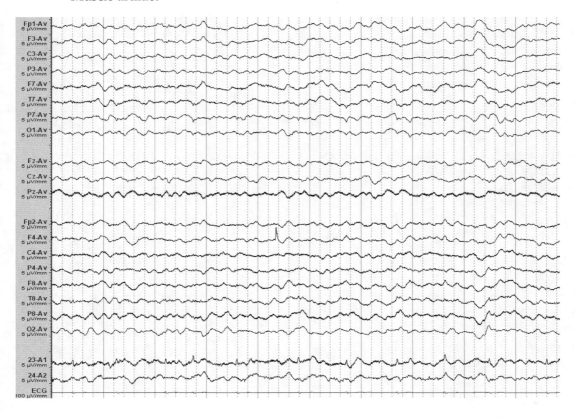

ADDITIONAL NOTES

CHAPTER 5

Movement Disorders

I. Classification

Hypokinetic movements	Hyperkinetic movements
Parkinsonism	Chorea (involuntary, irregular, purposeless, nonrhythmic, abrupt, rapid, unsustained movements that seem to flow from one body part to another)
Hypothyroid slowness	
Stiff muscles	Dystonia (twisting movements that tend to be sustained at the peak of the movement, frequently repetitive and often progress to prolonged abnormal postures)
Catatonia	
Psychomotor	Myoclonus (sudden, brief, shock-like involuntary movements caused by muscular contractions or inhibitions [negative myoclonus])
depression	
Blocking (holding) tics	Hemifacial spasm (unilateral facial muscle contractions)
	Hyperekplexia (excessive startle reaction to a sudden, unexpected stimulus)
	Ballism (very large amplitude choreic movements of the proximal parts of the limbs, causing flinging and flailing of limbs)
	Athetosis (slow writhing, continuous, involuntary movement)
	Akathisia (feeling of inner, general restlessness, which is reduced or relieved by walking about)
	Ataxia
	Tremors (an oscillatory, usually rhythmic and regular movement affecting one or more body parts)
	Myokymia (fine persistent quivering or rippling of muscles)
	Myorhythmia (slow frequency, prolonged, rhythmic or repetitive movement without the sharp wave appearance of a myoclonic jerk)
	Stereotypy (coordinated movement that repeats continually and identically)
	Tics (consist of abnormal movements or sounds; can be simple or complex)
	Restless legs (unpleasant crawling sensation of the legs, particularly when sitting and relaxing in the evening, which then disappears on walking)

Hypokinetic movements	Hyperkinetic movements
	Paroxysmal dyskinesias (choreoathetosis and dystonia that occur "out of the blue," lasting for seconds, minutes, or hours)

NB: Dopamine agonists are first-line treatment for restless legs syndrome.

II. Parkinsonism: core features: resting tremor, rigidity, bradykinesia, loss of postural reflexes
   A. *Etiologies*

Idiopathic parkinsonism	Parkinson's disease (PD)
Secondary parkinsonism	Drug induced (neuroleptics, antiemetics, reserpine, tetrabenazine, lithium, flunarizine, cinnarizine, diltiazem)
	Hydrocephalus
	Hypoxia
	Toxins (1-methyl-4-phenyl-1,2,3,6-tetrahydropyridine [MPTP], CO, manganese, cyanide, methanol)
	Infections (fungal, acquired immunodeficiency syndrome, subacute sclerosing panencephalitis, postencephalitic parkinsonism, Creutzfeldt-Jakob disease)
	Metabolic (hypo-/hypercalcemia, chronic hepatocerebral degeneration, Wilson's disease)
	Paraneoplastic parkinsonism
	Psychogenic
	Trauma
	Tumor
	Vascular
Parkinson-plus syndromes	Multiple system atrophy (striatonigral degeneration, Shy-Drager syndrome, olivopontocerebellar atrophy)
	Progressive supranuclear palsy
	Corticobasal ganglionic degeneration
	Progressive pallidal atrophy
	Lytico-Bodig
Heredodegenerative disease	Alzheimer's disease (AD)
	Dementia with Lewy bodies
	Pick's disease
	Huntington's disease
	Machado-Joseph's disease
	Hallervorden-Spatz disease
	Lubag (X-linked dystonia-parkinsonism)

B. **PD**

1. *Clinical: unilateral onset; rest tremor (in 80%);* absence of other neurologic signs (spasticity, Babinski signs, atypical speech); absence of lab or radiologic abnormalities (e.g., strokes, tumors); *slow progression; significant and sustained response to dopaminergic therapy;* usually with preservation of postural reflexes early in the illness; tremor, rigidity, bradykinesia, and, in later stages, postural instability; *autonomic dysfunction* (constipation, impotence, seborrheic dermatitis, bladder dyssynergia); *neuropsychiatric dysfunction* (**NB**: *depression* in up to 50%, *dementia* in up to 20%; *anxiety, panic attacks, hallucinations, delusions*); nearly all PD patients suffer from sleep disorders (e.g., insomnia, sleep fragmentation, excessive daytime sleepiness, nightmares, REM behavior disorder); insidious, often unilateral onset of subtle motor features; rate of progression varies; eventually symptoms worsen and become bilateral; treatment must be individualized and continually adjusted as the disease evolves

2. *Epidemiology of PD:* estimated prevalence: *500,000–1 million* patients in United States; incidence: 40,000–60,000 new cases per year; average age of onset is 60 years; affects up to 0.3% of general population, but 1–3% of those >65 y/o; PD is largely a disease of older adults: only *5–10% of patients have symptoms before 40 y/o (young-onset PD)*

3. *Genetic factors:* autosomal dominant (AD) and recessive patterns of inheritance have been identified

   a. *Park 1: chromosome 4q21-23;* alanine-53-threonine mutation in the α *synuclein gene; AD;* earlier disease onset (mean, age 45 years), faster progression, some with fluent aphasia

   b. *Park 2: chromosome 6q25.2-27;* the *parkin gene;* parkin; autosomal *recessive (AR);* relatively young-onset parkinsonism; early dystonia; symmetric involvement; good levodopa response; *absence of Lewy bodies* at autopsy

   c. *Park 3: chromosome 2p13; AD* but with 40% penetrance; all from northern Germany and southern Denmark; nigral degeneration and Lewy bodies at autopsy; dementia may be more common

   d. *Park 4: alpha synuclein triplications and duplications on chromosome 4p14-16.3; AD;* from a family known as the *Iowa kindred;* also younger age of onset (mean, 34 years), rapid clinical course, early-onset dementia; equivocal response to levodopa; some family members with only postural tremor resembling essential tremor; autopsy shows Lewy bodies in the nigra and hippocampus

   e. *Park 5: mutation in ubiquitin carboxy-terminal hydrolase L1 on chromosome 4; AD;* young-onset progressive parkinsonism

   f. *Park 6: mutation of the PINK1 gene on chromosome 1p35-36; AR;* early-onset parkinsonism, slow progression, and marked response to levodopa; gene not yet identified

   g. *Park 7: mutation of DJ-1 gene on chromosome 1p36;* early *AR* parkinsonism, slow progression, with levodopa responsiveness; mostly from the Netherlands

   h. *Park 8: mutation of the LRRK2 gene on chromosome 12cen; AD;* age of onset in the 60s with variable alpha synuclein and tau apathology

   i. *Park 9: mutation of ATP13A2 on chromosome 1q36; AR;* age of onset in the 30s

   j. *Park 10 and 11:* reported but inheritance is still unclear, probably AD, and gene mutation has not yet been identified

4. *Pathology:* many theories on cell death but no firm conclusions; apoptosis, mitochondrial dysfunction, oxidative stress, excitotoxicity, deficient neurotrophic support, immune mechanisms; *loss of pigmentation of the substantia nigra and locus ceruleus with decreased neuromelanin-containing neurons;* affected neurons contain large homogenous

eosinophilic cytoplasmic inclusions called *Lewy bodies,* which possess neurofilament, ubiquitin, and crystalline immunoreactivity

5. *Pharmacotherapy of PD*

   a. *Amantadine:* useful for newly diagnosed patients with mild symptoms and in some patients with advanced disease; provides mild-to-moderate benefit by decreasing tremor, rigidity, and akinesia; rarely effective as monotherapy for >1–2 years, may be continued as adjunctive agent; effective for levodopa-induced dyskinesias; adverse effects: anticholinergic effects, livedo reticularis, renal disease increases susceptibility to adverse effects, leg edema, neuropsychiatric effects—confusion, hallucinations, nightmares, insomnia; mechanism: ?N-methyl-D-aspartate antagonist

   b. *Anticholinergic agents:* option for young patients <60 y/o) whose predominant symptoms are resting tremor and hypersalivation; available agents—trihexyphenidyl and benztropine; adverse effects often limit use—memory impairment, confusion, hallucinations

   c. *Levodopa:* advantages—most efficacious antiparkinsonian drug, immediate therapeutic benefits (within 1 week), easily titrated, reduces mortality, lower cost; disadvantages—no effect on disease course, no effect on nondopaminergic symptoms (such as dysautonomia, cognitive disturbances, and postural instability), motor fluctuations and dyskinesia develop over time (especially in younger patients, those with more severe disease and those requiring higher doses); acute adverse effects—nausea/vomiting (carbidopa alleviates by inhibiting amino acid decarboxylase enzyme), confusion, psychosis, dizziness; chronic effects—hallucinations; motor fluctuations—peak dose or diphasic dyskinesias, wearing off, sudden off, delayed on, yo-yoing

   d. *Dopamine agonists*

Drug	Ergot derived	D1	D2	D3/D4	Half-life (hrs)
Bromocriptine	Yes	—	++	+	3
Pergolide*	Yes	+	++	++	27
Pramipexole	No	—	++	+++	12
Ropinirole	No	—	++	+	4
Cabergoline	Yes	—	++	+	65

+, least receptor affinity; +++, greatest receptor affinity.
* Withdrawn from the market due to increased risk of valvulopathy.

   i. Effective for initial monotherapy; also indicated in combination with levodopa to smooth clinical response in advanced disease; directly stimulate postsynaptic dopamine receptors; effective against key motor symptoms (tremor, bradykinesia, and rigidity); early use shows reduced risk of dyskinesia compared with levodopa therapy; antiparkinsonian effects consistently inferior to levodopa; adverse effects: slightly higher than levodopa—nausea/vomiting, sedation, orthostatic hypotension, hallucinations, dyskinesia in more advanced disease, leg edema, **NB:** sleep attacks; ergot-derived side effects—livedo reticularis, erythromelalgia, cardiac, pulmonary or retroperitoneal fibrosis, valvulopathy

   ii. *Apomorphine:* available in the United States as an injectable (subcutaneous) short acting dopamine agonist; U.S. Food and Drug Administration (FDA) approved as a "rescue therapy" for symptoms of wearing off in advanced PD patients; benefits take effect as early as 5 minutes from the time of injection, but lasts for only 1 to 1.5 hours

iii. *Rotigotine:* the latest dopamine agonist approved in the United States for monotherapy in early PD; used in other countries as an adjunct treatment for levodopa in advanced PD; available in patch form, but has been temporarily pulled out of the market because of crystallization observed in some of the patches which may lessen its potency; side effects, other than skin reactions, are similar to nonergot dopamine agonists, including somnolence, sleep attacks, nausea, vomiting, weight gain, hallucinations, etc.

iv. Increasing reports recently of impulse control disorders (e.g., hypersexuality, binge eating, pathological gambling, and compulsive shopping) associated with PD medications, especially dopamine agonists

e. **NB**: *Catechol methyltransferase inhibitors: inhibit levodopa catabolism to 3-O-methyldopa, increasing levodopa bioavailability and transport to brain;* extend duration of levodopa effect; indicated for treatment of patients with PD experiencing end-of-dose wearing off with levodopa; no role as monotherapy; used only in combination with levodopa; two available agents: *entacapone (Comtan®) and tolcapone (Tasmar®);* fatal fulminant hepatitis in four tolcapone-treated patients: requires liver function monitoring and signed patient consent; side effects: dyskinesias, diarrhea (4–10%), nausea

f. *Monoamine oxidase B (MAO-B) inhibitors*

i. *Selegiline:* selective monoamine oxidase-B inhibitor with doses ∂10 mg/day; Deprenyl and Tocopherol Antioxidative Therapy of Parkinsonism study showed unlikely neuroprotective effect and mild symptomatic benefit in early PD; with higher doses, avoid tyramine-rich food, meperidine, or selective serotonin reuptake inhibitor, as monoamine oxidase-B selectivity is lost predisposing to cheese effect

ii. *Rasagiline:* new selective, once per day, MAO-B inhibitor; FDA approved for monotherapy in early PD, and also for adjunctive treatment to levodopa in moderate-to-advanced PD; "off time" was decreased by 0.9 hours among PD patients with wearing off symptoms compared to placebo in the PRESTO trial and LARGO trials; the recently concluded ADAGIO trial showed that early, medication naïve PD patients placed on rasagiline at 1 mg per day immediately at study entry had a better average total Unified Parkinson Disease Rating Scale score after 3 years compared to those who received rasagiline 9 months later; unlike selegiline, this new MAO-B inhibitor is not broken down into amphetamine metabolites; however, dietary precaution on tyramine-rich foods is advised

g. *Management of dementia and hallucinations in PD:* eliminate medical causes of delirium (e.g., infection or dehydration); discontinue nonparkinsonian psychotropic medications, if possible; eliminate antiparkinsonian drugs in order of their potential to produce delirium (anticholinergics > amantadine > monoamine oxidase-B inhibitors > dopamine agonists > catechol methyltransferase inhibitor > levodopa); use regular levodopa formulation at lowest possible dose; use atypical antipsychotic agents (clozapine > quetiapine > other atypicals). *Rivastigmine:* for cognitive impairment, *the first FDA-approved medication for Parkinson's disease with dementia (PDD);* available orally and in patch form; may also improve mild hallucinations; most frequent side effects: nausea, vomiting, and tremors (usually mild and transient but can be bothersome in some); no worsening in the UPDRS motor scores in patients who were randomized to rivastigmine compared to placebo in the EXPRESS trial

h. *Surgical management of PD:* lesion vs. deep brain stimulation; *lesion* (thalamotomy—most effective for parkinsonian and essential tremor; pallidotomy—improves bradykinesia, tremor, rigidity, dyskinesia in PD) has the advantage of simplicity, no technology or adjustments required, no indwelling device; however, disadvantages include inability to do bilateral lesions without increased risk of dementia, swallowing dysfunction, etc., and side effects could be permanent; *deep brain stimulation surgery of globus pallidus internus or subthalamic nucleus* may improve most symptoms of PD and has the advantage of minimal to no cell destruction and the ability to perform deep brain stimulation on both sides and to adjust the stimulation settings as the disease progresses; however, deep brain stimulation is more expensive, requires technical expertise, and could be prone to hardware malfunctions (e.g., kinks, lead fractures) or infections; the *ideal surgical candidate: clear PD diagnosis with unequivocal and sustained levodopa response, relatively young, nondemented, nondepressed, nonanxious, emotionally and physically stable*

C. **Multiple system atrophy** (the term encompasses three overlapping entities: (1) **Shy-Drager syndrome,** (2) **striatonigral degeneration,** and (3) **olivopontocerebellar atrophy**)
  1. *Clinical manifestations*
     a. *Striatonigral degeneration:* a sporadic disorder with an insidious onset of neurologic symptoms in the 4th–7th decades of life; the mean age at onset is 56.6 years, and there is no sex preference; akinetic rigid syndrome, similar to PD; patients initially present with rigidity, hypokinesia, and sometimes unexplained falling; may be symmetric or asymmetric at onset; the course is relentlessly progressive, with a duration ranging from 2–10 years (mean, 4.5–6.0 years); eventually, patients are severely disabled by marked akinesia, rigidity, dysphonia or dysarthria, postural instability, and autonomic dysfunction; mild cognitive and affective changes with difficulties in executive functions, axial dystonia with anterocollis, stimulus-sensitive myoclonus, and pyramidal signs; respiratory stridor due to moderate to severe laryngeal abductor paralysis can sometimes occur; resting tremor is not common; cerebellar signs are typically absent; the majority do not respond to levodopa, except early in the course
     b. *Olivopontocerebellar degeneration:* essentially a progressive degenerative cerebellar-plus syndrome; male to female ratio is 1.8:1.0 in familial olivopontocerebellar atrophy and 1:1 in sporadic olivopontocerebellar atrophy; the average age of onset is 28 years for familial and 50 years for sporadic olivopontocerebellar atrophy; the mean duration of the disease is 16 years in familial and 6 years in sporadic olivopontocerebellar atrophy; cerebellar ataxia, especially involving gait, is the presenting symptom in 73% of patients; dysmetria, limb ataxia, and cerebellar dysarthria are characteristic; other initial symptoms include rigidity, hypokinesia, fatigue, disequilibrium, involuntary movements, visual changes, spasticity, and mental deterioration; as the disease progresses, cerebellar disturbances remain the most outstanding clinical features; dementia is the next most common symptom in familial olivopontocerebellar atrophy and is present in 60% of the patients; dementia occurs in 35% of sporadic olivopontocerebellar atrophy patients
     c. *Shy-Drager syndrome:* presence of parkinsonian features with prominent autonomic dysfunction, such as orthostatic hypotension, erectile dysfunction, bladder and bowel disturbance, etc.
  2. *Pathology:* striatonigral degeneration is characterized pathologically by cell *loss and gliosis in the striatum and substantia nigra;* macroscopically, the putamen is most affected with significant atrophy; the substantia nigra exhibits hypopigmentation; microscopically,

severe neuronal loss, gliosis, and loss of myelinated fibers are evident in the putamen, less on the caudate; gliosis is found, but Lewy bodies or neurofibrillary tangles are not commonly present; a recent finding in cases of multiple system atrophy is the presence of *argyrophilic cytoplasmic inclusions in oligodendrocytes and neurons*; the inclusions are composed of granule-associated filaments that have immunoreactivity with tubulin, τ protein, and ubiquitin; they seem to be specific for multiple system atrophy; there is considerable clinical and pathologic overlap among the three multiple system atrophy syndromes; *in olivopontocerebellar atrophy, neuronal loss with gross atrophy is concentrated in the pons, medullary olives, and cerebellum; in Shy-Drager syndrome, the intermediolateral cell columns of the spinal cord are affected as well*

3. *Differential diagnosis:* striatonigral degeneration is most frequently misdiagnosed as *PD*; features suggestive of striatonigral degeneration include initial presentation of unexplained falls, early appearance of autonomic symptoms, rapid progression of parkinsonian disability, lack of significant response to levodopa therapy, symmetric presentation, and minimal or no resting tremors; it is different from olivopontocerebellar atrophy because of the absence of prominent cerebellar symptoms and from Shy-Drager syndrome because of a lack of pronounced orthostatic hypotension; its relatively symmetric presentation will not be confused with *cortical-basal ganglionic degeneration*, and its intact oculomotor function distinguishes it from *progressive supranuclear palsy*; mentation is relatively preserved in striatonigral degeneration (less so in olivopontocerebellar atrophy) and is helpful in differentiating from dementing diseases, such as AD with parkinsonian features, *diffuse Lewy body disease, or Creutzfeldt-Jakob disease*; finally, multiple system atrophy should be distinguished from *acquired parkinsonism* by ruling out infectious, toxic, drug-induced, vascular, traumatic, and metabolic causes

NB: The orthostatic hypotension may be treated with fludrocortisone, midodrine, or erythropoietin.

D. **Progressive supranuclear palsy:** *Steele-Richardson-Olszewski syndrome*; clinical: supranuclear *ophthalmoparesis (especially downgaze) and falls within the 1st year of onset of parkinsonism* are mandatory criteria for probable progressive supranuclear palsy; 60–80% with subcortical form of dementia; pathology: widespread diencephalic and mesencephalic (leading to a Mickey Mouse midbrain), brain stem and cerebellar nuclear neuronal loss; with *globose neurofibrillary tangles* (exhibit paired helical filament, τ protein and ubiquitin immunoreactivity); marked midbrain atrophy

NB: Falls and aspiration cause the most frequent complications.

E. **Corticobasal ganglionic degeneration:** an *asymmetric* form of parkinsonism presenting with *unilateral dystonia, myoclonus, alien limb phenomena* plus parkinsonism; *dementia* is common; pathologically with *achromatic neuronal inclusions* but no classic Pick bodies; asymmetric findings on magnetic resonance imaging (MRI) or functional imaging

NB: Synucleinopathies: multiple system atrophy, PD, Lewy body dementia.

NB: Tauopathies: AD, Pick's disease, frontotemporal dementia with parkinsonism, progressive supranuclear palsy, and corticobasal ganglionic degeneration.

F. **Postencephalitic parkinsonism:** *von Economo's encephalitis*; this disease is now almost nonexistent but nevertheless an extremely important disease *after the 1914–1918 influenza pandemics*; some individuals developed encephalitis, and in the months to years after *recovery from the acute illness, they developed parkinsonism* with prominent *oculogyric symptoms*; condition was generally nonprogressive; pathology: depigmentation of the substantia nigra and locus ceruleus, *no classic Lewy bodies, with neurofibrillary tangles*

G. **Dementia-parkinsonism-amyotrophic lateral sclerosis complex of Guam:** exhibits gross atrophy of the frontotemporal regions, depigmentation of the substantia nigra, and loss of anterior roots; histologically, there are *neurofibrillary tangles* in the cortical neurons, loss of pigmented neurons in the substantia nigra without Lewy bodies, and loss of anterior horn cells with neurofibrillary tangles

H. **Acute parkinsonism:** *etiology: infectious, postinfectious, autoimmune (systemic lupus erythematosus), medication (typical side effects of antidopamine drugs, idiosyncratic effects—neuroleptic malignant syndrome, serotonin syndrome, chemotherapeutic drugs), toxic (carbon monoxide, cadmium, MPTP, ethanol withdrawal, ethylene oxide, methanol, disulfiram, bone marrow transplantation), structural (stroke, subdural hematoma, central and extra pontine myelinolysis, tumor, hydrocephalus), psychiatric (catatonia, conversion, malingering)*

 1. *Structural lesions:* obstructive hydrocephalus is a well-known cause of parkinsonism; may occur in adults and children, either due to shunt obstruction or at presentation of the hydrocephalus; obstructive hydrocephalus after meningitis or subarachnoid hemorrhage may also cause parkinsonism; normal pressure hydrocephalus often mimics parkinsonism, but the onset is insidious

 2. *Vascular parkinsonism:* previously called *atherosclerotic parkinsonism,* usually results from tiny lacunes in the basal ganglia; generally insidious in onset and slowly progressive, although sudden worsening may occur with new strokes; *frontal, cingulated gyrus, supplementary motor area strokes* have also caused acute parkinsonism; of interest, strokes in the lenticular nuclei do not cause parkinsonism; acute hemorrhage is a less common cause of acute parkinsonism.

 3. *Toxic/metabolic:* some, like *manganese,* develop subacutely or over long periods; parkinsonism may follow *carbon monoxide* poisoning after an acute, life-threatening poisoning after recovery from the coma; carbon monoxide poisoning is a persistent problem in some countries, notably Korea, where faulty oil-burning heaters are used; the globus pallidus is typically involved, but recent data suggest that white matter deterioration must also be present for parkinsonism to develop; *cadmium and ethylene oxide, disulfiram* (used to prevent alcoholics from imbibing), and *cyanide poisoning* are other uncommon causes

 4. *MPTP:* severe, acute parkinsonism in intravenous drug abusers in the San Francisco Bay area; the drug is taken up by glial cells and converted to MPP+, which is secreted and taken up by dopaminergic cells in the pars compacta of the substantia nigra; the first systemically administered drug that selectively targets these cells and, because it has a similar effect in other primates, it has been widely used to create animal models of PD; the onset of parkinsonism occurs after the first few doses

 5. *Neuroleptic malignant syndrome is variably defined but generally requires fever, alteration of mental status, and rigidity; many patients have extreme elevations of creatine phosphokinase* due to rhabdomyolysis; neuroleptic malignant syndrome may occur at any point once a patient is treated with neuroleptics, but it usually occurs relatively shortly after drug initiation and dose increase; the onset of neuroleptic malignant syndrome may be fulminant, progressing to coma over hours, but it usually develops over days; patients develop fever, stiffness, and mental impairment with delirium and obtundation; treatment: requires excluding infection, stopping the suspected offending drug, close monitoring of autonomic and respiratory parameters, and treatment with dopaminergic replacement (either levodopa or dopamine agonists)

 6. *Dopamine D2 receptor-blocking drugs* routinely cause parkinsonism; may also occur with *lithium or valproic acid;* syndrome usually develops over the course of weeks, but may

occasionally develop over days; in patients with a primary parkinsonian syndrome, a low-potency neuroleptic or even an atypical antipsychotic can induce acute parkinsonism; this is not uncommon when a patient with PD is treated with an antiemetic, such as prochlorperazine or metoclopramide

III. Chorea: irregular, nonrhythmic, rapid, unsustained involuntary movement that flows from one body part to another

A. *Etiology*

Primary	Essential chorea
	Senile chorea
Hereditary	Huntington's disease
	Neuroacanthocytosis
	Wilson's disease
	Lesch-Nyhan syndrome
	Metabolic disorders
Secondary	*Infectious:* subacute bacterial endocarditis, subacute sclerosing panencephalitis, acquired immunodeficiency syndrome, Lyme disease, tuberculosis, syphilis
	Sydenham's chorea
	Chemicals: CO, Hg, lithium
	Encephalitides
	Creutzfeldt-Jakob disease
	Systemic lupus erythematosus, antiphospholipid antibody syndrome
	Paraneoplastic
	Postvaccinal
	Vascular
	Polycythemia vera
	Henoch-Schönlein purpura
	Venous thrombosis
	Drugs: levodopa, neuroleptics, oral contraceptives, anticholinergics, antihistamines, phenytoin, methylphenidate (Ritalin®), pemoline, methadone, cocaine, etc.
	Kernicterus/ethyl alcohol
	Pregnancy
	Metabolic etiologies: hypoparathyroidism, hypomagnesemia, Addison's disease, hypernatremia, thyrotoxicosis, hypoglycemia, nonketotic hyperglycemia
	Anoxia
	Mitochondrial myopathies
	Tumors including metastasis
	Multiple sclerosis

NB: The primary treatment of any tardive syndrome (late onset chorea, dystonia, akathisia, after sustained exposure to dopamine receptor blocking agents such as antipsychotics and anti-emetics) is elimination of the precipitating medication

B. **Huntington's disease:** *AD disorder (with 100% penetrance) carried on chromosome 4*
   1. *Clinical:* combines *cognitive (subcortical dementia), movement disorders (chorea, dystonia, motor impersistence, incoordination, gait instability, and, in the young, parkinsonism: Westphal variant), and psychiatric disorders (depression, anxiety, impulsivity, apathy, obsessive compulsive disorders, etc.);* commonly manifest by age 20–40 years; usually progresses relentlessly to death in 10–15 years
   2. *Pathology:* the brain is atrophic, striking atrophy of the caudate nucleus, and, to a lesser degree, the putamen is seen; compensatory hydrocephalus may be seen *(box car-shaped ventricles);* microscopically: preferential *loss of the medium spiny striatal neurons accompanied by gliosis;* biochemically: decreased γ-aminobutyric acid, enkephalins, and substance P
   3. Genetics: *anticipation:* the age of onset occurs earlier with succeeding generations due to increase in trinucleotide repeat, and, because repeats may amplify between generations, anticipation may be seen
   4. *Trinucleotide repeat diseases*

Disease	Inheritance	Repeats	Chromosome	Protein
Huntington's disease	AD	CAG	4p16	Huntingtin
Fragile X	AD	CGG	X	FMR-1
Myotonic dystrophy	AD	CTG	19	Myotonin
SCA type 1	AD	CAG	6p23	Ataxin-1
SCA type 2	AD	CAG	12q24	Ataxin-2
SCA type 3 (Machado-Josephs disease)	AD	CAG	14q32	Ataxin-3
SCA type 6	AD	CAG	19p13	Voltage-dependent calcium channel
SCA type 7	AD	CAG	13p12	Ataxin-7
SCA type 12	AD	CAG	5q31-33	Regulatory subunit of protein phosphatase (PP2A)
SCA type 17	AD	CAG	6q27	TATA-binding protein
Spinobulbar muscular atrophy (Kennedy's)	X-linked recessive	CAG	Xq13	Androgen receptor
Dentatorubropal-lidoluysian atrophy	AD	CAG	12p13	Atrophin-1
Friedreich's ataxia	AR	GAA	9q13-21.1	Frataxin

SCA, spinocerebellar ataxia.

5. *Hereditary causes of chorea*

Disorder	Inheritance	Chromosome	Gene	Findings
Huntington's disease	AD	4p16.3	Huntingtin	See section III.B
Huntington's disease–like 1 (HDL1)	AD	20p	Prion protein gene (PRNP)	Almost like Huntington's disease; with seizures
HDL2	AD	16q23	Junctophilin 3 (JPH3)	Onset in the 4th decade, like HDL1 but no seizures; almost exclusively in blacks
HDL3	AR	4p15.3	—	Onset at 3–4 years with chorea, dystonia, ataxia, gait disorder, spasticity, seizures, mutism, mental decline
Neuroacanthocytosis	AR X-linked AD has also been reported	9q21 Xp21	CHAC gene XK gene	Behavioral and personality disorders, chorea, dystonia, dysphagia, dysarthria, seizures, motor axonopathy, high creatine phosphokinase
Neurodegeneration with brain iron accumulation type 1 or Hallervorden-Spatz disease	AR	20p12.3-p13	PANK-2	Childhood onset, progressive rigidity, dystonia, choreoathetosis, spasticity, optic nerve atrophy, dementia with acanthocytosis
Benign hereditary chorea	AD	14q13.1-q21.1		Slight motor delay with chorea, ataxia, usually self-limiting after adolescence
Dentatorubropallidoluysian atrophy	AD	12 (CAG repeat)	Jun NH(2)-terminal kinase (JNK)	Onset typically 4th decade; myoclonus, epilepsy, mental retardation (early onset); ataxia, choreoathetosis, dystonia, rest and postural tremor, parkinsonism, dementia (late onset)

Disorder	Inheritance	Chromosome	Gene	Findings
				Others: SCA 2, 3, and 17; Wilson's disease

6. *Treatment: chorea:* dopamine receptor-blocking agents (e.g., haloperidol, risperidone, reserpine, tetrabenazine), clonazepam, amantadine; *tetrabenazine has been recently approved for the treatment of chorea in HD; gait instability:* reassess if dopamine-blocking agents are causing parkinsonism, physical and occupational therapy; *depression and anxiety:* selective serotonin reuptake inhibitors, clonazepam; *speech and swallowing therapy; genetic counseling; family counseling*

C. **Neuroacanthocytosis**

1. *Clinical:* mean age of onset is 32 years (range, 8–62 years), and the clinical course is progressive but with marked phenotypic variation

   a. *Psychiatric:* behavioral, emotional disorders, and psychiatric manifestations are common; depression, paranoia, and obsessive-compulsive disorder, self-mutilative behavior; compulsive head banging or biting of tongue, lips, and fingers can lead to severe injury; dementia is often reported

   b. *Epilepsy:* a considerable proportion of patients have seizures

   c. *Involuntary movement disorders:* jerky movements of the limbs; sucking, chewing, and smacking movements of the mouth; shoulder shrugs, flinging movements of the arms and legs, and thrusting movements of the trunk and pelvis; wild lurching truncal and flinging proximal arm movements; oral-facial dyskinesias; tic-like, repetitive, and stereotyped movements; involuntary vocalizations are common; occasional patients have primarily dystonia

   d. *Disordered voluntary movements:* lack of ¯oral-facial coordination is prominent; dysarthria and dysphagia occur in most cases; many patients have a characteristic eating disorder in which food is propelled out of the mouth by the tongue—patients may learn to swallow with their head tipped back "facing the ceiling," or place a spoon over the mouth to prevent the food from escaping; bradykinesia in concert with chorea is also common; gait is disordered and features a combination of involuntary movements and poor postural reflexes

   e. *Neuromuscular weakness:* elevated creatine phosphokinase; peripheral neuropathy with distal sensory loss and hyporeflexia is common; electrophysiologic studies show increased duration and amplitude of motor unit potentials, indicative of chronic denervation

2. *Genetics:* considered to have a genetic basis, but the gene defect is unknown in most patients; some cases are *AD*, others are *AR (chromosome 9q21)*; in a subset of patients with a similar but *X-linked* clinical syndrome, the *lack of a common red blood cell antigen, Kx,* has been described; it is caused by mutations in the XK gene encoding the Kx protein, a putative membrane transport protein of yet unknown function; this X-linked illness, known as *McLeod syndrome,* is characterized by *hemolysis, myopathy, cardiomyopathy, areflexia, chorea, elevated creatine phosphokinase, liver disease, and chorea*

NB: Gene product: chorein.

D. **Dentatorubropallidoluysian atrophy:** rare disorder, more *common in Japan;* characterized by the presence of *progressive myoclonic epilepsy, ataxia, choreoathetosis, and dementia;* age of onset is broad, mostly in the 3rd or 4th decade, but juvenile form occurs in childhood; pathology:

degeneration of the dentate nucleus, red nucleus, globus pallidus, and subthalamic nucleus; a trinucleotide *CAG repeat mapped to chromosome 12p, producing the protein atrophin-1*

E. **NB: Pantothenate Kinase-Associated Neurodegeneration (PKAN); formerly Hallervorden-Spatz syndrome:** rare *AR* disorder pathologically associated with *iron deposition* and high concentration of lipofuscin and neuromelanin in the substantia nigra pars reticulata and the internal segment of the globus pallidus; mapped to *chromosome 20p12.3-13*; due to a mutation in the *gene for pantothenate kinase gene (PANK2)*; three presentations: early onset <10 y/o), late onset (10–18 y/o), and adult variant; characterized by progressive *personality changes, cognitive decline, dysarthria, motor difficulties, spasticity; dystonia is common but choreoathetosis tremor* may be present; retinitis pigmentosa, optic atrophy, and seizures may also occur; MRI: decreased T2-weighted signal in the globus pallidus and substantia nigra; some have a hyperintense area within the hypodense areas *("eye of the tiger" sign); hyperprebetalipoproteinemia, acanthocytosis, retinitis pigmentosa, and pallidal degeneration syndrome*

F. **Sydenham's chorea:** initial manifestation: usually disturbance in school function, daydreaming, fidgety, inattentiveness, and increased emotional lability; onset of chorea is rather sudden, lag time between streptococcal infection and chorea averages 6 months; serologic evidence is absent in one-third of patients; *risk of developing carditis with Sydenham's chorea is 30–50%; recurrent episodes of chorea are most common at the time of pregnancy in female patients;* lab findings: elevated erythrocyte sedimentation rate or C-reactive protein, prolonged PR interval; treatment for chorea: dopamine receptor-blocking agents, such as haloperidol, pimozide, phenothiazines, or amantadine; for acute rheumatic fever: penicillin V, 400,000 U (250 mg) tid for 10 days, followed by prophylaxis (benzathine penicillin G, 1.2 million U intramuscularly every 3–4 weeks, or penicillin V, 250 mg by mouth bid, or sulfisoxazole, 0.5–1.0 g by mouth qd)

G. **Lesch-Nyhan syndrome:** rare *X-linked; uricemia in association with spasticity and choreoathetosis* in early childhood with *self-mutilation*; normal at birth up to 6–9 months; self-mutilation (mainly lips) occurs early; spasticity, athetosis, and tremor later; mental retardation moderately severe; gouty tophi appear on ears, risk for gouty nephropathy; lab: serum uric acid, 7–10 mg/dL; *deficiency in hypoxanthine-guanine-phosphoribosyl transferase that lies on X chromosome* by DNA analysis; treatment: allopurinol (xanthine oxidase inhibitor) but no effect on central nervous system; transitory success with 5-hydroxytryptophan with L-dopa; fluphenazine/haloperidol for self-mutilation; behavior modification

H. **Paroxysmal dyskinesias:** a heterogeneous group of disorders that have in common *sudden abnormal involuntary movements* out of a background of normal motor behavior; may be *choreic, ballistic, dystonic, or a combination* of these

Features	Paroxysmal kinesogenic dyskinesia	Paroxysmal nonkinesogenic dyskinesia	Paroxysmal exertion-induced dyskinesia	Paroxysmal hypnogenic dyskinesia
Inheritance	AD or sporadic	AD or sporadic	AD	AD or sporadic
Male to female ratio	4:1	1.5:1.0	1:2	—
Age at onset	<1 1–40 yrs	<1–30 yrs	2–20 yrs	10–40 yrs

Features	Paroxysmal kinesogenic dyskinesia	Paroxysmal nonkinesogenic dyskinesia	Paroxysmal exertion-induced dyskinesia	Paroxysmal hypnogenic dyskinesia
Attacks				
Duration	<5 mins	2 mins–4 hrs	5–30 mins	Seconds to minutes
Frequency	100/day–1/mo	2/day–2/yr	1/day–2/mo	5/night–2/yr
Trigger	Sudden movement/startle, hyperventilation	None	Prolonged exercise, vibration, passive movement, cold	Nonrapid eye movement sleep
Precipitant	Stress	Alcohol, stress, caffeine, fatigue	Stress	Stress, menses
Treatment	Anticonvulsants, acetazolamide	Clonazepam, oxazepam	L-Dopa	Anticonvulsants, acetazolamide

IV. **Myoclonus:** sudden, brief, shock-like involuntary movements caused by muscular contraction (*positive myoclonus*) or inhibitions (*negative myoclonus*), usually arising from the central nervous system; stimulus sensitive myoclonus is termed *reflex myoclonus,* and action-sensitive myoclonus is termed *action* (or *intention*) *myoclonus;* can be classified according to the distribution: *focal or segmental* (confined to one particular region of the body), *multifocal* (different parts of the body affected, not necessarily at the same time), or *generalized* (whole body part affected in a single jerk); can also be broadly classified as symptomatic or essential myoclonus; may be rhythmic, in which case, it is referred to by some as *tremor,* but more *typically, it is arrhythmic*

   A. **Cortical myoclonus** (frequently multifocal, rather than focal): the jerks are usually more distal than proximal and more flexor than extensor; typically, stimulus sensitive and may be precipitated by sudden loud noise or a visual stimulus; *etiology:* any type of focal cortical lesion, including tumors, angiomas, and encephalitis, may be associated with focal cortical myoclonus, rarely, Huntington's disease; *epilepsia partialis continua* refers to repetitive focal cortical myoclonus with some rhythmicity; etiology: can occur in focal encephalitis (e.g., Rasmussen's syndrome), stroke, tumors, and, rarely, in multiple sclerosis

   B. **Palatal myoclonus:** usually rhythmic, continuous, independent of rest, action, sleep, or distraction; may occur unilaterally or bilaterally; may involve other muscles, including those of the eye, tongue, neck, and diaphragm; etiology: stroke, encephalitis, tumors, multiple sclerosis, trauma, and neurodegenerative disorders

NB: Palatal myoclonus usually is a result of a lesion affecting the dentatorubrothalamic tract!

   C. **Spinal myoclonus**
      1. *Spinal segmental myoclonus:* affecting a restricted body part, involving a few spinal segments
      2. *Propriospinal myoclonus:* producing generalized axial jerks, usually beginning in the abdominal muscles; etiology: inflammatory myelopathy, cervical spondylosis, tumors, trauma, ischemic myelopathy, and a variety of other causes

D. **Multifocal myoclonus:** individual jerks affecting different parts of the body; generalized myoclonus: each jerk affects a large area or the entire body; generalized myoclonus may be triggered by external stimuli and aggravated by action; *etiologies* (multifocal and generalized) include spinocerebellar degenerations, mitochondrial disease (myoclonic epilepsy with ragged red fibers), storage diseases (e.g., GM_2 gangliosidosis), ceroid lipofuscinosis, sialidosis, and dementias (e.g., Creutzfeldt-Jakob disease and AD), viral and postviral syndromes; multifocal myoclonus is frequently due to metabolic causes, including hepatic failure, uremia, hyponatremia, hypoglycemia, and nonketotic hyperglycemia; toxic encephalopathies causing myoclonus include bismuth, methyl bromide, and toxic cooking oil; *Lance-Adams syndrome* refers to action myoclonus occurring after hypoxic brain injury with associated asterixis, seizures, and gait problems

E. **Reflex myoclonus:** may be seen in PD, multiple system atrophy, cortical-basal ganglionic degeneration, and Rett's and Angelman's syndrome
  1. A variant of cortical reflex myoclonus is *cortical tremor,* which results in fine, shivering finger twitching provoked mainly by action and posture phenomenologically similar to essential tremor; cortical tremor may be familial
  2. *Reticular reflex myoclonus:* the origin of electrical discharge is usually in the brain stem, proximal muscles are more affected than distal ones, and flexors are more active than extensors; reflex myoclonus

F. **Progressive myoclonic epilepsies:** a combination of severe myoclonus, generalized tonic-clonic or other seizures, and progressive neurologic decline, particularly dementia and ataxia; in the *adult, dentatorubropallidoluysian atrophy* is a consideration; *in the young, the following five conditions* may cause progressive myoclonic epilepsy
  1. *Lafora body disease:* characterized by polyglucosan–Schiff-positive inclusion bodies in the brain, liver, muscle, or skin (eccrine sweat gland)
  2. *Neuronal ceroid lipofuscinosis (Batten disease):* presents with seizures, myoclonus, and dementia, along with blindness (in the childhood forms); characterized by curvilinear inclusion bodies in the brain, eccrine glands, muscle, and gut
  3. *Unverricht-Lundborg disease:* characterized by stimulus-sensitive myoclonus, tonic-clonic seizures, a characteristic electroencephalography (paroxysmal generalized spike-wave activity and photosensitivity), ataxia, and mild dementia with an onset at around age 5–15 years
  4. *Myoclonic epilepsy with ragged red fibers:* maternally inherited, diagnosed by increased serum and CSF lactate and ragged red fibers on muscle biopsy
  5. *Sialidosis:* a lysosomal storage disorder associated with a cherry-red spot by funduscopy and dysmorphic facial features

G. **Progressive myoclonic ataxias:** also known as *Ramsay-Hunt syndrome;* seizures and dementia being mild to absent, with myoclonus and ataxia as the major problems; has a much wider span of presentation, ranging from the 1st–7th decade; may be due either to recognizable etiology or to neurodegenerative disease; *etiology:* mitochondrial encephalomyopathy, celiac disease, late-onset neuronal ceroid lipofuscinosis, biotin-responsive encephalopathy, adult Gaucher's disease, action myoclonus renal failure syndrome, May-White syndrome, and Ekbom syndrome, neurodegenerative diseases (pure spinocerebellar degeneration, spinocerebellar plus dentatorubral degeneration, olivopontocerebellar atrophy, or dentatorubropallidoluysian atrophy)

H. **Opsoclonus-myoclonus syndrome:** results in random chaotic saccadic eye movements in association with multifocal and generalized myoclonus; *in adults: idiopathic in approximately 50% of cases; second most common cause is paraneoplastic,* usually from ovarian cancer, melanoma, renal cell carcinoma, and lymphoma; in younger patients, can be idiopathic, associated with viral infections, such as Epstein-Barr virus; *neuroblastoma is a major consideration in children,* mainly in tumors with diffuse and extensive lymphocytic infiltration and lymphoid follicles; other causes include drugs, toxins, and nonketotic hyperglycemia

I. **Myoclonus-dystonia syndrome:** a genetically heterogeneous *AD* disorder with reduced penetrance and variable expression; characterized by proximal bilateral myoclonic jerks, mainly involving the arms and axial muscles; a mild dystonia often presents as cervical dystonia or writer's cramp; the myoclonus can be rhythmic or arrhythmic, action provoked, asymmetric, and *may (or may not) be alcohol responsive*

J. **Startle syndromes:** characterized by an exaggerated startle response to a surprise stimulus; *hyperekplexia* refers to a familial condition in which symptoms start in infancy; enhanced startle response occurs to any type of stimulus, with generalized stiffening and falling to the ground

K. **Myoclonic seizures:** in children, major syndromes include *infantile spasms* and *Lennox-Gastaut syndrome;* it is important to distinguish infantile spasms from benign myoclonus of infancy in which electroencephalography is normal and the course is nonprogressive

L. **Asterixis:** results in lapses of maintained postures and is considered a form of negative myoclonus; usually occurs in conjunction with multifocal myoclonus in the setting of a metabolic encephalopathy and is generalized; focal asterixis may be seen in lesions of the thalamus, the putamen, and the parietal lobe

V. Dystonia: sustained muscle contractions, frequently causing twisting and repetitive movements or abnormal postures; distribution: *focal* (e.g., writer's cramp, blepharospasm, torticollis, spasmodic dysphonia), *segmental* (Meige's syndrome), *multifocal, generalized;* early onset usually starts in the leg or arm and frequently progresses to involve the other limbs or trunk; late onset: usually starts in the neck, cranial muscles, or arm and tends to remain localized with restricted spread to adjacent muscles

A. **Primary (idiopathic) torsional dystonia:** dystonia is the only sign; **child or adolescent limb onset:** often spreads to other limbs, may also involve the trunk, neck, and, more rarely, cranial muscles, many due *to TOR1A (DYT1) GAG deletion;* **mixed phenotype:** child or adult onset in limb, neck, or cranial muscles, dysarthria/dysphonia common; in Swiss Mennonite families: *chromosome 8 (DYT6);* **early-onset segmental cervical/cranial:** *chromosome 1p (DYT 13);* **adult cervical, cranial, or brachial onset:** *chromosome 18 (DYT 7)*

B. **Secondary dystonia**

1. *Dystonia-plus disorders:* dystonia is a prominent sign but associated with other features

   a. *Dopa-responsive dystonia* (GCHI mutations [DRD or DYT5], other biopterin-deficient states, tyrosine hydroxylase mutations, dopamine agonist-responsive dystonia due to decarboxylase deficiency)

   b. *Myoclonus dystonia:* many due to *epsilon-sarcoglycan mutations (DYT 11) on chromosome 7*

   c. *Rapid-onset dystonia-parkinsonism (DYT 12)*

2. *AD*

   a. Huntington's disease

   b. SCA type 3 (Machado-Joseph's disease)

   c. Dentatorubropallidoluysian atrophy

   d. Familial basal ganglia calcifications

   e. SCA type 1

3. *AR*

   a. Juvenile parkinsonism

   b. **NB: Wilson's disease:** can present with any movement disorder; *Kayser-Fleischer* rings (yellow-brown copper deposits in the cornea); *AR, mutation in the copper trans-*

porting P-type ATP7B gene on chromosome 13; diagnosis: decreased serum ceruloplasmin, increased 24-hour urine copper excretion, liver biopsy, slit lamp; affects mostly young patients (median age 8-20); half with liver disease; neurological manifestations: resting and intention tremors, spasticity, rigidity, dystonia, chorea; psychiatric disturbances are present in the majority of patients; penicillamine is the drug of choice (symptoms may worsen in the first months of treatment); trientine or zinc are alternatives

   c. Neuroacanthocytosis (can also be AD or X-linked)

   d. Glutaric aciduria

   e. Hallervorden-Spatz syndrome

   f. Methylmalonic aciduria

   g. Metachromatic leukodystrophy

   h. GM_1 and GM_2 gangliosidoses

   i. Homocystinuria

   j. Hartnup's disease

   k. Dystonic lipidosis

   l. Ceroid lipofuscinosis

   m. Ataxia telangiectasia

   n. Intraneuronal inclusion disease

  4. *X-linked recessive*

   a. **Lubag**: Filipino X-linked dystonia parkinsonism, DYT3

   b. Lesch-Nyhan syndrome

   c. Mitochondrial (myoclonic epilepsy with ragged red fibers, mitochondrial encephalomyopathy with lactic acidosis and stroke-like episodes, Leber's disease)

  5. *Acquired dystonias:* peripheral nerve injury, encephalitis, head trauma, pontine myelinolysis, primary antiphospholipid syndrome, stroke, tumor, multiple sclerosis, cervical cord injury, drugs (dopamine receptor-blocking agents, levodopa, and other antiparkinsonian agents), toxins, psychogenic, anoxia

C. *Genetics*

Dystonia type	Gene	Inheritance	Chromosome	Gene product/mutation
Early-onset generalized torsion dystonia	DYT 1	AD	9q34	GAG deletion in the DYT1 gene results in the loss of 1 glutamic acid residue in Torsin A
Autosomal recessive torsion dystonia	DYT 2	AR	Unknown	Unknown
X-linked dystonia parkinsonism	DYT 3	X-linked	Xq13.1	Unknown
Non-DYT1 torsion dystonia	DYT 4	AD	Unknown	Unknown
Dopa-responsive dystonia and parkinsonism (Segawa syndrome)	DYT 5	AD	14q22.1-22.2	Mutation in the GTP cyclohydrolasel gene
Adolescent and early adult torsion dystonia of mixed phenotype	DYT 6	AD	8p21-22	Unknown

Dystonia type	Gene	Inheritance	Chromosome	Gene product/mutation
Late-onset focal dystonia	DYT 7	AD	18p	Unknown
Paroxysmal nonkine-sogenic dyskinesia	DYT 8	AD	2q	Unknown
Paroxysmal choreoathetosis with episodic ataxia and spasticity	DYT 9	AD	1p21-13.3	Unknown
Paroxysmal kinesogenic dyskinesia	DYT 10	AD	16p11.2-12.1	Unknown
Myoclonus-dystonia	DYT 11	AD	7q21-31	Mutation in epsilon-sarcoglycan
Rapid-onset dystonia parkinsonism	DYT 12	AD	19q	Unknown
Early- and late-onset cervical cranial dystonia	DYT 13	AD	1p36.13	Unknown

VI. Ataxia

  A. **Friedreich's ataxia:** classic phenotype: *progressive gait disturbance, gait ataxia, loss of proprioception in the lower limbs, areflexia, dysarthria and extensor plantar responses* with an age of onset <25 years; electrocardiography: early repolarization; echocardiograms: hypertrophic cardiomyopathy; diabetes mellitus in fewer than one-half the patients; also with skeletal deformities, such as scoliosis and pes cavus; mutation is an *unstable expansion of a GAA repeat in the first intron of the gene X25 on chromosome 9q12-21.1, leading to deficiency of the protein frataxin;* treatment: coenzyme Q10 and vitamin E may improve cardiac and skeletal muscle bioenergetics, idebenone (a coenzyme Q10 analog) may have benefit on cardiomyopathy

NB: The clinical findings are secondary to involvement of spinocerebellar and corticospinal tracts, dorsal columns, and a peripheral neuropathy.

  B. **Ataxia-telangiectasia:** *(Louis-Bar syndrome): AR; chromosome 11q22-23; characterized by progressive cerebellar ataxia, oculocutaneous telangiectasia, abnormalities in cellular and humoral immunity, and recurrent viral and bacterial infections;* neurologic manifestations: cerebellar ataxia, nystagmus; chorea, athetosis, dystonia, oculomotor apraxia, impassive facies; decreased deep tendon reflexes and distal muscular atrophy; intelligence progressively deteriorates; polyneuropathy; other manifestations: immunodeficiency (thymic hypoplasia); patients lack helper T cells, but suppressor T cells are normal; immunoglobulin A is absent in 75% of patients, immunoglobulin E in 85%, immunoglobulin G is low; α-fetoprotein and carcinoembryonic antigen are elevated; ovarian agenesis, testicular hypoplasia, and insulin-resistant diabetes; malignant neoplasms in 10–15% of patients; most common are lymphoreticular neoplasm and leukemia; death by 2nd decade from neoplasia or infection

NB: Recurrent infections are frequently the presenting finding in ataxia-telangiectasia.

C. *AR ataxias with known gene loci*

Disease	Chromosome	Gene	Mutation
Friedreich's ataxia	9q13-21.1	X25/frataxin	GAA expansion
Ataxia-telangiectasia	11q22-23	ATM	Point mutations/deletions
Ataxia with isolated vitamin E deficiency	8q	α TTP	Point mutations
AR ataxia of Charlevoix-Saguenay	13q11	SACS	Point mutations
Ataxia with oculomotor apraxia	9p13	Aprataxin	Point mutations/deletions/insertions
Ataxia, neuropathy, high α fetoprotein	9q33-34	Unknown	Unknown
Infantile onset olivo-pontocerebellar atrophy	10q24	Unknown	Unknown
Ataxia, deafness, optic atrophy	6p21-23	Unknown	Unknown
Unverricht-Lundborg disease	21q	Cystatin B	Repeat expansion

D. **AD ataxias:** present between 3rd and 5th decades of life but with a wide range; male to male transmission is the sine quo non of AD inheritance; large clinical overlap between each type

Disease	Chromosome	Gene	Mutation	Additional features
SCA 1	6p23	Ataxin-1	CAG expansion	Young adult; upper motor neuron signs; late chorea
SCA 2	12q23-24.1	Ataxin-2	CAG expansion	Young adult; upper motor neuron signs (rare); parkinsonian; late chorea; very slow saccades; areflexia
SCA 3/Machado-Josephs disease	14q21	Ataxin-3	CAG expansion	Young adult; upper motor neuron signs; parkinsonian; late chorea
SCA 4	16q24	—	—	Areflexia
SCA 5	11p11-q11	—	—	—
SCA 6	19p	CACNA1	CAG expansion	Older adult; benign course; downbeat nystagmus
SCA 7	3p21.2-12	Ataxin-7	CAG expansion	Childhood onset; upper motor neuron signs; very slow saccades; vision loss; seizures

Disease	Chromosome	Gene	Mutation	Additional features
SCA 8	13q21	—	CAG expansion	Upper motor neuron signs
SCA 10	22q13	—	—	Seizures
SCA 11	15q14-21.3	—	ATTCT expansion	—
SCA 12	5q31-33	PP2R2B	CAG expansion	Action tremor
SCA 13	10q13.3-13.4	—	—	—
SCA 14	19q13.4	—	—	—
SCA 16	8q23-24.1	—	—	Action tremor
SCA 17	6p21	TBP	CAG expansion	Parkinsonian
Dentatorubro-pallidoluysian atrophy	12p	Atrophin	CAG expansion	Childhood onset; chorea; seizures
Episodic ataxia 1	12p	KCNA 1	Point mutations in ion channels	Short-lived intermittent ataxia; interictally with myokymia
NB: Episodic ataxia 2	19p	CACNA 1	Point mutations in ion channels	Longer-duration intermittent ataxia; downbeat nystagmus; similar to SCA 6; associated with migraine; aceta-zolamide reduces frequency of attacks

NB: Despite the motor findings seen in Machado-Josephs disease, cognitive function is usually not affected.

E. *Metabolic disorders:* maple syrup urine disease, Hartnup's disease, pyruvate decarboxylase deficiency, arginosuccinic aciduria, hypothyroidism, Leigh disease

VII. Tremors

Type	Characteristic	Frequency (Hz)
Parkinsonian tremor	Rest >> posture = action	3–6
Enhanced physiologic tremor	Action = posture	8–12
Essential tremor	Action > posture >> rest	4–10
Cerebellar tremor	Action	2–4
Rubral tremor	Posture = action > rest	2–5
NB: Orthostatic tremor	Only when standing still; relieved by walking or sitting	15–18
Dystonic tremor	Posture = action >> rest	4–8
Palatal tremor	Rest	1–6
Neuropathic tremor	Posture >> action	5–9

ADDITIONAL NOTES

CHAPTER 6

Demyelinating Disorders

I. Definition: The commonly accepted pathologic criteria for demyelinating disease are
  A. Destruction of myelin sheaths or nerve fibers.
  B. Relative sparing of other elements of nervous tissue, such as axis cylinders.
  C. Infiltration of inflammatory cells in a perivascular distribution.
  D. Distribution is perivenous, primarily in white matter.
  E. Lack of wallerian degeneration or secondary degeneration of fiber tracts (due to integrity of the axis cylinders).
  F. Caveat of criteria, *Schilder's disease* and *necrotizing hemorrhagic leukoencephalitis* may have *damage to axis cylinders as well as myelin.*
  G. Subacute combined degeneration, tropical spastic hemiparesis, progressive multifocal leukoencephalopathy, central pontine myelinolysis, and Marchiafava-Bignami disease were not included because of their known etiology—they are part of either viral or nutritional deficiency; metabolic deficiencies with white matter involvement are also excluded.

II. Neuroimmunology

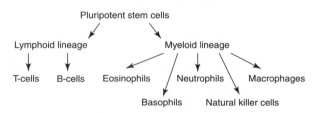

Figure 6-1. Differentiation of stem cells.

  A. **B-lymphocytes:** develop in the *bone marrow*; acquire immunoglobulin (Ig) receptors that commit them to a specific antigen; express IgM on the surface; after antigen challenge, T-lymphocytes assist B-lymphocytes either directly or indirectly through secretion of helper factors to differentiate and form mature antibody secreting plasma cells
  B. **Igs:** glycoproteins; secretory *products of plasma cells*; the heavy chain on Fc portion determines class: IgM, IgD, IgG, IgA, and IgE; *activates complement cascade: IgM, IgG1, and IgG3*
  C. **T-lymphocytes:** *thymus derived; CD4: helper cell; CD8: cytotoxic/suppressor cells;* specificity of T-cells is to the foreign major histocompatibility complex (MHC) antigens; *CD2 and CD3: T-cell activation*
  D. **Natural killer cells:** *lymphocytes; lack immunologic memory;* have the ability to kill tumor or virus-infected cells without any MHC restriction; ?role in tumor immunity
  E. **MHC and HLA:** HLA lies on the short arm of *chromosome 6*; four major loci: *class I* (on all nucleated cells; HLA-A, HLA-B, HLA-C) and *class II* (on macrophages, B-cells, activated T-cells; HLA-DR, -DQ, -DP); class I antigens regulate the specificity of cytotoxic T-cells (CD8) and act on viruses; class II antigens regulate the specificity of helper T-cells (CD4),

then CD4 regulates hypersensitivity and antibody response; examples: *HLA-DR2 (multiple sclerosis [MS] among white Northern Europeans), HLA-DR3 (young myasthenic without thymoma), HLA-DR2 (narcolepsy)*

F. **Regulation of immune response**
   1. Antigen cleared from immune system
   2. Formation of antigen-antibody complex, which inhibits B-cell differentiation and proliferation
   3. Idiotypic regulation: variable region on Ig molecule expresses proteins that are new and can act as antigens
   4. Suppressor T-cells

G. **Lymphokines** (cytokines): *secreted products of immune cells*
   1. *Growth factors:* interleukin-1, -2, -3, -4; colony-stimulating factors
   2. *Activation factors:* interferons (α, β, and γ)
   3. *Lymphotoxins:* tumor necrosis factors

III. MS

A. **Disseminated sclerosis, sclerose en plaques:** protean clinical manifestations; usually a course of remission and relapse, but occasionally intermittently progressive or steadily progressive (especially in those >40 y/o)

B. **Pathology:** grossly, numerous pink-gray (due to myelin loss) lesions scattered surrounding white matter; vary in diameter; do not extend beyond root entry zones of cranial or spinal nerves
   1. *Periventricular localization:* characteristic, in which subependymal veins line ventricles
   2. Other favored structures: *optic nerves, chiasm, spinal cord;* distributed randomly through brain stem, spinal cord, cerebellar peduncles
   3. Astrocytic reaction: *perivascular infiltration with mononuclear cells and lymphocytes; sparing of axis cylinders* prevents wallerian degeneration

C. *Etiology and epidemiology:* prevalence is <1 per 100,000 in equatorial areas, 6–14 per 100,000 in southern United States, 30–80 per 100,000 in Canada, northern Europe, and northern United States; in southern hemisphere: less well defined; in the United States: blacks at lower risk; few "epidemics" reported
   1. *Migration:* before age 15 years, carries risk from native land
   2. *Familial tendency* also now established: 15% have an affected relative; *HLA-DR2, DQW1, b1, a1, to a lesser extent -DR3, -B7, and -A3,* on chromosome 6 are over-represented in MS; low conjugal incidence (supports disease occurring early in life); 1st-degree relatives have a 10–20-fold greater risk
   3. Low incidence in children, peak at age 30 years, falling sharply in the 6th decade; two-thirds with onset between ages 20 and 40 years; ?greater in rural than urban dwellers
   4. Popular view is that initial event is a viral infection of the nervous system with secondary activation by autoimmune reaction; role of *humoral system* is evident by presence of *oligoclonal immune proteins in cerebrospinal fluid (CSF)* that are produced by B-lymphocytes
   5. *Cellular factor* is demonstrated by abundance of *helper T-cells (CD4$^+$)* in MS plaques; T-cells react to antigens presented by MHC class II on macrophages and astrocytes → stimulate T-cell proliferation, activation of B-cells, macrophages → secretion of cytokines (e.g., interferon β) → breakdown of blood-brain barrier, destruction of oligodendrocytes and myelin
   6. *Physiologic effects of demyelination:* impede saltatory conduction; temporary induction by heat or exercise of symptoms (*Uhthoff phenomenon*); rise of 0.5°C can block electrical

transmission; smoking, fatigue, and rise in environmental temperature all can cause worsening of symptoms

D. ***Clinical manifestations:*** weakness and numbness, both in one or more limbs, are the initial symptoms in one-half the patients; useful adage that patient with MS presents with symptoms of one leg with signs in both; *Lhermitte sign:* passive flexion of the neck induces a tingling, electric-like feeling down the shoulders and legs; two particular syndromes are among the most typical modes of onset

1. **Optic neuritis**: in 25% of all MS patients, this is the initial manifestation; characteristically, rapid evolution over several hours to days of partial or total loss of vision, pain within the orbit, worsened by eye movement and palpation

   a. *Cecocentral scotoma* (macular area and blind spot) can be demonstrated, as well as other field defects.

   b. Evidence of swelling/edema of nerve head (*papillitis*) in one-half of cases (distinguished from papilledema by severe vision loss).

   c. One-third recover completely, most improve significantly; dyschromatopsia is a frequent persistent finding; one-half or more who present with optic neuritis eventually develop MS; risk is lower in childhood.

   d. *Uveitis and sheathing of retinal veins* (due to T-cell infiltration) are other ophthalmologic findings in MS.

NB: After an episode of optic neuritis, the best predictor of subsequent MS is an abnormal MRI of the brain (and not CSF findings)!

2. **Acute transverse myelitis**: transverse is imprecise: usually asymmetric and incomplete; clinically: *rapidly evolving* (several hours to days) paraparesis, sensory level on the trunk, sphincteric dysfunction, bilateral Babinski signs; CSF: may show modest increase in lymphocytes and protein

NB: Patients with transverse myelitis are at risk for developing MS. However, the presence of partial rather than complete myelitis puts a patient at higher risk for progression to MS! The strongest predictor of subsequent MS is the presence of subclinical lesions on imaging at the time of initial presentation.

3. Other patterns of MS: unsteadiness in walking, brain stem symptoms (diplopia, vertigo, vomiting), disorders of micturition; discrete manifestations: hemiplegia, trigeminal neuralgia, pain syndromes, facial paralysis, deafness, or seizures, or (in the elderly) slowly progressive cervical myelopathy; *Charcot's triad:* nystagmus, scanning speech, intention tremor; *one-and-a-half syndrome:* intranuclear ophthalmoplegia in one direction and horizontal gaze paresis in the other

NB: The paramedian pontine reticular formation is usually involved in the one-and-a-half syndrome, besides the medial longitudinal fasciculus.

4. *Symptoms and signs of established stage of disease:* one-half manifest with a mix of generalized type (involvement of optic nerves, brain stem, cerebellum, and spinal cord); 30–40% with spinal form; 5% each have predominantly cerebellar or pontobulbar-cerebellar form or amaurotic form; some have euphoria (stupid indifference, morbid optimism), but larger group has depression; global dementia (more subcortical, with prominent frontal lobe syndrome and abulia) or confusional-psychotic state in advanced stage; 2–3% have seizures

5. *Clinical course*

Type	Percent
Benign	30
Malignant	10
Neurologic dysfunction	60
Relapsing remitting	35
Relapsing progressive	45
Chronic progressive	20

E. **Variants**
   1. *Acute MS:* highly *malignant* form; combination of cerebral, brain stem, spinal manifestations evolves over a few weeks, rendering the patient stuporous, comatose, or decerebrate; death in a few weeks to months, without remission; lesions are of macroscopic dimensions, typical of acute plaques—only difference: plaques are of the same age and more prominent confluence; CSF: shows a brisk cellular response

NB: The malignant form of MS is also known as the Marburg's variant.

   2. *Neuromyelitis optica:* simultaneous or successive involvement of *optic nerves and spinal cord;* acute or subacute blindness of one or both eyes preceded or followed within days or weeks by transverse or ascending myelitis; sometimes, the spinal cord lesions are necrotizing rather than demyelinating (i.e., more permanent); usually children, only one episode of illness; usually a form of MS, but acute disseminated encephalomyelitis, acute MS, acute necrotizing hemorrhagic leukoencephalitis and leukomyelitis may conform with this pattern; *corticosteroid or plasma exchange* for active neuromyelitis optica relapses; antiplatelets and anticoagulant should be considered in neuromyelitis optica cases with IgG antiphospholipid antibodies
F. **Lab findings**
   1. One-third of patients with MS with slight to moderate mononuclear pleocytosis (<50); in rapidly progressive, may reach or exceed 100–1000; hyperacute cases may have polymorphonucleocytes; 40% have slight increase in total protein in CSF; proportion of γ globulin (IgG) is increased >12% to the total protein in two-thirds; *IgG index:* ratio of >1.7 indicates the probability of MS; IgG index and oligoclonal bands are also increased in syphilis and subacute sclerosing panencephalitis; high concentrations of *myelin basic protein* during acute exacerbations; at present, measurement of γ *globulins and oligoclonal bands are the most reliable chemical tests for MS*

NB: Neuromyelitis optica usually does not present with oligoclonal bands in CSF.

   2. Other tests: *visual-evoked potentials* (80% in clinical features of definite MS, 60% in probable); *somatosensory evoked* (69% in definite and 51% in probable); *brain stem auditory-evoked responses* (47% in definite and 20% in probable); on *magnetic resonance imaging (MRI),* several asymmetric, well-demarcated lesions, immediately adjacent to the ventricular surface; display contrast enhancement when acute
G. **Diagnosis**
   1. *Schumacher's criteria*
      a. Two separate central nervous system lesions
      b. Two separate attacks or 6 months progression

    c. Objective findings on examination

    d. White matter disease

    e. Usually 10–50 y/o

    f. No other disease that explains the constellation of signs and symptoms

  2. Lab and imaging serve as confirmatory tests

  3. McDonald Criteria for MS

Disease episodes	Objective lesions	Additional requirements
2 or more	2 or more	None
2 or more	1	Dissemination is space by MRI or + CSF AND 2 or more MRI lesions consistent with MS, OR another attack involving a different site
1	2 or more	Dissemination in time by MRI OR another clinical attack
1	1	Dissemination in space AND time by MRI, OR another attack, OR MRI space dissemination AND + CSF
0 (progressive from onset)	1	+ CSF and specific MRI dissemination in space criteria AND MRI dissemination in time OR continuous progression for 1 year

H. *Differential diagnosis*

  1. Acute disseminated encephalomyelitis

  2. Elsberg sacral radiculopathy

  3. Vitamin B$_{12}$ deficiency

  4. Rheumatoid arthritis (collagen vascular disease)

  5. Sarcoid

  6. Human T-cell lymphotrophic virus (tropical spastic paraparesis)

  7. Adult-onset adrenoleukodystrophy

  8. Primary lateral sclerosis

I. *Treatment*

  1. *Adrenocorticotropic hormone, methylprednisolone, prednisone, cyclophosphamide* may be beneficial; however, there is no strong evidence that steroids alter the ultimate course of MS or prevent relapses; high dose often used initially to be effective; attempt to limit the period of corticosteroid administration to <3 weeks but prolong the taper if neurologic signs return.

  2. *For optic neuritis, intravenous methylprednisolone* for 3 days followed by oral prednisone for 11 days speeds the recovery from vision loss (compared to placebo or 14 days of oral prednisone), although there was no significant difference after 6 months as compared with placebo (The Optic Neuritis Treatment Trial).

  3. *For chronic, progressive phase* of the disease, MS study group reports modest benefit from *prednisolone plus cyclophosphamide* (however, burdensome and with potentially serious complications).

  4. Interferons: several mechanisms—antiproliferative effect, blocking of T-cell activation, apoptosis of autoreactive T cells, interferon gamma antagonism, cytokine shifts, antiviral effect.

    a. **Interferon β-1b (Betaseron®):** reduces the number and severity of exacerbations; reduces lesion load on MRI; for secondary progressive MS, interferon β-1b showed minor effect on delaying disability for a few months despite clear evidence of durable effect on reducing relapses; dosage: *8 million U subcutaneously every other day;* complete blood cell count, liver function tests every 3 months; side effects: local skin reaction (inflammation, thickening, and necrosis), flu-like symptoms (usually within the first 2 weeks), fatigue, decreased white blood cell count, platelets, and hematocrit, increased γ-glutamyltransferase, serum glutamic-oxaloacetic transaminase, depression

b. **Interferon β-1a (Avonex®):** slows accumulation of physical disability and decreases frequency of exacerbation; dosage: *30 mg intramuscularly every week;* complete blood cell count, platelets, fluid balance profile at least every 6 months; side effects: flu-like symptoms, injection site reactions, myalgias, fever, chills, headache, depression, bronchospasm, anxiety; Interferon β-1a (Rebif®): Early Treatment Of Multiple Sclerosis trial, even very low doses of **Rebif** (22 μg *subcutaneously three times a week*) delays the second event

5. **Glatiramer acetate (copaxone/copolymer-1):**
   a. Act by blocking autoimmune T cells, induction of energy, induction of anti-inflammatory Th2 cells, bystander suppression, possibly neuroprotection
   b. Reduces frequency of relapses; dosage: *20 mg subcutaneously daily;* side effects: injection site reactions, immediate postinjection reaction (10%), transient chest pain (26%), anxiety, arthralgias, asthenia, vasodilatation, hypertonia

6. **Mitoxantrone**: Mitoxantrone In Multiple Sclerosis study led to U.S. Food and Drug Administration (FDA) indication for use in aggressive MS; dosage: *5 mg/m² or 12 mg/m² every 12 weeks for 24 months (eight infusions).*

NB: Risk of cardiomyopathy.

NB: Mitoxantrone is the only FDA-approved drug for the treatment of secondary progressive MS and for relapsing progressive MS.

7. *Natalizumab:* recombinant monoclonal antibody; first selective immunomodulator in the treatment of MS; blocks the molecular interaction of alpha-4-beta-1 intergin with vascular cell adhesion molecule-1 on vascular endothelial cells, thus preventing adhesion of activated T-cells to endothelium and prevents transmigration of lymphocytes to the CNS; AFFIRM study demonstrated the rate of clinical relapse was reduced by 68% and number of new MRI lesions was reduced by 83%; SENTINEL trial suggested that combination therapy is nearly as effective as natalizumab alone; however, two reported cases of PML has restricted its use.

8. *Other immunomodulators: azathioprine, methotrexate, cyclophosphamide* (pulse monthly treatments were associated with a small but significant reduction in progression in >30% of patients), *cyclosporine, linomide* (may cause cardiotoxicity and myocardial infarction), *sulfasalazine, cladribine (Leustatin®); monoclonal antibody therapy using anti-CD11/CD18:* no difference with placebo; *intravenous Ig:* a large phase III trial failed to demonstrate a treatment benefit of intravenous Ig in secondary progressive MS.

9. *Plasma exchange:* seven alternate-day plasma exchanges hasten at least a moderate clinical improvement in 40% of steroid-unresponsive patients with *acute catastrophic demyelinating illness;* complications: anemia, sepsis, hypotension, heparin-induced thrombocytopenia with hemorrhage.

10. *General measures:* adequate bed rest, prevention of fatigue, infection, use of all rehabilitative measures to postpone bedridden stage; *fatigue* responds to amantadine, 100 mg morning and noon, and pemoline, 20–75 mg each morning, or modafinil, 100 mg once

or twice daily; *bladder dysfunction:* urinary retention use bethanecol chloride; residual urine up to 100 mL are generally well-tolerated; for spastic bladder, propantheline or oxybutynin may relax detrusor muscle; *spastic paralysis:* intrathecal baclofen; oral baclofen, tizanidine, clonazepam, botulinum toxin type A; *surgical procedures:* rhizotomy, myelotomy, crushing of obturator nerves; *disabling tremor:* ventrolateral thalamotomy; isoniazid, 300–1200 mg with 100 mg of B_6 (for severe postural tremor); limited success with carbamazepine and clonazepam.

11. *Specialized, multidisciplinary team approach* to patient with active treatment issues; outpatient and intensive inpatient programs, combined with postdischarge outpatient services improve patient outcomes.

IV. Diffuse Cerebral Sclerosis of Schilder *(Schilder's disease, encephalitis periaxialis diffusa)*: more frequent in children and adolescent life; nonfamilial, run a progressive course, either steady or punctuated by a series of rapid worsening; dementia, homonymous hemianopia, cerebral blindness, deafness, hemiplegia/quadriplegia, pseudobulbar palsy; CSF: often no oligoclonal bands, but myelin basic protein found in large quantity; lesion: large, sharply outlined, asymmetric focus of demyelination involving the entire lobe or cerebral hemisphere, crosses the corpus callosum

A. **Concentric sclerosis of Baló:** probably a *variant of Schilder's* disease; distinguishing feature: *alternating* bands of destruction and preservation of myelin

B. **Adrenoleukodystrophy:** may be clinically indistinguishable from Schilder's disease, but *sex-linked* and *adrenal atrophy* are unique

V. Acute Disseminated Encephalomyelitis *(Postinfectious, Postexanthem, Postvaccinal Encephalomyelitis)*: acute, demyelination scattered throughout brain and spinal cord, surround small- and medium-sized veins; axons and nerves are intact; perivenular inflammation and meningeal infiltration; may *precede respiratory infection* (Epstein-Barr, cytomegalovirus, mycoplasma rarely, after influenza and mumps), within a few days of onset of exanthem of measles, rubella, smallpox, chickenpox; after rabies, smallpox, and, rarely, tetanus vaccine

A. *Prognosis:* significant death rate and persistent deficits to those who survive; acute stage is followed by behavioral problems or mental retardation, epilepsy in children; adults make good recoveries; more benign *cerebellitis* clears over several months

B. *Pathogenesis:* unclear; probably immune-mediated complication rather than direct central nervous system infection; lab model: *experimental allergic encephalomyelitis* produces pathology between the 8th and 15th day after sensitization

C. *Clinically:* acute onset of confusion, somnolence, convulsions, headache, fever, neck stiffness; sometimes with ataxia, myoclonus, and choreoathetosis; in myelinic form: partial or complete paraplegia, quadriplegia, loss of bladder and bowel control, generally no fever; in postexanthem encephalomyelitis: 2–4 days after appearance of rash

D. *Treatment:* high-potency steroids (1g/d for 5 days followed by oral prednisone taper over 1 to 2 weeks); plasma exchange (daily for 5 days) and intravenous Ig (0.4 g/kg/d for 5 days) has been anecdotally successful in fulminant cases; use of embryonated duck eggs for rabies vaccine is free of neurologic complications; chemotherapy used as a last resort for severe, fulminant ADEM, based on anecdotal evidence

VI. Acute Necrotizing Hemorrhagic Encephalomyelitis *(Acute Hemorrhagic Leukoencephalitis of Weston Hurst)*: *most fulminant* of demyelinating diseases, affects mostly young adults but also children; almost invariably preceded by respiratory infection; neurologic symptoms appear abruptly with headache, fever, stiff neck, confusion, followed by seizures, hemiplegia, pseudobulbar paralysis, progressively deepening coma; many cases terminate fatally in 2–4 days

A. *Lab:* leukocytosis, elevated erythrocyte sedimentation rate; increased CSF pressure, pleo-cytosis (lymph or poly), increased protein, normal glucose; computed tomography/MRI shows massive lesion in cerebral white matter
B. *Pathology:* white matter is destroyed almost to the point of liquefaction; resembles disseminated encephalomyelitis but with widespread necrosis
C. *Treatment:* corticosteroids; ?plasma exchange

ADDITIONAL NOTES

CHAPTER 7

Infections of the Nervous System

I. Bacterial Meningitis

A. **Pathophysiology**

1. Acute bacterial infection of the leptomeninges, subarachnoid space, underlying cortical tissue, and structures passing through the subarachnoid space

2. Routes of infection
   a. Nasopharynx (most common)
   b. Open trauma/surgical procedure
   c. Sinus infection
   d. Communicating congenital defect

3. Epidemiology
   a. More common in winter
   b. Annual incidence: Overall: 10/100,000; <6 y/o: 90/100,000; ≥6 y/o: 2/100,000
   c. Immunization against *Haemophilus influenzae* has produced a significant reduction in the United States, but *H. influenzae* is a common etiology in developing countries

4. *Etiology*

Neonate (<1 mo)	Infant to young child (1 mo–5 yrs)	Adult (15–60 y/o)	Elderly (>60 y/o)
Gram-negative rod (50–60%)	Group B streptococcus	*Streptococcus pneumoniae* (50%)	*S. pneumoniae* (50%)
Group B streptococcus (30%)	*S. pneumoniae* (20%)	*Neisseria meningitidis* (25%)	*N. meningitidis*
Listeria (2–10%)	*H. influenzae* (50%)	*Staphylococcus* (15%)	*Listeria*
Staphylococcus			Gram-negative bacilli

5. Clinical
   a. Fever
   b. Stiff neck
   c. Diminished level of awareness
   d. Seizures
   e. Focal neurologic deficits
   f. Kernig/Brudzinski sign
   g. Petechial rash *(N. meningitidis)*
   h. Infant: lethargy, seizures, extended fontanel
   i. Complications

       i. Stroke
      ii. Hydrocephalus
     iii. Cranial nerve (CN) palsies
     iv. Disseminated intravascular coagulation (with *N. meningitidis*)
      v. Syndrome of inappropriate secretion of antidiuretic hormone
     vi. Abscess/subdural empyema
  j. Prognosis: fatality in those >15 y/o: 20–25%; fatality in neonates 20%: gram-negative > gram-positive infection

6. Diagnostic testing
  a. Lumbar puncture
    i. Initial cerebrospinal fluid (CSF)
      (A) White blood cell count, 100–10,000 cells/mL, predominantly polymorpho-nuclear cells
      (B) Glucose, <20 mg/dL
      (C) Protein usually elevated
    ii. Gram stain
    iii. Culture: within 48–72 hours after institution of antibiotic therapy, the CSF culture is usually negative
    iv. Detection of bacterial antigen with counterimmunoelectrophoresis, latex agglutination, and limulus lysate

7. Treatment
  a. Supportive
  b. Antibiotics
    i. Always administer immediately if cannot readily perform spinal tap; administration may produce sterile cultures but associated changes in CSF (if necessary, may need to follow CSF parameters)
    ii. Empiric treatment
    (A) Typical empiric treatment
      (1) Ceftriaxone, 2 g q12h, or cefotaxime, 2 g q4h

NB: With the emergence of resistant strains, vancomycin has become part of the initial empiric treatment in meningitis.

        (a) *If* Listeria *suspected (in those <3 months old or >60 y/o; immunosuppressed, alcoholic), add ampicillin*
        (b) *If* Staphylococcus, *add vancomycin*
        (c) *If gram-negative rod, add aminoglycosides*
      (B) **NB**: Role of corticosteroids: a large, randomized trial showed the beneficial effects of 0.15 mg/kg IV q 6 hours for 4 days, in conjunction with antibiotics, of suspected or proven meningitis due to *S. pneumoniae; in kids: dexamethasone, 0.15 mg/kg/day, q6h for 4–7 days should be used in conjunction with antibiotics for suspected or proven Haemophilus influenzae type B to reduce hearing loss*
      (C) *If meningococcal meningitis, prophylaxis with rifampin*
    iii. *Antibiotics for specific bacterial meningitis*

H. influenzae	*S. pneumoniae*	*N. meningitidis*	Gram-negative bacilli	*Staphylococcus species*	*Listeria*
Ampicillin	Penicillin G	Penicillin G	Cefotaxime	Nafcillin	Ampicillin
Cefuroxime	Ampicillin	Ampicillin	Ceftazidime	Oxacillin	

H. influenzae	S. pneumoniae	N. meningitidis	Gram-negative bacilli	Staphylococcus species	Listeria
Ceftriaxone	Chloramphenicol	Chloramphenicol	Ceftriaxone	Cefuroxime	
Cefotaxime	Cefotaxime	Cefuroxime	Amikacin	Vancomycin	
Chloramphenicol	Ceftriaxone	Ceftriaxone		Rifampin	
	Cefuroxime				
	Vancomycin				

8. *Recurrent meningitis*
   a. Evaluate for cranial or spinal defect permitting re-entry
   b. Evaluate for immune deficiency (i.e., human immunodeficiency virus [HIV])
   c. Differential diagnosis
      i. *Behcet's syndrome*
      ii. *Sarcoidosis*
      iii. *Mollaret's meningitis*

II. Viral Infections of the Nervous System
A. **General**
   1. Pathophysiology
      a. Etiologies of aseptic meningitis
         i. Enterovirus: 90% of aseptic meningitis
         ii. Echovirus and coxsackie: late summer and early fall
         iii. Mumps: usually winter and early spring
   2. Clinical
      a. Signs/symptoms
         i. Malaise, anorexia, myalgia, low-grade fever, vomiting, or headache
         ii. Physical examination reveals photophobia, somnolence or irritability, and meningeal irritation
         iii. Systemic features to assess include rash, pharyngitis, lymphadenopathy, arthritis, parotid gland enlargement, or hepatosplenomegaly
         iv. Transverse myelitis with flaccid weakness, reduced/absent reflexes, sensory loss, and bladder dysfunction
   3. Diagnostic procedures
      a. Neuroimaging
         i. Computed tomography (CT)
            (A) May be normal in encephalitis
            (B) 50% of infants with congenital cytomegalovirus (CMV) infection have intracranial (periventricular) calcifications
         ii. Magnetic resonance imaging (MRI)
            (A) More sensitive than CT
            (B) Herpes simplex virus 1 (HSV-1) encephalitis: T2 prolongation or enhancement of the mesial temporal lobe, insular cortex, and cingulate gyrus
            (C) Distinguish viral encephalitis from acute disseminated encephalomyelitis
            (D) Transverse myelopathy: T2 prolongation or cord swelling
      b. Electroencephalography (EEG)
         i. Viral meningitis: normal or nonspecific abnormalities

      ii. Encephalitis: slowing of background rhythms and focal or diffuse epileptiform discharges

         (A) *HSV-1 encephalitis often exhibits temporal slowing or periodic lateralizing epileptiform discharges*

    c. Lumbar puncture for CSF

      i. Viral: lymphocytic pleocytosis ($10–1000/mm^3$), mildly elevated protein, and normal glucose

      ii. Polymerase chain reaction (PCR) available

         (A) HSV

         (B) HIV

         (C) CMV

         (D) Enteroviruses

         (E) Adenoviruses

         (F) Epstein-Barr virus (EBV)

         (G) Varicella zoster virus (VZV)

         (H) Flaviviruses

  4. *Specific antiviral treatment*

Virus	Medication
HSV	Acyclovir
VZV	Acyclovir, valacyclovir, famciclovir
CMV	Ganciclovir, foscarnet, cidofovir
Subacute sclerosing panencephalitis	Isoprinosine
HIV	Highly-active antiretroviral therapy regimen (see section II.B.10)

B. **Specific viral infections of the nervous system**

  1. Herpes viruses

    a. **HSV-1 and HSV-2**

      i. HSV-1

         (A) Usually adolescent/adult

         (B) Transmitted via oral mucosa

         (C) Most common nonepidemic encephalitis

         (D) Latently infects the trigeminal ganglia with reactivation and retrograde transmission to the central nervous system (CNS)

         (E) Exhibits propensity for the frontotemporal regions

      ii. HSV-2

         (A) Usually neonate

         (B) Transmitted sexually or via birth canal to infant

         (C) Involves the brain diffusely via hematogenous transmission

         (D) Causes 70% of neonatal HSV infections

         (E) Common cause of aseptic meningitis in adult women

      iii. Clinical

         (A) HSV encephalitis

            (1) Prodrome of headache, fever, malaise, or vomiting followed by dysphasia, short-term memory dysfunction, hemiparesis, visual field deficits, or partial seizures

        (2) Two presentations
           (a) Can be rapidly progressive with coma and death within 2 weeks
           (b) Indolent, with hallucinations, headache, memory loss, and behavioral disturbances
    (B) Other HSV infections
        (1) Bell's palsy
        (2) Acute myelitis
        (3) Rhombencephalitis
        (4) Aseptic meningitis
        (5) Mollaret's meningitis
    (C) Diagnosis
        (1) CSF
           (a) Lymphocytic pleocytosis and elevated protein content
           (b) HSV PCR
        (2) Neuroimaging
           (a) HSV-1: frontotemporal edema
           (b) HSV-2: diffuse changes
        (3) EEG: slowing, periodic lateralizing epileptiform discharges, or frank epileptiform discharges
        (4) Pathology
           (a) Hemorrhagic encephalitis with neuronal destruction
           (b) Predilection for frontal and temporal regions
           (c) Cowdry A inclusions
               (i) Intranuclear, solitary large viral inclusions with halo due to margination of chromatin
              (ii) Seen in HSV, VZV, CMV, and subacute sclerosing panencephalitis
    (D) Treatment
        (1) HSV-1 encephalitis: acyclovir, 10 mg/kg q8h for minimum of 14–21 days
        (2) HSV-2 in neonates: acyclovir, 20 mg/kg q8h for 3 weeks
    (E) Prognosis
        (1) Mortality of acyclovir-treated neonates still 15%
        (2) Remaining survivors usually have permanent neurologic complications
b. **VZV**
  i. *Chickenpox (varicella)*
    (A) Peak incidence between ages 5 and 9 years
    (B) Respiratory transmission
  ii. *Shingles (herpes zoster)*
    (A) After primary VZV infection, the virus persists in a latent state in the dorsal root ganglia
    (B) Virus reactivates and migrates via axon to the skin, producing shingles (erythematous, maculopapular rash that progresses to vesicles)
    (C) More common among the elderly or immunocompromised
    (D) T5-T10 most commonly affected
    (E) Ramsay-Hunt syndrome: lower CN VII palsy with associated vesicular eruption in the auditory canal
    (F) Diagnosis: Tzanck prep positive
  iii. CNS complications
    (A) Cerebellar ataxia
    (B) Encephalitis

(C) Aseptic meningitis

(D) Brachial plexus neuritis

(E) Acute transverse myelitis

(F) Cortical stroke (associated with herpes zoster ophthalmicus)

(G) Reye syndrome

(H) Acute inflammatory demyelinating polyneuropathy (AIDP)

(I) Basal ganglia infarction

iv. Diagnosis

(A) Isolation of VZV from the oropharynx or skin lesions

(B) VZV-specific antibodies in the CSF

(C) PCR studies of CSF or vesicular fluid

v. Treatment

(A) Immunocompetent

(1) Supportive care

(2) Oral acyclovir can shorten the duration of cutaneous lesions in either herpes zoster or primary varicella infection

NB: Prompt treatment may also reduce the development and potential severity of postherpetic neuralgia if it occurs.

(B) Immunocompromised or herpes zoster ophthalmicus

(1) Intravenous (i.v.) or oral acyclovir

(2) Newer agents: *famciclovir, valacyclovir; both have better* oral bioavailability compared to acyclovir

c. **EBV**

i. 50% of children have EBV infection by age 5 years

ii. 90% of adults have had EBV infection

iii. Neurologic complications in <1%.

iv. Clinical

(A) Encephalitis: most common acute neurologic complication

(B) Bell's palsy

(C) AIDP

(D) Acute transverse myelitis

(E) Optic neuropathy

(F) Aseptic meningitis

(G) CNS lymphoma

v. Diagnostic testing

(A) MRI may be normal or show T2 prolongation involving the basal ganglia, thalamus, white matter, or cerebral cortex

(B) Diagnosis of EBV infection is usually established serologically but can also be detected in the CSF, oropharynx, or brain tissue by culture or PCR

vi. Treatment.

(A) Supportive care

(B) Corticosteroids for optic neuritis or acute disseminated encephalomyelitis

d. **CMV**

i. Acquired by body fluid transmission, blood transfusion, etc.

ii. Common in immunocompromised, including after transplantation (>40–90% of transplant recipients), and HIV patients have high rates

iii. Clinical

(A) Congenital CMV infection

(1) Ranges from asymptomatic infections to disseminated disease
(2) Systemic: jaundice, petechial rash, hepatosplenomegaly, or intrauterine growth retardation
(3) Neurologic: microcephaly, seizures, abnormal tone, and/or sensorineural hearing loss

NB: CMV infection is the most common cause of congenital deafness.

(4) May have disorders of neuronal migration (cortical dysplasia, lissencephaly) or absence of the corpus callosum
(5) Neuroimaging: intracranial calcification in 50% of infected infants (worse prognosis)
    (a) CT: periventricular Ca^{2+}; also Ca^{2+} in BG, cortical, and subcortical regions
    (b) MRI: disruption of gyral pattern and delayed myelination
(B) Postnatal CMV infection
  (1) Systemic: similar to mononucleosis syndrome
  (2) Neurologic
    (a) AIDP
      (i) 10–20% are CMV positive before onset
      (ii) More commonly also have cranial neuropathies and sensorineural hearing loss
    (b) Encephalitis
    (c) Usually only in immunocompromised when CD4 <50
    (d) Acute myelitis
    (e) Polyradiculopathy
    (f) Retinitis
      (i) 5–10% of persons with acquired immunodeficiency syndrome (AIDS)
      (ii) Unilateral vision loss followed by bilateral vision loss if untreated
      (iii) Ganciclovir, foscarnet, and cidofovir may reduce extent of vision loss
iv. Diagnosis
  (A) Isolated from urine, saliva, CSF, amniotic fluid
  (B) CMV-specific immunoglobulin M (IgM): strongly supports infection, but CMV IgG not useful because of the high prevalence of CMV in the general population
  (C) PCR
  (D) Pathology: microglial nodules especially periventricular on cortical biopsy/autopsy
v. Treatment
  (A) Acute: ganciclovir, 5 mg/kg q12 h for >2–4 weeks
  (B) Prophylactic: ganciclovir, 5 mg/kg/day for 5 days per week
2. *Arthropod-borne infections*
  a. Families
    i. *Alphaviruses*
      (A) **Western equine encephalitis (EE) virus**
        (1) Potential cause of encephalitis in United States
        (2) *Principal mosquito vector,* Culex tarsalis
        (3) Birds and other wild vertebrates serve as the natural reservoir for the virus

(4) Usually occurs late spring to early fall
(5) Clinical: headache, myalgias, malaise, vomiting, stiff neck, fever, irritability, coma, or seizures
(6) Diagnosis: lab diagnosis established serologically (>4× rise in virus-specific antibodies)
(7) Treatment: supportive care only
(8) Prognosis
   (a) Mortality: 5–15%
   (b) Most survivors recover completely
   (c) Potential complications: seizures and paralysis

(B) **Eastern EE virus**
(1) Exhibits the highest mortality rate (>30%)
(2) *Transmitted to humans and equines by* Aedes *mosquitoes*
(3) Typically occurs during the summer months
(4) Clinical: fever, headache, lethargy, vomiting, and seizures; deteriorate rapidly within 24–48 hours
(5) Diagnosis: confirmed by isolating the virus from brain tissue or by detecting characteristic serologic responses in paired sera; rapid diagnosis by detecting virus-specific IgM in serum or CSF
(6) Treatment: supportive care only
(7) Prognosis
   (a) Highest mortality rate
   (b) Complications: survivors often with neurologic deficits, including focal-motor deficits, behavioral disturbances, seizures, or cognitive impairments

(C) **Venezuelan EE virus**
(1) Mosquitoes and small mammals are reservoirs
(2) Clinical: headache, myalgias, malaise, vomiting, stiff neck, fever, irritability, coma, or seizures
(3) Diagnosis: confirmed by detecting serologic responses
(4) Treatment: supportive care only
(5) Prognosis: usually good with low mortality rate (0.4%)

ii. *Flaviviruses*
(A) **St. Louis encephalitis virus**
(1) *Midwest and southeast United States*
(2) Bird reservoir
(3) Culex *mosquito species transmit the virus to humans*
(4) Disease severity correlates with advancing age
(5) Clinical
   (a) Encephalitis (60%)
   (b) Aseptic meningitis (15%)
   (c) Influenza-like illness
   (d) Nonconvulsive status epilepticus may occur more frequently than with other arbovirus infections
(6) Diagnosis: St. Louis encephalitis virus-specific IgM in serum or CSF or PCR
(7) Prognosis: mortality (10–20%); 10% of survivors have persistent neurologic dysfunction

(B) West Nile virus

(1) Initially predominantly found in Africa, Europe, and Asia; in North America since 1999
(2) Reservoir: bird
(3) Vectors: *Culex, Aedes,* and *Coquillettidia* mosquitoes
(4) Human-to-human transmission has occurred via blood transfusion and other body fluid transmission, including breast-feeding
(5) Clinical
    (a) Usually asymptomatic
    (b) Prodrome of fever, malaise, headache, nausea, and vomiting followed by meningitis, encephalitis (60% of symptomatic cases), and myelitis

NB: A polio-like syndrome that includes lower motor neuron findings may also occur with West Nile infection.

(6) Diagnosis: virus-specific serology, CSF, or PCR
(7) Prognosis: mortality (5–10%); 30–40% of survivors have persistent neurologic dysfunction

(C) **Japanese encephalitis virus**
(1) Most common arboviral encephalitis worldwide
(2) Vaccination has reduced incidence
(3) Most common encephalitis in eastern Asia
(4) Affects approximately 50,000 persons annually
(5) Late spring through early fall
(6) Reservoir: birds and pigs
(7) Clinical: headache, fever, anorexia, malaise, convulsions, and coma; symptoms/signs similar to AIDP have been reported
(8) Diagnosis: virus-specific IgM serology or CSF
(9) MRI: abnormalities within thalamus, brain stem, basal ganglia, and cerebellum
(10) Treatment: supportive care only
(11) Prognosis: mortality 20–40%; 30% of survivors have persistent neurologic dysfunction, including parkinsonism

iii. *Bunyaviruses*
(A) **California (La Crosse) encephalitis virus**
(1) *Vector:* Aedes *mosquito*
(2) *Hosts: small animals, including squirrel*
(3) Usually infects children in the *midwest and eastern United States*
(4) Usually occurs in summer and early fall
(5) Clinical: fever, vomiting, headache, and abdominal pain with CNS signs 2–4 days later; 50% of children have seizures; 20% have focal CNS dysfunction; 10% of children have aseptic meningitis
(6) Diagnosis: >4× increase in virus-specific serology or CSF
(7) Treatment: supportive care only
(8) Prognosis: majority of children survive without CNS complication

3. *Tick-borne viruses*
  a. **European tick-borne encephalitis viruses**
  b. **Powassan encephalitis virus**
    i. Rare cause of human encephalitis in United States
    ii. Clinical: fever, headache, vomiting, and somnolence followed by cognitive dysfunction, ophthalmoplegia, diffuse or focal weakness, ataxia, and seizures

     iii. Diagnosis: virus-specific IgM in CSF or serum and elevations of the virus-specific IgG in convalescent sera

     iv. Treatment: supportive care

     v. Prognosis: mortality (10–15%)

  c. *Colorado tick fever virus*

     i. *Orbivirus transmitted by the wood tick* Dermacentor andersoni

     ii. Typically mountainous regions of the western United States

     iii. Usually occur during summer and early fall

     iv. Clinical: fever, headache, myalgia, anorexia, nausea, and rash (similar to symptoms of Rocky Mountain spotted fever), followed by aseptic meningitis

     v. Treatment: supportive care only

     vi. Prognosis: mortality rare

Vectors

Mosquito-borne	Tick-borne
Western EE	Russian spring-summer/central European
Eastern EE	Powassan
Venezuelan EE	Colorado tick fever
California EE	
St. Louis encephalitis	
Japanese encephalitis	
West Nile virus	

Animal Host

Birds	Equine	Rodents
Western EE	Venezuelan EE	California encephalitis
Eastern EE		Russian spring-summer/central European
Venezuelan EE		Powassan
St. Louis encephalitis		Colorado tick fever
Japanese encephalitis (also pigs)		
West Nile virus		

4. **Rabies**

  a. Reservoirs: skunks (most common), dogs, raccoons, and bats

  b. 50,000–60,000 die annually worldwide (but only 1–5 per year in United States)

  c. Pathogenesis: virus enters *peripheral nerves followed by axonal transport of the virus to the cell bodies of neurons, where the virus replicates and disseminates throughout the CNS*

  d. Clinical

     i. Incubation: 1 week to years (shortest after infection to the head and neck)

     ii. Prodrome: headache, malaise, sore throat, nausea/vomiting, and/or abdominal pain

      iii. *Furious = encephalitis*
- (A) 80% of human rabies cases
- (B) Confusion; anxiety; agitation; hallucinations; dysphagia, causing hydrophobia, hypersalivation, and seizures
- (C) Death secondary to muscle spasms involving diaphragm or accessory respiratory muscles leads to respiratory arrest (or) patient's lapse into a fatal coma

      iv. *Dumb = paralytic signs predominate*
- (A) Similar course as AIDP
- (B) The most frequent initial symptoms are pain and paresthesias at the site of infection followed by motor weakness affecting the same extremity and rapid diffuse
- (C) Death secondary to respiratory arrest

e. Diagnosis
- i. Neuroimaging: abnormalities of the basal ganglia
- ii. Diagnosis confirmed by
  - (A) Isolating the rabies virus from saliva
  - (B) Pathology
    - (1) Negri bodies: eosinophilic intranuclear inclusions in pyramidal cells and cerebellar Purkinje cells
    - (2) Babès nodules: focal microglial nodules
  - (C) Serologic responses
  - (D) Rabies virus antigen by immunofluorescent staining of full-thickness skin biopsy specimens
  - (E) Rabies virus-specific antibodies can be detected in serum or CSF by day 15
  - (F) PCR in saliva or brain tissues by day 5

f. Treatment
- i. Postexposure prophylaxis
  - (A) Begin with cleaning of the wound with soap and water
  - (B) If animal suspected of having rabies, immediately vaccinate with human diploid cell rabies vaccine and consult local public health officials
- ii. Symptomatic
  - (A) Supportive care only
  - (B) Place in isolation because rabies virus present in body fluids

g. Prognosis: death usually within 2 weeks of onset of symptoms

5. Progressive multifocal leukoencephalopathy (PML)
   a. Caused by the JC virus and simian virus 40
   b. Opportunistic CNS infection due to reactivation of latent JC virus
   c. Virus replication begins in tonsils
   d. Invariably in conjunction with immunodeficiency (5% of AIDS patients have PML), hematologic malignancies, organ transplantation, inflammatory or connective tissue disorders
   e. Pathogenesis: infection of oligodendrocytes (demyelination) > astrocytes (neuronal dysfunction)
   f. Clinical
      - i. Neurologic: dementia, headache, visual dysfunction, cranial neuropathies, sensory deficits, paralysis, speech disturbances, ataxia, seizures
      - ii. Invariably progressive, resulting in long-term complete disability and death
   g. Diagnosis
      - i. Confirmed by detecting JC virus particles or antigens in brain tissue, isolating the virus from brain, or PCR

    ii. MRI: focal or multifocal white matter lesions with T2 prolongation, typically within cerebral subcortical white matter > brain stem

    iii. Pathology: *oligodendrocytes contain eosinophilic intranuclear inclusions;* bizarre astrocytes

  h. Treatment: supportive care; cytarabine, 2 mg/kg/day for 5 days, each month may be of benefit

    i. Prognosis: mortality: 80% usually die within 9 months

6. *Picornaviruses*

  a. *Enteroviruses*

    i. **Polioviruses**

      (A) Clinical

        (1) Usually limited symptoms or asymptomatic

        (2) Neurologic sequelae

          (a) *Aseptic meningitis*

          (b) *Paralytic poliomyelitis*

            (i) Usually due to poliovirus type 1

            (ii) Prodrome of fever, headache, vomiting, myalgia, and meningeal signs

            (iii) Paralysis appears within 1–2 days

          (c) *Bulbar poliomyelitis*

            (i) Involves the motor CNs of the medulla or pons (usually CNs IX, X, and XI) with dysphagia, dysphonia, and upper airway compromise

          (d) *Polioencephalitis*

      (B) Diagnosis

        (1) Confirmation of poliovirus requires isolation from feces, CSF, or throat

        (2) Detected in feces or CSF by using PCR

      (C) Treatment

        (1) Prophylactic

          (a) *Salk vaccine*

            (i) *Inactivated poliovirus vaccine*

          (b) *Sabin vaccine*

            (i) *Attenuated, live-virus oral vaccine*

            (ii) *No longer distributed in the United States*

        (2) Acute treatment

          (a) Supportive care

          (b) Immunocompromised: i.v. immunoglobulin

      (D) Prognosis

        (1) Mortality high (50%)

        (2) Mild paralytic poliomyelitis: frequently recover but may have residual fatigue, myalgia, arthralgia, or progressive muscle weakness and atrophy later in life (postpolio syndrome)

    ii. **Coxsackieviruses**

      (A) Summer or fall

      (B) Either coxsackievirus A or B groups

      (C) *Coxsackievirus B has more complications with involvement of the heart, liver, and CNS*

      (D) Clinical

        (1) Range from mild febrile illnesses to severe disseminated multiple organ infections

(2) Commonly includes pharyngitis, herpangina, pleurodynia, gastroenteritis, neonatal sepsis, or the hand-foot-and-mouth syndrome

(3) CNS: aseptic meningitis, encephalitis, poliomyelitis-like illnesses, Guillain-Barré syndrome, acute cerebellar ataxia, or opsoclonus-myoclonus

(E) Diagnosis

(1) Isolated from feces, CSF, or throat washings

(2) Feces, serum, or CSF PCR

(3) Treatment: supportive only

iii. **Echoviruses**

(A) Infect humans *by fecal-oral or respiratory routes (less common)*

(B) Usually late summer or fall

(C) Clinical: similar to coxsackie; may also produce disseminated intravascular coagulation; 10% maculopapular or petechial rash

(D) Diagnosis: virus isolation from feces, throat washings, or CSF; detected in CSF or feces by PCR

(E) Treatment: supportive care only

7. **Reye syndrome**

a. *VZV and influenza viruses have roles in Reye syndrome*

b. *Develops between ages 2 and 15 years*

c. *Strong correlation with aspirin*

d. Clinical

i. *<72 hours after viral illness*

ii. Begins with continuous vomiting followed by increasing lethargy, hypoglycemia, and hyperammonemia with liver failure (and dysfunction of clotting factors)

iii. Death and neurologic sequelae are related to increased intracranial pressure (ICP)

e. Treatment

i. Supportive with strict control of electrolytes and treatment of clotting dysfunction

ii. Observation/treatment of increased ICP

f. Prognosis: depends on severity of increased ICP; mortality: 10–30%

8. **Measles virus**

a. Spreads via *respiratory droplets*

b. Measles vaccination has been linked with acute encephalopathy and permanent neurologic deficits

c. Clinical (CNS involvement)

i. *Encephalomyelitis*

(A) 1/1000 cases of measles

(B) Begins 2–5 days after the rash appears

(C) Usually <10 y/o

(D) Headache, irritability, seizures, somnolence, or coma; occasionally paralysis, ataxia, choreoathetosis, or incontinence

(E) Treatment: supportive care

(F) Prognosis: mortality (10–15%); neurologic sequelae (20–60%)

ii. *Subacute measles virus encephalopathy*

(A) Progressive neurodegeneration

(B) Usually have deficiency of cell-mediated immunity or immunocompromised

(C) Occurs in conjunction with measles infection or vaccination

(D) Begins insidiously with ataxia, dementia, and/or seizures followed by coma and often death

(E) Reports of temporary improvement with ribavirin

      iii. *Subacute sclerosing panencephalitis*
- (A) Defective measles virus replication in the brain
- (B) Rare since development of vaccination
- (C) Affects young (50% have had measles before 2 y/o)
- (D) Clinical
  - (1) Etiology: measles (rubeola) before 2 y/o
  - (2) Stage 1: mental status changes followed by myoclonus (usually focal)
  - (3) Stage 2: persistent mental status changes with generalization of myoclonus, followed by ataxia, language difficulties; apraxias, and spasticity
  - (4) Stage 3: vision also begins to deteriorate with worsening myoclonus; patients become nonambulatory; may have facial involvement requiring tube feeding
  - (5) Stage 4: myoclonus stops and patients persist in vegetative state
- (E) Diagnosis
  - (1) Virus-specific IgG in CSF and serum
  - (2) EEG: *bilateral synchronous high-amplitude spike or slow-wave bursts that correlate with myoclonus; EEG progresses to burst-suppression pattern*
  - (3) Pathology
    - (a) Patchy demyelination
    - (b) Intranuclear eosinophilic inclusions
- (F) Treatment: supportive care and treatment of clinical symptoms
- (G) Prognosis: usually death within 1–3 years

9. **Congenital rubella syndrome**
   - a. Risk to fetus directly correlates with time of maternal infection
     - i. <16th week: fetal loss, cataracts, and/or heart disease
     - ii. >17th week: asymptomatic
     - iii. Clinical
       - (A) *Classic*
         - (1) *Cataracts*
         - (2) *Sensorineural hearing loss*
         - (3) *Congenital heart disease (patent ductus arteriosus or septal defects)*
       - (B) *Other*
         - (1) *Microcephaly*
         - (2) *Developmental delay*
         - (3) *Seizures*
         - (4) *As adults, may develop diabetes mellitus and thyroid disease*
     - iv. Diagnosis: prenatal diagnosis possible via amniotic fluid or rubella-specific IgM in fetal blood

10. *Retroviruses*
    - a. *Contain an RNA-dependent DNA polymerase (reverse transcriptase) and replicate through a DNA intermediary*
    - b. *Lentiviruses (HIV-1 and HIV-2)*
      - i. **HIV-1:** About 33.2 million people living with HIV as of 2007; the incidence of AIDS-defining illness has decreased in countries with access to highly active anti-retroviral therapy (HAART); approach is defined by the CD4 T lymphocyte count (> 500 cells/uL—normal range; 200–500 cells/uL—increased risk for cognitive changes and tuberculosis; <200 cells/uL—most neurological complications occur)

(A) Systemic
  (1) Range from asymptomatic infection to overt AIDS
  (2) Lymphadenopathy, malaise, fever, weight loss, diarrhea, or night sweats
  (3) Opportunistic infections (*Pneumocystis carinii*, CMV, PML, fungal) or neoplasms
(B) CNS complications of AIDS
  (1) AIDS dementia
     (a) Most common complication
     (b) 20–75% with advanced HIV
     (c) Usually subcortical dementia with bradykinesia, short-term memory deficit, apathy, and decreased concentration (note: no signs of cortical dementia [i.e., no aphasia])
     (d) MRI: diffuse atrophy
  (2) HIV encephalopathy
     (a) Perinatal HIV infections have a static encephalopathy
     (b) In children, resembles the HIV dementia of adults
     (c) 20% have associated seizures
  (3) HIV meningitis
  (4) Toxoplasma meningoencephalitis
     (a) 5–15% of AIDS
     (b) Usually CD4 of 100–500
     (c) Ring-enhancing lesions on CT or MRI (predilection to hemispheres and basal ganglia)
     (d) Treatment: pyrimethamine plus folinic acid + sulfadiazine or clindamycin for 6 weeks

NB: Bactrim can be given to AIDS patients for *Toxoplasma* prophylaxis.

  (5) Cryptococcal meningitis: IV amphotericin B + oral fluconzaole x 14 days, then oral fluconazole for 8 weeks; may need daily LPs/lumbar drain/shunt to relieve increased ICP
  (6) PML: caused by JCV, a polyomavirus; typically lesions lack enhancement or mass effect; usually asymmetric multifocal white matter lesions; HAART is the only effective therapy for PML with survival improving from 10% to 50%
  (7) Primary CNS lymphoma
     (a) 2% of AIDS patients
     (b) Second most common focal CNS lesion in AIDS

NB: The most common focal lesion is toxoplasmosis.

     (c) B cell
     (d) Usually CD4 <100
     (e) Imaging characteristics: can be solitary, usually uniform enhancement; more likely to "cross the midline" and involve deep white matter (as opposed to toxoplasmosis where lesions tend to be multiple, with heterogeneous or ring enhancement); SPECT and PET also with greater uptake than toxoplasmosis
     (f) Steroids "melt" away lesions but without long-term improvement in prognosis; brain irradiation may prolong life 3–6 months

      (8) CMV encephalitis

          (a) Usually only when CD4 <50

      (9) Vacuolar myelopathy

          (a) 20% of AIDS patients

          (b) May appear similar to subacute combined degeneration

     (10) Polyradiculopathy: usually CMV mediated

     (11) AIDP

     (12) Chronic inflammatory demyelinating polyneuropathy

     (13) Sensory neuropathies

     (14) Mononeuritis multiplex

     (15) Myopathy

          (a) HIV associated

          (b) Zidovudine induced with ragged-red fibers secondary to mitochondrial toxicity

     (16) Stroke

  (C) Diagnosis

     (1) Positive enzyme-linked immunosorbent assay for HIV and confirmed by Western blot analysis

     (2) Detection of HIV by PCR

     (3) HIV loads used for monitoring response to therapy

     (4) Lab and imaging for opportunistic infections

     (5) Pathology: microglial nodules especially periventricular on cortical biopsy/autopsy

  (D) Treatment

     (1) Antiretroviral therapy

          (a) Nucleoside/nucleotide reverse transcriptase inhibitors

             (i) Zidovudine: inhibits HIV replication; treatment of HIV-infected pregnant women and their newborns substantially reduces the infection rate among infants born to HIV-infected women; postexposure prophylaxis; resistance develops frequently

            (ii) Abacavir

           (iii) Didanosine

           (iv) Emtricitabine

            (v) Lamivudine

           (vi) Stavudine

          (vii) Tenofovir DR

        (viii) Zalcitabine (withdrawn)

          (b) Nonnucleoside reverse transcriptase inhibitors

             (i) Delavirdine

            (ii) Efavirenz

           (iii) Nevirapine

          (c) Protease inhibitors

             (i) Amprenavir

            (ii) Atazanavir

           (iii) Indinavir

           (iv) Lopinavir + ritonavir

            (v) Nelfinavir

           (vi) Ritonavir

          (vii) Saquinavir

        (d) Fusion inhibitors
            (i) Enfuvirtide
        (e) Highly active antiretroviral therapy protocol
            (i) *Two nucleoside reverse transcriptase inhibitors plus protease inhibitor (or) nonnucleoside reverse transcriptase inhibitor*
            (ii) Produces immunologic and neurocognitive improvement
            (iii) Goal: reduce/eliminate HIV viral load
            (iv) Potential complications: immune restoration disease characterized by paradoxic exacerbation of secondary infections during the initial several months of highly active antiretroviral therapy

Summary of Neurologic Complications of HIV

Muscle	HIV myopathy
	Zidovudine myopathy
Nerve and nerve roots	HIV distal sensory polyneuropathy
	Antiretroviral drug toxic polyneuropathy
	CMV polyradiculopathy
	CIDP
	HIV or HZV cranial neuropathy
	HIV or CMV mononeuropathy multiplex
Spinal cord	HIV vacuolar myelopathy
	Myelitis due to VZV, HSV, CMV, Toxoplasma
Meninges	HIV meningitis
	Neurosyphilis
	Tuberculous meningitis
	Crytococcal meningitis
Brain-focal	Bacterial abscess from atypical organisms
	HIV-associated stroke
	Toxoplasmic encephalitis
	Primary CNC lymphoma
	PML
Brian-diffuse	HIV-associated dementia
	Postinfectious encephalomyelitis
	CMV encephalitis
	VZV encephalitis

    c. *Oncoviruses*
        i. **Human T-cell leukemia virus type 1**
            (A) Clinical
                (1) Progressive myelopathy (only 0.25% of human T-cell leukemia virus type 1 infections)

          (a) Progressive spastic paraparesis

          (b) Urinary incontinence

          (c) Variable sensory loss

     (2) Uveitis

     (3) Infective dermatitis

     (4) Nonneoplastic inflammatory conditions

     (5) Three females to one male

  (B) Diagnosis

     (1) Human T-cell leukemia virus type 1-specific IgG in serum or CSF

     (2) PCR (666)

  (C) Transmission via contact with body fluids

  (D) Treatment: supportive care: corticosteroids may produce some improvement

III. Encephalitis

  A. *Viral encephalitis* (see section II for specific infections)

    1. General clinical presentation

      a. Alterations of awareness, including somnolence and coma

      b. Fever

      c. Seizures (30–60%)

      d. Examination: hyperreflexia; ataxia; cognitive disturbances, including short-term memory dysfunction, seen particularly with herpes encephalitis; or focal deficits

      e. Increased ICP

  B. *Other etiologies of encephalitis*

    1. **Rickettsiae**

      a. *Typhus group*

        i. *Epidemic typhus*

        (A) Pathophysiology and epidemiology

          (1) Caused by *Rickettsia prowazekii*

          (2) Acquired by the inoculation of infected louse feces into the skin or mucous membranes

          (3) Pathology: typhus nodule consisting of mononuclear inflammatory cells and proliferating astrocytes surrounding small blood vessels

        (B) Clinical

          (1) Incubation: 1 week

          (2) Initial fever, headache, and malaise followed by a generalized macular rash (day 5) that begins in the axillary folds and the upper trunk and spreads centrifugally

          (3) Neurologic

            (a) Appear at the end of 1st week

            (b) Begin with an agitated delirium associated with pyramidal tract signs and neck stiffness followed by seizures and brain stem dysfunction

            (c) May die in the 2nd week owing to peripheral vascular collapse

          (4) *Brill-Zinsser disease*

            (a) *Reactivation of* R. prowazekii *that remains in the lymph nodes after bout of typhus*

            (b) *Less severe clinical course*

        (C) Diagnosis: *Weil-Felix reaction*

        (D) Treatment

          (1) Doxycycline (200 mg/day)

        (2) Chloramphenicol (50 mg/kg/day)

        (3) Tetracycline (25 mg/kg/day)

        (4) Antibiotics must be continued for 2 or 3 days after fever subsides

ii. *Endemic (murine) typhus*

  (A) Pathophysiology and epidemiology

      (1) Caused by *Rickettsia typhi*

      (2) Acquired by the inoculation of infected flea or louse feces into the skin or mucous membranes

  (B) Clinical

      (1) Similar to epidemic typhus but not as acute, and neurologic manifestations tend to be less severe

  (C) Treatment

      (1) Doxycycline (200 mg/day)

      (2) Chloramphenicol (50 mg/kg/day)

      (3) Tetracycline (25 mg/kg/day)

      (4) Antibiotics must be continued for >24 hours after fever subsides

b. *Spotted fever group*

  i. *Rocky Mountain spotted fever*

    (A) *Caused by* Rickettsia rickettsii

    (B) Transmitted from domestic animals to humans by tick

    (C) *Tick vectors:* wood tick, *D. andersoni*

    (D) More prevalent between May and September

    (E) Pathology: generalized angiitis of the vascular endothelium, and every organ can be involved

    (F) Clinical

      (1) Incubation period of 2–12 days

      (2) Initial complaints include fever, chills, generalized muscle pain, and headache followed by rash (more prominent on distal extremities)

      (3) Neurologic: headache with agitation followed by progressive lethargy, stupor, and coma; may also develop a transverse myelitis, a sensory neuropathy, or AIDP-like syndromes

      (4) Serology: thrombocytopenia, hyponatremia, increased liver function tests and creatinine

      (5) Electrocardiography may demonstrate myocarditis

    (G) Diagnosis: confirmed by serologic tests or by isolation of *R. rickettsii* from the blood

    (H) Treatment

      (1) Doxycycline (200 mg/day)

      (2) Chloramphenicol (50 mg/kg/day)

      (3) Tetracycline (25 mg/kg/day)

c. *Other Rickettsial diseases*

  i. *Q fever*

    (A) Caused by *Coxiella burnetii*

    (B) Spreads from animals to humans by inhalation of the infected dust or by handling infected animals

    (C) Primarily an occupational disease, mainly affecting shepherds and farmers

    (D) Pathology: endothelial damage or vasculitis

    (E) Clinical

      (1) Incubation period of 3 weeks

        (2) Begins abruptly with chills, fever, and headache and is self-limited

        (3) May also develop involvement of lungs, liver (hepatitis), heart (myocarditis or endocarditis)

        (4) Neurologic: rare but may cause severe encephalitis similar to HSV; other acute neurologic manifestations of Q fever include optic neuritis, CN palsies, AIDP, and aseptic meningitis

        (5) Chronic phase: valvular heart disease, granulomatous disease of the liver, osteomyelitis, or bone marrow necrosis

    (F) Treatment

        (1) Doxycycline (200 mg/day)

        (2) Chloramphenicol (50 mg/kg/day)

        (3) Tetracycline (25 mg/kg/day)

IV. Brain Abscess

  A. **Pathophysiology**

    1. Arises from

      a. Direct extension of sinusitis (40%)

      b. Generalized septicemia (30%): usually multiple abscesses

      c. Cryptogenic (20–25%)

      d. Direct extension of otitis, facial or dental infection (5%)

      e. Penetrating and closed head injury

      f. Meningitis

  B. Clinical

    1. Onset subacute cases within 1 month of initial manifestation

    2. Infectious symptoms

      a. Fever

      b. Meningeal signs (one-third of cases)

    3. Neurologic symptoms

      a. Seizures (one-third of cases)

      b. Focal neurologic deficits (two-thirds of cases)

      c. Movement disorders (e.g., *Toxoplasma* often localizes to the basal ganglia)

    4. Complications usually arise from increased ICP or abscess rupture, particularly into the ventricles causing an empyema

    5. Immunocompromised patient more susceptible

    6. Differential diagnosis

      a. Meningitis

      b. Stroke

      c. Neoplasm

      d. Mycobacteria (*Mycobacterium tuberculosis*)

      e. Fungi

      f. Parasites (cysticercosis)

  C. Diagnostic procedures

    1. Neuroimaging: CT/MRI

      a. Ring-enhancing lesion radiologic differential diagnosis: primary glial tumors, lymphoma, metastatic tumor, resolving hematoma, subacute infarct, thrombosed aneurysm, acute demyelinating process, focal infections other than abscess (e.g., granuloma)

    2. Do not perform lumbar puncture, owing to risk of herniation and/or rupture of abscess

D. Treatment
  1. Dexamethasone, 4–6 mg q6h
     a. Disadvantages: retards the capsule formation, may suppress the immune system, and may decrease penetration of the antibiotics
     b. Should be used for short periods
  2. Antimicrobial treatment

Predisposing condition	Common pathogens	Antimicrobial agents
Dental abscess	Streptococci	Penicillin + metronidazole
	Bacteroides fragilis	
Chronic otitis media	*B. fragilis*	Ceftriaxone + metronidazole
	Pseudomonas	Add ceftazidime or cefepime for *Pseudomonas*
	Proteus	
	Klebsiella	
Sinusitis	Streptococci	Ceftriaxone + metronidazole
	Haemophilus	
	Staphylococcus	
Penetrating trauma	Staphylococci	Vancomycin + ceftriaxone + metronidazole
Postcraniotomy	*Pseudomonas*	Vancomycin + ceftazidime + metronidazole
	Enterobacter	
	Streptococci/ Staphyloccici	
Bacterial endocarditis	Mixed flora	Vancomycin + ceftriaxone + metronidazole
Drug use	Streptococci	
	Staphylococci	
Congenital heart disease	Streptococci	Ceftriaxone
Pulmonary infection	*Nocardia*	Penicillin + metronidazole + trimethoprim-sulfamethoxazole
	B. fragilis	
	Streptococci	
	Mixed flora	

Note: May substitute nafcillin for vancomycin.

  3. Surgical intervention
     a. Aspiration for culture diagnosis
     b. Resection/drainage if superficial or aggressive organisms
     c. Surgical mortality rates 20–40%

E. *Other types of CNS abscess*
  1. *Toxoplasmosis abscess*
     a. Diagnosis by the demonstration of tachyzoites
     b. Pyrimethamine and sulfadiazine
     c. Supplement with folate
     d. Prophylactic therapy to prevent relapse
        i. Pyrimethamine plus sulfadiazine and leucovorin
        ii. If sulfa allergy, pyrimethamine plus clindamycin
  2. *Fungal abscess*
     a. Best treatment with combined surgical aspiration and antibiotics
     b. Immunosuppressed: high mortality
     c. ***Candida* brain abscess**
        i. Amphotericin B and 5-flucytosine
        ii. Fluconazole may be an alternative to flucytosine
     d. ***Aspergillus* brain abscess**
        i. Poor prognosis
        ii. Amphotericin B plus 5-flucytosine

V. Other Bacterial Infections of the Nervous System
  A. **Botulism**
  1. Pathophysiology
     a. Caused by the neurotoxins of Clostridium botulinum *and, in rare cases,* Clostridium butyricum *and* Clostridium baratii
     b. Gram-positive spore-forming anaerobes
     c. Three forms
        i. *Food-borne botulism*
           (A) 1000 cases per year worldwide
           (B) Associated with home-canned vegetables
           (C) Most associated with type A spores
        ii. *Wound botulism*
           (A) Injection drug use with black tar heroin
           (B) Post-traumatic
        iii. *Infant botulism*
           (A) Most common in children aged 1 week to 11 months
           (B) Usually neurotoxins types A and B
           (C) Death in <2% of cases in United States but higher worldwide
     d. The most common form now is wound botulism and then subcutaneous heroin
     e. *Neurotoxins types A, B, and E are most frequently responsible for disease in humans, whereas types F and G have been reported only occasionally.*
     f. Irreversible binding to the presynaptic membrane of cholinergic nerve endings in the peripheral nervous system, blocking release of acetylcholine at the neuromuscular junction
        i. Three-step process
           (A) Toxin binds to receptors on the nerve ending
           (B) Toxin molecule is then internalized
           (C) Within the nerve cell, the toxin interferes with the release of acetylcholine
        ii. Cleavage of one of the SNARE (soluble N-ethylmaleimide-sensitive factor attachment protein receptor) proteins by botulinum neurotoxin inhibits the exocytosis of acetylcholine from the synaptic terminal

2. Clinical
   a. Blurred vision, dysphagia, dysarthria, pupillary response to light, dry mouth, constipation, and urinary retention
   b. Tensilon® (edrophonium chloride) test: positive in 30% cases
   c. Infant botulism: constipation, lethargy, poor sucking, weak cry
   d. Electrophysiologic criteria for botulism
      i. ↓Compound muscle action potential amplitude in at least two muscles
      ii. 20% facilitation of compound muscle action potential amplitude
      iii. Persistent facilitation for 2 minutes after muscle contraction
      iv. No postactivation exhaustion
      v. Single fiber electromyography—↑jitter and blocking
   e. Prognosis
      i. Most patients recover completely within 6 months
3. Treatment
   a. Supportive care
   b. Antibiotics
      i. Local antibiotics, such as penicillin G or metronidazole, may be helpful in eradicating *C. botulinum* in wound botulism
      ii. Antibiotics are not recommended for infant botulism, because cell death and lysis may result in the release of more toxin
   c. Horse serum antitoxin
      i. Types A, B, and E
      ii. Side effects of serum sickness and anaphylaxis
B. **Brucellosis**
   1. Pathophysiology and epidemiology
      a. Also known as *Malta fever*
      b. Caused by facultative intracellular bacilli of the genus *Brucella* (*B. melitensis, B. abortus, B. suis,* and *B. canis*)
      c. Mainly a disease of domestic animals
      d. Humans acquire the disease via close contact with infected animals (through skin abrasions), by contaminated aerosols, or by consumption
      e. Incidence: <0.5 cases per 100,000
   2. Pathology
      a. Systemic: primary involvement of lymph nodes, spleen, and bone marrow, but almost every organ may be involved
      b. Neuropathology: granulomas, demyelination, thickening of leptomeninges, angiitis, mycotic aneurysms, and degeneration of anterior horn cells
   3. Clinical
      a. Systemic: chills, fever, headache, generalized weakness, muscle pain, and arthralgias with lymphadenopathy
      b. Neurologic
         i. 5% of patients
         ii. Usually acute encephalitis with drowsiness, seizures, and signs and symptoms of increased ICP
         iii. Mononeuritis
         iv. Acute inflammatory polyradiculoneuritis
   4. Diagnosis: identification of the presence of *Brucella* species from blood or CSF
   5. Treatment
      a. Doxycycline (200 mg/day) plus rifampin (600–900 mg/day) for 6 weeks

     b. Parenteral gentamicin (5 mg/kg/day) or streptomycin (1000 mg/day) may be used instead of rifampin for patients with acute symptoms

     c. Trimethoprim-sulfamethoxazole is an alternative for doxycycline

     d. CNS involvement: antibiotics given for 3–6 months

C. **Leprosy (Hansen's disease)**

  1. Pathophysiology and epidemiology

     a. Caused by *Mycobacterium leprae (obligate intracellular acid-fast bacillus)*

     b. Acquire the disease from *skin-to-skin contact or through nasal secretions of infected individuals*

     c. Differences in the host's susceptibility to infection result in marked differences in the severity of disease

     d. *M. leprae* only replicates in body areas where the temperature is low (i.e., skin, distal peripheral nerves)

  2. Clinical

     a. Major forms

       i. *Tuberculoid*

         (A) Intense immune reaction reduces organism proliferation but causes circumscribed acute peripheral nerve and skin damage

         (B) Cell-mediated immune reaction results in development of an epithelioid granuloma (hypopigmented, anesthetic skin lesion) at the portal of entry of organisms, usually the skin of the face, the chest, or upper limbs

         (C) Skin lesions and peripheral neuropathy with involvement of a single nerve (usually ulnar = claw-hand, radial = wristdrop, peroneal = footdrop, and/or facial nerves)

       ii. *Lepromatous*

         (A) Do not mount an adequate immune reaction and more generalized

         (B) Skin lesions and peripheral neuropathy with symmetric loss of pain and temperature sensations in the distal portions of the extremities and relative preservation of deep sensation

         (C) Anesthetic hands are prone to repeated trauma and infection, leading to ulcerated skin lesions, bone destruction, finger loss, and deformities

         (D) Trigeminal nerve involvement leads to facial hypoalgesia with associated corneal ulcerations and blindness

     b. Skin lesions and peripheral neuropathy

  3. Diagnosis: identification of *M. leprae* in skin or peripheral nerve biopsy

  4. Treatment

     a. Tuberculoid leprosy: rifampin (600 mg/day) for 6 months plus dapsone (100 mg/day) for 2 years

     b. Lepromatous leprosy: clofazimine (50–300 mg/day) plus rifampin (600 mg/day) for 2 years plus dapsone (100 mg/day) for 2 years

D. **Rheumatic fever**

  1. Pathophysiology and epidemiology: *Group A β-hemolytic streptococci*

  2. Clinical

     a. Systemic

       i. Usually begins 1–5 weeks after an acute episode of streptococcal pharyngitis

       ii. May present in acute migratory polyarthritis or subacute/chronic carditis

       iii. Begins with subcutaneous nodules and erythema marginatum

       iv. May cause congestive heart failure and valvular heart disease

   b. Neurologic complications
      i. Sydenham's chorea: chorea, dysarthria, and obsessive-compulsive behavior
      ii. Delirium
      iii. Seizures
      iv. Stroke due to valvular disease
   3. Treatment for acute rheumatic fever
      a. Aspirin (100 mg/day)
      b. Prednisone (1 mg/kg/day)
E. **Whipple's disease**
   1. Pathophysiology and epidemiology
      a. Caused by *Tropheryma whippelii*
      b. Impaired cell-mediated immunity
      c. Pathology: *infiltration of tissues with foamy macrophages containing periodic acid–Schiff-positive bacilli in the cytoplasm (rectal or jejunal biopsy)*
   2. Clinical
      a. Systemic: chronic migratory arthralgias followed by abdominal pain, diarrhea with steatorrhea, and weight loss
      b. Neurologic
         i. Triad
            (A) Slowly progressive dementia
            (B) Supranuclear vertical-gaze palsy
            (C) Myoclonic jerks
         ii. Other
            (A) Oculomasticatory myorhythmia
               (1) Due to hypothalamic involvement
               (2) Pendular vergent oscillations of the eyes with synchronous rhythmic contractions of the masticatory muscles
            (B) Dysarthria
            (C) Ataxia
            (D) Seizures
            (E) Deafness
            (F) Tinnitus
            (G) Visual field loss
            (H) Motor deficits
   3. Treatment
      a. Trimethoprim (320 mg)-sulfamethoxazole (1600 mg) daily for 6–12 months
      b. Penicillin G (12–24 million U/day)
      c. Ceftriaxone (50–100 mg/kg/day)

VI. Fungal Infections of the Nervous System
A. **Cryptococcosis**
   1. Pathophysiology
      a. Caused by *Cryptococcus neoformans:* inhabits the soil and pigeon feces and enters the human body by the respiratory tract
      b. Opportunistic infections of cell-mediated immunity (AIDS, lymphoreticular malignancy, chronic steroids)
      c. Most common CNS fungal infection
   2. Clinical
      a. Neurologic
         i. Arachnoiditis

        ii. Chronic basilar meningitis

       iii. Brain abscesses

       iv. Granulomas causing focal CNS lesions

        v. Hydrocephalus (due to occlusion of foramina by granulomas or other lesions)

   3. Treatment

     a. Non-CNS cryptococcosis or immunocompetent meningeal cryptococcosis

        i. Amphotericin B (0.3–1.0 mg/kg/day) for 2–3 months

       ii. Fluconazole (200–400 mg/day) for 2–3 months

     b. AIDS-associated cryptococcal meningitis: amphotericin B (0.7 mg/kg/day) plus flucytosine (100 mg/kg/day) for 2 weeks, followed by fluconazole (400 mg/day) or itraconazole (400 mg/day) for 8 weeks

B. **Aspergillosis**

   1. Pathophysiology

     a. Aspergillus fumigatus *(85–90% of cases): septated hyphae*

     b. Acquired by inhalation of airborne spores

     c. May occur in immunocompetent hosts but usually opportunistic infection

     d. Pathology: mucosal invasion of the nose and paranasal sinuses by *Aspergillus* is followed by spreading to contiguous structures, causing abscess formation and tissue necrosis due to vascular infiltration

   2. Clinical

     a. Most common in patients with chronic sinusitis

     b. *Aspergillus meningitis*

     c. Parenchymal granulomas

     d. Brain abscess (classic fungus ball)

     e. Ophthalmoplegia

     f. Cranial neuropathies

     g. Mortality: 80–90%

   3. Treatment: amphotericin B, 0.80–1.25 mg/kg/day intravenously, for a total dose of 1.0–1.5 g; renal function and serum potassium levels should be closely monitored

C. **Candidiasis**

   1. Pathophysiology

     a. Various species of *Candida*

     b. Typically opportunistic infection

     c. Most cases of CNS candidiasis are caused by *Candida albicans*

   2. Clinical

     a. Neurologic

         i. Meningitis

       ii. Parenchymal microabscesses

      iii. Granulomas

   3. Treatment: amphotericin B, 0.80–1.25 mg/kg/day intravenously, for a total dose of 1.0–1.5 g; renal function and serum potassium levels should be closely monitored

D. **Coccidioidomycosis**

   1. Pathophysiology

     a. Caused by *Coccidioides immitis*

     b. *Inhabits dry acidic soil endemic in southwest United States*

     c. Acquired via inhalation of arthroconidia that is transformed into nonbudding spherules composed of hundreds of endospores

     d. Elicits a caseating granulomatous reaction

     e. CNS involvement occurs in <1%

2. Clinical
  a. Neurologic
    i. Arachnoiditis
    ii. Chronic basilar meningitis
    iii. Brain abscesses
3. Treatment
  a. Pulmonary disease
    i. Fluconazole (400–800 mg/day)
    ii. Itraconazole (400 mg/day)
    iii. Ketoconazole (400–800 mg/day)
  b. Coccidioidal meningitis
    i. Fluconazole
    ii. Amphotericin B
      (A) i.v.
      (B) Intrathecal (Ommaya reservoir) amphotericin B
        (1) Begin with 0.01 mg of the drug. The dose must be progressively increased up to 1.0–1.5 mg every other day, to a total dose of 50–100 mg
        (2) Hydrocortisone (25–50 mg) should be given together with every intrathecal dose of amphotericin B to ameliorate adverse reactions
        (3) Continuing for 12–18 months for cerebral abscesses is advised
E. **Mucormycosis (zygomycosis)**
  1. Pathophysiology
    a. Rhizopus arrhizus (*90% of cases with CNS involvement*)
    b. Inhabits soil, plants, and certain foods in a mold form
    c. Causes disease in patients with diabetic ketoacidosis or in those who are acidemic from other causes
    d. Infection acquired by the inhalation of airborne spores or through direct inoculation of fungi into subcutaneous tissue or bloodstream
    e. Pathology: *broad hyphae invade arteries and veins, causing tissue necrosis*
  2. Clinical
    a. Sinusitis
    b. Orbital cellulitis
    c. Thrombophlebitis with stroke
    d. Focal CNS involvement via direct extension of infection
    e. Rhinocerebral form usually begins with fever and a painful swelling of the nose and fronto-orbital area, which rapidly progresses to the striking necrotic lesions
    f. Usually fatal disease
  3. Treatment
    a. Amphotericin B, 1.5 mg/kg/day intravenously, for a total dose of 1.0–1.5 g; renal function and serum potassium levels should be closely monitored
    b. Surgical debridement of necrotic tissue
F. **Blastomycosis**
  1. Pathophysiology
    a. Caused by *Blastomyces dermatitidis*
    b. Acquire the infection by inhalation of spores found in soil and vegetation; can cause disease readily in immunocompetent host
    c. Pathology: affects lungs, skin, bones, retina, urinary tract, and CNS (25% of patients)
  2. Clinical
    a. Systemic: nonspecific fever, malaise, etc.

   b. Neurologic
      i. Arachnoiditis
      ii. Focal intracranial or paraspinal abscess
      iii. Cranial neuropathies due to skull base lytic lesions
   3. Treatment: amphotericin B, 0.6–1.0 mg/kg/day intravenously, for a total dose of 1–2 g; renal function and serum potassium levels should be closely monitored
G. Miscellaneous
   1. Fungal infection in normal host
      a. *Coccidioides*
      b. Histoplasmosis
      c. Blastomycosis

VII. Lyme Disease
A. Pathophysiology
   1. Caused by *Borrelia burgdorferi*
   2. Vector: via *Ixodes dammini* tick
   3. Early summer most common
B. Clinical
   1. Acute form: more severe signs and symptoms and often with CN palsy (facial palsy most common)
   2. Presentations
      a. Erythema chronicum migrans
      b. Headache
      c. Myalgias
      d. Meningismus
      e. Cranial neuropathy (CN VII most common)
      f. Radiculopathy
      g. Mononeuritis multiplex
      h. Peripheral neuropathy (one-third have neuropathies)
   3. Diagnosis: sural biopsy demonstrates perivascular inflammation and axonal degeneration
   4. Treatment
      a. Facial palsy: doxycycline, 100 mg bid for 3 weeks
      b. CNS involvement
         i. Third generation i.v. cephalosporin (e.g., ceftriaxone, 2 mg intravenously q12h)
         ii. Penicillin, 3.3 million units intravenously q4h
         iii. Treatment for 2–3 weeks

VIII. Prion Infections of the Nervous System
A. **Creutzfeldt-Jakob disease (CJD)**
   1. Pathophysiology and epidemiology
      a. Prevalence: 0.5/1,000,000
      b. More common in men
      c. Most cases sporadic
      d. 10–15% are familial (autosomal dominant)
      e. Genetics: variable mutations or repeats in the *PrP* gene
      f. Prion destroyed by autoclave 132°C or bleach for >1 hour
   2. Clinical
      a. Begins insidiously with apathy, followed by incoordination and visual dysfunction (diplopia, vision loss) and evolves within several weeks to significant neurologic involvement (rigidity, motor dysfunction, and cognitive dysfunction)

   b. Characteristically have rapidly progressive dementia (Heidenhaim dementia) and exhibit startle or stimulation myoclonus
   c. May also have other movement disorders, pyramidal signs, and seizures
3. Diagnosis
   a. Definitive diagnosis: detecting CJD-specific mutations by prion gene analysis

NB: Detection of the 14-3-3 protein in CSF in the appropriate setting may aid with the diagnosis.

   b. *Pathology: diffuse spongiform encephalopathy with widespread neuronal loss, gliosis, and amyloid plaques*
   c. *EEG: 80% have periodic sharp wave complexes by 12 weeks, which evolves to diffuse slowing*
   d. *MRI: increased T2 signal in basal ganglia and thalamus*
4. Pathology: vacuolization of the cortex
5. Prognosis: 90% die within 1 year
B. **Gerstmann-Straüssler-Scheinker syndrome**
   1. Pathophysiology and epidemiology
      a. *Probable autosomal dominant disorder*
      b. *Genetics: codon 102 (proline for leucine) or mutations at codons 105, 117, 198, or 217*
      c. Can be transmitted to nonhuman primates and rodents
      d. Prevalence: 0.1/1,000,000
   2. Clinical
      a. Usually begins gradually after age 40 years
      b. Hallmark clinical sign: progressive ataxia and insomnia
      c. Early signs/symptoms: dysphonia, dysphagia, dysarthria, nystagmus, tremor, and visual disturbances
      d. Later signs/symptoms: dementia, behavioral disturbances, spasticity, rigidity, paralysis, and muscle atrophy
      e. Myoclonus is variable
   3. Pathology: atrophy and amyloid plaques
   4. Diagnosis
      a. EEG: diffuse slowing
      b. MRI: cerebellar atrophy or T2 prolongation involving the basal ganglia (iron deposition)
      c. Confirmed by detection of prion gene mutations
      d. Pathology: spongiform encephalopathy and demyelination
   5. Prognosis: most die within 1–10 years
C. **Kuru**
   1. Pathophysiology and epidemiology
      a. Tribes in New Guinea (particularly in women and children) secondary to consumption of brain and/or mucosal and cutaneous contact with neural tissues
      b. Very rare because of discontinuation of cannibalism
      c. Long incubation period (>5–20 years)
      d. Genetics: mutation of methionine homozygosity at codon 129 is a risk factor
   2. Clinical
      a. First symptoms are tremor and ataxia followed by dysarthria, dementia, and progressive neurologic deterioration
      b. May have pain in lower extremities
      c. Loss of facial motor control
      d. Euphoria
      e. Development of dementia is late in course

   3. Diagnosis/Pathology: neuronal loss in cortex and cerebellum: kuru plaques in cere-
      bellum
   4. Prognosis: death within 1 year
 D. **Fatal familial insomnia**
   1. Clinical features
      a. *Dysautonomia and loss of dream-like state with dream enactment in patients with degener-*
         ative lesions of dorsomedial and anterior nucleus of thalamus
      b. Typically begins between ages 30 and 60 years
      c. Death within 6–36 months of onset
      d. Progressive loss of sleep associated with other autonomic and somatomotor mani-
         festations, worsening within a few months to almost total lack of sleep <2 hours per
         night)
      e. May have abnormal galvanic sympathetic skin response
      f. Plasma epinephrine and norepinephrine may increase
      g. Neurophysiologic and polysomnographic features
      h. EEG: background EEG demonstrates α rhythm that becomes progressively slower
         and more diffuse; may develop spike complexes that recur every 1–2 seconds
      i. Evoked potentials: normal
      j. Sympathetic skin response: diminished or absent
      k. Polysomnography: physiologic sleep (spindles, K complexes, and other nonrapid
         eye movement features) is absent or decreased to only a few minutes' duration;
         rapid eye movement sleep may occur briefly but usually has incomplete muscle ato-
         nia and may have dream-enacting behavior (similar to rapid eye movement sleep
         behavior disorder); late in course, myoclonic jerks may accompany periodic slow
         waves (similar to CJD)
      l. Administration of benzodiazepine and barbiturates provokes transition to coma but
         does not trigger activity typical of pharmacologically induced sleep
   2. Neuropathology and DNA studies
      a. Spongiform degeneration with severe neuronal loss and reactive gliosis in anterior
         and dorsomedial thalamic nuclei (other thalamic nuclei were less frequently noted)
      b. Moderate gliosis of deep layers of cortex (more prominently in frontal and temporal
         regions), inferior olives, and cerebellar cortex
      c. Hypothalamus and reticular activating center are spared
      d. Prion fragments differ from those of CJD
      e. DNA
         i. The PRNP (prion protein) D178N/129M genotype must be present for the dis-
            ease to occur
        ii. Autosomal dominant inheritance (very rare, with two families in Italy and one in
            France identified, and at least three other families in the United States) associated
            with prion disease due to a mutation in codon 178 of the PRNP gene
       iii. Sporadic cases do occur with selective spongiform thalamic degeneration that
            appears to affect methionine at codon 129 of the mutant allele (a site common for
            methionine/valine polymorphism)

IX. Parasitic Infections of the Nervous System
 A. **Primary amebic meningoencephalitis**
   1. Caused by *Naegleria fowleri* that inhabits soil and water (especially warm climates)
   2. Enters the nasal cavity and migrates through cribriform plate via olfactory nerves to
      the CNS

3. Rapidly progressive with mortality >90%
4. Pathology: hemorrhagic meningoencephalitis
5. Diagnosis: motile trophozoites in CSF on wet mount
6. Treatment: supportive only

B. **Cerebral amebiasis**
  1. Caused by *Entamoeba histolytica*
     a. Common intestinal parasite
     b. Infects almost 10% of the world population, causing 100,000 deaths every year
     c. May become aggressive and enter the bloodstream to cause systemic disease and CNS involvement
  2. Diagnosis: demonstration of parasites in biopsy
  3. Treatment
     a. Metronidazole (2000 mg/day) for 10 days
     b. Surgical resection of accessible lesions

C. **Toxoplasmosis**
  1. Caused by *Toxoplasma gondii* (intracellular parasite)
  2. Humans are infected by eating undercooked meat or by ingestion of contaminated cat feces.
  3. Seropositive in 30–75% of the general population
  4. *Congenital toxoplasmosis.*
     a. Transmission of the infection from mother to fetus when women acquire the infection during pregnancy
     b. Clinical: hydrocephalus, microcephalus, intracranial calcifications, mental retardation, seizures, deafness, blindness, and hepatomegaly
     c. CT: periventricular Ca^{2+} or diffuse parenchymal Ca^{2+}
  5. *Acquired toxoplasmosis*
     a. May occur in immunocompetent (usually asymptomatic and without CNS involvement) or immunocompromised (frequent opportunistic infection)
     b. CT with contrast: ring-enhancing lesions (diffuse focal lesions with predilection for basal ganglia and deep gray matter)
  6. Pathology: cerebral abscesses consisting of a necrotic center and a periphery in which multiple tachyzoites and cysts are seen together with patchy areas of necrosis, perivascular cuffing of lymphocytes, and glial nodules composed of astrocytes and microglial cells
  7. Treatment
     a. Cerebral toxoplasmosis: pyrimethamine (100–200 mg the first day, followed by 50–75 mg/day) plus sulfadiazine (4–6 g/day) for >2 months
     b. Supplement with folate, 8–10 mg/day, to avoid the toxic effects of pyrimethamine
     c. Clindamycin (2400 mg/day) is an alternative drug in AIDS patients developing skin reactions to sulfadiazine

D. **Trypanosomiasis**
  1. *Chagas' disease (American trypanosomiasis)*
     a. *Caused by* Trypanosoma cruzi
     b. In South and Central America, affects more than 15 million people
     c. Transmitted by the bite of *Triatoma*
     d. Myocarditis and hepatosplenomegaly may occur during the acute stage
     e. Meningoencephalitis with multiple areas of hemorrhagic necrosis, glial proliferation, and perivascular infiltrates of inflammatory cells
     f. May go into latent phase, but this is not associated with primary neurologic complications

    g. Treatment
       i. Nifurtimox (8–10 mg/kg/day)
       ii. Benznidazole (5–10 mg/kg/day)
       iii. Itraconazole (400 mg/day)
2. *Sleeping sickness (African trypanosomiasis)*
    a. *Caused by subspecies of* Trypanosoma brucei
    b. Painful erythematous nodules associated with regional lymphadenopathy that disappear spontaneously
    c. *Winterbottom's sign: fever, cervical lymphadenopathy, and hepatosplenomegaly (aka stage I)*
    d. Stage II: somnolence, apathy, involuntary movements, cerebellar ataxia, delayed hyperesthesia with eventual progression to dementia, stupor, coma, and death if untreated
    e. Treatment
       i. Suramin (1 g weekly for 1 month)
       ii. Pentamidine (4 mg/kg/day in two doses given 4 days apart)

E. **Cysticercosis**
1. Humans are intermediate hosts of the pork tapeworm, *Taenia solium*
2. Acquired by ingesting its eggs from contaminated water/food or by the fecal-oral route
3. After 1–3 months, eggs hatch into oncospheres in the human intestine that cross the intestinal wall into the bloodstream and spread mainly to eye, skeletal muscles, and the CNS, where the larvae (cysticercus) develop
4. Considered the most common helminthic disease of the CNS in the developing world
5. Clinical
    a. Seizures
       i. Epilepsy is most common presentation
       ii. Most common cause of epilepsy in Central America
    b. Focal neurologic deficits from CNS lesions
    c. Neuroimaging
       i. Migrating intraventricular cyst is pathognomonic
       ii. MRI T1 = target lesion, which is scolex
6. Treatment
    a. Calcified lesions: only symptomatic treatment (i.e., antiepileptic drugs)
    b. Viable cysts
       i. Albendazole (10 mg/kg/day divided in 2 doses) for 15 days; better CNS penetration, more effective cyst destruction
       ii. Praziquantel (three doses of 25–30 mg/kg given every 2 hours)
       iii. If > 50 cysts or with subarachnoid or ventricular involvement, treat for increased ICP/edema prior to initiation of antihelminthics

F. **Trichinosis**
1. *Intestinal nematode infection due to undercooked pork containing encysted larvae of* Trichinella spiralis
2. After initial gastroenteritis, may have invasion of skeletal muscle, but weakness is mainly limited to muscles innervated by CNs (e.g., tongue, masseters, extraocular muscle, oropharynx, etc.)
3. Rarely, in acute phase may have cerebral symptoms due to emboli from trichinella myocarditis

4. Lab findings: eosinophilia/bentonite flocculation assay, muscle biopsy
5. Treatment
   a. Symptoms usually subside spontaneously
   b. If severe
      i. Thiabendazole, 25 mg/kg bid
      ii. Mebendazole (200 mg/day)
      iii. Add prednisone, 40–60 mg/day, to decrease inflammatory response

ADDITIONAL NOTES

CHAPTER 8

Neurotoxicology and Nutritional Disorders

I. Heavy Metals
A. **Arsenic**
1. Pathophysiology: a primary source is pesticides; reacts with sulfhydryl groups of proteins and interferes with several steps of exudative metabolism in the neuron, producing dying back type axonal degeneration, particularly in myelinated fibers
2. Clinical
   a. Axonal sensory neuropathy begins within 5–10 days.
   b. *Acute gastrointestinal symptoms followed by painful paresthesia with progressive distal weakness.*
   c. Central nervous system (CNS) symptoms may develop rapidly in acute poisoning, with drowsiness and confusion progressing to stupor or delirium.
   d. Hyperkeratosis and sloughing of the skin on the palms and soles may occur several weeks after acute poisoning followed by a chronic state of redness and swelling of the distal extremities.
   e. *Nail changes (Mees' lines).*
   f. Chronic poisoning may develop aplastic anemia.
3. Diagnosis
   a. Acute intoxication: renal excretion >0.1 mg arsenic in 24 hours
   b. Chronic intoxication: hair concentrations >0.1 mg/100 g of hair
4. *Treatment*
   a. *Acute oral ingestion*
      i. *Gastric lavage followed by instillation of 1% sodium thiosulfate*
      ii. *British anti-Lewisite (BAL) given parenterally in a 10% solution*
5. Prognosis
   a. Once neuropathy occurs, treatment is usually ineffective
   b. Mortality: >50–75% in severe cases
B. **Gold**
1. Pathophysiology: used in the treatment of inflammatory conditions
2. Clinical
   a. Chronic distal axonal sensory > motor neuropathy
   b. Painful, involving palms or soles
   c. Myokymia
   d. Brachial plexopathy
   e. Acute inflammatory demyelinating polyradiculopathy
3. Pathology: loss of myelin as well as active axonal degeneration
4. Treatment: chelation therapy with BAL has been used but usually is not necessary

C. **Mercury**
 1. Clinical
   a. Acute: salivation and severe gastrointestinal dysfunction followed by hallucinations and delirium
   b. Chronic
      i. Chronic axonal sensory neuropathy
      ii. Constriction of visual fields, ataxia, dysarthria, decreased hearing, tremor, and dementia
      iii. Parkinsonism
      iv. Children may have acrodynia
 2. Treatment
   a. Chelating agents (e.g., D-Penicillamine, BAL, ethylenediaminetetraacetic acid)
D. **Thallium**
 1. Pathophysiology: found in rat poison; thallium ions act interchangeably with potassium in respect to their transport by the Na/L ATPase system
 2. Clinical
   a. *Hallmark: alopecia; sometimes with cranial nerve and autonomic involvement*
   b. Acute
      i. Gastrointestinal symptoms within hours of ingestion.
      ii. Moderate doses produce neuropathic symptoms in <48 hours consisting of pain and paresthesia followed by ascending sensory loss and distal weakness.
      iii. May produce acute inflammatory demyelinating polyradiculopathy-like syndrome.
      iv. Large doses (>2 g) produce cardiovascular shock, coma, and death within 24 hours.
   c. Chronic: chronic axonal sensorimotor neuropathy
 3. Treatment
   a. Chelating agents
      i. Prussian blue (potassium ferric hexacyanoferrate)
      ii. BAL
      iii. Dithiozone
      iv. Diethyldithiocarbamate
   b. If acute, can also perform gastric lavage
E. **Lead**
 1. Pathophysiology
   a. Diminishes cerebral glucose supplies
   b. Intoxication results in inhibition of myelin synthesis with demyelination

NB: Lead has direct effects on porphyrin metabolism, by inhibiting gamma-aminolevulinic acid dehydrase.

   c. Adults
      i. Use of exterior paints and gasoline
      ii. More likely to present with neuropathy, predominantly, but not exclusively, the radial nerve
   d. Children
      i. Pica and eating lead-based paints
      ii. More likely to present with encephalopathy
 2. Clinical
   a. *Neuropathy*

      i. *Chronic axonal motor neuropathy*
     ii. *Classic neurologic presentation: wristdrop*
    iii. *Typical clinical triad*
        (A) *Abdominal pain and constipation*
        (B) *Anemia*
        (C) *Neuropathy*
  b. CNS toxicity
      i. Adult
        (A) Prodrome: progressive weakness and loss of weight
        (B) Ashen color of the face
        (C) Mild persistent headache
        (D) Fine tremor of the muscles of the eyes, tongue, and face
        (E) Progression into encephalopathic state
        (F) May have focal motor weakness
     ii. *Children: prodrome usually nonspecific evolving into encephalopathy (50%)*
3. *Diagnosis*
  a. *Lead lines on gums*
  b. *Serum: microcytic anemia and red blood cell basophilic stippling*
  c. *X-rays may demonstrate lead lines of long bones*
4. Treatment
  a. Chelating agents (e.g., BAL, ethylenediaminetetraacetic acid, penicillamine)
5. Prognosis
  a. Mild intoxication: usually complete recovery
  b. Severe encephalopathy: mortality high but lessened by the use of combined chelating agent therapy
  c. Residual neurologic sequelae: blindness or partial visual disturbances, persistent convulsions, personality changes, and mental retardation
  d. Prognosis worse in children than in adults

F. **Manganese**
  1. Pathology: diffuse injury to ganglion cells, *primarily of globus pallidus*
  2. Clinical
    a. *Extrapyramidal signs/symptoms, including dystonia, bradykinesia, tremor, and gait dysfunction*
    b. Personality changes consisting of irritability, lack of sociability, uncontrollable laughter, tearfulness, and euphoria
  3. Treatment: supportive therapy

G. **Iron**
  1. Acute iron toxicity
    a. Symptoms occur in 30–60 minutes
    b. Initially, bloody vomiting followed by bloody diarrhea
    c. Severe cases: coma or convulsions
    d. Treatment
      i. Supportive: induction of vomiting, gastric lavage, maintenance of adequate ventilation, correction of acidosis, and control of vital signs
     ii. Chelation: deferoxamine, 5–10 g
    e. Mortality: 45%
  2. Iron deficiency can lead to restless legs syndrome

H. **Tin:** Triethyltin exposure acutely results in white matter vacuolation; and with chronic exposure, demyelination and gliosis are seen

II. Organic Solvents
A. **Methyl alcohol (e.g., methanol, wood alcohol)**
1. Pathophysiology
   a. Component of antifreeze and alcoholic drinks.
   b. Methanol itself is only mildly toxic, but its oxidation products (formaldehyde and formic acid) induce a severe acidosis.
   c. Methanol may cause bilateral hemorrhagic necrosis of the caudate, putamen, pons, optic nerves, cerebellum, and subcortical white matter.
2. Clinical
   a. *Visual disturbance and ocular manifestations*
      i. Amblyopia
      ii. Scotomas
      iii. Total blindness
   b. Extrapyramidal signs (bradykinesia, masked facies, tremor)
3. Treatment: three-part approach—ethanol, bicarbonate, dialysis (in severe cases)
B. **Ethylene glycol**
1. Pathophysiology: used as antifreeze, tobacco moistener, and in paint; toxic dose > 100 mL
2. Clinical
   a. Restless and agitated followed by somnolence, stupor, coma, and even convulsions
   b. Death due to cardiopulmonary failure
   c. Characteristic metabolic findings: metabolic acidosis with large anion gap, hypocalcemia, and calcium oxalate crystals in the urine
3. Treatment
   a. Supportive care
   b. Correct metabolic acidosis and hypocalcemia
   c. Infuse ethanol at 5–10 g/hour
   d. Dialysis may be necessary to remove ethylene glycol and to treat uremia

III. Gases
A. **Carbon monoxide poisoning**
1. Pathophysiology
   a. *Most common cause of death by poisoning in the United States*
   b. Damages the brain by three mechanisms
      i. Production of carboxyhemoglobin that causes hypoxemia
      ii. Decreased release of oxygen to tissues
      iii. Direct mitochondrial toxicity
   c. Pathology
      i. Bilateral necrotic lesions involving the *globus pallidus*
      ii. Hippocampal damage
      iii. Supratentorial demyelination
      iv. Cortical damage (watershed distribution)
2. Neuroimaging
   a. Magnetic resonance imaging (MRI): lesions usually appear hypointense on T1 and hyperintense on T2 involving globus pallidus
   b. May also involve the thalamus, caudate, putamen, and cerebellum
   c. Differential diagnosis of bilateral basal ganglia lesions
      i. Carbon monoxide
      ii. Cyanide

     iii. Ethylene glycol
     iv. Methanol (more putamen)
      v. Aminoacidopathies
     vi. Infarction
    vii. PKAN (formerly Hallervorden-Spatz disease)
   viii. Leigh disease
     ix. Wilson's disease
      x. Mitochondrial disorders
     xi. Neoplasm
    xii. Multiple systems atrophy
  3. Clinical
    a. Hypoxia without cyanosis (cherry-red appearance)
    b. ± Myocardial infarction
    c. Retinal hemorrhages
    d. Neurologic: lethargy that progresses to coma followed by brain stem dysfunction and movement disorders
  4. Treatment
    a. Oxygen 100%
    b. Hyperbaric chamber (if severe)
  5. Prognosis: residual movement disorders are common

IV. Organophosphates
  A. **Pathophysiology**
    1. Irreversible acetylcholinesterase inhibitors.
    2. Organophosphates are found in insecticides (e.g., parathion, malathion), pesticides, and chemical warfare agents (e.g., tabun, sarin, soman).
    3. Highly lipid soluble.
    4. May be absorbed through the skin, mucous membranes, gastrointestinal tract, and lungs.
  B. **Clinical**
    1. Symptoms occur within a few hours of exposure
    2. Neuromuscular blockade; autonomic and CNS dysfunction, including headache, miosis, muscle fasciculations, and diffuse muscle cramping; weakness; excessive secretions; nausea; vomiting; and diarrhea
    3. Excessive exposure: seizures and coma
    4. Delayed neuropathy or myelopathy beginning 1–3 weeks after acute exposure
    5. Electrophysiology
      a. Increased spontaneous firing rate and amplitude of the miniature end-plate potentials
      b. Depolarization block
  C. **Treatment**
    1. Supportive care: clean patient completely
    2. Lavage
    3. Atropine, 1–2 mg
    4. Pralidoxime, 1 g intravenously
      a. Cholinesterase reactivator
      b. Reversal of peripheral acetylcholinesterase for proportion of enzyme that has not irreversibly bound the inhibitor

V. Other Industrial Toxins
  A. **Cyanide intoxication**

1. Pathophysiology: inhibition of ferric ion-containing enzymes, including cytochrome oxidase (produces tissue hypoxia by inhibiting the action of respiratory enzymes)
2. Clinical
   a. Acute: excessive dose: loud cry with generalized convulsions and death within 2–5 minutes
   b. Chronic: agitation, salivation, anxiety, confusion, and nausea followed by vertigo, headache, and ataxia followed by sudden loss of consciousness and seizures ± opisthotonos
3. Treatment
   a. Supportive care with respiratory assistance, if needed
   b. Sodium and amyl nitrite
   c. Methylene blue: for excessive methemoglobinemia
   d. Commercially available cyanide antidote kit
B. **Acrylamide:** impairs axonal transport causing accumulation of neurofilaments and para-noidal swelling mostly in large myelinated axons, producing a dying back axonopathy, affecting bother peripheral nerves and central tracts (e.g., dorsal spinocerebellar and gracile tract)

VI. Animal Toxins
A. **Snake venoms**
   1. Pathophysiology
      a. In the United States, estimated 50,000 snakebites annually
      b. Individuals are often drunk
      c. Families
         i. Viperidae
            (A) True vipers, pit vipers, rattlesnakes, moccasins, cottonmouths, and copperheads
            (B) 95% of the annual snakebites in the United States
         ii. Elapidae
            (A) Cobras, kraits, mambas, and coral snakes
         iii. Hydrophiidae
            (A) Sea snakes in Asian and Australian waters
      d. Potent toxins to cardiac muscle, coagulant pathways, and neurologic system
      e. Neurotoxicity
         i. Associated with action on neuromuscular junction, either presynaptically or postsynaptically
         ii. Presynaptic toxins
            (A) *α-Bungarotoxin, notexin, and taipoxin*
            (B) *Act to inhibit the normal release of acetylcholine (ACh) from the presynaptic cell of the neuromuscular junction*
         iii. *Postsynaptic neurotoxins: produce variable degrees of nondepolarizing neuromuscular block*
   2. Clinical
      a. Local evidence of envenomation: bite site pain and swelling
      b. Preparalytic signs and symptoms: headache, vomiting, loss of consciousness, pares-thesia, ptosis, and external ophthalmoplegia
      c. Paralytic signs and symptoms
         i. Paralysis develops within 1–10 hours
         ii. Facial and jaw paresis compromises swallowing

iii. Progressive diaphragmatic, oropharyngeal, intercostal, and limb weakness followed by loss of consciousness and seizures

iv. Death due to circulatory arrest if not stabilized

d. Other systemic effects: relate to coagulation deficits, including cerebral and subarachnoid hemorrhage

3. Treatment: supportive care, antivenoms

B. **Ciguatoxin toxin**

1. Found in the Pacific and Caribbean
2. Produced by a marine dinoflagellate (*Gambierdiscus toxicus*) that attaches to algae and is passed up the food chain
3. Carried by numerous fish, but only humans are adversely affected
4. Mechanism: tetrodotoxin-sensitive sodium channel resulting in membrane depolarization
5. Clinical: begins >3–5 hours after ingestion, with perioral and distal paresthesia followed by weakness, myalgia, dizziness, and dry mouth; may also have ptosis, dilated pupils, photophobia, transient blindness
6. Treatment: supportive

C. **Saxitoxin**

1. Similar in action and structure to the sodium channel blockers (i.e., tetrodotoxin found in puffer and sunfish)
2. Found in clams and mussels
3. Produced by dinoflagellates of the genus *Gonyaulax*
4. Clinical: acute paralysis within 30–60 minutes; may have paresthesia and cerebellar ataxia
5. Mortality: 1–10%
6. Treatment: supportive

D. **Latrodectism**

1. Clinical syndrome that follows black widow spider bite
2. More potent than pit viper venom, but lower volume
3. Mechanism: forced release of ACh from the presynaptic neuromuscular junction and also stimulation of sympathetic and parasympathetic cholinergic systems
4. Clinical
   a. Acute: pain with severe local muscle spasm occurs immediately
   b. Subacute: headache, fatigue, weakness
5. Mortality: <1% (fatal if cardiovascular complications)
6. Treatment: usually supportive care only; antivenom is available but usually not used due to higher risk of adverse effects of sera

VII. Plant Toxins

A. **Mushrooms**

1. Most often abundant in summer and fall, resulting in higher rates of intoxication during those seasons

Scientific name	Toxin	Clinical presentation	Treatment
Amanita muscaria	Cyclic polypeptides	Strong anticholinergic effects, including agitation, muscle spasms, ataxia, mydriasis, convulsions, and hallucinations	No treatment Atropine of minimal benefit

Scientific name	Toxin	Clinical presentation	Treatment
Amanita pantherina	Atropine-like toxins	Strong anticholinergic effects, including agitation, muscle spasms, ataxia, mydriasis, convulsions, and hallucinations	No treatment Atropine of minimal benefit
		Mortality: 10%	

B. **Lathyrism**
1. *Consumption of the chickpea,* Lathyrus: associated with toxic neurologic signs when *Lathyrus* accounts for > one-third of calories
2. Three neurotoxins
   a. Amino-β-oxalyl aminopropionic acid
   b. Amino-oxalyl aminobutyric acid
   c. β-N-oxalyl amino-L-alanine: responsible for corticospinal dysfunction by inducing neurodegeneration through excitotoxic actions at the AMPA receptor
3. Pathology: anterolateral sclerosis in the thoracolumbar cord with loss of axons and myelin
4. Clinical: spastic paraplegia
5. Treatment: supportive only

VIII. Bacterial Toxins
A. **Diphtheria**
1. Caused by *Corynebacterium diphtheriae*
2. Rare in the United States but may occur with travel, particularly to Eastern Europe
3. Pathology: *noninflammatory demyelinating, primarily affecting muscle and myelin*
4. Clinical
   a. Two clinical forms
      i. Oropharyngeal
      ii. Cutaneous
   b. Often begins with cranial neuropathies, particularly involving oropharyngeal and eye muscles
   c. Over weeks, may develop predominantly sensory polyneuropathy or a proximal motor neuropathy
   d. May be misdiagnosed as acute inflammatory demyelinating polyradiculopathy, but diphtheria has more prominent visual blurring and palatal dysfunction
5. Treatment
   a. Supportive care
   b. Antitoxin administration
6. Mortality
   a. Without antitoxin: 50%
   b. With antitoxin: <10%
B. *Tetanus*
1. *Produced by* Clostridium tetani *under anaerobic conditions of wounds*
2. Mechanism: retrograde axonal transport to nervous system and blocks exocytosis via interaction with synaptobrevin
3. Clinical
   a. Rapidly progressive axonal peripheral neuropathy
   b. Asymmetric sensory and motor responses
   c. May also have CNS involvement

     d. Death in <1 week of symptoms

4. Treatment

    a. Removal of the toxin source

    b. Supportive care

    c. Neutralization of circulating toxin via human tetanus immune globulin

C. **Botulism**

1. *Pathophysiology*

    a. *Caused primarily by* Clostridium botulinum, *which is a gram-positive anaerobe*

    b. Three forms

       i. *Food-borne botulism*

         (A) 1000 cases per year worldwide

         (B) Usually home-canned vegetables

         (C) Most associated with type A spores

       ii. *Wound botulism*

         (A) Injection drug use

         (B) Post-traumatic

       iii. *Infant botulism*

         (A) Most common in children aged 1 week to 11 months

         (B) Usually neurotoxins types A and B

         (C) Death in <2% of cases in the United States, but higher worldwide

    c. The most common form now is wound botulism resulting from illicit drug use

    d. Neurotoxins types A, B, and E are usual cause, but, rarely, types F and G can also be symptomatic

    e. *Irreversible binding to the presynaptic membrane of peripheral cholinergic nerves blocking ACh release at the neuromuscular junction*

       i. Three-step process

         (A) Toxin binds to receptors on the nerve ending

         (B) Toxin molecule I then internalized

         (C) Within the nerve cell, the toxin interferes with the release of ACh

      ii. Cleavage of one of the SNARE (soluble N-ethylmaleimide-sensitive factor attachment protein receptor) proteins by botulinum neurotoxin inhibits the exocytosis of ACh from the synaptic terminal

2. Clinical

    a. Blurred vision, dysphagia, dysarthria, papillary response to light, dry mouth, constipation, and urinary retention

    b. Tensilon® (edrophonium chloride) test: positive in 30% of cases

    c. Infant botulism: constipation, lethargy, poor sucking, weak cry

    d. *Electrophysiologic criteria for botulism*

       i. *↓Compound muscle action potential amplitude in at least two muscles*

       ii. *20% facilitation of compound muscle action potential amplitude*

       iii. *Persistent facilitation for 2 minutes after activation*

       iv. No postactivation exhaustion

       v. Single fiber electromyography—↑jitter and blocking

    e. Prognosis

       i. Most patients recover completely in 6 months

3. Treatment

    a. Supportive care

    b. Antibiotics

       i. Wound botulism: penicillin G or metronidazole.

       ii. Antibiotics are not recommended for infant botulism because cell death and lysis may result in the release of more toxin.
   c. Horse serum antitoxin
      i. Types A, B, and E
      ii. Side effects of serum sickness and anaphylaxis

IX. Miscellaneous
  A. *Marchiafava-Bignami disease*
    1. Clinical
      a. Insidious cerebral dysfunction
      b. Dementia
      c. Depression
      d. Apathy
      e. Delusions
      f. Slow progression with death in 3–6 years
    2. Pathology: necrosis of corpus callosum; no evidence of inflammation
  B. *Tryptophan:* may cause eosinophilic myalgic syndrome
  C. *Drugs/toxins causing peripheral neuropathy*
    1. Nitrofurantoin
    2. Vincristine
    3. N-hexane
    4. Methyl butyl ketone
    5. Disulfiram (Antabuse®)
    6. Arsenic
    7. Lead
    8. Mercury
    9. Thallium
  D. *Medications associated with myopathy*
    1. Alcohol
    2. Colchicine
    3. Lovastatin
    4. Zidovudine (AZT)
    5. Diazacholesterol
    6. Clofibrate
    7. Steroids
    9. Rifampin
   10. Kaluretics
   11. Chloroquine
  E. **Toxins that cause seizures**
    1. Alcohol toxicity or withdrawal
    2. Barbiturate toxicity or withdrawal
    3. Benzodiazepine toxicity or withdrawal
    4. Cocaine
    5. Phencyclidine
    6. Amphetamines
    7. Common medications that cause seizures
      a. Antidepressants (tricyclic antidepressants, bupropion)
      b. Antipsychotics (chlorpromazine, thioridazine, trifluoperazine, perphenazine, haloperidol)

    c. Analgesics (fentanyl, meperidine, pentazocine, propoxyphene, topiramate [Ultram®])

    d. Local anesthetics (lidocaine, procaine)

    e. Sympathomimetics (terbutaline, ephedrine, phenylpropanolamine)

    f. Antibiotics (penicillin, ampicillin, cephalosporins, metronidazole, isoniazid, pyrimethamine)

    g. Antineoplastic agents (vincristine, chlorambucil, methotrexate, bischloronitrosourea, cytosine arabinoside)

    h. Bronchodilators (aminophylline, theophylline)

        i. Immunosuppressants

        i. Cyclosporine

        ii. Muromonab-CD3 (Orthoclone OKT3®)

    j. Others (insulin, antihistamines, atenolol, baclofen, cyclosporine)

F. *Specific action of toxins/agents*

    1. *α-Bungarotoxin: irreversible postsynaptic receptor blockade*

    2. *Curare and vecuronium: competitive postsynaptic nicotine receptor blockade*

    3. *Succinylcholine: postsynaptic receptor blockade causing depolarization*

G. **Ethanol**

    1. **Acute alcohol intoxication features are related to the blood level dose of the toxin.**

      a. 0.05–0.1 mg/dL: disinhibited

      b. 0.1–0.3 mg/dL: inebriated, ataxic

      c. 0.3–0.35 mg/dL: very intoxicated

      d. >0.35 mg/dL: potentially lethal (especially when drinking takes on a competitive quality such as chugging contests, etc.)

    2. Chronic alcohol use can lead to

      a. *Wernicke's encephalopathy* (arising from nutritional deficiency of vitamin B_1)

        i. Spongy degeneration

        ii. Petechiae hemorrhage involving mamillary bodies, hypothalamus, thalamus (dorsal and anterior medial nuclei, pulvinar), periaqueductal gray matter, floor of the fourth ventricle, dorsal nuclei, vestibular nuclei

        iii. Characterized by confusion, ataxia, ophthalmoplegia

        iv. Mortality can be up to 10–20%

        v. Treatment: thiamine

      b. *Korsakoff disease*

        i. Chronic phase of Wernicke's syndrome

        ii. There is atrophy of the mamillary bodies, dorsomedial nucleus of the thalamus

        iii. Presents with retrograde and anterograde amnesia

      c. *Nutritional polyneuropathy:* typically a sensorimotor neuropathy

      d. *Hepatic failure* (hepatic encephalopathy or non-Wilsonian hepatocerebral degeneration)

        i. Asterixis with altered level of consciousness

        ii. Alzheimer's type 2 cells ("watery cells")

        iii. Pseudolaminar necrosis, microcavitation of the lenticular nuclei

        iv. Electroencephalogram: general slowing, triphasic waves

        v. Serum NH_3 may not correspond to symptoms

      e. *Central pontine myelinolysis*

        i. From rapid correction of hyponatremia

        ii. Characterized by progressive paresis, cranial nerve paresis, preserved mental responsiveness

        iii. The demyelination is often M- or W-shaped in the pons

  f. *Anterior superior vermal cerebellar degeneration*
   i. Predominantly in alcoholic men, presenting with truncal ataxia
   ii. Loss of Purkinje > granule cells
  g. *Marchiafava-Bignami disease:* central necrosis of the corpus callosum presenting with a disconnection syndrome

H. **Neurologic complications associated with chemotherapy**

Altretamine	Peripheral neuropathy
	Ataxia
	Tremor
	Visual hallucinations
Amsacrine	Seizures
Azacitidine	Muscle pain and weakness
Bleomycin	Raynaud's phenomenon
Busulfan	Seizures
	Venous thrombosis
Carboplatin	Peripheral neuropathy
	Hearing loss
	Transient cortical blindness
Cladribine	Peripheral neuropathy
Cisplatin	Peripheral neuropathy
	Ototoxicity (high frequency is affected; tinnitus)
	Encephalopathy
Cytarabine	Cerebellar dysfunction
	Somnolence
	Encephalopathy
	Personality changes
	Peripheral neuropathy
	Rhabdomyolysis
	Myelopathy
Dacarbazine	Paresthesia
Etoposide	Peripheral neuropathy
5-Fluorouracil	Acute cerebellar syndrome
	Encephalopathy
	Seizures
Fludarabine	Visual disturbances
Interleukin-2	Parkinsonism
	Brachial plexopathy
Isotretinoin	Pseudotumor cerebri

Altretamine	**Peripheral neuropathy**
L-Asparaginase	Central vein thrombosis
	Headache
Levamisole	Peripheral neuropathy
Methotrexate	Leukoencephalopathy
	Chemical arachnoiditis (if given intrathecally)
Nitrourease (Carmustine [BCNU])	Encephalopathy
Paclitaxel (Taxol®)	Peripheral neuropathy
Procarbazine	Peripheral neuropathy
	Autonomic neuropathy
	Encephalopathy
	Ataxia
Suramin	Peripheral neuropathy
Tamoxifen	Decreased visual acuity
Teniposide	Peripheral neuropathy
Thiotepa	Myelopathy
Trimexetrate glucoronate	Peripheral neuropathy
Vinblastine	Peripheral neuropathy
	Myalgias
	Cranial neuropathy
	Autonomic neuropathy
Vincristine	Peripheral neuropathy
	Autonomic neuropathy
	Decreased antidiuretic hormone secretion
Vinorelbine	Peripheral neuropathy
	Autonomic neuropathy

I. **Conditions and associated vitamin deficiencies**

Disease	**Vitamin deficiency**	**Clinical features**
Alcoholism	Thiamine	Wernicke-Korsakoff syndrome
Combined system disease	B_{12}; also reported in folate deficiency	Peripheral neuropathy, sensory loss, ataxia, anemia; pathology: spongy degeneration of dorsal and lateral columns; demyelinating peripheral neuropathy; with or without pernicious anemia
Methylmalonic aciduria	B_{12}	Recurrent lethargy, Reye-like disease, aciduria
Not applicable	Biotin	Alopecia, thrush, recurrent encephalopathy

Disease	Vitamin deficiency	Clinical features
Multiple carboxylase deficiency	Biotin	Recurrent encephalopathy with aciduria
Pellagra	Niacin	3 Ds = *di*arrhea, *de*mentia, *der*matitis; peripheral neuropathy; pathology: central chromatolysis; if severe, with degeneration of the dorsal and lateral columns of the spinal cord but without the spongy appearance that is characteristic of B_{12} deficiency
Hartnup's disease	Niacin	Recurrent ataxia and aminoaciduria
Lactic acidosis	Thiamine lipoate	Recurrent ataxia, lethargy, acidosis
Mitochondriopathies	Riboflavin	Recurrent encephalopathy, muscle disease
Bassen-Kornzweig disease	Vitamin E	Neuropathy, ataxia, acanthocytosis
Cholestatic liver disease	Vitamin E	Neuropathy, ataxia
Friedreich-like ataxia	Vitamin E	Ataxia, sensory neuropathy

NB: Nitrous oxide abuse can produce myeloneuropathy that is clinically indistinguishable from vitamin B_{12} deficiency: paresthesias of the hands and feet, gait ataxia, and leg weakness, with reverse Lhermitte's sign (shock-like sensation from feet upwards with neck flexion). Serum B_{12} and Schilling test are usually normal.

ADDITIONAL NOTES

CHAPTER 9

Sleep and Sleep Disorders

I. Neurobiology of Sleep

A. *Sleep-wake regulation*

1. Wake is associated with high monoaminergic and cholinergic projection systems.
2. Nonrapid eye movement (NREM) is associated with low monoaminergic and cholinergic projection systems.
3. Rapid eye movement (REM) is associated with low monoaminergic and high cholinergic projection systems.
4. The reticular activating center uses neurotransmitters that act slowly as neuromodulators.

	Wake state	NREM sleep	REM sleep
Monoaminergic	Increased	Decreased	—
Cholinergic	Increased	Decreased	Increased

B. *Arousal*

1. Activity of the postmesencephalic neurons that modulate arousal is modulated by afferents from the sensory paths, cortex, and hypothalamus.
2. The thalamus provides selective attention by enhancing or attenuating stimuli.
3. *Wakefulness.*
   a. *Modulated by*
      i. Reticular formation (RF).
      ii. Posterior hypothalamus.
      iii. Basal forebrain (nucleus basalis of Meynert or substantia innominata, nucleus of diagonal band, septal nucleus).
      iv. Subthalamic nucleus.
      v. Reticular thalamic nuclei (ventromedial, intralaminar, midline thalamic nuclei).
      vi. Catecholamine- and acetylcholine-containing neurons modulate brain activity in wakefulness.
4. *Ascending pathways mediating arousal.*

	Site of origin	Major cortical projection sites
Norepinephrine	Locus ceruleus (LC) and lateral tegmentum	Diffuse with greater innervation of structures involved in visuomotor response and spatial analysis
Dopamine (DA)	Ventral tegmentum	Primary motor cortex and prefrontal cortex; sensory association areas
Serotonin	Dorsal and median raphe nuclei	Diffuse with some laminar and topographicspecificity
	Dorsolateral medulla	

	Site of origin	Major cortical projection sites
Acetylcholine	Basal forebrain; brain stem, including pedunculopontine tegmental and lateral dorsal tegmental nuclei	Diffuse
Histamine	Posterior hypothalamus	Diffuse

a. *Noradrenaline:* noradrenergic neurons via LC are almost always active during wake state; these neurons become less active in NREM and relatively inactive in REM sleep.

b. *Serotonin:* facilitates sleep onset; raphe nuclei fire most frequently during wake state, decrease in NREM, and are nearly silent in REM; raphe nuclei act as pacemaker by changing firing rates before a change in behavioral state, such as at the end of REM sleep, at which time the dorsal raphe nuclei increase firing before return of muscle tone; therefore, raphe nuclei are integral in control and timing of state changes, especially between REM and NREM sleep; serotonin neurons of raphe nuclei inhibit sensory input and reduce motor activity, facilitating slow-wave sleep (SWS); serotonin antagonists (i.e., phencyclidine inhibits serotonin synthesis by blocking tryptophan hydroxylase) can produce severe insomnia.

c. *DA:* effect of DA on sleep-wake cycle is predominantly wake/arousal.
   i. Mesencephalic DA system has two main paths
      (A) Substantia nigra—projects to the corpus striatum (involved in motor).
      (B) Mesocorticolimbic system, which projects from the ventral tegmentum to the nucleus accumbens, septal nuclei, and frontal lobes (involved in maintaining wakefulness).
   ii. Alerting effects of amphetamines work largely through enhanced release and inhibition of reuptake of DA.
   iii. D1 receptor antagonists desynchronize electroencephalogram (EEG).
   iv. D2 autoreceptors mediate sleep through autoinhibition of ventral tegmental dopaminergic neurons.
   v. DA receptors become supersensitive with REM sleep deprivation.

d. *Histamine:* drowsiness induced by antihistamines; produced mainly within posterior hypothalamus.

e. *Acetylcholine:* muscarinic and nicotinic agonists can induce wake state via cortical activation; brain stem cholinergic neurons are more active in wake state than in NREM sleep, but lesions only cause transient loss of consciousness, suggesting that they are involved but not essential for wakefulness.

f. *Adenosine:* adenosine neurons are located in the hypothalamus; adenosine receptors are blocked by xanthines and caffeine.

g. *γ-Aminobutyric acid (GABA):* neurons located in—reticular nucleus of thalamus, anterior hypothalamus, basal forebrain; GABA is the neurotransmitter within the geniculohypothalamic tract that conveys nonphotic information to the suprachiasmatic nucleus (SCN).

h. Glutamate: conveys information via the retinohypothalamic tract to the SCN.

C. **NREM sleep**
   1. Structures involved in NREM sleep
      a. Basal forebrain (preoptic area)
      b. RF

      c. Anterior hypothalamus

      d. Thalamus

  2. Sleep onset

      a. Regions involved: ascending reticular-activating system (ARAS), thalamus, basal forebrain.

      b. Neurons in preoptic and basal forebrain are critical for initiation of sleep, with stimulation of these regions inducing sleep and lesions causing reduction of SWS and REM sleep.

      c. Neurotransmitters involved in sleep initiation: histamine, serotonin (and its precursor L-tryptophan), adenosine.

D. REM sleep

  1. Generated by mesencephalic (caudal midbrain) and pontine cholinergic neurons.

  2. Receptors associated with REM sleep: muscarinic cholinergic receptors (M1 receptors).

  3. Neurotransmitters that promote REM: cholinergic cells of median and dorsolateral pons increase their firing rates during REM.

  4. Neurotransmitters that suppress REM: brain stem serotonergic neurons of the raphe nuclei.

  5. Pontine tegmentum lesions will abolish REM sleep.

  6. REM-on cells: pontine laterodorsal and pedunculopontine tegmental (cholinergic); pontine RF (cholinergic).

  7. REM-off cells: pontine serotonin neurons of raphe nucleus; pontine noradrenergic neurons of LC; histamine neurons of posterior hypothalamus; medulla.

  8. Events comprising REM sleep

      a. Desynchronized cortical EEG with low-voltage fast activity that arises from activation of midbrain RF; EEG desynchronization is associated with miosis, REMs, middle-ear movement, nocturnal penile tumescence, and poikilothermia.

      b. Hippocampal highly synchronized θ (4–8 Hz) generated by CA1/dentate gyrus neurons.

      c. *Sawtooth waves:* bilateral synchronous frontocentral symmetric positive waves at 2–5 Hz of trains of >3 waves; origin unknown.

      d. *Muscle atonia*

        i. Regulated by pontine neurons associated with intraspinal glycine.

        ii. Probable cholinergic neurons just outside the LC area, aka LC-α, locus subceruleus, and peri-LC-α (whole group aka small-cell reticular group).

        iii. Note: Active motor inhibition only occurs in stage 1 sleep.

      e. *Pontine-geniculate-occipital waves/spikes*

        i. Generated by pedunculopontine and laterodorsal tegmental neurons.

        ii. Nicotinic blockers decrease amplitude.

        iii. Muscarinic blockers decrease incidence.

        iv. Inhibited by neurons within the raphe system.

        v. Responsible for phasic REM sleep.

        vi. May be pacemaker of myoclonic activity, variation of blood pressure and heart rate, and respirations (in cats).

        vii. Associated with increase in medullary respiratory activity during REM sleep.

      f. *REMs*

        i. Horizontal REMs: generated by saccade generators of the paramedian pontine RF.

        ii. Vertical REMs: presumably generated by mesencephalic RF neurons.

      g. *Myoclonia:* stimulus for phasic muscle twitches originate in reticular nucleus pontis caudalis and nucleus gigantocellularis.

    h. *Dream generation:* pontine-geniculate-occipital waves traveling to lateral geniculate nucleus of thalamus and forebrain.

E. *Sleep factors and other related serum levels*

    1. *Melatonin:* secreted by pineal gland from tryptophan; serotonin is the immediate precursor of melatonin; sleep-promoting affects and reduces sleep latency; important in circadian rhythmicity by effects on SCN; light inhibits melatonin secretion; darkness promotes melatonin secretion; peak secretion is between 2 and 4 a.m.

    2. *Benzodiazepines:* hypnotic effects are result of inhibitory effects of increased GABAergic transmission on neurons of the ARAS.

    3. *Cortisol:* marker of adrenocorticotropic hormone release; release occurs at night, peaking in early a.m.

    4. *Growth hormone:* largest secretion occurs at night associated with onset of SWS (approximately 60 minutes after falling asleep).

    5. *Thyroid-stimulating hormone:* release is inhibited during sleep.

    6. *Tryptophan:* effects on sleep include—decreased sleep latency, decreased REM latency, increased REM activity, increased total sleep time (TST).

    7. *Substance P:* peptide associated with wakefulness.

    8. *Prolactin:* secreted at sleep onset.

    9. *Progesterone:* increases during pregnancy and late luteal phase, causing hyperventilation.

F. *Neuroanatomic correlates*

    1. *Thalamus*

        a. In cats, ablation leads to insomnia.

        b. In humans, diffuse lesion leads to ipsilateral decrease or abolition of sleep spindles.

        c. *Dorsomedial nucleus implicated in sleep.*

        d. Bilateral paramedian thalamic lesions lead to hypersomnolence; polysomnograph (PSG): reduced stage 3 and stage 4 sleep (disrupts SWS); most sleep is stage 1 and stage 2.

        e. **Fatal familial insomnia.**

            i. Clinical features

                (A) *Dysautonomia and loss of dream-like state with dream enactment in patients with degenerative lesions of dorsomedial and anterior nucleus of thalamus.*

                (B) *Autosomal dominant inheritance* (very rare, with two families in Italy and one in France identified, and at least three other families in the United States) associated with prion disease due to a mutation in codon 178 of the prion protein gene.

                (C) Sporadic cases do occur with selective spongiform thalamic degeneration, which appears to affect methionine at codon 129 of the mutant allele (a site common for methionine/valine polymorphism); thus, the ^{129}Met, ^{178}Asn haplotype must be present for the disease to occur.

                (D) Progressive loss of sleep associated with other autonomic and somatomotor manifestations worsening within a few months to almost total lack of sleep (less than 2 hours per night).

            ii. *Neuropathology*

                (A) *Spongiform degeneration with severe neuronal loss and reactive gliosis in anterior and dorsomedial thalamic nuclei* (other thalamic nuclei were less frequently noted).

                (B) Moderate gliosis of deep layers of cortex (more prominently in frontal and temporal regions), inferior olives, and cerebellar cortex.

(C) Hypothalamus and reticular activating center are spared.

(D) Prion fragments differ from those of Creutzfeldt-Jakob disease.

2. *Basal ganglia:* descending output from internal globus pallidus and pars reticulata of the substantia nigra reaches pedunculopontine nucleus-laterodorsal tegmental region.

   a. Provides supratentorial modulation of REM, muscle atonia, and other REM sleep activity.

   b. *These pathologies link sleep disorders of REM sleep with Parkinson's disease (PD), Parkinson-plus syndromes, schizophrenia, obsessive-compulsive disorder (OCD), attention-deficit/hyperactivity disorder (ADHD), and Tourette's syndrome.*

3. *Diencephalon and hypothalamus*

   a. Decreased wakefulness is due to lesions of: posterior hypothalamus; basal forebrain (substantia innominata nucleus basalis of Meynert, nucleus of diagonal band septum).

   b. **Von Economo's encephalitis lethargica:** *lesions of posterior hypothalamus and mesencephalic tegmentum result in lethargy/hypersomnia; lesions of anterior hypothalamus result in insomnia.*

   c. *Hypothalamic tumor results in hypersomnia.*

   d. *Diencephalic lesion results in: sleep attacks, sleep-onset REM periods (SOREMPs), cataplexy.*

4. *Brain stem*

   a. *Mesencephalon*

      i. *Reticular activating system lesion (at level of cranial nerve III):* decreased alertness, vertical gaze paresis, pupillary dysfunction

      ii. *Rostral brain stem lesion* involving floor of the third ventricle: cataplexy, sleep paralysis, sleep attacks

      iii. *Lesion of lower mesencephalon/upper pons involving peri-LC:* REM sleep without atonia, motor behavior driven by a dream (aka phantasmagoria), cardiorespiratory dysfunction

      iv. May have hallucinations (due to alteration of dreams/REM)

   b. *Pons:* locked-in syndrome; lose REM and NREM stage differentiation

   c. Medulla: medullary lesion can result in

      i. REM sleep without atonia

      ii. Motor behavior driven by a dream (aka phantasmagoria)

      iii. Cardiorespiratory dysfunction

      iv. Sleep apnea symptomatology from Arnold-Chiari malformation compression medulla

G. *Chronobiology of the circadian rhythm*

1. *Circadian distribution of sleep and sleepiness*

   a. For typical sleep pattern (11 p.m. to 7 a.m.), circadian rhythm has bimodal pattern.

   b. Sleepiness: greatest during early morning hours (4–6 a.m.) when body temperature is lowest; second peak in afternoon (3:30 p.m.) when body temperature is high.

   c. Alertness: highest in morning (8–11 a.m.), and again in the evening (8–10 p.m.).

   d. Sleep deprivation studies show correlation between alertness and body temperature.

2. *Neuroanatomy of the circadian timing system*

   a. *SCN*

      i. Located in anterior hypothalamus

      ii. Primary circadian pacemaker

      iii. Two major subdivisions

(A) Ventrolateral—neurons contain vasoactive intestinal peptide and neuropeptide Y

(B) Dorsomedial—neurons contain vasopressin

    iv. Primary afferent tract of SCN: retinohypothalamic tract—axons from retinal ganglion cells via lateral geniculate nucleus

    v. Although in mammals the effect of light on circadian rhythms is mediated almost exclusively via the retina (enucleated animals do not respond to light), certain birds and reptiles have encephalic photoreceptors that permit entrainment

    vi. Efferents of SCN: project to the periventricular nuclei and other areas of the hypothalamus, thalamus, and basal forebrain

    vii. Exert effect on excretion of melatonin from the pineal gland via multisynaptic pathway

3. *Effects of the circadian pacemaker on sleep and wakefulness:* most people have temperature rhythms of 25.0–25.5 hours and adopt a similar sleep-wake schedule if environmental cues are absent.

4. *Polysomnographic findings based on conceptual age (CA)*

CA	PSG findings
26 wks	EEG consists of high-voltage slow waves and runs of low-voltage α (8–14 Hz) separated by 20- to 30-sec intervals of nearly isoelectric background with independent activity over each hemisphere (aka hemispheric asynchrony).
	The discontinuous pattern, aka *trace discontinu,* is accompanied by irregular respiration and occasional eye movement.
27–30 wks	Hemispheric asynchrony and discontinuous EEG is common; temporal sharp waves are common; Δ brush present (Δ with superimposed 14–24-Hz activity with posterior prominence); differentiate QS (EEG discontinuous and eye movement is rare) from AS (continuous Δ or Δ–θ activity).
30–33 wks	EEG of AS is nearly continuous with low-voltage mixed-frequency patterns; EEG of QS remains discontinuous; Δ brushes and temporal sharp waves remain prominent; amount of indeterminate sleep decreases and NREM-REM cycle becomes more evident with a duration of 45 mins by wk 34 and increases to 60–70 mins by term delivery; state rhythms are more prominent.
	AS demonstrates increased muscle tone compared to QS; QS has more regular cardiac and respiratory rhythms than AS.
33–37 wks	AS develops additional features, including REMs, smiles, grimaces, and other movements; third state develops that is similar to AS, but eyes are open and it is considered a step toward wake state.
37–40 wks	By 37 wks CA, AS is well developed with low-to-moderate–voltage continuous EEG, REMs, irregular breathing, muscle atonia, and phasic twitches; QS demonstrates respiration that is regular, extraocular movements are sparse/absent, and body movements are few; the discontinuous EEG pattern seen at earlier ages evolves to *trace alternant* (1–10-sec bursts of moderate-to-high–voltage, mixed-frequency activity alternates with 6–10-sec bursts of low-voltage mixed-frequency activity); Δ brush: becomes less frequent and disappears between 37 wks CA and 40 wks CA; periods of continuous slow-wave activity begin to occur during QS at approximately 37 wks CA, becoming more prevalent with increasing age.

AS, active sleep; QS, quiet sleep.

H. *Term neonates through infancy*
  1. At term: one-third wake, one-third NREM, one-third REM.
  2. At birth, have *trace alternant* (but usually disappears by age 2–3 months and is replaced by continuous slow-wave activity that evolves to SWS characteristic of stages 3 and 4 sleep).
  3. Lack sleep spindles and α rhythm, making staging impossible until later in infancy.
  4. AS represents 35–45% of TST, and QS represents 55–65% of TST.
  5. Sleep approximately 17.5 hours per 24-hour period; sleep is evenly distributed throughout the day and night.
  6. Development of circadian sleep-wake rhythms: begins at approximately 4–6 weeks; during first 3 months, clock begins to run in tandem with core body temperature rhythm.
  7. Definite sleep spindles are usually evident by age 3–4 months.
  8. K complexes are usually evident from age 6 months onward.
  9. SOREMPs usually disappear after age 3–4 months.
  10. TST decreases to 12–13 hours by age 12 months almost entirely due to decrease in REM sleep from 7–8 hours at term, to 6 hours by age 6 months, to 4–5 hours by age 12 months (associated with decrease in frequency of SOREMPs from 65% of cycles at term to 20% by age 6 months, and only occasionally by age 12 months).
  11. Specific EEG changes.
    a. Background rhythm: mixed frequencies diffusely seen initially, evolving to posterior rhythm of 3–4 Hz by age 3 months, 5 Hz by 5 months, 6 Hz at 1 year, 7 Hz at 2 years, 8 Hz at 3 years, and 9–10 Hz by age 6–10 years.
    b. Sleep spindles: initially develop by 6–8 weeks; asynchronous during 1st year, but by 1 year, approximately 70% are synchronous, and by age 2 years, nearly all are synchronous.
    c. Vertex waves and K complexes: evident during NREM by age 3–6 months.
    d. Light sleep and SWS can be differentiated by age 6 months.
I. **Early childhood**
  1. By age 1 year, α rhythm and sleep spindles are fully developed, with subsequent conversion from AS/QS to NREM/REM sleep.
  2. Nocturnal sleep shows high levels of both stage 3 and stage 4 SWS (30–40% of TST) and REM sleep (30–45% of TST).
  3. SWS (stages 3 and 4): important feature during 1st decade is evolution of SWS; first appears at 3–5 months; increases to 50% of NREM by 1 year and remains high for several years; SWS declines after 1st few years, and by age 9 years, makes up only 22–28% of TST (in boys slightly more than in girls); kids are difficult to arouse during SWS (up to 123 dB).
  4. Naps: decrease to one nap per day by age 2 years (68% take one nap, 25% take two naps); by age 2–3 years, 25% do not nap; by age 6 years, nearly all kids do not nap.
J. *Late childhood and adolescence:* amounts of SWS and REM sleep steadily decrease with corresponding increases in light sleep (stages 1 and 2 NREM sleep); with increased light sleep, increased wake after sleep onset occurs; length of REM cycle also continues to increase (to 60–75 minutes by age 6 years and to adult levels of 85–110 minutes by adolescence)
K. *Adult:* monophasic sleep period; normal sleep time in the adult; percentage of TST devoted to REM sleep is age dependent (full term = 50% TST; by age 1 year, decreases to 25%); normal adult has five to seven sleep cycles
L. *Elderly:* naps again become more prominent; the daytime naps taken by elderly individuals also show relatively low amounts of SWS and are more fragmented than those of

younger subjects; in the elderly, the amount of SWS is markedly suppressed; the number of awakenings increases: normal REM latency shortens, indicating a phase advance of the ultradian REM cycle probably secondary to weakened SWS in the first third of the night; sleep also lightens behaviorally, as reflected in a lowered threshold for awakening stimuli: many normal elderly patients perceive this normal sleep fragmentation and lengthening as insomnia: contributors to decreased sleep in older patients

1. Degenerative central nervous system changes
2. Reduced amplitude of circadian rhythms
3. Decreased light exposure
4. Inactivity and bed rest
5. Increased daytime sleep
6. Use of hypnotics and ethanol (EtOH)
7. Illness (medical and psychiatric)
8. Retirement and loss of social cues; loss of time cues
9. Increased prevalence of sleep disorders, such as sleep apnea and periodic limb movements of sleep

M. **Alertness:** most alert age group with longest average sleep latency on Multiple Sleep Latency Test (MSLT) = prepubertal child/adolescent; elderly have shortest average sleep latency on MSLT

II. Normal Human Sleep (See Chapter 10: Clinical Neurophysiology)

III. Epidemiology of Sleep Disorders

A. *Psychophysiological insomnia:* makes up 15% of insomnias
B. *Sleep state misperception:* makes up 5% of insomnias
C. *Idiopathic hypersomnia:* makes up 5–10% of excessive daytime sleepiness (EDS)
D. **Obstructive sleep apnea (OSA):** 1–2% of general population have OSA
E. **Restless legs syndrome**

In general population	5–15%
In pregnancy	11%
In uremia	15–20%
In rheumatoid arthritis	30%

F. **Parasomnias**
1. *Sleepwalking:* prevalence in kids, 10–30%; in adults, 1–7%
2. **NB:** *Sleep terrors:* occur occasionally in 20–30% of kids; occurs frequently in 1–4% of kids, only 1% of adults; pavor nocturnus; arousal during the SWS and characteristically occur during the first half of the night (30 minutes after the onset of sleep); the child often cries out and is uncommunicative; treatment is not necessary.
3. *Hypnic jerks* occur in 60–70% of population.
4. *Nightmare* prevalence is frequent in 10–50% of 3–5 y/o, and 50% of adults have occasional nightmares.
5. *Bruxism:* 90% of population (especially in infants); 50% of normal infants

G. **Enuresis prevalence**

4 y/o	30%
6 y/o	10%

12 y/o	3%
18 y/o	1–2%

H. **Apnea of prematurity (AOP) prevalence**

31 wks CA	50–80%
32 wks CA	12–15%
34–35 wks CA	7%

I. **Sudden infant death syndrome (SIDS):** incidence, 1–2 per 1000; 90% of SIDS occurs in those <6 months old; eskimos are at 4–6× increased risk; risk increases with sleeping prone before age 6 months, possibly because infant cannot turn over.

J. **Sleep disorders with increased familial incidence**
   1. Narcolepsy
   2. OSA
   3. Restless legs syndrome
   4. Insomnia
   5. Arousal disorders
   6. Enuresis
   7. Sleep terrors
   8. Fatal familial insomnia

IV. Disorders of the Circadian Sleep-Wake Cycle
A. *General*
   1. *Circadian timing system:* "Circadian" pacemaker—SCN of the hypothalamus: site of mammalian circadian clock (may be only site).
   2. Internal pacemaker endogenous rhythm is 24.2 hours; internal pacemaker is nearly always longer than 24 hours.
   3. *Tau* refers to the natural period of circadian rhythmicity evident on free-running conditions; Tau in humans is 25.3 hours based on time isolation experiments and, therefore, a small daily phase advance is necessary to synchronize with the environmental 24-hour day.
   4. Largest phase shift produced by light is given at 11–13 hours of the 0–24-hour circadian cycle.
   5. Free-running circadian rhythms are noted in the blind and in Alzheimer's disease (AD).
   6. Only a few stimuli can cause a phase shift of circadian clocks.
      a. Light: most potent of such stimuli.
      b. Exercise: along with social stimuli, it may have a role in the daily resetting process.
      c. Social stimuli: blind people may be free-running (sleeping and waking as if they were in a time isolating experiment) and may have difficulty in conforming to a 24-hour schedule; this suggests that social interactions may have only a minor role in the circadian cycle and light is the most important.
   7. Melatonin: pineal gland hormone; precursor: L-tryptophan; in pineal gland, tryptophan converted to serotonin; role in daily synchronization; secreted only in darkness, and secretion is suppressed by light acting via the SCN; administration of melatonin causes phase shifting effects opposite those of light stimuli.
   8. Humans can tolerate up to 24 months of chronic sleep deprivation.

9. Kleitman's research on sleep deprivation noted that performance decrements were maximal after 61 hours of sleep deprivation.

10. Marian's research with the heliotrope plant demonstrated that some plants have an endogenous 24-hour rhythm that exists apart from external cues.

B. *Delayed sleep phase syndrome*

1. Clinical symptomatology

   a. *Severe difficulty initiating sleep at conventional hour of night and cannot go to sleep until early morning hours (therefore complains of sleep-onset insomnia)*

   b. *Difficulty awakening on time in morning (for school, work, etc.); fall to sleep at school in morning, but get good grades in afternoon classes*

   c. *After falling to sleep, they will usually have normal sleep and will awaken approximately 7–8 hours later if undisturbed (but if they must awaken in the morning to go to work, they will have sleep deprivation symptomatology)*

   d. Prevalence in school-aged kids, 7%, in middle-aged adults, 0.7%

   e. Sleep log often shows normal amount of sleep for age (7.5–9.5 hours), but sleep onset is between 2 a.m. and 6 a.m. and awaken at noon

2. Management

   a. Chronotherapy: original/early method consists of daily 3-hour delays at bedtime and arising time until sleep schedule is realigned to desired social schedule; usually can be accomplished in 5–7 days, but to be successful, it must be adhered to indefinitely; small phase advances of 30–60 minutes can also be performed but require more time to achieve effect.

   b. Sleep deprivation on first night and following day of a weekend, followed by bedtime and waking times each 90 minutes earlier continuing the next night onward; process is repeated on successive weekends until the desired schedule is achieved.

   c. Enhancement of morning light cue with bright lights (2500 lux) may be helpful.

   d. Melatonin, 2.5–10.0 mg, at desired bedtime.

C. *Advanced sleep phase syndrome*

1. Clinical symptomatology

   a. Much less common than delayed sleep phase syndrome.

   b. Sleepiness and sleep onset occur earlier in evening than desired (between 6 and 9 p.m.), with awakening well before dawn (between 2 and 5 a.m.).

   c. Unlike in depression, patients with advanced sleep phase syndrome obtain normal amounts of consolidated sleep without mood disturbances.

   d. Elderly reflect characteristics of advanced sleep phase syndrome.

2. Management

   a. 3-hour phase advance regimen (variable success)

   b. 15- to 30-minute phase advances with evening bright light exposure, followed by maintenance of new schedule 7 days per week

D. *Non–24-hour sleep-wake syndrome* (aka *hypernychthemeral syndrome*)

1. Clinical: *chronic pattern of daily delays in sleep onsets and wake times because internal pacemaker is not entrained to 24-hour cycle*

2. Etiology

   a. Majority of these patients are congenitally blind (usually is total and prechiasmatic and, therefore, theoretically deprives the SCN of synchronizing light info); up to 70% of the blind have sleep disorders.

   b. May be due to optic or retinal pathology, interruption of retinohypothalamic tract, lack of SCN responsiveness to transmitted impulses, or failure of the SCN to entrain sleep-wake rhythms.

   c. Circadian rhythms of melatonin and cortisol secretion are free running in blind people.

3. Management
    a. Unresponsive to sedatives or stimulants.
    b. Oral vitamin B_{12} has been helpful in some cases.
    c. Oral melatonin, 0.5–7.5 mg, in evening has been helpful in some cases.
E. **Irregular sleep-wake cycle**
    1. Clinical
        a. Temporarily irregular sleep and waking with normal or near normal average amounts of total daily sleep.
        b. Sleep logs show irregular sleep onset or wake times, although there may be fairly consistent broken sleep between 2 and 6 a.m. and a daily period of agitation and wandering, especially in the evening (known as *sundowning*).
    2. Etiology
        a. In degenerative central nervous system (CNS) disease, may result from damage connecting to or of the SCN, of systems mediating arousal, or both.
        b. Prolonged bed rest may alter normal circadian sleep cycle due to ↓social and environmental cues.
    3. Management
        a. Sleep hygiene (minimize time in bed to <7–8 hours, ↑environmental cues such as light and social interactions, instituting regular meal times and sleep-wake times).
        b. Both morning and evening bright light (3000 lux for 2 hours) have been shown to improve nocturnal sleep in institutionalized patients and reduce agitation in some demented patients.
        c. Melatonin, 2.5–10.0 mg, at desired sleep time.
F. *Zone change (jet lag)*
    1. Clinical
        a. 80% of business travelers complain of sleep disturbances.
        b. Besides distance/time zones traveled, factors such as high altitude, low humidity, secondary smoke, and reduced barometric pressure also contribute to jet lag.
        c. Generally greater after eastward flights.
        d. Symptoms include insomnia, EDS, decreased subjective alertness; may also have somatic complaints, including dyspepsia, constipation, eye irritation, nasal discharge, nausea, headaches, cramps, dependent edema, and intermittent dizziness.
    2. Etiology
        a. Caused by desynchronization of person's intrinsic circadian rhythm (internal clock) and local environmental time (external clock).
        b. Associated with relationship between sleep and core body temperature rhythms.
        c. Circadian rhythm will adjust at rate of 60 minutes per day after eastbound flights and 90 minutes per day for westbound flights.
        d. Range of entrainment: the range of which the circadian rhythm can adjust to environmental time; it is no more than 1–2 hours (may be up to 3–4 hours) in either direction of the individual's intrinsic circadian rhythm.
        e. Sleep deprivation before trip and EtOH may worsen symptoms.
    3. Management
        a. Approach to management depends on number of time zone changes and length of stay.
        b. For fewer than four time zone changes, best treatment for long stays is rapid adjustment to new time zone schedule; this would include sleep deprivation on first night following an eastward flight rapidly adhering to the new time zone.
        c. May also attempt adjustment to new time zone before flight.

      d. Daytime napping hinders synchronization.

      e. Pharmacologic treatment

         i. Short-acting benzodiazepines can help insomnia (but may cause amnestic effects).

        ii. Melatonin, 2–5 mg: may ameliorate symptoms when taken at what would be midnight of the new time zone for 1 or 2 days before departure, and then at bedtime in the new time zone for about 3 days after arrival (i.e., eastbound flight: 10 mg in evening).

       iii. Light exposure reduces the duration of symptoms, with timing of light critical (>10,000 lux for >30 minutes; can be attained by sitting 2 ft in front of 40-W bulb).

       iv. Modafinil 100-200 mg per day.

G. *Shift work sleep disorder*

  1. Clinical

      a. In the United States, 21 million shift workers (one-sixth of employed women and one-fourth of employed men).

      b. Because of poor health, 20–30% leave shift work within 3 years.

      c. Often revert to societal "norm" sleep patterns on weekends, thus making it difficult to keep biorhythms entrained.

      d. *Shift maladaptive syndrome:* chronic sleep disturbance (insomnia) and waking fatigue; gastrointestinal symptoms (dyspepsia, diarrhea, etc.); EtOH or drug abuse; higher accident rates; psychological changes (depression, malaise, personality changes); difficult interpersonal relations.

      e. Factors related to shift work coping problems.

>40–50 y/o
Heavy domestic workload
History of sleep disorder
EtOH or drug abuse
Epilepsy
Heart disease
Second job ("moonlighting")
Morning-type person ("larks")
Psychiatric illness
History of gastrointestinal complaints
Diabetes

      f. Factors associated with work systems and work that are likely to cause shift work problems.

         i. More than five third shifts in a row without off-time days

        ii. More than four 1-hour night shifts in a row

       iii. 1st shift starting before 7 a.m.

       iv. Rotating hours that change once per week

        v. Less than 48 hours off-time after a run of third shift work

       vi. Excess regular overtime

      vii. Backward rotating hours (first to third to second shift)

     viii. 12-hour shifts, including critical morning tasks

      ix. 12-hour shifts involving heavy physical work

       x. Excess weekend work
      xi. Long commuting times
     xii. Split shifts with inappropriate break period lengths
    xiii. Shifts lacking appropriate shift breaks
    xiv. 12-hour shifts with exposure to harmful agents
     xv. Complicated schedules making it difficult to plan ahead

  g. Permanent night shift workers sleep an average of 6 hours per night (1 hour less than day workers); rotating shift workers average only 5.5 hours per night.

  h. Shift rotations from days to evenings and evenings to nights (forward) are better tolerated than moving shifts backward.

  i. PSG: daytime sleep is more fragmented (in part due to environmental light and noise); may have SOREMPs; dissociated REM sleep may also occur.

2. Etiology

  a. Work schedules are typically 90–120 degrees (6–8 hours) out of line with environmental cues for sleep-wake cycle; never completely synchronizes even after years of shift work.

  b. Domestic and social factors: confounded by night shift worker attempting to conform to "normal" sleep-wake cycles of society on days off work (i.e., weekend).

  c. Night shift workers get approximately 5–7 hours less sleep per week (and comes primarily from reduction in stage 2 sleep and REM sleep, with SWS relatively unaffected; sleep latency is also reduced; some studies also suggest reduced REM latency).

3. Management

  a. If working night shift for extended period, patient should maintain same sleep schedule 7 days per week if possible (often difficult due to societal obligations).

  b. Splitting daily sleep into two long naps (2–3 hours in afternoon, and 4–6 hours at night before work) may help.

  c. Sleeping in absolute darkness using shades, mask, etc., with excess bright light (>7000 lux) while awake.

  d. Modafinil, 100–400 mg/day, on waking (U.S. Food and Drug Administration [FDA] approved in 2004).

V. Sleepiness and Sleep Deprivation

A. **Clinical features of sleepiness/EDS**

1. EDS occurs in 4–15% of population; women slightly > men; young adults > middle-aged adults; increases in elderly > 60 y/o.
2. More than one-half of patients with EDS have automobile or industrial accidents.
3. Sleep deprivation: deprivation of as little as 1-hour reduction per night can lead to EDS.
4. Insufficient sleep syndrome: likely most common cause of EDS in Western civilization.

B. **MSLT**

	Mean sleep latency (mins)
Preadolescent	15–20
Young adult	10
Middle-aged adult	11–12
Elderly >60 y/o	9
One night's sleep deprivation	5
Two nights' sleep deprivation	<1

C. **Human studies**
   1. Incentives can overcome diminished cognitive abilities secondary to sleep deprivation during the first 36 hours, but have little effect at >60 hours.
   2. Disorientation and altered time perception occur after 48 hours.
   3. Bodily function is less impaired during the first 3 days of sleep deprivation, with slight drop in body temperature and circadian rhythm amplitude; endocrine and organ studies are usually normal.
   4. Longest documented time without sleep is 264 hours (Randy Gardner).
D. **Animal studies**
   1. The increase in energy expenditure appears to be the result of: increased heat loss—related mainly to REM sleep deprivation, and increase in the preferred body temperature—related to loss of SWS
   2. With extended sleep deprivation, rats may demonstrate: 2°C decrease in body temperature, 25% increase in activity, appear emaciated with skin lesions, have increased plasma norepinephrine
E. *Insufficient sleep syndrome*
   1. Clinical features
      a. Well-educated and above average income—trying to get ahead results in self-induced sleep deprivation
      b. EDS usually afternoon or evening
   2. Psychobiologic basis
      a. Impaired vigilance is noted after just 2 nights with only 5 hours of sleep
      b. With partial sleep deprivation, SWS is relatively well preserved, with most of reduced sleep in stages 1 and 2 and REM sleep

VI. Sleep Apnea
A. **Clinically**
   1. Three types of apneas
      a. **Central apnea:** cessation of both airflow and abdominal/thoracic respiratory movements, with both falling below 20% of basal value; due to failure of the medullary centers responsible for respiratory drive; arousal need not follow the respiratory irregularities; oxygen desaturation is not essential
      b. **Obstructive (or upper airway) apnea:** no airflow despite continued abdominal/thoracic respiratory effort resulting in paradoxic breathing (thoracoabdominal movements are out of phase); treatment: positive airway pressure is standard therapy (continuous positive airway pressure [CPAP], bilevel positive airway pressure (BiPAP), or acetaminophen (APAP); if unable to tolerate: weight reduction, sleep hygiene, positional therapy, and oxygen therapy

NB: Modafinil is now approved by the FDA for the treatment of excessive sleepiness associated with obstructive sleep apnea/hypopnea syndrome and shift-work sleep disorder; mechanism is unknown but orexin neurons are activated with its administration.

      c. **Mixed apnea:** evidence of both central and obstructive apnea (essentially central apnea that evolves into obstructive apnea); characterized by cessation of airflow and absence of respiratory effort early, and followed by later resumption of respiratory effort that eventually appears obstructive
   2. Sudden relief of obstruction is what causes the characteristic inspiratory guttural snort.
   3. Restoration of respiratory effort is likely due to resultant hypoxia or hypercapnia by activating the medullary RF.

4. If untreated, it may cause resultant pulmonary and then systemic hypertension and cardiac arrhythmias.

5. *Sleep-related respiratory disorders*

   a. *Upper airway resistance syndrome (UARS)*

      i. Definition and etiology: narrowed upper airway fails to cause easily identifiable apneas or hypopneas but instead results in increased work required to move air through the constricted airway; the increased effort causes repetitive brief arousals, just as increased work of breathing rather than decreased oxygen saturation or hypercapnia.

      ii. Clinical features: younger and thinner than patients with OSA, especially kids and women with narrow airways; symptoms are similar to OSA except complaints not as severe.

      iii. Diagnosis: often remains undetected because PSG scoring at most centers is not designed to detect UARS; PSG often shows brief, unsustained arousals; documentation of UARS requires correlation between arousals and abnormally negative intrathoracic pressures during inspiration (more negative than -10 cm H_2O).

      iv. Treatment: similar to OSA

6. Primary snoring

   a. 44% of middle-aged men and 28% of middle-aged women

   b. Believed to be produced by vibration of the uvula, soft palate, and narrowed upper airway as turbulent air passes

   c. Likely that snoring, UARS, and OSA are on a continuum, and exacerbating factors such as age and weight gain may promote progression

   d. Unknown whether snoring is associated with hypersomnolence and cardiovascular complications

   e. Treatment: dental devices, CPAP, surgery (laser-assisted uvulopalatopharyngoplasty [UPPP]), weight loss, sleep hygiene

B. **Nocturnal PSG**

   1. *Apnea:* defined as cessation of airflow at the level of the nose/mouth for at least 10 seconds with >4% oxygen desaturation; measured from the end of exhalation to the beginning of the next exhalation

   2. Hypopnea: irregular respiratory event characterized by a decrease in respiratory airflow to one-third of its basal value and parallel reduction in amplitude of thoracic/abdominal movements associated with a decrease in oxygen saturation

   3. Apnea/hypopnea index (AHI) = (total apneas and hypopneas/TST [in minutes]) × 60 minutes

      a. Aka respiratory distress index.

      b. AHI of ≤5 is within normal limits in adults.

      c. AHI of ≤1 is within normal limits in young children <12 y/o.

      d. Sleep apnea syndrome is diagnosed by having respiratory distress index ≥5 in normal middle-aged adults.

   4. General indications for treatment of OSA

      a. Altered daytime performance (EDS)

      b. AHI ≥20

      c. Oxygen desaturation <90%

      d. Arrhythmia and hemodynamic changes associated with obstruction

5. *Sleep apnea severity*

	AHI	Apnea duration (secs)	O_2 saturation (%)	Electrocardiogram
Mild	5–20	<20	>85	Mild tachybradycardia
Moderate	20–40	20–40	75–85	Prominent tachybradycardia or asystole <3 secs
Severe	>40	>40	<75	Asystole >3 secs or ventricular tachycardia

C. **Treatment**
   1. General recommendations
      a. Goals: return both nocturnal respiration and sleep to normal to eliminate EDS and reduce risk of cardiovascular complications
      b. If specific upper airway abnormality is found
         i. Nasal obstruction: anatomic = surgical referral; allergic rhinitis = inhaled nasal steroids for 1 month ± oral antihistamine
         ii. Enlarged tonsils or adenoids: UPPP, tonsillectomy, and adenoidectomy
         iii. Facial skeletal abnormality
      c. If no specific upper airway obstruction is found
         i. Weight loss (including surgery for weight loss)
         ii. CPAP/BiPAP
         iii. UPPP
         iv. Medications
         v. Sleep hygiene
         vi. Abstain from sedative hypnotics
      d. When CPAP therapy fails: check compliance and correct use of device; if CPAP and devices fail, surgery (UPPP followed by maxillofacial surgery) may be necessary
      e. Positive airway pressure (PAP) devices
         i. Mechanism of upper airway obstruction: when patient is awake, muscle tone prevents collapse of oropharyngeal tissue with inspiration; during sleep, tongue and soft palate are sucked against the posterior oropharyngeal wall
         ii. Mechanism of PAP: pneumatic positive pressure splint to keep upper airway open; may have some minor effects on reflex mechanisms, but these are of little clinical significance
      f. CPAP constant pressure throughout, where BiPAP has adjustable pressure for both inspiration and expiration (can often maintain upper airway patency at lower expiratory than inspiratory pressure)
      g. Indications for use of CPAP and BiPAP
         i. OSA
         ii. Central sleep apnea
         iii. Sleep apnea with chronic lung disease
         iv. Nocturnal asthma
         v. Heavy snoring
         vi. Neuromuscular disorders: used in end-stage amyotrophic lateral sclerosis and myasthenic syndromes to relieve burden of skeletal muscle effort
      h. Long-term effects of PAP: improved cognitive abilities and Minnesota Multiphasic Personality Inventory; reversal of reduced testosterone and somatomedin C levels

associated with OSA; improved cardiovascular function, especially in patients with systemic hypertension or right-sided heart failure

  i. BiPAP

    i. Higher pressure during inspiration (IPAP) and a lower but still positive pressure during expiration (expiratory PAP).

    ii. BiPAP is beneficial if inspiratory CPAP pressures are of significantly high pressure that is intolerable to the patient.

    iii. Benefit is due to comfort of negative pressure effect during expiration so that the pharyngeal tissue does not collapse on exhaling; also recommended if frequent central apneas are present at baseline or if central apneas significantly increase during CPAP titration.

  j. Pressure of CPAP/BiPAP is determined during PSG by starting at lowest pressure (5 cm H_2O) and gradually increasing until apneas and hypopneas are essentially eliminated (AHI <5) and snoring is eliminated (if snoring persists, it is likely that the patient will have apneas or hypopneas during some portion of the night); must have adequate sleep recording, including REM sleep at optimal levels of PAP

  k. Higher PAP pressure required with: supine position typically will require higher PAP than a lateral posture; REM sleep usually requires higher pressure than NREM, secondary to skeletal muscle atonia during REM sleep; higher CPAP is usually necessary if sedatives are taken (including EtOH), and, typically, the patient abstains from these on the night of the PSG; therefore, higher doses of CPAP should be advised to patients who are alcoholics or use sedatives if the initial CPAP titration during PSG is performed in a sober state

  l. Compliance with CPAP/BiPAP is major problem

    i. Comfort with mask, leaks, nasal congestion, skin abrasion (25%); allergic reaction (5–10%); conjunctivitis due to air leak (10%); expense ($1200–$2000 for CPAP, and twice as much for BiPAP)

    ii. Overall compliance is approximately 40–80% (with most patients using the device suboptimally even though they report appropriate use; nonetheless, even these patients show benefit)

    iii. Mask comfort: single most important compliance factor

    iv. Nasal congestion: 10% with persistent stuffiness

  m. Most immediate evidence of benefit is reflected in PSG by increased quantities (rebound) of stages 3 and 4 NREM sleep and REM sleep

  n. Rebound sleep phase of treatment: within seconds of securing an open upper airway, patients with severe sleep apnea begin to have long periods of REM and stage 4 NREM sleep, which lasts about 1 week (trends downward after first night); patients will have decreased arousability due to these factors and, therefore, may be at higher risk for hypoxemia

2. Surgery

  a. Surgical procedures for OSA

    i. Bypass all upper airway obstruction: tracheostomy—the first/initial treatment for OSA, but has been replaced by cosmetically superior alternatives with less risk for medical complications

    ii. Selectively eliminate one or several specific abnormalities

      (A) Nasal reconstruction

      (B) UPPP

        (1) Indications for UPPP

          (a) Long soft palate

          (b) Redundant lateral pharyngeal wall
          (c) Excess tonsillar tissues
       (2) Although commonly performed, has variable effectiveness in improving nocturnal breathing, with significant improvement in only 50% of patients; typically will have only a 20–50% reduction of apneas; rarely a "cure" for moderate to severe OSA
       (3) Many still require CPAP to eliminate residual apneas
       (4) May reduce snoring but not apneas
       (5) Airway obstruction at the base of the tongue is reason apneas do not improve
       (6) Complication: 10% have nasal reflux of liquids; inflammation/pain after procedure
     (C) Inferior mandibular sagittal osteotomy with geniohyoid advancement
     (D) Bimaxillary advancement
  b. Phased surgical protocols

Phase I

  Nasal reconstruction

  UPPP

  Inferior mandibular sagittal osteotomy with geniohyoid advancement

Phase II (typically have base-of-tongue obstruction)

  Bimaxillary advancement

  Subapical mandibular osteotomy

  Base-of-tongue surgery

---

3. Dental devices
  a. Used to modify mouth and upper airway by positioning forward the lower jaw, increasing the pharyngeal airway passage; stabilizing anterior placement of the mandible; advancing the tongue or soft palate; and, possibly, changing genioglossus muscle activity
  b. Mild to moderate benefit for snoring but minimal for OSAS
  c. Side effects include increased salivation, gingival discomfort, temporomandibular joint (TMJ) discomfort, and changes in occlusion
  d. Poor compliance
4. Medications (little, if any, clinical benefit)
  a. Tricyclic antidepressants (TCAs): protriptyline has been studied the most; may exert effect by: increasing tone of upper airway muscles, suppressing REM sleep states
  b. Medroxyprogesterone: respiratory stimulant; little long-term benefit; can be used in patients with obesity hypoventilation syndrome (hypoventilation while awake as demonstrated by a $PaCO_2$ greater than 48 mm Hg with a forced expiratory volume in 1 second greater than 1 L; dose, 60 mg/day); typically does not benefit obese patients with OSA
  c. Fluoxetine
  d. Nicotine
  e. Theophylline
  f. Acetazolamide

   g. Modafinil: FDA approved as adjunctive therapy for residual EDS despite PAP therapy; should not be used as alternative, as only improves EDS symptoms and not underlying OSA
   5. Adjuvant treatments
      a. Weight loss: dramatic weight loss (>50 kg) may lead to abolition of OSA
      b. Sleeping supine (sewing tennis ball onto back of pajamas serves as reminder)
      c. Improve sleep hygiene: avoid sleep deprivation and EtOH and sedatives before sleep (therefore, insomnia should not be treated with sedatives unless the OSA is under excellent control)

VII. Idiopathic Hypersomnia
   A. **Clinically**
      1. Sleep is markedly lengthened, often up to 10–16 hours or even up to 20 hours per day.
      2. Deep sleep from which it is difficult to arouse.
      3. Approximately 50% have sleep "drunkenness" on awakening.
      4. Awaken unrefreshed from daytime naps.
      5. No true sleep attacks.
      6. Many cases are familial, but may also be sporadic.
   B. **PSG:** marked sleep extension with normal cyclicity; very few awakenings
   C. **MSLT:** sleep latency <5–10 minutes; lack of SOREMP

VIII. Narcolepsy
   A. *Clinically (tetrad)*
      1. *Inappropriate and irresistible sleep attacks*
      2. *EDS*
      3. *Cataplexy*
      4. *Hypnagogic hallucinations*
   B. **Idiopathic narcolepsy**
      1. Narcolepsy with cataplexy
      2. Narcolepsy without cataplexy
         a. Narcolepsy with two or more SOREMPs on MSLT with or without sleep paralysis and hypnagogic/hypnopompic hallucinations
         b. Narcolepsy with one or no SOREMPs in MSLT with or without sleep paralysis and hypnagogic/hypnopompic hallucinations
   C. **Symptomatic narcolepsy:** associated with tumor, cerebrovascular accident, infection, multiple sclerosis, head trauma, or neurodegenerative disease
   D. **May have associated:** increased apneas, periodic limb movements of sleep (in 9–59% of narcoleptics), REM behavior disorder (in 12%)
   E. **Prevalence:** 0.1% of population; familial form exists; nearly 100% association with HLA-DR2 (DW 15)
   F. **Genetics**
      1. Haplotypes
         a. *HLA-DR15 (subtype of DR2)*
         b. *HLA-DQ6 (subtype of DQ1)*
      2. Diagnostic benefit is overestimated
         a. >99% with either DR15 or DQ6 do not have narcolepsy.
         b. DR15 (in whites and Japanese) and DQ6 (in all races) may be absent in 1–5% of patients with classic narcolepsy (in patients without cataplexy, this is even higher).
   G. **Nocturnal PSG**
      1. In monosymptomatic narcolepsy (without cataplexy)

      a. Daytime sleep attacks consist of sustained NREM sleep.

      b. Nocturnal sleep tends to be normal or extended.

  2. In narcolepsy-cataplexy

      a. Decreased sleep-onset REM latency

      b. Nocturnal sleep is usually disturbed and unrestorative with frequent awakenings

      c. Even distribution of stages 3 and 4 throughout the night

      d. Frequent stage shifts

      e. Fragmentation of sleep (especially REM sleep)

      f. Poor REM cyclicity

H. MSLT in narcolepsy-cataplexy

  1. Sleep attacks or naps frequently have SOREMPs or short REM latencies of ≤5 minutes.

  2. 85% of narcoleptics have MSLT of ∂5 minutes, two or more SOREMPs, or both (but only 61% of narcoleptics present with both on their initial MSLT).

  3. Up to 44% of patients presenting with EDS and two or more SOREMPs have a condition other than narcolepsy.

  4. 20–100% of sleep attacks begin with REM sleep (depending on study).

IX. Periodic Limb Movements of Sleep

A. Clinically

  1. May lead to EDS if associated with frequent microarousals noted on EEG.

  2. Movement is classically a triple flexion response of the toe/ankle/knee/hip.

  3. Duration is 0.5–2.0 seconds.

  4. Movements are usually pseudorhythmic, occurring every 20–80 seconds over an extended period.

  5. Due to sleep fragmentation, may also have insomnia as main complaint.

X. Parasomnias

Three types occur preferentially in stages 3 and 4 SWS, including: (1) confusional awakenings, (2) sleepwalking, and (3) sleep terrors.

  A. *Confusional arousals* (*nocturnal sleep drunkenness*): on awakening, patient will have confusion, disorientation, poor coordination, automatic behavior, and varying degrees of amnesia; typically occur with arousal in the first part of the night, during stages 3 and 4; especially common in kids; must be distinguished from morning sleep drunkenness, which occurs in approximately 50% of patients with idiopathic hypersomnia.

  B. *Sleepwalking* (*somnambulism*): typically occurs with arousal in the first third of the night, during stages 3 and 4; if awakened, the patient is amnestic for the event (but may recall fragmentary imagery); may be precipitated if patient is awakened during SWS; if awakened during sleepwalking, patient can be highly combative; PSG: attacks begin in stages 3 and 4 SWS; during the attack, the EEG becomes relatively desynchronized and shows fragments of stage 1 sleep with mixed (mainly θ) frequencies, or a continuous (substage 1A[3]) nonreactive α.

  C. **Sleep terrors** (aka *pavor nocturnus*, incubus attack)

    1. Clinically

      a. Piercing scream with inconsolable fear on awakening

      b. Typically occur with arousal in the first part of the night, during stages 3 and 4

      c. On exam → tachycardia and tachypnea, often profuse sweating, and dilated pupils

      d. Full consciousness is usually not attained for 5–10 minutes

      e. Feelings of choking or being crushed are common

      f. PSG: arise during stages 3 and 4 SWS; associated with rapid desynchronization to low-voltage fast waking patterns; evidence of arousal with tachycardia, tachypnea, increased muscle tone; if multiple attacks occur, they may also begin in stage 2 sleep

2. Treatment: usually respond well to diazepam qh

D. **Terrifying dreams** (dream anxiety attacks)

1. Clinically: dreams are often threatening to patient's life; not accompanied by confusion or as marked systemic changes as in night terrors

a. PSG: attacks usually occur in second half of night (night terrors are usually in first third); associated with REM sleep (night terrors with SWS)

E. **REM sleep behavioral disorders**

1. Clinically: unusually aggressive behavior during sleep; most common in older patients with underlying pathology, or in chronic alcoholics; also seen in a variety of neurologic pathologies, including dementia, subarachnoid hemorrhage, olivopontocerebellar atrophy, Guillain-Barré syndrome, and PD

2. PSG: arise from REM sleep; marked phasic REM bursts and myoclonic potentials (on peripheral electromyography) plus movement artifacts associated with continuing REM sleep patterns or EEG of wakefulness after REM sleep

F. *Sleep-related head banging* (*jactatio capitis nocturna*)

1. Clinically: seen occasionally in normal kids, especially in times of stress or family disharmony, but more frequent in mentally retarded (mentally retarded children are more prone to dormitional form)

2: PSG: may occur at sleep onset in stages 1A and 1B drowsiness (predormitional form) or throughout all sleep stages; interferes little or not at all with ongoing sleep

XI. Sleep-related epileptic seizures

A. 20–25% of epileptics have seizures exclusively during sleep, and another 30–40% have seizures in both sleep and wake periods (remaining 35–50% of epileptics have seizures only during wakefulness).

B. Evidence that tonic-clonic, tonic, and myoclonic generalized epilepsies are activated in NREM sleep.

C. Evidence that typical absences are activated in REM sleep.

D. Partial seizures have a more complex relationship with sleep and may be dependent on the location of their epileptogenic focus.

XII. Childhood Sleep Disorders

A. *Specific types of pediatric sleep disorders*

1. *Insomnia*

a. Main causes

i. Habits and associations: often, the only difference between a child sleeping through the night and one that is having frequent awakenings is the ability of the former to go back to sleep readily without intervention; child should be put to sleep alone to help train the child to readily go back to sleep on his or her own if he or she awakens at night and notes being alone

ii. Nighttime feedings: by 5–6 months, full-term healthy infants should be able to sleep through the night without requiring nighttime feedings; nighttime feedings may also affect circadian rhythms by altering vascular flow and changes in body temperature; some infants become trained to need feeding to fall back to sleep; this can be treated by slowly reducing and subsequently eliminating nighttime feedings carried out over the course of a week

iii. Poor limit setting

iv. Improper schedules

v. Medical triggers

vi. Neurologic dysfunction

vii. Fears and anxieties

2. *Schedule disorders*
   a. Early awakenings may be caused by early sleep cycles and excessive daytime naps, which may also cause difficulty with sleep onset.
   b. It is important to correlate sleep time with in-bed time.
3. *Arousal disorders*
   a. Confusional arousals (see section X).
   b. Sleepwalking (somnambulism): typically occurs with arousal in the first third of night, during stages 3 and 4; if awakened, the patient is amnestic for the event (but may recall fragmentary imagery); may be precipitated if patient is awakened during SWS; if awakened during sleepwalking, patient can be highly combative.
   c. Sleep terrors (aka *pavor nocturnus*, incubus attack): piercing scream with inconsolable fear on awakening; typically occur with arousal in the first part of the night, during stages 3 and 4; on exam → tachycardia and tachypnea, often profuse sweating, and dilated pupils; full consciousness is usually not attained for 5–10 minutes; feelings of choking or being crushed are common; PSG: arise during stages 3 and 4 SWS, associated with rapid desynchronization to low-voltage fast waking patterns, evidence of arousal with tachycardia, tachypnea, increased muscle tone; if multiple attacks occur, they may also begin in stage 2 sleep.
   d. Terrifying dreams (dream anxiety attacks): dreams are often threatening to patient's life: not accompanied by confusion or marked systemic changes as in night terrors: PSG: attacks usually occur in second half of night (night terrors are usually in first third), associated with REM sleep (night terrors with SWS); most often occur when children are overly tired, or when sleep is disrupted (stuffy nose, etc.).
4. *Enuresis*
   a. Definition
      i. Primary: inability to maintain urinary control from birth
      ii. Secondary: inability to maintain urinary control once control has been achieved
      iii. Must be at least two episodes per month in children 3–6 y/o, and at least one episode per month in older children
   b. Genetics
      i. Prevalence in family members
         (A) Father: 40–55%
         (B) Mother: 35–40%
         (C) Siblings: 40%
         (D) 77% of children will have enuresis when both father and mother have enuresis
      ii. More common in males
   c. Incidence

Age (yrs)	Incidence (%)
4	30
6	10
12	3
18	1–2

   d. Treatment: behavior modification, alarm devices, medications to enhance urinary retention

5. *Landau-Kleffner syndrome*
   a. Characterized by: continuous spike-wave activity in kids during sleep, hyperkinesias, seizures, neuropsychological disturbances, progressive aphasia
6. *Sleep apnea syndromes in infancy and childhood*
   a. *AOP*
       i. Excessive periodic breathing with pathologic apnea in a premature infant.
       ii. Almost 50% of premature infants have periodic breathing, and increases in frequency with lower-gestational-age premature infants.

CA (wks)	Incidence of AOP
<28	Noted in almost all
31	50–80%
32	12–15%
34–35	7%

       iii. AOP occurs in one-half of infants, with periodic breathing.
       iv. Likely caused by immature respiratory brain stem centers, central and peripheral chemoreceptors, and pulmonary reflexes.
       v. Most pauses are central apneas (but nearly one-half will also have obstructive or mixed apneas).
       vi. Treatment
           (A) AOP is responsive to medical treatment.
               (1) Methylxanthines: most commonly used medication
               (2) Theophylline: shown to reduce number of apneic episodes and less risk of respiratory failure
               (3) Caffeine: increases ventilation (by increasing central respiratory drive), tidal volume, and mean inspiratory flow
           (B) May require CPAP or oxygen, or mechanical ventilation.
   b. *SIDS*
       i. Prevalence of 1/1000.
       ii. Highest incidence between 2 and 4 months; by age 5–6 months, baby can roll over, which is likely reason for lower incidence.
       iii. In <10%, apneas are noted before death.
       iv. Risk factors for SIDS
           (A) Prone sleeping position: increases risk of SIDS by 3–7×
           (B) Young, unwed mothers
           (C) Maternal smoking or substance abuse
           (D) Maternal depression
           (E) Short interpregnancy interval
           (F) Low socioeconomic status
           (G) Deficient prenatal care
           (H) One or more siblings with SIDS, or near-SIDS
           (I) Preterm birth
           (J) Low birth weight
           (K) Formula feeding/no breast-feeding
           (L) Excessively warm sleeping environment
           (M) Winter months

(N) Preceding gastrointestinal symptoms

(O) Infection with *Campylobacter jejuni*

v. Biologic basis

(A) Although bradycardia may occur during apnea, most likely associated with apnea rather than cardiac arrest.

(B) Occurrence of apnea in normal infants suggests that an abnormal or absent response to apnea is cause (rather than apnea itself).

(C) Arousal responses to apneas are underdeveloped before birth because of lack of need to breathe in utero.

(D) Accidental suffocation.

(E) Infection may trigger SIDS (especially respiratory infection; risk for SIDS twice as high in winter).

vi. Prognosis and management of infant with apparent life-threatening event

(A) 30–50% have additional episodes of prolonged apnea

(B) 3–7% die of SIDS

(C) Monitors to evaluate chest movement, heart, and oxygenation

(D) Parental training in cardiopulmonary resuscitation

vii. Possible indications for apnea monitors

(A) Congenital central hypoventilation syndrome

(B) Two or more siblings with SIDS

(C) Tracheostomy

(D) Severe bronchopulmonary dysplasias

XIII. Medications: Effect on Sleep and Wakefulness

A. **Antidepressants**

1. Sleep changes associated with depression: difficulty falling asleep, early morning awakening, intermittent wakefulness, reduced SWS, reduced REM latency, increased duration of REM sleep

2. Antidepressants may: suppress REM sleep, impair daytime performance due to EDS

3. Most potent REM suppressing group is monoamine oxidase inhibitors (MAOIs) (i.e., phenelzine)

4. Effect of TCAs on sleep: suppress REM, moderately improve sleep continuity, slightly increase SWS

B. *Lithium:* sleep changes associated with lithium: increases REM latency, suppresses REM sleep, increases SWS, wake and drowsy sleep states may be reduced

C. *Neuroleptics:* sleep changes associated with neuroleptics: decrease wakefulness, increase SWS, chlorpromazine may increase REM sleep (possibly due to α-2 antagonism); but with larger doses, it may reduce REM sleep (due to effects on α-1 receptors)

D. *Stimulants*

1. Central action of the xanthines is likely due to adenosine receptor antagonism

2. Sleep changes associated with amphetamines: increased wakefulness, delayed onset and duration of REM sleep, amphetamines function by DA releaser and norepinephrine reuptake inhibitor

E. **Meds that cause suppression of SWS:** benzodiazepines

F. **Suppression of REM sleep:** amphetamines, antipsychotics, lithium, MAOIs, nicotine, TCAs, opiates

XIV. Sleep and Psychiatric Disorders

A. *Mood disorders*

1. *Depression*

a. Most common complaint is insomnia

b. PSG of depressed patient demonstrates three general abnormalities

   i. Decreased sleep continuity (prolonged sleep latency, increased wake time during sleep, early morning awakening, decreased sleep efficiency, and reduced TST)

   ii. Reduced SWS: preferential loss of SWS in first NREM period

   iii. REM abnormalities

     (A) Shortened REM latency: possibly most important marker for mood disorders

     (B) Increased phasic REM measurements for both REM activity and REM density

     (C) Increased duration of first REM period, increased total minutes of REM sleep

     (D) Increased REM percentage of total sleep

2. Treatment of sleep disturbances associated with mood disorders

a. Major depression

   i. Antidepressants (most) will suppress REM sleep (including reducing REM latency and total REM sleep time); these include selective serotonin reuptake inhibitors, TCAs, and MAOIs.

   ii. MAOIs may cause almost complete loss of REM sleep.

   iii. Antidepressants without significant REM-sleep suppression.

     (A) Nefazodone: 5-Hydroxytryptamine type 2 receptor antagonist and 5-hydroxytryptamine reuptake inhibitor; decreases wake time and increases stage 2 sleep without effect on REM

     (B) Trimipramine/iprindole/amineptine

   iv. An important related side of antidepressants (especially TCAs and selective serotonin reuptake inhibitors) is that they may cause primary sleep disorders, including periodic limb movements of sleep and REM sleep behavior disorder.

b. Seasonal affective disorder: light therapy

   i. 10,000 lux for 30 minutes per day (40-W bulb 2–3 ft from face), or 2500 lux for 2 hours

   ii. More effective in morning

   iii. Improves symptoms in 60% of seasonal affective disorder cases (especially in cases with hypersomnia and hyperphagia)

   iv. Middle range of visible wavelengths is optimal (ultraviolet is not necessary, especially since may cause retinal damage)

ADDITIONAL NOTES

Neurophysiology

CHAPTER 10

Clinical Neurophysiology

I. Electromyography (EMG) and Nerve Conduction Velocity (NCV) Studies
  A. *Basic neurophysiology*
    1. *Action potential (AP) generation*
      a. Definition: a self-propagating regenerative change in membrane potential
      b. Originally found to be the result of sodium/potassium channels via voltage clamp experiments on giant squid axons; involves maintaining membrane potential at a fixed value and then using channel blockers to test current changes
        i. *tetrodotoxin blocks Na^+ channels*
        ii. *tetraethylammonium blocks K^+ channels*
      c. *Three phases: resting, depolarizing, repolarizing*
      d. Myelinated are faster than unmyelinated nerves
        i. Myelin decreases membrane capacitance and conductance and the time constant
        ii. Increases the space constant of the segment of axon between the nodes of Ranvier

NB: AP propagation in myelinated fibers is known as saltatory conduction.

        iii. Velocity is proportional to axon radius
    2. *Neuromuscular junction*
      a. Presynaptic components
        i. Motor neuron
        ii. Axon
        iii. Terminal bouton: synaptic vesicles contain 5,000–10,000 molecules (1 quanta) of acetylcholine; release based on voltage-gated calcium channels
      b. Synaptic cleft: 200–500 μm
      c. Positive-synaptic components
        i. Motor end plate
        ii. Acetylcholine receptors
        iii. Voltage-gated sodium channels
    3. *Volume conduction*
      a. Definition: spread of current from the potential source through a conducting medium.
      b. May cause considerable differences in waveforms when a potential travels from one medium to a different medium.

    c. The interstitial fluid and body tissues possess a finite resistance capable of attenuating the magnitude of a potential at a distance from the current source. This diminution in potential magnitude is directly proportional to the square of the distance from the current source and falls approximately 20% in 6.25 cell diameters in neural tissue.

    d. *The amplitude of the recorded potential is dependent on*
      i. Membrane's charge density.
      ii. The orientation of the recording electrode and active portion of the membrane.
      iii. Distance between the membrane and recording electrode.
      iv. Type of recording electrode used.

    e. *The amplitude is also directly proportional to a defined portion of the membrane's surface area and indirectly proportional to the square of the distance between the membrane and the electrode.*
      i. The amplitude increases if the membrane's surface area increases or the distance to the membrane decreases.
      ii. *The amplitude of sensory nerve AP (SNAP) or compound muscle AP (CMAP) is the composite of the amplitudes of the individual nerve fibers, some faster or slower than others, resulting in a final amplitude that is less than would be seen if all were summated together in phase.*

    f. The triphasic waveform results from the negative cathode receiving a wave of depolarization that changes in polarity as it passes and subsequent repolarization occurring later.

4. *Far-field recording:* recording electrical activity of biologic origin generated at a considerable distance from the recording electrodes
    a. Usually implies stationary rather than propagating signals recorded at a distance.
    b. Tissue of different density can distort the potential into a complex waveform with latencies that are different from the actual latencies measured near the generator.
    c. Changes in extracellular resistance caused by anatomic inhomogeneities and/or by conductivity changes give rise to far-field components.

5. Filters and gain
    a. High and low frequencies
      i. High- (low pass) frequency filters (HFFs) exclude high frequencies
      ii. Low- (high pass) frequency filters (LFFs) exclude low frequencies
    b. *Gain:* recorded in microvolts per centimeter

6. *Artifacts*
    a. *Physiologic*
      i. *Temperature: most negative factor; conduction velocity slows 1.5–2.5 m per second for every 1°C drop in temperature, and distal latency prolongs by approximately 0.2 millisecond per degree*
      ii. *Age: newborns have 50% of normal adult NCV; age 1 year: 75% of normal adult NCV; normal velocities by age 3–5 years when complete myelination occurs; SNAP amplitude drops by up to 50% by age 70 years; motor unit AP duration is longer in older patients*
      iii. *Height:* taller individuals have slower NCVs due to longer nerves (adjust to normative data)
      iv. *Proximal vs. distal nerve segments: distal segments have slower NCVs due to smaller diameter nerve segments*
    b. *Nonphysiologic:* electrode impedance mismatch and 60 Hz interference
      i. Electrode impedance: minimize by using same electrodes, cleaning skin, using conducting jelly
      ii. 60 Hz: if problematic, may be faulty ground

    c. *Stimulus artifact*
       i. Cathode position: may not stimulate directly over the nerve (submaximal stimulation); may stimulate other nerves
      ii. Supramaximal stimulation: all nerve fibers must be depolarized (suboptimal stimulation will give lower amplitude)
     iii. Costimulation of adjacent nerves brings in other nerves as artifacts superimposed on desired nerve
     iv. Electrode placement: if too distant, may result in distortion from far-field effect
      v. *Antidromic vs. orthodromic: antidromic* advantage is higher amplitude potentials; disadvantage is volume-conducting motor potential after the SNAP
     vi. Distance between recording and referencing electrodes must be >4 cm
    vii. Make sure accurate distance

B. *Equipment*
  1. Principle
    a. Clinical EMG is recorded extracellularly from muscle fibers embedded in tissue (conducting medium)
    b. *Muscle fiber: motor unit ratio variable—1:3 in ocular muscles, 100:1 in axial muscles*
  2. *Sources of wave generators*
    a. *Fibrillation and positive sharp waves are from the spontaneous depolarization of a muscle fiber (i.e., myopathic).*
    b. *Fasciculation, doublets, multiplets, cramps, and myokymic discharges are from the motor neuron and its axon (i.e., neuropathic).*
    c. *Complex repetitive discharge: recurrent loops of muscle fibers that fire sequentially (i.e., denervation).*
  3. Techniques of EMG
    a. Four steps: insertion, spontaneous activity, minimal contraction to assess different motor unit potentials (MUPs), and maximal contraction to assess recruitment
    b. Sensitivity: 50–100 µV/cm for spontaneous activity; 200 µV/cm to 1 mV/cm to assess voluntary activity
    c. Filter: low, 10–20 Hz; high, 10 kHz
    d. Muscles typically assessed of upper and lower extremities
       i. Upper extremities
         (A) 1st dorsal interosseus
         (B) Extensor indicis proprius
         (C) Flexor pollicis longus
         (D) Pronator teres
         (E) Biceps brachii
         (F) Triceps
         (G) Deltoid
         (H) Cervical paraspinal muscles
      ii. Lower extremities
         (A) Adductor hallucis
         (B) Extensor digiti brevis
         (C) Tibialis anterior and posterior
         (D) Vastus lateralis
         (E) Gluteus maximus and medius
         (F) Lumbar and sacral paraspinals
  4. *Single fiber EMG*
    a. *To determine fiber density and jitter*

    b. Record 300-μm radius

    c. Amplifier: higher impedance ≥100 megaohms

    d. Sweep faster, higher gain, high frequency allowed filter

C. *Clinical EMG of normal muscle*

  1. *EMG of normal muscle*

    a. *Insertional activity*

      i. Produced by mechanic stimulation of the muscle fibers by the penetrating electrode with muscle at rest

      ii. Typically persists for a few hundred milliseconds

      iii. Duration slightly exceeds the movement of the electrode

      iv. Divided into normal, increased, and decreased insertional activity

      v. An isolated positive wave may be present at the end of insertional activity in normal muscle

      vi. *Prolonged insertional activity occurs in two types of normal variants and in denervated muscle and myotonic discharges*

        (A) *Normal variants:* short trains of regularly firing positive waves—may be familial or subclinical myotonia; short recurrent bursts of irregularly firing potentials—most often seen in muscular individuals, especially in calf muscles

        (B) *Reduced insertional activity:* occurs in *periodic paralysis* (during paralysis) and with replacement of muscle by connective tissue or fat in myopathies and neurogenic disorders

        (C) *Increased insertional activity:* needle movement resulting in any waveform that lasts >300 milliseconds; needle movement may provoke positive waves; *may be seen in neuropathic and myopathic conditions: denervated muscle, myotonic disorders, polymyositis, myopathies*

    b. Motor end-plate activity

      i. The end-plate region is the usual place normal resting muscle shows electrical activity when the needle is held in a stationary position

      ii. *Consists of end-plate noise and end-plate spikes*

        (A) *End-plate noise*

          (1) Monophasic, irregular negative potentials with low amplitude (10–50 μV) and 1–2 milliseconds in duration.

          (2) "Ocean"/"sea shell" sound due to depolarization caused by spontaneous release of acetylcholine.

          (3) Biphasic potentials with a negative onset are also a constituent of end-plate noise and have duration of 3–5 milliseconds and amplitude of 100–200 μV.

          (4) Biphasic potentials represent muscle fiber APs arising sporadically at the neuromuscular junction or intramuscular nerve fibers.

        (B) *End-plate spikes*

          (1) Amplitude: 100–200 μV

          (2) Duration: 3–4 milliseconds

          (3) Frequency: 5–50 Hz irregularly firing

          (4) Initially negative amplitude (as opposite to fibrillations)

          (5) Possibly originate in intrafusal muscle fibers

    c. *MUP*

      i. Waveform

        (A) *Composed of a group of muscle fibers innervated by a single anterior horn cell*

        (B) *The spatial relation between the needle and the individual muscle fibers plays the greatest role in determining the waveform of the MUP*

(C) *Composite of the compound potential of the sum of individual APs generated in the few muscle fibers of the unit that are in the range of the EMG needle*

(D) Cooling of the muscle (from 37° to 30°C): increase in the duration; decrease in the amplitude; marked increase in the percentage of polyphasic potentials

(E) The MUP is made up of <20 muscle fibers lying within a 1-mm radius from the electrode tip

(F) *MUP waveform*

    (1) *Amplitude: typically 200 μV to 3 mV; determined largely by the distance between the recording electrode and the active fibers that are closest to it;* computer simulations have suggested that MUP is determined by less than eight fibers situated within 0.5 mm of the electrode

    (2) *Rise time*

        (a) Time lag from the initial positive peak to the subsequent negative peak

        (b) Should be <500 microseconds

        (c) Area of negative spike depends on number and diameter of muscle fibers closest to electrode and their temporal dispersion

        (d) Produces a crisp sound

        (e) Distance units have a slower rise time

    (3) Duration

        (a) It relates to anatomic scatter of end plates of the muscle fibers in the units studied

        (b) Measured from the initial takeoff to the return to the baseline

        (c) Indicates the degree of synchrony among many individual muscle fibers

        (d) Varies from 2–15 milliseconds depending on the muscle, temperature, and age: decreased temperature causes increased duration and number of polyphasic potentials; increases with age due to increased width of territory of end plates that are scattered

        (e) Duration is a more negative parameter in assessing MUP size, and it reflects more accurately all the muscle fibers within the motor unit

        (f) Pathologic findings

            (i) Long duration: seen in lower motor neuron disorders and chronic myositis

            (ii) Short duration: seen in all myopathies, occasionally in neuromuscular junction disorders and early phases of reinnervation

            (iii) Polyphasia: five or more phases, seen in myopathic and neurogenic disorders

    (4) *Phases*

        (a) Determined by counting the negative and positive peaks to and from the baseline

        (b) Normal: less than four

        (c) More than four suggests desynchronization of discharges or drop out of fibers

        (d) May see polyphasic potential in normal muscles but should not exceed 5–15%

        (e) Desynchronization may be suggested by complex or pseudopolyphasic potentials (potentials that have several turns but do not cross the baseline)

d. *Recruitment patterns of MUPs*
  i. *Recruitment pattern:* relationship between the number of MUPs firing and their firing rate varies between muscles but is constant for a particular muscle
  ii. *Recruitment frequency:* frequency at which a particular unit must fire before another is recruited; 5–20 Hz; ratio of the number of active motor units to the firing frequency of individual units is generally <5 and is relatively constant for individual muscles
  iii. *Motor units are activated according to Henneman's size principle: early recruited units are usually small type I, larger type 2 fibers are activated later during strong voluntary contractions*
  iv. Increase in muscle force results in: recruitment of previously inactive units; increased firing rate of already active units
  v. Number of active units >10 are indicative of loss of motor unit
  vi. *Interference pattern*
    (A) *Simultaneous activation of multiple motor units precludes the identification of individual motor units–interference pattern*
    (B) The spike density and the average amplitude are determined by several factors, including descending input, number of motor units capable of firing, firing frequency, waveforms, and phase cancellation
    (C) Provides a simple quantitative means of evaluating the relationship between the number of firing units and the muscle force exerted with maximal effort
    (D) *Decreased recruitment (interference) pattern*
      (1) *Characterized by a rapid rate of firing of MUPs disproportionate to the number of units firing*
      (2) *Caused by any disorder that: destroys motor axons or neurons, blocks conduction along motor axons, devastates (or blocks) a large number of muscle fibers so that many motor units are practically lost*
      (3) *Can be seen in: acute neuropathic conditions (trauma, infarction, Guillain-Barré syndrome [GBS]), acute demyelinating and axonal loss lesions, Kugelberg-Welander disease; in uncooperative patients, the interference pattern may be reduced during maximal voluntary effort (but CMAPs are normal in configuration)*
e. *Clinical applications*
  i. *Denervation*
    (A) Conditions: acquired neuropathy, hereditary neuropathy, plexopathy, radiculopathy
    (B) *Typically long duration, large amplitude (reinnervation), poor recruitment, ± polyphasic*
  ii. *Myopathy*
    (A) Conditions: acquired myopathies, hereditary myopathies
    (B) *Typically short duration, small amplitude, increased or normal recruitment, polyphasic*
  iii. *Spontaneous discharges*
    (A) *Fibrillation potentials and positive waves: APs of single muscle fibers that are twitching spontaneously in the absence of innervation*
      (1) *Fibrillations*
        (a) *Triphasic or biphasic, 1–5 milliseconds in duration, and 20–200 μV in amplitude; duration, <5 milliseconds; firing rate, 2–20 Hz; high pitched, bi- or triphasic; first phase is positive except when recorded in end plate*

(b) *Muscle fibers that show fibrillation potentials:* denervated muscle fibers 3–5 weeks after acute lesions (may persist for months or years until muscle fibers are reinnervated or are degenerated); regeneration; never innervated; normal patients

(c) Grading

   (i) Fibrillations that are not persistent (continuous)

   (ii) One or more fibrillations persistent in at least two areas

   (iii) Two or more persistent fibrillations of moderate numbers in three or more areas

   (iv) Three or more persistent fibrillations of large numbers but not obscuring the baseline

   (v) Four or more persistent fibrillations of large numbers that obscure the baseline

(2) *Positive waves*

   (a) Biphasic: 10–30 milliseconds in duration and 20–200 μV in amplitude

   (b) Arising from single fibers that are injured

   (c) Same significance as fibrillation: indicates early denervation, chronic denervation, rapidly progressive degeneration of muscle fibers

(B) *Myotonia*

   (1) APs of the muscle fibers that are firing spontaneously in a prolonged fashion after external excitation

   (2) Regular in rhythm but vary in frequency between 40 and 100 per second

   (3) *Occur as brief spikes or positive waveforms*

   (4) *Sounds like a dive-bomber*

   (5) *Conditions: myotonic disorders, hyperkalemic periodic paralysis, polymyositis, acid maltase deficiency, myotonia congenita*

(C) *Myokymia*

   (1) *Spontaneous muscle potentials associated with the fine, worm-like motoric movement*

   (2) Appear as normal MUPs that fire with a fixed pattern and rhythm

   (3) Burst of 2–10 potentials

   (4) Rate of 40–60 Hz

   (5) Bursts that recur at regular intervals of 0.1–10.0 seconds

   (6) Firing pattern of one potential is unrelated to other potentials

   (7) Hyperexcitability of lower motor neuron, peripheral nerves, ephaptic excitation, axons

   (8) Unaffected by voluntary activity

   (9) In tetany, similar findings are seen but under voluntary control

   (10) *Conditions: radiation-induced plexopathy or myelopathy, multiple sclerosis (MS),* acute inflammatory demyelinating polyradiculopathy, *chronic radiculopathy, entrapment neuropathy, gold intoxication, facial myokymia (MS, brainstem tumor)*

(D) *Complex repetitive discharges*

   (1) *APs of groups of muscle fibers discharging spontaneously in near synchrony*

   (2) *May be the result of ephaptic activation of groups of adjacent muscle fibers*

   (3) *Characterized by abrupt onset and cessation*

   (4) Uniform frequency from 3–40 Hz

   (5) Typically polyphasic with 3–10 spike components with amplitudes from 50–500 μV and durations up to 50 milliseconds

   (6) *Conditions: periodic paralysis, hypothyroidism, certain glycogen storage diseases*

(E) *Cramp potentials*
   (1) Distinguished from other potentials for their firing pattern
   (2) Fire rapidly from 40–60 Hz, usually with abrupt onset and cessation
   (3) May fire in a sputtering pattern, but typically appear as increasing numbers of potentials that fire at similar rates as the cramp develops and then drop out as the cramp subsides
   (4) Common in normal patients and usually occur when a shortened muscle is strongly activated
(F) *Neuromyotonia*
   (1) *MUPs associated with some forms of continuous muscle fiber*
   (2) Fire at frequencies of 10–300 Hz
   (3) May decrease in amplitude because of the inability of muscle fibers to maintain discharges at rates >100 Hz
   (4) May be continuous or recur in bursts
   (5) Unaffected by voluntary activity and are commonly seen in neurogenic disorders
   (6) *Conditions: peripheral neuropathy, sporadic or hereditary muscle stiffness, other neuromuscular symptoms without evidence of neuropathy (Isaacs' syndrome)*
(G) *Fasciculations*
   (1) *APs of a group of muscle fibers innervated by an anterior horn cell that discharges in a random fashion*
   (2) *Conditions: normal patient, chronic partial denervation, including lower motor neuron disease*

D. *Pathologic conditions*
   1. **Myopathic disorders**
      a. Similar findings are that of reinnervation after severe nerve damage
      b. Assess proximal muscles (e.g., iliacus, glutei, spinati, and paraspinous muscle) and midlimb muscles (brachioradialis and tibialis anterior)
   2. **Muscular dystrophies (MDs)**
      a. Decreased insertional activity when muscle replaced by fatty tissue
      b. Increased insertional activity, positive waves, fibrillations, and complex repetitive discharges may occur owing to segmental necrosis of muscle fiber or regeneration of fibers
      c. Conditions: Duchenne's MD, Becker's MD, Limb-girdle MD, Fascioscapulohumeral MD, Emery-Dreifuss MD: both myopathic and neuropathic patterns
   3. **Inflammatory myopathy**
      a. Important EMG findings are patchy
      b. EMG myopathic findings especially common in paraspinal muscles
      c. Conditions: polymyositis, Human immunodeficiency virus myopathy, zidovudine-related myopathy, inclusion body myositis
   4. **Endocrine and metabolic myopathies**
      a. *Hypokalemic periodic paralysis*
         i. Normal between attacks
         ii. During attacks: no spontaneous activity, decreased duration and amplitude of CMAP, decreased interference pattern, complete electrical silence in severe cases
      b. *Hyperkalemic or normokalemic periodic paralysis*
         i. Increased insertional activity
         ii. Myotonic discharges
   5. **Drug-related myopathy**
      a. Both myopathic and neuropathic findings
         i. Cimetidine

      ii. D-Penicillamine
      iii. Colchicine
      iv. Chloroquine
  b. Myopathic findings only
      i. Clofibrate
      ii. Lovastatin
      iii. Gemfibrozil
      iv. Niacin
  c. Acute rhabdomyolysis
      i. Lovastatin
      ii. Gemfibrozil
6. **Critical illness myopathy**
  a. Myopathy
  b. ± Fibrillations
  c. Decreased CMAP
  d. Decreased SNAP
  e. Decreased response in repetitive nerve stimulation
7. **Neuropathic disorders**
  a. Immediately after acute neuropathic lesion
      i. Decreased CMAP under voluntary control
      ii. No complete interference pattern
      iii. Increased firing rate of individual units
      iv. No electrical activity in severe cases
  b. Reinnervation
      i. Decreased spontaneous activity and amplitude of CMAP
      ii. Variable in size and configuration of CMAP
      iii. Increased duration of CMAP and polyphasia

Recruitment	MUP appearance	Disorders
Normal	Normal	*Normal*
		Endocrine and metabolic myopathies
		Myasthenia gravis
		Myasthenic syndrome
Normal	Short duration, polyphasic	*Primary myopathies*
		Severe myasthenia
		Botulinum intoxication
		Reinnervation (neurogenic or myositis)
Normal	Mixed short duration and long duration	*Chronic myositis*
		Inclusion body myositis
		Rapidly progressing neurogenic disorder (i.e., amyotrophic lateral sclerosis)
Poor	Normal	*Acute neurogenic lesion*
Poor	Long duration, polyphasic	*Chronic neurogenic atrophy*
		Progressing neurogenic atrophy

Recruitment	MUP appearance	Disorders
Poor	Short duration, polyphasic	*Severe myopathy (end-stage, neurogenic atrophy)*
		Early reinnervation after severe nerve damage

E. **Clinical NCV studies**
   1. Miscellaneous: maximum difference of NCV latencies between right vs. left
      a. Motor: 0.7 millisecond
      b. Sensory: 0.5 millisecond
   2. *Neuropathy*
      a. *Axonal: decreased amplitude;* mild slowing; reduced recruitment; giant MUPs; fibrillations

Motor NCV

Amplitude	Decreased
Duration	Normal
Shape	Normal
Velocity	Normal or decreased (>60% normal)

Sensory NCV

Amplitude	Decreased
Duration	Normal
Shape	Normal
Velocity	Normal or decreased (>60% normal)
H-reflex	Increased (<150% normal) or absent
F-wave	Increased (<150% normal) or absent

   b. *Demyelinating:* NCV <60% of normal; conduction block; temporal dispersion; latency prolonged

Motor NCV

Amplitude	Variable
Duration	Dispersion
Shape	Normal or multiphasic
Velocity	Decreased (<60% normal)

Sensory NCV

Amplitude	Variable
Duration	Increased
Shape	Decreased
Velocity	Decreased (<60% normal)
H-reflex	Increased (>150% normal)
F-wave	Increased (>150% normal)

3. Reinnervation
   a. May begin as early as 1–2 weeks after injury
   b. Reinnervation progresses at 1 mm per day
4. Motor nerves typically degenerate at faster rates than sensory nerves
5. Sensory NCVs are typically better preserved than motor NCVs
6. Lesion proximal to dorsal root ganglion will produce sensory loss but preservation of sensory NCV

F. *H-reflex studies*
   1. Technique
      a. Stimulating cathode proximal to avoid anodal block
      b. Stimulus pulse with long duration (1 millisecond)
      c. Submaximal stimulus
      d. Frequency = 0.2 Hz to allow full recovery before next stimulus
      e. Late response must be larger than the preceding direct motor response
      f. *Lower extremity H-reflex: posterior tibial nerve at popliteal fossa (PF) recorded on soleus muscle*
      g. *Upper extremity H-reflex: flexor carpi radialis muscle via median nerve stimulated at cubital fossa*
   2. *Neurophysiologic significance*
      a. *H-reflex involves fast conducting afferent (Ia) fibers via monosynaptic reflex*
      b. H-reflex and Achilles' reflex are interchangeable
      c. Uses
         i. It is a normal test available within the routine EMG test to evaluate the preganglionic segment of the sensory fibers of the S1 root
         ii. Upper limit of normal latency: soleus—35 milliseconds; flexor carpi radialis—21 milliseconds
         iii. Side-to-side difference of latency: 2 milliseconds between lower extremities; 1.5 milliseconds between upper extremities
         iv. Side-to-side difference of amplitude: ≤3 milliseconds for both upper and lower extremities
         v. Note: may be absent in elderly
      d. *Disorders of peripheral nervous system: absence early in GBS; important in plexopathies and radiculopathies; important in C6, C7, or S1 radiculopathies; useful in radiculopathies—showing the injury to the anterior rami even when EMG is unrevealing owing to sparing the ventral roots*
      e. *Disorders of central nervous system (CNS): important in CNS lesion with upper motor neuron signs*
      f. *Other uses of H-reflex: decreased in cataplexy and acute spinal cord lesion*

G. *F-response*
   1. Physiology: F-waves are produced by *antidromic activation (reflected impulse) of motor neuron; useful to estimate conduction in proximal motor nerves by testing length of entire motor nerve; no synapse is tested*
   2. Technique
      a. Cathodes—proximal
      b. Supramaximal stimulation
      c. No need of long duration
      d. Rate <0.5 Hz
      e. Gain amplifier, 200–500 µV; sweep, 5–10 milliseconds
   3. *Clinical application of F-wave*

a. Normal range
    i. Upper limits of F-wave latency
       (A) Hand: 31 milliseconds
       (B) Calf: 36 milliseconds
       (C) Foot: 61 milliseconds
    ii. Maximal side-to-side difference
       (A) Hand: 2 milliseconds
       (B) Calf: 3 milliseconds
       (C) Foot: 4 milliseconds
    iii. >70% of normal patients do not have peroneal nerve F-wave, but most should have normal tibial nerve F-waves
    iv. *Disorders of peripheral nervous system*
       (A) Prolonged F-wave latencies
          (1) Polyneuropathies
          (2) Amyotrophic lateral sclerosis
          (3) Myotonic dystrophy
          (4) GBS and chronic inflammatory demyelinating polyradiculoneuropathy: prominent F-wave slowing compared to distal motor NCV
          (5) Syringomyelia
          (6) S1 radiculopathy
    v. *Disorders of CNS*
       (A) Absent in spinal shock
       (B) Disorders of upper motor neurons

II. Electroencephalography (EEG)

A. *Physics and biology of electricity*
  1. *Ion fluxes and membrane potentials*
    a. Most of the charge movement in biologic tissue is attributed to passive properties of the membrane or changes in ion conductance
    b. Positive cations: K^+, Na^+, Ca^{2+}
    c. Negative anions: Cl^-, proteins
    d. Resting membrane potential: –75 mV (due to difference in permeability of ions and sodium-potassium pump forcing K^+ in and Na^+ out)
  2. *AP:* an AP normally develops if the depolarization reaches the threshold determined by the voltage-dependent properties of the sodium channels; sodium channels are also time dependent, staying open for a limited period
  3. *Synaptic transmission*
    a. Intraneuronal negative polarity of 70 mV noted with intracellular recording.
    b. Resting membrane potential is based on outward K^+ current through passive leakage channels.
    c. If resting membrane potential is diminished and threshold is surpassed, the AP is generated.
    d. AP is based on sodium inward currents and potassium outward current through voltage-dependent channels.
    e. When AP reaches presynaptic region, it causes release of neurotransmitter (NT).
    f. NT binds to positive-synaptic receptors, opening positive-synaptic membrane channels.
    g. *Depending on the ionic currents flowing through the transmitter (ligand)-operated channels, two types of positive-synaptic potentials are generated.*

    i. *Excitatory positive-synaptic potentials (EPSPs)*
      (A) Occurs when sodium inward current prevails
      (B) Increases the probability that AP will be propagated
    ii. *Inhibitory positive-synaptic potentials (IPSPs)*
      (A) Occurs when potassium outward current or chloride inward current prevails
      (B) Causes hyperpolarization of the positive-synaptic membrane, making it more difficult to reach the threshold potential
h. *Summation*
    i. *EPSPs and IPSPs interact to determine whether AP is propagated positive-synaptically*
    ii. *Temporal summation:* EPSPs/IPSPs sequentially summate at a monosynaptic site
    iii. *Spatial summation:* EPSPs/IPSPs simultaneously evoke an end-plate potential polysynaptically
i. Depolarization of the nerve terminal results in opening of all ionic channels, including those for calcium; calcium entry causes release of NT from the presynaptic terminal that binds to positive-synaptic receptor sites.
j. *Chemical transmission is the main mode of neuronal communication and can be excitatory or inhibitory* (if positive-synaptic binding opens sodium channels and/or calcium channels → EPSP; if opens potassium channels and/or chloride channels → IPSP); most common excitatory NT is glutamate, common inhibitory NTs are γ-aminobutyric acid and glycine.
k. Several EPSPs may be necessary to generate depolarization.
l. Summation of EPSPs in the cortex occurs mainly at the vertically oriented large pyramidal cells.
m. EEG is generated by the summation of EPSPs and IPSPs that are synchronized by the complex interaction of large populations of cortical cells (but, rhythmic cortical activity is believed to arise from subcortical pacemakers, including the thalamus).

4. *Field potentials and volume conduction*
  a. The influx of sodium during an AP is effectively an inward current (an intracellular electrode notes the interior becoming more positive than it was at rest), whereas an extracellular electrode sees this as a negative potential.
  b. The extracellular potential can be recorded at a considerable distance from the cell and is known as a field potential; near-field potentials are recorded close to the cell membrane, whereas far-field potentials are recorded from a distance.
  c. The movement of charge from excitable tissue to surrounding tissue is called *volume conduction.*

5. *Generation of EEG rhythms*
  a. *Cortical potentials*
    i. Electrical activity in the deep cortical nuclei produces surface potentials of low amplitude.
    ii. The largest neurons are involved in efferent outflow and are oriented perpendicular to the cortical surface, producing a vertical columnar orientation of the cortex.
    iii. Influx of positive ions into the efferent neurons results in a negative extracellular field potential; electrotonic depolarization of the soma and axon hillock results in a positive field potential; because of the vertical orientation of the large efferent neurons, the negative field potential is usually superficial to the positive field potential forming a dipole.
    iv. *In humans, the thalamus is believed to be the main site of origin of EEG rhythms;* oscillations at the thalamic level activate cortical neurons; EPSPs acting on the dendrites mainly in layer 4 (the main site of depolarization) create a dipole with

negativity at layer 4 and positivity at more superficial layers; scalp electrodes detect a small but perceptible far-field potential that represents the summed potential fluctuations.

b. *Scalp potentials*

   i. Estimated that 4–6 cm^2 of cortex must be synchronously activated for a potential to be recorded at the scalp (note: potentials must be volume conducted through the meninges, skull, and skin before being detected by scalp electrodes).

   ii. Scalp potentials are determined by the vectors of cortical activity; if the superficial layer 4 of the cortex is a positive field potential and deeper layers are negative, then there is a vertical vector produced with the positive end pointing toward the scalp electrode; the amplitude of the vector depends on the total area of activated cortex and the degree of synchrony among the neurons.

   iii. Scalp electrodes can record a few millimeters deep and are not able to detect deep nuclei; scalp EEG, therefore, records approximately one-third of cortical activity.

6. *Generation of epileptiform activity*

   a. *Generated when depolarization results in synchronous activation of many neurons*

   b. **Spikes and sharp waves**

      i. Duration: spikes, <70 milliseconds.

      ii. Sharp wave, 70–200 milliseconds.

      iii. Spike potentials are the summation of synchronous EPSPs and APs in the cortex; the foundation for the bursting spike potential is the paroxysmal depolarization shift.

      iv. The negative end of the epileptiform dipole points toward the cortical surface, resulting in a negative deflection at the scalp electrode.

      v. The distribution of the epileptiform potential across the cortical surface is called the field.

      vi. Occasionally, is surface positive (and in normal patterns of positives and 14- and 6-Hz–positive spikes).

   c. **Paroxysmal depolarization shifts**

      i. Extracellular field potentials characterized by waves of depolarization followed by repolarization.

      ii. High amplitude afferent input to the cortex produces depolarization of cortical neurons sufficient to trigger repetitive APs, which in turn contribute to the potentials recorded at the scalp rhythmicity, and is likely due to a mechanism inherent of neurons to be unable to sustain prolonged high-frequency discharges (termination of the sustained depolarization is likely due to activation of K$^+$ channels and inactivation of Ca^{2+} channels).

      iii. Ultimately, termination of epileptiform discharges is due to inhibitory feedback to neurons.

      iv. Note: the above is for partial seizures ± secondary generalization; for primary generalized seizures, the generator is likely a loop between the cortex and thalamus (possibly also responsible for sleep spindles).

B. ***The EEG machine, electrodes, and their derivations***

1. Input board: channel—formed by the two selected electrodes, amplifier, and recording unit to form a system to display the potential differences between two electrodes

2. *Filters*

   a. Filters selectively reduce the amplitude of voltage changes or signals of selected frequencies

   b. *Types of EEG filters*

    i. LFF (aka high-pass filter)
       (A) Allows frequencies higher than designated
       (B) Typically maintained between 0.5 and 1.0 Hz
    ii. HFF (aka low-pass filter)
       (A) Allows frequencies lower than designated
       (B) Standardly, should not have HFF <30 Hz on scalp EEG because high-frequency epileptiform discharges may be filtered
    iii. 60-Hz filter
  3. *Amplifiers*
     a. Amplifier sensitivity is typically 7 μV/mm.
     b. Two main functions of the amplifier: discrimination and amplification
     c. Each amplifier has two inputs connected to the input selector switches.
     d. EEG amplifiers are differential amplifiers (increase the difference in voltage between the two input terminals, with identical inputs of the two terminals being rejected); this serves to distinguish cerebral potentials that are likely to have different amplitude, shape, and timing at electrodes in different regions and allows rejection of potentials that will be similar at all electrodes (e.g., 60 Hz) if impedance is equal at all electrodes; failure to reject artifact, such as 60 Hz, may occur if impedance is different at the two input electrodes or there is absence of an effective ground to the patient.
  4. *Calibration*
     a. Square-wave calibration: square-wave pulse of 50-μV amplitude is delivered to the inputs of each amplifier at rate of 1-second intervals from square-wave pulse
     b. Biocalibration: assesses the response of the amplifiers, filters, et cetera, to complex biologic signals
  5. Paper speed: typically 30 mm per second
  6. *Electrodes*
     a. Usually made of gold, silver chloride, or other material that does not interact chemically with the scalp; skin is prepared by abrasion to remove excess oils and dead skin containing low levels of electrolytes that may alter impedance; electrode gel (usually NaCl) is used to reduce resistance and improve contact of the electrode to the skin.
     b. Impedance between the scalp and electrode must be <1,000 Ω.
     c. *Electrode placement*
        i. *Standard 10–20 international system*
           (A) Measuring the head
               (1) Measure from nasion to inion and mark at 50% point
               (2) Measure between the two preauricular points and mark at 50%; the intersection with step 1 is Cz
        ii. *Intracranial electrodes*
           (A) Depth electrodes
           (B) Subdural/epidural grids and strips
C. **Montage**
  1. **Referential**
     a. Localizes epileptiform potentials by amplitude and complexity (sharpness) of the waveform.
     b. Interelectrode distance alters amplitude; usually CZ or CPz (midline posterior electrodes) are used as reference electrodes or ipsilateral (IL)/contralateral (CL) ear electrodes.
     c. Digital EEG allows for average of electrodes as reference.

2. **Bipolar:** Phase reversal—localization based on positive deflection in one channel with negative deflection in adjacent channel (epileptiform potentials on scalp recordings are typically electronegative)

D. **Rhythm and frequency**
  1. *Frequency categories*
    a. Δ: *1.0–3.9 Hz*
    b. θ: *4.0–7.9 Hz*
    c. α: *8.0–12.9 Hz*
    d. β: *≥13 Hz*
  2. *Normal awake rhythm in adult*
    a. Rhythm and frequency differ in that rhythm is a subcortical generation (likely thalamus) of continuous activity, whereas frequency describes that rate at a given time for recorded activity.
    b. α Rhythm with attenuation/reactivity with eye opening.

E. **Artifact**
  1. *Physiologic artifacts:* usually due to movement, bioelectric potentials, or skin resistance changes
    a. Eye movement: cornea approximately 100-mV positive compared to retina
    b. Cardiovascular: often noted in temporal electrodes
    c. Perspiration: causes slow waves usually >2 seconds in duration (0.5 Hz) owing to changes in impedance between electrode and skin
    d. Muscle: usually ≥35 Hz
    e. Galvanic skin response: slow waves of 1–2 Hz that last for 1–2 seconds with two to three prominent phases; represents an autonomic response of sweat glands and changes in skin conductance in response to sensory stimulus or psychic event
  2. *Nonphysiologic artifacts*
    a. *Two main sources*
      i. *External electrical signal:* 60-Hz electrical input; factors that reduce 60-Hz artifact:
        (A) Proper ground
        (B) Keeping electrode impedance low and approximately equal
        (C) Keeping power lines away from electrodes
        (D) Shielded room to reduce artifact from electricity
      ii. *EEG equipment:* Electrode pops
        (A) Spike-like potentials that occur in random fashion and are caused by sudden changes in junction potentials.
        (B) Small movements or alterations of the electrode-gel interface may temporarily short out the junction potential, and the sudden change in junction potential is seen in all channels with that electrode in common.
        (C) Dissimilar metals build up large junction potentials that are discharged into the amplifier.
        (D) High electrode impedance and loose electrodes predispose to pops.

F. *Activation procedures*
  1. *Hyperventilation (HV)*
    a. Duration: at least 3 minutes of adequate effort (5 minutes if absence seizure is suspected)
    b. Useful in primary generalized seizure disorders; HV will elicit seizure activity in 75% of patients with absence seizures

    c. HV not performed in elderly or other patients with possible cardiovascular/atherosclerotic disease owing to the risk of vasoconstriction with resultant cardiac or cerebral hypoperfusion

  2. *Photic stimulation*

    a. Useful in primary generalized seizure disorders

    b. May demonstrate occipital driving (typically at photic frequency near baseline background cortical frequencies)

  3. Sleep deprivation

    a. Potential for increased epileptiform activity in light sleep

    b. Useful in primary generalized seizure disorders and partial seizure disorders

G. Normal EEG findings

  1. *Normal background cortical activity*

    a. During the *awake state, the patient demonstrates a well-modulated, well-developed 8–10-Hz posterior predominant* α *rhythm.*

    b. *Attenuates with eye opening.*

  2. *Sleep patterns* (see section IV.J)

  3. μ *Rhythm*

    a. *7–11 Hz*

    b. α *Variant, arch shaped*

    c. Noted with immobility

NB: μ Rhythm attenuates with CL hand movement.

  4. *Normal EEG in premature infant* includes

    a. Occasional sharps in temporal and central regions

    b. Δ Brush (which appears between 33 and 35 weeks' gestational age [GA])

    c. Trace alternans (common between 33 and 35 weeks' GA)

    d. Multifocal sharp transients (common between 33 and 35 weeks' GA)

  5. *EEG of neonates and infants*

    a. *Preterm*

      i. <29 weeks' GA

        (A) Discontinuous with periodic bursts of moderately high amplitude activity on suppressed background recurring every 6 seconds

        (B) Δ Brush (which occasionally may also be seen in term infants) at 0.3–1.5 Hz in posterior quadrant

      ii. 32–34 weeks' GA: multifocal sharp transients can been seen as normal variant (and may persist until 44 weeks' GA)

      iii. 37–42 weeks' GA: continuous θ and Δ activity

    b. *Full term*

      i. Trace alternans with mild asynchronies

      ii. Sleep spindles do not occur until 6–8 weeks post-term

      iii. At 3 months post-term, vertex waves present

Conceptual age	EEG findings
26 wks	EEG consists of high-voltage slow waves and runs of low-voltage α (8–14 Hz) separated by 20–30-sec intervals of nearly isoelectric background with independent activity over each hemisphere (aka hemispheric asynchrony)

Conceptual age	EEG findings
	The discontinuous pattern, aka, *trace discontinu,* is accompanied by irregular respiration and occasional eye movement
27–30 wks	Hemispheric asynchrony and discontinuous EEG are common; temporal sharp waves are common; Δ brush present (Δ with superimposed 14–24-Hz activity with posterior prominence); differentiate quiet sleep (QS) (discontinuous EEG and eye movement is rare) from active sleep (AS) (continuous Δ or Δ-θ activity)
30–33 wks	EEG of AS is nearly continuous with low-voltage mixed frequency patterns; EEG of QS remains discontinuous; Δ brushes and temporal sharp waves remain prominent; amount of indeterminate sleep decreases and nonrapid eye movement (NREM)–rapid eye movement (REM) cycle becomes more evident with a duration of 45 mins by wk 34 and increases to 60–70 mins by term delivery; state rhythms are more prominent
	AS demonstrates increased muscle tone compared to QS; QS has more regular cardiac and respiratory rhythms than AS
33–37 wks	AS develops additional features, including REMs, smiles, grimaces, and other movements; 3rd state develops that is similar to AS but eyes are open and is considered a step toward wake state
37–40 wks	AS by 37 wks' conceptual age is well developed with low- to moderate-voltage continuous EEG, REMs, irregular breathing, muscle atonia, and phasic twitches; QS demonstrates respiration that is regular, extraocular movements are sparse/absent, and body movement is few; the discontinuous EEG pattern seen at earlier ages evolves to trace's alternant (1–10-sec bursts of moderate- to high-voltage mixed frequency activity alternates with 6–10-sec bursts of low-voltage mixed frequency activity; Δ brush: become less frequent and disappear between 37–40 wks' conceptual age; periods of continuous slow-wave activity begin to occur during QS at approximately 37 wks' conceptual age, becoming more prevalent with increasing age

    c. By 6 months old, 6-Hz background
    d. By 3 y/o, typically achieve α background (8 Hz) activity
H. **Important EEG findings (for the boards)**
    1. *EEG of increased intracranial pressure*
      a. Rhythmic slow activity in Δ-θ range
      b. EEG not changed by ↑intracranial pressure until >30 mm Hg
    2. α *Coma (8–13 Hz)*
      a. *Hypoxia*
      b. *Drug overdose*

NB: α *Coma* pattern can be seen in comatose patients with pontine infarctions

      c. *Pontomesencephalic lesion*

3. **Cerebral death:** Technical aspects of EEG recording for cerebral death
   a. Interelectrode distance: 10 cm
   b. Impedance: 100–10,000 Ω
   c. Sensitivity: 2 μV/mm
   d. Electrocardiography (EKG) monitoring
   e. Minimum of eight scalp electrodes
   f. LFF <1 Hz
   g. HFF >30 Hz
4. **Triphasic waves**
   a. *Hepatic/renal encephalopathy*
   b. *Generalized frontal maximal discharge with 0.2–0.5-second major positive wave preceded and followed by minor negative waves*
   c. *Have a frontal to posterior lag in the positive wave*

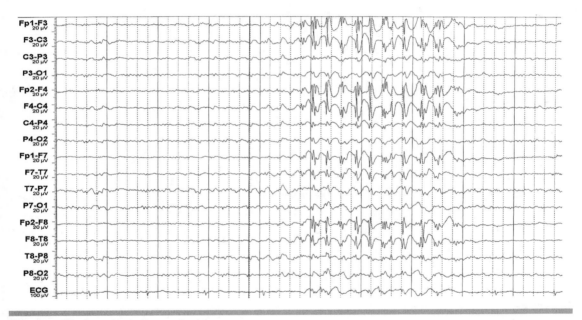

Figure 10-1. 3-Hz spike and wave pattern.

5. **Periodic lateralized sharp waves and spikes (periodic lateralizing epileptiform discharges):** u*sually positive-anoxic or ischemic state (i.e., stroke) > infection > tumor; frequency, 0.5–2.0 Hz*
6. **Epileptiform activity** (see Chapter 4)
   a. *3-Hz spike and wave* (see Figure 10-1) *facilitated by*
      i. HV
      ii. Alkalosis
      iii. Hypoglycemia
      iv. Drowsiness

b. Occurrence of 3-Hz spike and wave and other epileptiform is diminished during REM sleep

c. *Spikes and sharp waves* (see Figure 10-2): duration—spikes <70 milliseconds: sharp wave, 70–200 milliseconds

d. *Focal epileptiform potentials:* localization: temporal, 70%; frontal, 20%; occipital/parietal, 10%

e. *Spike and slow wave:* spike represents excitatory potential; slow wave represents inhibitory potential

f. In 20–30% of patients with epilepsy, no epileptiform potentials may be seen during four separate sleep-deprived EEGs

g. *Hypsarrhythmia = infantile spasm*

h. Slow spike and wave EEG and generalized seizure = Lennox-Gastaut syndrome

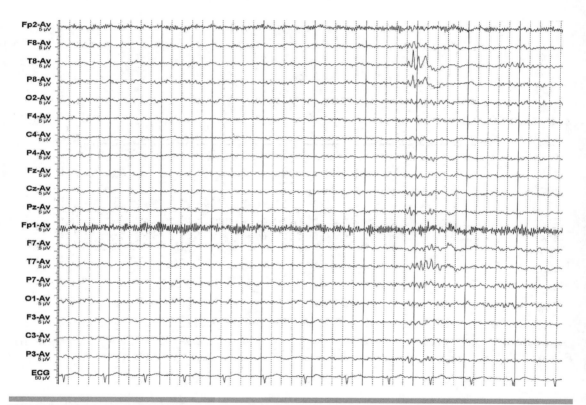

Figure 10-2. Temporal lobe spike and wave discharges.

7. **Burst suppression**

a. *Due to anoxic/ischemic injury or medication effect*

b. *Intermittent sharp complexes interspersed with low amplitude Δ or minimal activity*

III. Evoked Potentials (EPs)

A. **Brain stem auditory-evoked responses (BAERs)**

Classification of BAERs According to Latency

Type	Latency (msecs)	Presumed source
Early (short latency)	<12	
Electrocochleogram	1–4	Auditory nerve compound AP
BAERs	1–12	Wave I = auditory nerve AP
		Waves II–V = brain stem
Middle	12–50	Myogenic vs. neurogenic source
Transient		
Steady-state		
Slow or Late	>50	
Late	50–250	Cortical (N100, P150, N200)
Long	>250	Cortical (P300)

1. *Early AEPs*
   a. *Electrocochleogram*
      i. Sound waves travel via the external auditory canal to the tympanic membrane, in which they produce changes in air pressure and displacement of the tympanic membrane → displacements of the tympanic membrane are transmitted via the ossicular chain (malleus, incus, and stapes) to the oval window of the cochlea.
      ii. The cochlea contains the cochlear duct, an endolymphatic epithelial tube; the endolymph is suspended within another space, the perilymphatic space, which is a spiral tube enclosed at one end by the footplate of the stapes in the oval window and at the other end by the round window; it is continuous with the vestibular labyrinth and cerebrospinal fluid; within the cochlear duct are the basilar membrane and organ of Corti; vibration or displacement of the stapedial foot plate causes change in perilymphatic pressure; vibrations transmitted at the stapedial foot plate are transmitted into a traveling wave at the basilar membrane; high-frequency vibes produce maximum displacement at the base of the cochlea, whereas low-frequency vibes produce maximum displacement at the apex; organ of Corti contains sensory cells: inner and outer hair cells that carry cilia of graded length, with longest embedded in tectorial membrane; when the basilar membrane vibrates, hair cell cilia bend against the tectorial membrane and are moved by the endolymphatic displacement, which produces electrical depolarization of hair cells (receptor potential); inner hair cells transmit to afferent nerve fibers of spiral ganglion cells (the first order afferents of the auditory system) and from there form the cochlear nerve; a separate set of spiral ganglion fibers innervates the outer hair cells.
      iii. Occurs within 2.5 milliseconds of stimulus.
2. *BAERs*
   a. Physiology

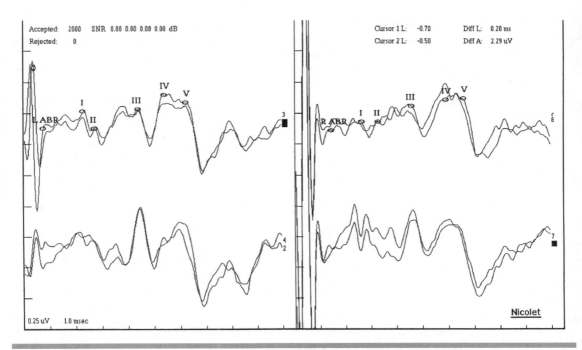

Figure 10-3. Brain stem auditory-evoked potentials. Wave legend: I = acoustic nerve; II = cochlear nuclei (medulla); III = superior olivary complex (pons); IV = lateral lemniscus (pons); V = inferior colliculus (midbrain).

Origin of BAER Waves

Wave	Generator/source
I	Compound AP recorded from the distal end of the *acoustic nerve* or graded potential of dendritic terminals of the acoustic nerve; approximately 2 msecs positive-stimulus
II	Changes in current flow at the acusticus internus, or compound AP of the auditory nerve at the entrance into the brain stem, or graded potentials from *cochlear nucleus*
III	Cochlear nucleus and trapezoid body or *superior olivary complex* and trapezoid body
IV	*Lateral lemniscus,* ventral lemniscus cells, or superior olivary complex or ascending auditory fibers in the pons
V	Generated by projections from the pons to the midbrain, including the ventrolateral *inferior colliculus* and ventrolateral lemniscus; approximately 6 msecs positive-stimulus; first wave whose falling edge goes below baseline; last wave to disappear as stimulus intensity is dropped
VI, VII	Higher brain stem structures (medial geniculate body)

    i. All waves used for assessment are negative potentials
  b. *Recording and stimulus parameters*
    i. Earphones must completely envelope the ears to reduce ambient noise; for infants and young kids, tubes placed in auditory canal because headphones may collapse the external canals.

ii. Three types of sounds are produced:
   (A) Clicks: most frequently used for routine testing; produced by square wave pulse with the rising phase moving the diaphragm in one direction and the fall of the phase returning it to the origin; condensation = initial movement of diaphragm toward eardrum, refraction = away from eardrum (refraction is used predominantly); duration approximately 100 microseconds (producing a sound complex approximately 2 milliseconds in duration)
   (B) Pure tone: delivers exact frequency; most commonly used for pure tone audiometry to test hearing
   (C) White noise: composed of all audible frequencies; delivered into nonstimulated ear to mask ambient noise and avoid bone conduction of the click to the CL ear
iii. Stimulus rates: 8–10 seconds (waves I, II, VI, and VII have reduced amplitudes at higher frequencies).
iv. Each acoustic stimulus can be broken down to three components:
   (A) Frequency (hertz): relates to the location of physical stimulation along the basilar membrane of the cochlea and along the tonotopic representation of the central auditory pathways
   (B) Intensity (decibel): refers to the loudness of the stimulus
   (C) Time: includes duration, rise-fall time, repetition rate, and phase of onset of the stimulus; the phase of onset refers to the initial direction of the basilar membrane displacement
v. Intensity of an acoustic stimulus is measured in three ways:
   (A) Hearing level: average threshold in decibels measured in normal adults (0 dB hearing level); ≈30 dB per sound pressure level (SPL)
   (B) Sensation level: subject's individual threshold (decibel sensation level)
   (C) SPL: acoustic stimuli are measured in decibels peak equivalent SPL (dB SPL); SPL uses as a standard reference level of 20 micropascals
vi. Recording electrodes should be placed over vertex and bilateral ears and/or bilateral mastoids.
vii. BAERs are relatively independent of level of consciousness and affected little by sedatives.
viii. Refraction clicks are recommended because patients with high-frequency hearing loss may have cancellation of out of phase responses by condensation and refraction.
ix. BAER latencies decrease in a quasi-linear pattern with increasing stimulus intensities; waves I and V latencies increase as intensity decreases, whereas the I–V interpeak interval remains essentially unchanged; normative values for latency-intensity functions have been derived allowing for comparative analysis.
x. *Age is another negative variable:*
   (A) In premies → waves II, IV, and VI are less well defined than I and V, and the I–V interpeak interval is longer than in adults.
   (B) Latencies reach adult level by age 1 year.
   (C) Latencies also increase as age increases, but the I–V interval usually remains the same; most of the changes are likely related to wave I owing to associated cochlear dysfunction.
xi. Gender: females with shorter latencies (presumably owing to body and brain size).
c. *Clinical applications*
   i. *BAERs are useful for*
   (A) Hearing assessment in infants.
   (B) Assessing hearing loss in uncooperative adult.
   (C) Evaluating hearing in functional deafness.

(D) Evaluating brain stem function.
   (1) Possible MS
   (2) In central pontine myelinolysis: prolonged waves I–V and III–V latencies (damage to pontine region) with normal wave I (peripheral cochlear nerve/nucleus input)
(E) Evaluating neuro-otologic disorders.
   (1) Acoustic neuromas
   (2) Cerebellopontine angle tumors
   (3) Brain stem lesions
  ii. Interpretation usually requires measurement of waves I, II, and V and also I–III and I–V interpeak intervals.
 iii. *Use of latency-intensity functions allows differentiation of four types of pathology:*
   (A) *Latency-intensity functions indicating conductive hearing loss: prolonged waves I and V with latency-intensity curves parallel to the normal curve; I–III and I–V intervals are normal.*
   (B) *Latency-intensity functions indicating cochlear hearing loss: associated with high-frequency hearing loss; recruiting curve for wave I (i.e., normal or mildly prolonged wave I latencies with loud clicks and greater delays decreased intensity, resulting in a steep curve); wave V not markedly affected, and this curve less steep, resulting in a shortened I–V interval.*
   (C) *Latency-intensity functions indicating retrocochlear deficit type I: wave I prolonged with steep latency-intensity function; wave V prolonged; therefore, I–V interval prolonged; associated with lesions of cranial nerve VIII.*
   (D) *Latency-intensity functions indicating retrocochlear deficit type II: wave I latency-intensity curve is normal; wave V and I–V interval prolonged.*
  iv. *Prolonged I–V interpeak interval is most sensitive indicator of brain stem lesion; prolongation of the III–V interval alone suggests at or after the superior olivary complex (in either the high pons or low midbrain).*
   v. **NB:** Normal wave V latency practically rules out any peripheral or central lesions in auditory path.
  vi. Most common cause of impaired BAERs is demyelinating disease.
 vii. ↑Age → ↑hearing loss in high frequency (>1 kHz).
viii. In brain death, may have complete absence of BAERs or wave I and/or II (wave II noted in 10% of brain dead patients, which reinforces theory that wave II is generated by intracranial portion of cranial nerve VIII).
  ix. Important interpeak intervals may occur in metabolic derangements: B_{12} deficiency, meningitis, epilepsy, alcoholism, diabetes mellitus; diabetes mellitus, and meningitis have findings consistent with damage to acoustic nerve.
   x. *Neurologic disorders that cause important transient BAERs:*
   (A) *Intramedullary brain stem tumors*
      (1) Wave I: usually preserved because acoustic nerve usually not involved
      (2) Increased interpeak latency (IPL) I–III if pontomedullary
      (3) Increased IPL III–V if pontomesencephalic or midbrain
   (B) *Cerebellopontine angle tumors*
      (1) Absence, increased latency, or increased duration of wave I, and subsequent waves are either distorted or absent but may be present and delayed.
      (2) IPL I–III is often prolonged (if waves I and III are preserved), which is a sensitive indicator for cerebellopontine angle tumors.
   (C) *MS:* no particular BAER impairment is specific for MS

xi. General interpretation of BAERs:
  (A) Absent IL with CL normal: severe unilateral hearing loss due to unilateral cochlear or acoustic nerve lesion
  (B) Absent bilaterally: bilateral acoustic nerve lesions, brain death, rule out technical problems
  (C) Absent wave I with normal III and V: peripheral hearing disorder with normal central conduction
  (D) Absent peaks after normal wave I: IL proximal acoustic nerve, IL pontomedullary lesion
  (E) Absent wave III with normal I and V: normal variant
  (F) Absent wave V with normal I and III: IL lesion of brain stem (i.e., caudal pons)
  (G) Low amplitude or prolonged latency of entire BAER bilaterally: peripheral hearing loss (especially conductive), distal acoustic nerve lesion, rule out reduced stimulus intensity, in distal acoustic nerve lesions, there may be prolonged latencies of entire BAERs but will have normal IPL I–V.
  (H) Prolonged wave I latency and of all subsequent waves but normal IPL III–V: lesion of distal acoustic nerve, peripheral hearing loss
  (I) Prolonged I–V IPL: most sensitive indicator of brain stem lesion
  (J) Increased I–III IPL (but normal III–V): defect from between proximal acoustic nerve to inferior pons; most common impairment with acoustic neuromas
  (K) Prolonged III–V IPL but normal I–III latencies: if only impaired, suggests lesion at or after the superior olivary complex in caudal pons or midbrain
  (L) Increased I–III and III–V IPLs: IL lesion of lower and upper brain stem
  (M) Increased BAERs threshold: suspect peripheral hearing loss; distal acoustic nerve lesion
  (N) Parallel upward shift of latency-intensity curve: conductive hearing loss
  (O) Shift of latency-intensity curves upward especially at low frequencies: sensorineural hearing loss
xii. *Intraoperative BAERs monitoring:*
  (A) During surgery in posterior and middle fossa.
  (B) Useful for acoustic nerve and brain stem surgery because BAERs are not affected by ordinary anesthetics (i.e., halothane, thiopental; the exceptions are enflurane and imipramine overdose, which increase IPLs).
  (C) During acoustic neuroma surgery, the most common changes are loss of waves II–V or increased I–III IPL.
  (D) Good but not perfect relation between deterioration of intraoperative BAERs and subsequent postoperative hearing deficits.
xiii. *Coma:*
  (A) May help differentiate coma due to structural vs. metabolic factors (because metabolic/toxic processes usually do not cause important BAERs unless it inflicts irreversible structural damage).
  (B) Body temperature <32°C may alter BAERs.
xiv. *Conditions that may have normal BAERs:* supratentorial lesions, spinocerebellar degeneration, Huntington's chorea, vestibular neuronitis, Meniere's disease, labyrinthitis
xv. *BAERs in infants and children:*
  (A) All high-risk newborns (<1,500 g and infants in neonatal intensive care unit) should have BAERs within 1st month.

(B) If normal, nearly 100% will have normal hearing; if impaired, initiate rehabilitation but be cautious because a small percentage will have significant hearing loss.

xvi. *BAERs and audiometry:*

(A) Wave V is plotted vs. stimulus intensities of 20, 40, 60, and 80 dB greater than hearing threshold, producing a semilog plot with an inverse linear relationship between intensity and latency in normal adults ($\uparrow$ stimulus $\rightarrow$ $\uparrow$ latency).

(B) Effect of hearing loss on threshold and latency:
   (1) Hearing loss increases threshold of BAERs, specifically that of wave V if the loss involves the frequencies 1–4 kHz through which click stimuli exert their effect.
   (2) Increases of threshold <30 dB above normal hearing threshold cannot be taken as important hearing.
   (3) Increases latency of wave V.

(C) Conductive hearing loss:
   (1) Prolongs latency for all intensities producing an upward shift of the curve but no change in slope.
   (2) Interferes with the conduction of sound waves from the ear canal to the cochlea; therefore, acts like a reduction of stimulus intensity that produces a lower amplitude and longer latency of all waves of the BAERs.
   (3) At low stimulus intensities, the latency of wave I is more increased than that of other waves in conductive hearing loss, so that IPL I–III and I–V are shortened.
   (4) Does not apply to conductive hearing loss caused by ossicular chain disorders.
   (5) Impedance audiometry is just as effective as BAERs in assessment of conductive hearing loss.
   (6) Latency-intensity curve:
      (a) Increases the latency of wave V over the range of all intensities, and therefore causes a parallel shift in the curve equivalent to the amount of hearing loss.
      (b) The possibility of a central defect must be ruled out by determining that the I–V IPL is normal.

(D) Sensorineural hearing loss:
   (1) Produces a curve with two slopes; at low intensity, there is decreased responsiveness of end-organs so that for any given intensity $\rightarrow$ the latency is prolonged; with increased intensity, there is greater than normal recruitment of nerves, so that the curve is steeper; at exceedingly high intensities, there has been sufficient recruitment such that the latency may be normal with the remainder of the slope parallel to the slope of a normal patient (although usually shifted upward).
   (2) BAER amplitude is reduced (at least at moderate stimulus intensities).
   (3) Amplitude ratio V to I is usually increased.
   (4) Latency of wave V is increased (in keeping with the degree of hearing loss at 4 kHz).
   (5) Wave I (if visible) is at least equally increased in latency, causing a normal or importantly short IPL I–V.
   (6) Latency-intensity curve:
      (a) Greatest deviation from normal latency and amplitude at low stimulus intensities (the more the stimulus strength exceeds threshold, the

less disparity between the normal and important curve; at high intensities, the latency may be normal, which causes the characteristic steepening of the latency-intensity curve becoming L-shaped).

3. *Middle latency AEPs*
   a. Occur 12–50 milliseconds after stimulation.
   b. Middle-latency AEPs uncontaminated by muscle potentials (older theory discusses myogenic etiology as source) probably include components of Heschl's gyrus, thalamocortical projections, posterior temporal gyrus, angular gyrus, and the insula and claustrum.
   c. Lesions of the thalamus or midbrain are more likely to affect the middle latency AEPs.

4. Late AEPs
   a. >50 milliseconds postauditory stimulation.
   b. Subdivided into exogenous components N1, P1, and P2 that are primarily dependent on the external stimulus, and into endogenous components P300, N400, CNV, and the mismatch negativity (which are more dependent on internal cognitive processes).
   c. Exogenous late AEPs are best elicited by tone bursts and have the highest amplitude over the vertex; N100 may be generated in a posterior-superior temporal plane and adjacent parietal cortex, whereas the later waves may arise from the auditory cortex and frontal association cortex.
   d. N400 is a potential obtained to linguistic stimuli when there is semantic incongruity.

B. **Somatosensory EPs (SSEPs)**
   1. *Stimulation parameters*
      a. Unilateral stimulation of a motor/sensory nerve trunk sufficient to produce a moderate motor response is required.
      b. Duration: stimulus artifact is reduced by shorter duration (approximately 100 microseconds); no more than 500 microseconds.
      c. Rate: between 1 and 10 per second (faster than 10 per second is highly painful) and results in low-amplitude somatosensory response; faster rates prolong all absolute and interpeak latencies and suppress cortical amplitudes by 20–30% but produce little or no difference on subcortically generated potentials; thus, in short-latency (SSEPs) and AEPs, there is a direct relationship between rate and latency and an inverse relation between rate and amplitude.
      d. Stimulators: either constant voltage or constant current.
   2. *Recording:* important aspect of recording EPs: replication of waveforms
   3. *Generators*
      a. Overview of stimulus and waveform patterns
         i. Near-field: cortically generated N20 is a near-field response with maximum voltage between the CL central and parietal electrodes on the scalp.
         ii. Far-field: in contrast, far-field component is generated by subcortical structures that reach the scalp relatively rapidly via conduction by fluid (i.e., cerebrospinal fluid) mediums (and not via neural paths); typically smaller (microvolts), and faster in frequency and latencies; topographic nonspecificity at scalp.
      b. Most events of SSEPs are from dorsal column–lemniscal system (cuneate neurons not only project to CL thalamus, but also to other brain stem structures, including dorsal and medial accessory olives, portions of the inferior and superior colliculi, thalamic nuclei not in the specific projection system, etc.).
   4. *General clinical interpretation*
      a. *The undiagnosed patient:* owing to the nonspecific nature of SSEPs, they make little clinical relevance to the already diagnosed patient, but, in the undiagnosed patient, may have substantial benefit

b. **MS**

    i. *In patients with clinically definite MS, at least one of the EPs is positive in >75–90%; thus, if all EPs are normal, diagnosis of MS should be questioned.*

    ii. *33–50% of SSEPs find clinically silent lesions.*

    iii. *Diagnostic yield: visual EPs (VEPs) > SSEPs > BAERs.*

    iv. Magnetic resonance imaging (MRI) tends to be more sensitive than trimodality EP testing for evaluation of MS.

c. **Peripheral nerve disorders**

    i. SSEPs are absent with severe peripheral nerve disease or lesion

    ii. May be useful notably to evaluate proximal nerve pathology (i.e., GBS)

5. *Median nerve SSEPs*

a. *Median nerve response components*

    i. *Obligate waveforms*

        (A) *Erb's point potential (EP; P9)*

            (1) Near-field triphasic (positive-negative-positive) potential; the prominent negative peak usually occurs at 9 milliseconds (P9) after stimulation at the wrist.

            (2) Orthodromic sensory and antidromic motor APs ascending from peripheral nerve stimulation generate EP.

            (3) The recording derivation includes negative input potential over the brachial plexus at Erb's point (2 cm superior to the clavicular head of the

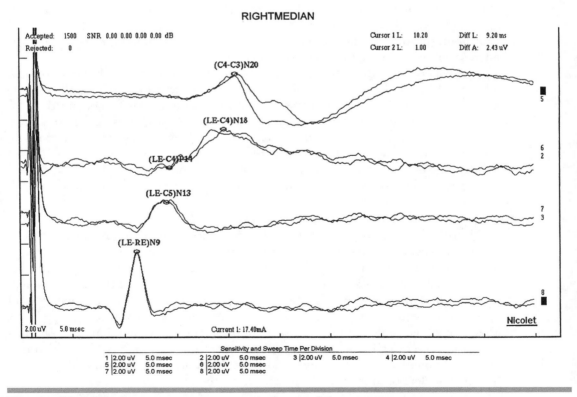

Figure 10-4. Median somatosensory-evoked potential.

sternocleidomastoid), and the positive input reference electrode is placed over the CL Erb's point or shoulder.
- (B) *N13*
  - (1) Near-field negative potential recorded over the dorsum of the neck (usually at 13 milliseconds after stimulation).
  - (2) Can be recorded referentially to any distal point, with Erb's point being a good location because it provides in-phase cancellation of a superimposed slow potential seen at the neck and Erb's point.
  - (3) Origin is dorsal horn neurons.
- (C) *P14*
  - (1) A far-field positive peak present broadly over the scalp (approximately 14 milliseconds after stimulation).
  - (2) Subcortically generated and probably reflects activity in the caudal medial lemniscus (brain stem).
  - (3) In-phase cancellation if recorded scalp-to-scalp, and, therefore, should be referenced to Erb's point or torso.
- (D) *N18*
  - (1) Far-field relatively slow potential present broadly over the scalp.
  - (2) Subcortically generated probably from postsynaptic activity from multiple brain stem generators.
  - (3) Inhalation anesthetics have little effect on N18 (as compared to N20).
- (E) *N20*
  - (1) Near-field negative peak
  - (2) Generated by the primary cortical somatosensory receiving area
  - (3) When recorded referentially, the N20 is preceded by the far-field P9, P11, and P14 and is superimposed on the coincidental N18
  - (4) Origin from thalamocortical radiations
- (F) *Late potentials*
  - (1) Include P25, N30, P45.
  - (2) Largely state dependent.
  - (3) Typically, these are unsuitable for neuronal evaluation.
  - (4) Generators of these are believed to be associated with cortical association areas.

ii. *Median nerve SSEP interpeak latencies*
- (A) EP-N20, EP-P14, P14-N20, and spinal lumbar potential (LP)-P37 (tibial SSEPs).
- (B) Much more reliable than absolute latencies.
- (C) Eliminate most of the peripheral effects, as described earlier.
- (D) Not appreciably affected by age/gender in the adult population, but SSEPs of newborns differ substantially from adults owing to immaturity of myelination of the peripheral nervous system and CNS.
  - (1) In term neonates, median SSEPs reliably show subcortical potentials but do not demonstrate cortical response (N20) in more than one-third of neonates.
  - (2) Cortical response (N20) is not reliably seen until 2–3 months old.

b. *Clinical interpretation*

N9	N13	P14	N20	N9-P14 interval	P14-N20 interval	Clinical interpretation
Normal	—	Normal	Normal	Normal	Normal	Normal; amyotrophic lateral sclerosis; anterior spinal artery syndrome because posterior columns spared; usually normal in cervical radiculopathy but may have delay at N9 and N13; Charcot-Marie-Tooth
↑	—	↑	↑	Normal but may ↑	Normal	Lesion of somatosensory nerves at or distal to brachial plexus (peripheral neuropathy); hypothermia and chronic renal failure should also be considered, particularly if delay noted in all SSEPs
Normal	—	↑	↑	↑	Normal	Lesion between Erb's point and lower medulla
Normal	—	Normal	↑	Normal	↑	Lesion between lower medulla and cortex
Normal	—	—	Ab or ↑	—	—	Brain death; persistent vegetative state; perinatal asphyxia; hemispherectomy; Minamata disease; parasagittal parietal lesion; thalamic lesion
Ab	—	Ab	Ab	N/A	N/A	Peripheral nerve lesion; rule out technical problem
Ab	—	Normal	Normal	N/I	Normal	Normal
↑	—	↑	↑	↑	Normal	Peripheral nerve lesion
—	↑	—	—	↑	Normal	Brachial plexus lesion
Normal	Ab or ↑	—	↑	—	↑	Cervical cord lesion; cervical spondylitic myelopathy; subacute combined degeneration due to B$_{12}$ deficiency; syringomyelia/hydromyelia; tumor
—	—	—	—	—	↑	Hepatic encephalopathy
—	Ab or ↑	—	—	—	Ab or ↑	Leukodystrophies
Normal	Normal	↑	↑	↑	↑	MS

↑ = increased; Ab = absent; N/A = not applicable; N/I = noninterpretable.

c. **Brachial plexopathy**
   i. Criteria for impairment are decreases of 40% or more in amplitude of N13 or Erb's point potential responses.
   ii. If the N13 were absent or reduced to a greater extent than Erb's point potential, then the lesion is more likely preganglionic.
   iii. If the EP response was reduced to an equal or greater degree than N13, then the lesion is more likely postganglionic.
d. **Radiculopathy/spondylosis/myelopathy**
   i. *Radiculopathy without myelopathy:* SSEPs are of little clinical benefit.
   ii. *Myelopathy due to cervical spondylosis.*
      (A) Usually seen and are attenuated or absent N13 and N20, a prolonged EP-N13 interval
      (B) Usually little clinical benefit
   iii. An increase in the clavicular-cervical (N9-N13) and the clavicular-scalp (N9-N20) conduction time combined with normal NCVs → is a reliable indicator of root involvement *or cord involvement below the medulla.*
   iv. *Cervical root lesions* are characterized by preservation of the clavicular EP and of SNAPs (unless there is additional involvement of the brachial plexus).

NB: Preganglionic lesions show normal SNAPs because of the integrity of the dorsal root ganglion.

   v. *Postganglionic (but not preganglionic) root damage* is followed by retrograde degeneration of sensory nerve fibers and eventual disappearance of SNAPs.
   vi. Cervical and scalp SSEPs are absent in complete avulsions of the nerve root and delayed or reduced in incomplete lesions (e.g., spondylitic radiculopathy).
6. *Ulnar nerve SSEPs:* similar to median nerve SSEPs except stimulation of distal ulnar nerve just above wrist
7. *Tibial nerve SSEPs*
   a. Most normative data are for ankle stimulation.
   b. Responses to femoral stimulation are approximately 20 milliseconds earlier, and popliteal are approximately 10 milliseconds earlier (than ankle stimulation); thus, the tibial P37 is similar to the common peroneal P27 and the femoral P17.
   c. Tibial nerve supplies the gastrocnemius and soleus muscles of the leg, as well as the small intrinsic muscles of the foot.
   d. The proximal stimulus electrode (cathode) is placed at the ankle between the medial malleolus and the Achilles' tendon, and the anode is placed 3 cm distal to the cathode.
   e. Stimulus produces a small amount of plantar flexion of the toes.
      i. Afferent nerve volley in the PF
      ii. LP: potential recorded over lumbar spine
   f. Obligate waveforms:
      i. PF potential
         (A) Traveling potential recorded over the midline of the PF.
         (B) Near-field potential.
         (C) Triphasic with positive-negative-positive waveform; the negative predominates.
         (D) When spinal, cortical, and subcortical responses are absent, it is important to demonstrate this potential to assess preservation of peripheral nerve.
      ii. LP
         (A) Recorded referentially over the broad spinal areas but with highest amplitude at approximately T12 level

LEFT TIBIAL

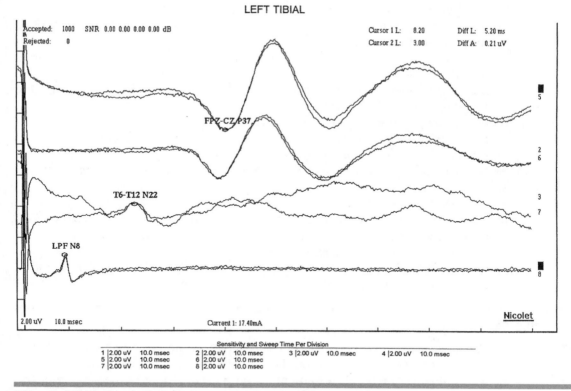

Figure 10-5. Tibial somatosensory-evoked potentials.

    (B) Reflect primarily positive synaptic activity in the lumbar cord with possible origin being dorsal roots and entry zone

  iii. N34

    (A) Subcortically generated far-field potential.

    (B) Distribution is broad and can be recorded from several scalp electrode sites.

    (C) N34 is recorded in isolation referentially from the Fpz electrode and is thought to be analogous to N18 after median nerve stimulation.

    (D) Likely represents postsynaptic activity from multiple generator sources in the brain stem.

    (E) N34 is preceded by a small P31 (probably analogous to P14 of median nerve SSEPs).

    (F) Typically not used for clinical assessment.

  iv. P37

    (A) Represents primary somatosensory cortex

    (B) Paradoxical lateralization: P37 is maximal at midline and centroparietal scalp IL to the stimulated leg

    (C) Major positive wave in the CPi and CPz-Fpz derivations

 g. *Clinical interpretation*

PF	LP	P37	LP-P37 Interval	Clinical interpretation
Ab	Ab	Ab	N/I	Peripheral nerve lesion
				Rule out technical problem

PF	LP	P37	LP-P37 Interval	Clinical interpretation
↑	↑	↑	Normal	Peripheral nerve lesion
				Possibly cauda equina
				Inaccurate measurement
				Hypothermia
Normal	Normal	↑	↑	Between cauda equina and brain (note: if median SSEPs are normal, this may help localize lesion to spinal cord below the midcervical cord)
↑	↑	↑	↑	Suggests two lesions involving both peripheral nerve and central conduction, or may have single lesion of cauda equina
Normal	Normal	Ab	N/I	Suspected defect above the cauda equina and at or below the somatosensory cortex

↑ = increased; Ab = absent; N/A = not applicable; N/I = noninterpretable.

8. *Surgical monitoring using SSEPs*
   a. Loss of median SSEP during surgery is highly predictive of subsequent neurologic deficit.
   b. Anesthetics, such as enflurane, halothane, and isoflurane, may cause a reduction in the amplitude of cortical SSEP (N20); nitrous oxide has little effect.
   c. Subcortical potentials are affected to a lesser extent.
C. **VEPs**
   1. Anatomy
      a. Retinal function

Properties of Rods and Cones

	Rods	Cones
Operating conditions	Dim (scotopic)	Daylight (photopic)
Visual acuity	Low	High
Sensitivity	High	Low
Pathway	Convergent	Direct
Spatial resolution	Poor	Good
Temporal resolution	Poor	Good
Rate of dark adaption	Slow	Fast
Color vision	Absent	Present

   i. Presume normal optic function to assess retinal function (i.e., cataract alters optic function).

    ii. The opening in the iris diaphragm, the pupil, determines the amount of light reaching photoreceptors.

    iii. Retina has five layers: outer nuclear layer (contains cell bodies of the photoreceptors); outer synaptic layer (aka outer plexiform layer); inner nuclear layer (contains cell bodies of horizontal, amacrine, and bipolar neurons and the cell bodies of the glial cells of Müller); inner synaptic layer; and the ganglion cell layer.

    iv. Visual pigment.

      (A) Rhodopsin: visual pigment for the rods

      (B) Iodopsin: visual pigment for the cones

    v. Three subtypes of cones that are sensitive to a particular wavelength of blue, red, or green.

    vi. Ganglion cells: three types → (1) Y cells: produce bursts of spikes (APs) in response to stimuli placed in their receptive field and have high conduction velocity and fire preferentially to edge movement; (2) X cells: fire continually in response to visual stimuli and have a small receptive field and are slow conducting and provide fine spatial discrimination; and (3) W cells: very slow conducting and are either excited or inhibited by contrast.

  b. *Function of anterior visual pathways*

    i. Optic nerve: approximately 50 mm long and comprises nerve fibers originating in the ganglion cells; optic nerve fibers are small, myelinated fibers (92% are <2 μμ in diameter).

    ii. Nasal fibers cross to CL cortex and temporal fibers remain IL.

    iii. The functional integrity of the visual pathway, once they enter the optic nerve, can be measured by VEPs recorded from the occipital region; it is presumed these are near-field potentials from the visual cortices.

    iv. It has been determined that full-field stimulation with patterned stimuli is best suited to evaluate anterior pathway function.

  c. Anatomy and function of retrochiasmal pathways

    i. From lateral geniculate nucleus, *all* fibers pass to area 17 and then area 18 and 19.

    ii. Positron emission tomography combined with magnetic resonance imaging has demonstrated that visual stimulation not only activates areas 17, 18, and 19, but also the lateral temporal cortex.

2. *VEP procedure*

  a. *Pattern-reversal stimulus*

    i. Several parameters influence the response, including

      (A) Size of checks: affects amplitude and latency of VEP; size is measured in minutes of visual field arc with 60 minutes (60′) per degree arc; max response between 15′–60′; smaller check causes increased latency and reduced amplitude; fovea stimulated better by small checks and the periphery better by large checks; therefore, the recommended size is 28′–32′

      (B) Size of the visual field stimulated: should be at least 8 degrees of the visual field arc (because approximately 80% of the response is generated by the central 8 degrees of vision)

      (C) Frequency of pattern reversal

      (D) Luminance: low luminance causes increased latency in P100 and decreased amplitude; pupillary diameter also affects retinal illuminance

      (E) Contrast between background and foreground: contrast between light and dark squares must be >50% (usually are much larger in routine studies); low contrast may cause increased latency and decreased amplitude P100

   (F) Fixation: helpful but not essential for reproducible responses; intentionally poor fixation does not affect P100 in most patients but can cause decreased amplitude that may be sufficient to make P100 not identifiable
  b. *VEP normative data*
     i. *Two most frequent are N70 (negative wave occurring 70 milliseconds after stimulation) and P100 (positive wave at approximately 100 milliseconds ± 10 milliseconds); often a positive wave P50 (at 50 milliseconds) precedes N70.*

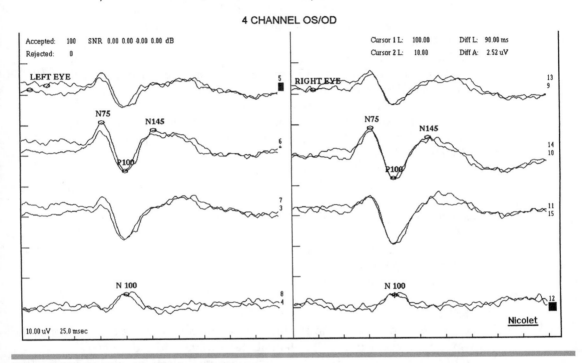

Figure 10-6. Visual-evoked potentials.

     ii. N70 and P100 change with age, and delay is most evident after 45 y/o (likely to ↓ conduction velocities due to defective myelin regeneration or axonal dystrophy, corpora malacia in optic nerve and chiasm, degeneration of retinal ganglion cells, changes in NT function and increased synaptic delay, and/or neuronal loss in the lateral geniculate nucleus or striatal cortex).
     iii. Absolute latency of the P100 is important if >117 milliseconds.
     iv. Gender affects latency: women with slightly shorter latency, which may be related to smaller brain size and therefore shorter pathways in women.
     v. P100 also affected by: luminance, stimulus field size, acuity, level of alertness.
     vi. Pupillary diameter also affects latency with evidence that small pupils cause delayed latency owing to decreased retinal illuminance; it is estimated that P100 latency increases by 10–15 milliseconds per log unit of decreased retinal illuminance.
  3. *Clinical applications*
    a. *General conditions*
       i. *Optic neuritis: in optic neuritis, absent or significantly reduced electroretinograms (ERGs) suggest poor prognosis, likely due to progressive development of optic nerve atrophy.*
       ii. *Papillitis*

     iii. *Ischemic optic neuropathy*
     iv. *Toxic and metabolic optic neuropathy*
      v. *Optic nerve compression*
     vi. *Optic atrophy*
    vii. *Early macular disease*
       (A) Funduscopic examination appears normal and, therefore, concurrent use of ERG and VEPs helps to elucidate presence of macular component.
         (1) If demyelinating → pattern ERG (P-ERG) is normal
         (2) If maculopathy → ERG is delayed or severely depressed
  b. *Specific disease processes*
      i. Simultaneous P-ERG and VEPs *in patients with MS detect three abnormalities*
       (A) Normal ERG/delayed VEP/prolonged retinocortical transient time (RCT) (indicate demyelination).
       (B) Normal P-ERG and absent VEP indicate complete block of optic nerve.
       (C) Absent P-ERGs and VEPs, impaired ERGs, and delayed VEPs suggest severe axonal damage with retrograde ganglion cell degeneration.
     ii. *VEPs in cortical blindness*
       (A) Surprisingly, VEPs present in most cases.
       (B) Responses to small checks or gratings may be important but larger often remain constant.
    iii. *Bilateral P100 impairment: bilateral disease of posterior visual pathways*
       (A) Bilateral cataracts
       (B) Bilateral optic nerve disease
       (C) Binocular pathology
    iv. *Reduced P100 on one side is most likely owing to ↓visual acuity*
4. *ERGs*
  a. Flash ERGs
      i. The flash ERG represents the algebraic summation of four basic components: the a wave, a direct current (DC) potential, the b wave, and the c wave.
     ii. The ERG to flashes consists of negative-positive deflections labeled a wave (the photoreceptor potential), b wave, and c wave.
    iii. a Wave: negative; results from rising phase of photoreceptor potential.
    iv. b Wave: large positive wave; originates in Müller's cells and is related to K^+-mediated current flow; reflects the activity of depolarizing bipolar cells.
     v. DC potential: unknown origin.
    vi. c Wave: originates in pigmented epithelium.
    vii. ERG morphology varies in relation to light and dark, and, therefore, ERG can differentiate between rod and cone systems.
   viii. Rods can only detect stimuli at <20 Hz, and background light >8 Lambert can eliminate rod response.
    ix. *Useful in diagnosis of retinal pigmentary degeneration (i.e., retinitis pigmentosa that primarily affects the rods early with impaired night vision [nyctalopia], and normally in advanced stages are cones affected).*
     x. *Congenital nyctalopia:* nonprogressive autosomal dominant disorder characterized by abnormal night vision and normal day vision and normal fundi; ERG → normal cone function but abnormal rod function with absent or severe reduction of b wave in dark adapted studies.
    xi. *Oguchi's disease:* night blindness; ERG 26 low amplitude or absent dark responses of b wave with diffuse graying of fundus.

xii. *Congenital achromatopsia:* normal dark response but no cone oscillations to red flashes and no light-adapted responses (mediated by cones).
  b. P-ERG
    i. Predominantly a foveal response that originates in the proximal retina.
    ii. Dependent on the integrity of the ganglion cells with contribution from amacrine cells.
    iii. P-ERGs to transient stimuli consist of a negative a wave followed by positive b wave.
    iv. May be used to assess RCT, which, when P-ERG is performed with VEPs, allows assessment of activity outside the retina in the visual pathway; two RCTs have been recorded → RCT (b-N70) and RCT (b-P100).
    v. Delayed P-ERGs occur only in macular diseases: absent or markedly depressed P-ERG in either maculopathies or severe optic nerve disease associated with axonal involvement and retrograde retinal ganglion cell degeneration.

IV. Polysomnography (PSG)
A. **Recording**
  1. To visually stage sleep adequately, the basic monitoring must be at least
    a. IL central and occipital referential (usually to an earlobe or mastoid) EEG linkages
    b. An oculogram for REM
    c. Submental EMG for axial muscle tone
  2. May also place additional EEG electrodes, superficial EMG of upper and lower extremities for evaluation of restless legs syndrome, intercostal EMG for respiratory status, upper airway exchange (thermistors or thermocouplers), monitors of important chest or abdominal patterns, arterial blood gases or O_2 saturation, EKG, and nocturnal penile tumescence
  3. *Standard PSG recording parameters*

Parameter	Sensitivity (µV)	LFF (Hz)	HFF (Hz)
EEG	5–7	0.3	70
Electro-oculography (EOG)	5–7	0.3	70
EMG	2	10	100
EKG	50	0.3	70
Air-flow with effort	Variable	0.15	0.5
Oximetry	50	DC	15

B. *EEG monitoring*
  1. Colloid provides better contact for long-term monitoring.
  2. Resistance should be kept <5,000 Ω.
  3. Basic 10–20 international electrode placement.
  4. Only C3 and C4 are used to record sleep in adults (with referential to IL ear); in infants, O1 and O2 are frequently added.
  5. A single central channel (either C3-A1 or C4-A2) is necessary to stage sleep, but six or more channels are recommended, including a combo of any of the following electrodes (FP1, FP2, C3, C4, O1, O2, T3, T4); O1 and O2 provide analysis of prominent waking rhythms, whereas central channels are best for V waves, spindles, and/or K complexes.

6. Electrodes to measure eye movement (EOG) are placed at the outer canthus of both eyes; there is a small electrical dipole of the eye with the cornea positive in relation to the retina.
7. EMG from chin also recorded.
8. Standard paper speed is 10 seconds with 30-second epochs, which results in compression of cerebral activity.

C. *EOG*
1. Commonly recommended to have referential electrode recording from the lateral canthus to the IL ear (provides out-of-phase recording for horizontal eye movements); disadvantage is marked artifact, especially slow-wave sleep (SWS) when the EEG reaches max amplitude; this also applies to the referential supra- and infraorbital electrodes for evaluation of vertical eye movements.
2. REMs usually last approximately 50–200 milliseconds and have a frequency of >1 Hz.
3. Slow rolling eye movements usually have a frequency between 0.25 and 0.50 Hz, with the duration of the sharpest slope >0.5 seconds.

D. *EMG monitoring*
1. Placed submentally on the skin over the mylohyoid muscle, and second electrode is usually placed 3 cm posterior and lateral (in case first electrode is defective).
2. Tonic EMG activity usually decreases from stage 1–4 NREM sleep and is absent in REM.
3. Limb EMG is used to evaluate periodic leg movements of sleep (PLMS)/restless legs syndrome, and electrodes are placed over the anterior tibialis muscle (identified by having the patient dorsiflex against resistance); a bipolar derivation is obtained by recording from one electrode on each leg.
4. Intercostal EMG may assist in respiratory monitoring.

E. *Respiratory monitoring*
1. Useful in determining between central, obstructive, and mixed apnea (see Chapter 9: Sleep and Sleep Disorders, section VI for details).
2. By definition, an apnea is a lack of upper airway exchange that must last >10 seconds with >4% oxygen desaturation.
3. All measures of upper airway airflow and of chest/abdominal movement use a bandpass of DC to 0.5 Hz.
4. Recordings of oxygen saturation, oxygen tension, and systemic pulmonary artery or other pressure requires DC recording.
5. *Upper airway breathing:*
   a. *Thermistor*
      i. Thermistor resistor fluctuations are induced by temperature changes in air passing in and out of the mouth/nostrils.
      ii. Useful only for evaluation of respiratory rate.
   b. *Thermocouple*
      i. Thermoelectric generators constructed of dissimilar metals (e.g., constantan and copper)
      ii. Generate a potential in response to temperature change
      iii. Usually, two thermocouplers are attached to the nostrils
   c. *Capnography:* uses carbon dioxide monitor to document CO_2 retention
   d. *Pneumotachography*
      i. Only technique that allows direct quantification of ventilation during sleep
      ii. Can measure flow rate, tidal volume, and other respiratory variables
      iii. Disadvantage: uses uncomfortable airtight mask and, therefore, rarely used

6. *Thoracoabdominal movement:*
   a. *Strain gauge*
      i. Most consist of a silicone tube filled with a conductor (e.g., mercury or packed graphite), the resistance of which varies with core diameter
      ii. Inspiration: stretches tube → decreases the core diameter → increases resistance (vice versa for expiration)
      iii. Piezoelectric crystals of quartz or sapphire strain gauges: distortion by inspiration or expiration creates a current; these are more sensitive to movement artifact
   b. *Inductive plethysmography*
      i. It is essentially an improved method of spirometry that separates chest and abdominal movement and adds them together, thus mimicking total spirometric volume.
      ii. Sensors are two wire coils (one placed around the chest and the other around the abdomen).
      iii. A change in mean cross-sectional coil area produces a proportional variation in coil conductance, which is converted into a voltage change by a variable frequency oscillator.
      iv. Three output channels: rib cage movement, abdominal movement, and total volume.
   c. *Impedance plethysmography:* rarely used method involving changes in impedance based on abdominal/chest movement
7. *Snoring monitors:*
   a. Snoring suggests reduced upper airway diameter and/or hypotonia
   b. Bursts of loud guttural inspiratory snorts after quiescent periods are characteristic of obstructive sleep apnea syndrome
8. *Arterial oxygen:* transcutaneous oxygen tension for measurement of desaturation with respiratory distress events.

F. **EKG**
1. Obstructive sleep apnea syndrome patients often may have sinus arrhythmias or extra-asystoles; may have more serious problems, such as prolonged asystole, atrial fibrillation, or ventricular fibrillation.

G. **Esophageal pH:** patients may have insomnia due to esophageal reflux from a hiatal hernia, etc.

H. **Penile tumescence**
1. Strain gauges are placed at the tip and base.
2. Buckling resistance (rigidity) is measured by a technician during the maximal penile circumference during an erection by applying a force gauge to the tip of the penis; force is gradually increased until the penis buckles (or a force of 1,000 g is reached); buckling pressure of >500 g is considered normal (because this has been determined to be the minimal force required to achieve penetration during intercourse).

I. **Technical parameters**
1. Must be performed under conditions conducive to natural sleep.
2. A nocturnal sleeper must be tested at night (note: a shift worker must be tested during the period of his/her longest sleep time); for a nocturnal sleeper, daytime testing is not acceptable because there is a circadian distribution of REM and SWS with REM sleep peaking between 3 a.m. and 6 a.m. and SWS peaking between 11 p.m. and 2 a.m.
3. Must avoid prior sleep deprivation (alters arousal threshold) and pharmacologic medications for sleep.

J. **Sleep staging**
1. Basic sleep staging

a. Most labs use the guidelines set by Rechtschaffen and Kales in 1968.
b. Usually done at a paper speed of 10 mm per second.
c. Sleep is divided into epochs of 60, 30, or 20 seconds; each epoch is scored as the stage that occupies >50% of the epoch.
d. Minimum of 6–8 recording hours is recommended.
e. Sleep architecture is commonly altered in patients undergoing initial PSG owing to unusual environment/conditions (1st night effect); findings associated with the 1st night effect include prolonged sleep latency and REM latency, reduction in sleep efficiency, increased unexplained arousals and awakenings, and reduced or absent stage 3/4 and REM sleep (often accompanied by an increase in stage 1 sleep).

2. *Sleep parameters and scoring*

Stage 1	May be subdivided into stages 1A (α rhythm diffuses to anterior head regions, often slows by 0.5–1.0 Hz, and then fragments before disappearing) and 1B (when EEG contains <20% diffuse slow α [>40 µV] and the EEG consists of medium amplitude mixed frequency [mostly θ] activity with occasional vertex waves); scored when >50% of epoch consists of relatively low voltage, mixed frequencies (mainly 2–7 Hz) with relative reduction in EMG activity; other features include slow rolling eye movements and vertex waves (vertex waves may persist into stage 2 and SWS; diphasic sharp transients having initial surface negativity followed by a low-voltage positive phase that is maximum at C3 and/or C4 and with phase reversal over the midline; present by 8 wks post-term)
Stage 2	Characterized by ≥1 sleep spindle, K complexes, and <20% of the epoch containing Δ; spindles are 11.5–15.0-Hz central bursts that must last >0.5 secs and have an amplitude >15 µV to be scored, and appear as rhythmic sinusoidal waves of progressively increasing amplitude followed by progressively decreasing amplitude; K complexes are diphasic waves that must contain two of three features (negative vertex sharp wave maximal over central regions, a following negative slow wave maximally frontal, and/or a sleep spindle maximal centrally); K complexes usually occur in trains either spontaneously or after a stimulus; K complexes may appear in infants as early as 5 mos old; may also have vertex waves (see Figure 10-7)
Stage 3	Scored when 20–30% of epoch contains Δ waves of 0.5–2.5 Hz and >75 µV; sleep spindles may be present but are less frequent than in stage 2 and of lower frequency (10–12 Hz)
Stage 4	Scored when >50% of epoch contains Δ of <2 Hz and amplitude >75 µV; spindles may be present but are rare (note: stages 3 and 4 are collectively also known as SWS; predominates in the first third of night) (see Figure 10-8)
REM	Contains medium amplitude mixed frequency (mainly θ and Δ), low voltage activity, associated with REM and relative absence of EMG; bursts of saw-toothed waves at 2–6 Hz may appear in frontal or midline regions (generally just before REM bursts); initial REM period may contain some low-voltage spindles, but generally sleep spindles and K complexes are absent; may also demonstrate α frequencies at rate 1–2 Hz slower than patient's waking background rhythm; also may have autonomic instability; although there is relative muscle atonia, bursts of phasic EMG activity may be noted in conjunction with REM; REM stage predominates in the last third of night (see Figure 10-9)
Sleep latency	Time from lights out to the first epoch of sleep (in minutes)

REM latency   Time from sleep onset to the first epoch of REM sleep (in minutes); significantly reduced in certain sleep disorders, sleep-deprivation, drug withdrawal; REM latency is usually 60–120 mins

Time in bed   Total time in bed; from time of lights out to lights on

Total sleep time   Total time from sleep onset to final awakening (note: some authors do not include stage 1 sleep)

Sleep efficiency   Percentage of time spent in bed asleep (i.e., total sleep time/time in bed)

Arousals   Defined as an abrupt shift in EEG frequency, including θ, α, and/or frequencies >16 Hz (but not spindles) that meet the following criteria: (1) at least 10 secs of sleep of any stage must precede an arousal and must be present between arousals; (2) at least 3 secs of EEG frequency shift must be present; (3) arousals in REM also necessitate a concurrent increase in chin EMG amplitude, because bursts of θ and α are found intrinsically during REM sleep; (4) arousals are not scored based on chin EMG alone; (5) artifacts, K complexes, and Δ are not scored as arousals unless accompanied by EEG frequency shift of >3 secs; (6) pen-blocking artifact is only considered an arousal when contiguous with an arousal pattern and then may be included toward the 3-sec duration criteria; (7) nonconcurrent but contiguous EEG and EMG changes that are <3 secs but together are >3 secs are not scored as arousals; (8) intrusion of α in NREM sleep is scored as arousal only if >3 secs in duration and preceded by >10 secs of α-free sleep; and (9) transitions between sleep stages are not scored as arousals unless they meet the above criteria; arousals are scored using EEG alone with the exception of REM sleep arousals that also require simultaneous increase in chin EMG amplitude

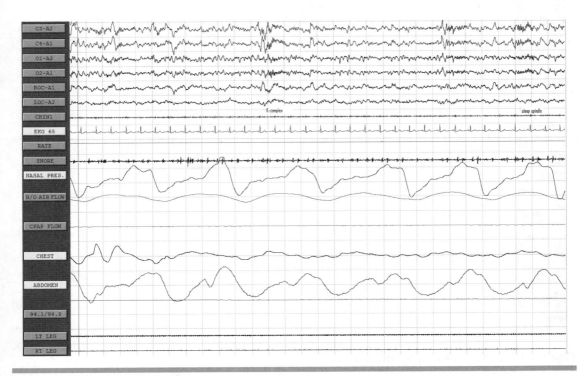

Figure 10-7. Stage 2 sleep.

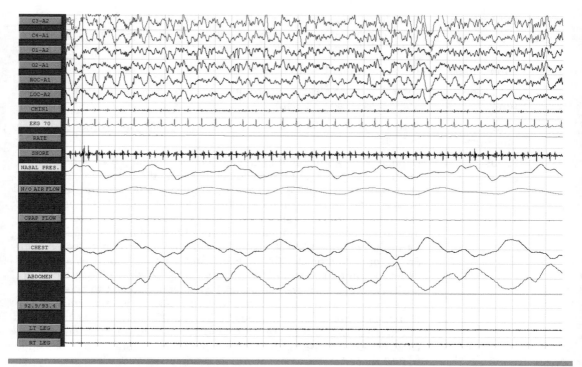

Figure 10-8. Stage 4 slow-wave sleep.

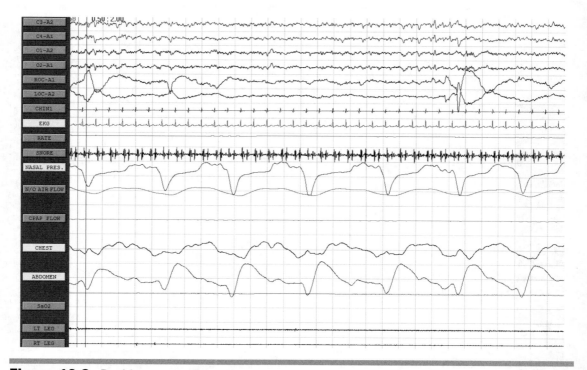

Figure 10-9. Rapid eye movement sleep.

3. *Sleep onset and sleep cycles*
   a. *Sleep onset*
      i. No definitive parameters signifying sleep onset
      ii. Three basic PSG assessments
         (A) EMG: gradual diminution but without discrete change
         (B) EOG: slow asynchronous rolling eye movement
         (C) EEG: change from normal background α to low-voltage mixed frequency pattern (stage 1 sleep), which usually occurs within seconds to minutes of rolling eye movements; patient, if aroused during stage 1 sleep, typically state they were awake, and, therefore, sleep onset recognized by EEG is taken at stage 2 (presence of K complexes and sleep spindles)
   b. *The 1st sleep cycle*
      i. Stage 1: in normal adults, the 1st sleep cycle begins with stage 1 NREM sleep lasting only a few minutes (1–7 minutes on average).
      ii. Stage 2: follows stage 1 and usually lasts 10–25 minutes; progressive increase in frequency of SWS is noted denoting evolution to stage 3.
      iii. Stage 3: SWS (20–50% of EEG) that usually persists normally a few minutes and evolves into stage 4.
      iv. Stage 4: SWS (>50% of EEG) with higher voltage; lasts 20–45 minutes during first cycle; if body movements occur, there is transient return to lighter sleep (stages 1 or 2); often there is transition from stage 4 to stage 2 sleep just before patient entering REM sleep.
      v. REM: transition from NREM to REM is not abrupt; REM sleep cannot be identified until the first REM; REM period during first cycle is short (between 2 and 6 minutes); REM sleep often ends with a brief body movement, and a new cycle begins.
      vi. The first NREM-REM cycle usually lasts approximately 70–100 minutes.
   c. *Later sleep cycles*
      i. The average length for later sleep cycles is 100–120 minutes; the last sleep cycle is usually the longest.
      ii. As the night progresses, REM sleep generally becomes longer; stages 3 and 4 occupy less time in the second cycle and may nearly disappear in later cycles, with stage 2 expanding to make up the majority of NREM sleep.
   d. *Dissociated or otherwise atypical sleep patterns*
      i. α-Δ Sleep
         (A) Characterized by presence of α and Δ waves in stages 3 and 4 SWS
         (B) May be induced in healthy individuals without awakening them by using auditory stimuli
         (C) Associated with a number of nonrestorative sleep disorders, especially fibromyalgia
      ii. *REM-spindle sleep*
         (A) Due to breakdown of barriers between NREM and REM sleep
         (B) May occur in up to 8% of normal patients
         (C) Increases in a number of sleep disorders, including increased frequency in the daytime sleep of hypersomniacs and nocturnal sleep of schizophrenics and narcoleptics
      iii. *REM sleep without atonia*
         (A) Common in patients taking tricyclic antidepressants, monoamine oxidase inhibitors, and phenothiazines
         (B) Disorders include REM behavior disorder

    iv. *REM burst during NREM sleep:* patients being treated with clomipramine (depression, narcolepsy), which is a medication that suppresses REM-based activity

    v. *Isolated REM atonia*

      (A) Cataplexy represents the selective triggering, during wakefulness and by emotional stimuli, of REM sleep atonia.

      (B) Sleep paralysis is the isolated appearance of REM sleep atonia associated with full wakefulness either before entry into REM sleep or during awakenings from REM sleep.

    vi. *Sleep-onset REM periods*

      (A) *Sleep-onset REM period is usually defined as entry into REM sleep within 10 minutes of sleep onset.*

      (B) *Presence is highly suggestive of diagnosis of narcolepsy-cataplexy* and characterizes approximately 50% of onsets of night sleep in these patients (but sleep deprivation, alcoholism, drug withdrawal, irregular sleep-waking habits, and/or severe depression must be ruled out).

4. *Respiratory parameters and scoring*

  a. Apneas and hypopneas represent decrements in airflow that may or may not be associated with arousals and/or oxygen desaturation.

  b. *Apnea: cessation or >90% reduction of nasal/oral airflow with >4% oxygen desaturation.*

  c. Brief central apneas that occur during transitional periods from wakefulness to sleep are believed to have no clinical significance.

  d. *Hypopnea:*

    i. *No consensus agreement of what constitutes a hypopnea*

    ii. *Defined as >50% reduction of airflow lasting >10 seconds and also reductions of airflow between 30% and 50%, which are associated with arousal or desaturation of at least 4%*

  e. Hypopneas and apneas have the same clinical significance as apneas (i.e., apneas and hypopneas are combined to give a total number divided by number of hours of sleep = apnea-hypopnea index or respiratory distress index.

5. *Leg movement (LM) parameters and scoring*

  a. LMs can be periodic (PLMS) or aperiodic/random (after arousals, respiratory events, snoring, etc.).

  b. An *LM* is defined as

    i. A burst of anterior tibialis muscle activity with a duration from onset to resolution of 0.5–5.0 seconds, and an amplitude of >25% of the bursts recorded during calibration.

    ii. Do not include hypnic jerks that occur on transition from wake to sleep, aperiodic activity during REM, phasic EMG during REM sleep, other forms of myoclonus, or restless legs.

  c. When scoring LMs, must document whether there are arousals, awakenings, or respiratory events; arousals attributed to LMs should occur no >3 seconds of termination of LM.

  d. PLMS:

    i. Characterized by rhythmic extension of the great toe and dorsiflexion of the ankle with occasional flexion of the knee and hip (similar to triple flexor response).

    ii. Lasting from 0.5–5.0 seconds.

    iii. Occur at intervals of 20–40 seconds.

    iv. Occur intermittently in clusters lasting minutes to hours throughout the night.

    v. Typically, the total number of LMs are reported with a breakdown of the number associated with arousals or awakenings and respiratory events.

vi. PLMS arousal index of >5 is important in middle-aged adults (but a cutoff of 10–15 should be used in elderly.

vii. If associated with arousals, patient may present with hypersomnia/excessive daytime sleepiness.

viii. Also commonly will have restless legs syndrome (may be associated with anemia due to folate or iron deficiency, renal failure, and a variety of neurologic disorders).

ix. A PLMS sequence or epoch is a sequence of four or more LMs separated by at least 5 seconds and not by >90 seconds (measured from LM onset to LM onset).

x. *PLMS are more abundant in stages 1 and 2 and less frequent in stages 3 and 4 and REM sleep.*

V. Multiple Sleep Latency Test (MSLT) and Maintenance of Wakefulness Test

A. *MSLT*

1. Use

   a. Developed by Carskadon and Dement (1977) and first tested on excessive daytime sleepiness patients by Richardson (1978)

   b. *Used to evaluate*

      i. *Excessive daytime sleepiness (by quantifying the time required to fall asleep)*

      ii. *REM latency (to evaluate specific disorders, e.g., narcolepsy, etc.)*

   c. Must perform urine toxicology screen for narcotics, psychotropics, stimulants, hypnotics, etc.

2. General procedures

   a. Standard montage using the Rechtschaffen and Kales (1968) guidelines

   b. Monitored for five 20-minute nap periods with 2 hours between each period; the first is standard set up for between 9:30 a.m. and 10:00 a.m.; first nap is performed at least 90 minutes after wake up time

   c. MSLT is usually performed on the night after PSG so that sleep disorders that might artifactually produce short daytime sleep latencies are ruled out (note: important nocturnal PSG will negate the usefulness of MSLT); patient must have at least 360 minutes of sleep on night before MSLT

   d. General considerations for MSLT

      i. 2 weeks of sleep diaries preceding MSLT

      ii. PSG on night before MSLT to evaluate habitual sleep and quantitate possible sleep-confounding deprivation before MSLT

      iii. Consideration of drug schedule (both prescribed and illicit drugs) with stable regimen for at least 2 weeks before testing (especially benzodiazepines, barbiturates, etc.)

      iv. Minimum of four tests at 2-hour intervals beginning 1.5–3.0 hours after waking

      v. Quiet, dark, controlled-temperature room

      vi. No alcohol or caffeine for at least 2 weeks before MSLT

3. Scoring

   a. *Sleep onset* is defined by any of the following parameters:

      i. The first three consecutive epochs of stage 1 NREM sleep

      ii. A single epoch of stage 2, 3, or 4 NREM sleep

      iii. REM sleep

   b. *Sleep offset* is defined as two consecutive epochs of wakefulness after sleep onset

   c. A nap is terminated after one of the following:

      i. No sleep has occurred after 20 minutes

    ii. After 10 minutes of continuous sleep as long as sleep criteria are met (if sleep onset is at 20 minutes, the sleep is allowed to continue until 30 minutes, etc.)

    iii. After 20 minutes or any point thereafter if the patient is awake

  d. Sleep latency is measured from the time of lights out to first sleep epoch; usually an average sleep latency of four or five naps is calculated

  e. REM latency: time of sleep onset to first epoch of REM sleep

4. Interpretation of MSLT

  a. *Normal sleep latency on MSLT*

Age	Sleep latency
Young adult (21–35 y/o)	10 mins
Middle-aged adult (30–49 y/o)	11–12 mins
Older adults (50–59 y/o)	9 mins

  b. *Decreased REM onset latencies during MSLTs can occur with:*

    i. *Sleep pathology (i.e., narcolepsy, severe obstructive sleep apnea, etc.)*

    ii. Sleep deprivation

  c. *MSLT interpretation of sleep onset latency*

Severity of sleepiness	Sleep latency on MSLT	Clinical correlation
Severe	<5 mins	Presence of pathologic or significant sleepiness; sleep episodes are present daily during times that require moderate attentiveness, such as eating, driving, etc., resulting in impairment of normal daily function
Moderate	5–10 mins	Excessively sleepy; sleep episodes occur daily during times that require moderate attentiveness, such as watching a movie/performance or attending a meeting
Mild	10–15 mins	Sleep episodes occur normally during times of relaxation, requiring little attentiveness, such as a passenger in a car or watching television

  d. 85% of narcoleptics have mean sleep latency of <5 minutes

  e. Patients with mild to moderate obstructive sleep apnea syndrome or sleep deprivation may have borderline sleep latency between 5 and 10 minutes

  f. Sleep latency may be affected by several factors, including:

    i. Sleep deprivation: causing a shortened sleep-onset latency

    ii. Sleep-wake schedule: must assess during patients' normal sleep schedule (e.g., shift worker)

    iii. Medications

    iv. Environment: if noisy, etc., may cause prolonged sleep latency

B. **Maintenance of wakefulness test**

1. An alternative to MSLT

2. Requires subject to sit in dark room with eyes closed reclining at a 45-degree angle

3. Required to attempt to stay awake for 20 minutes

4. Three to four testing periods every 2 hours

ADDITIONAL NOTES

Pediatric Neurology

CHAPTER 11

Pediatric Neurology

I. Development
A. Primitive reflexes

Reflex	Description	Appears (gestational age)	Disappears (age)
Moro	A triple response to sudden head movement: opening of palms, abduction of the arms, flexion of hips; cry	34 wks	3–4 mos
Tonic neck	When supine, turning of the head causes ipsilateral arm and leg extension and contralateral flexion (fencing position); normal infants can overcome after a few seconds	34 wks	6 mos
Crossed adductor	Knee jerk results in bilateral hip adduction	2–3 mos after birth	7–8 mos
Ankle clonus	Up to 8–10 beats; should not be sustained		2 mos
Babinski	Great toe dorsiflexion when lateral aspect of the foot is stroked	Birth	10–12 mos
Neck righting response	When supine, shoulders and trunk follow head turning	8–10 mos after birth	
Grasp reflex (hand)	Grasps objects with hand stimulation	32–34 wks	4–6 mos
Grasp reflex (foot)	Grasps objects with foot stimulation	32–34 wks	10 mos
Parachute	Horizontal dip results in arm extension, spreading of fingers (as if to break the fall)	6–7 mos after birth	Persists
Suck	Suck when finger or pacifier is placed in mouth	32–34 wks	4 mos

Reflex	Description	Appears (gestational age)	Disappears (age)
Landau reflex	With ventral suspension, head, trunk, and hips should extend, legs should flex at knees	*3 mos after birth*	*24 mos*
Placing reflex	When dorsal foot is brushed by bed/table, the knee should flex and foot lift as if to step	*35 wks*	*6 wks*

B. **Normal developmental milestones**

Age	Fine motor	Gross motor	Social/verbal
1 mo			Smiles
2 mos			Visual tracking to 180 degrees; coos
3 mos	Reaches for objects	Head control; chin up when prone; rolls over	Babbling and cooing
4 mos	Reaches with whole hand; holds and shakes rattle		Laughs out loud
5 mos		Will hold up head and straighten back with horizontal suspension	
6 mos	Transfers objects between hands	Sits with support; turns over	
8 mos	Thumb finger grasp	Sits unsupported	
9 mos	Transfers objects	Stands; creeps, crawls	Says "mama," "dada"
10 mos		Crawls; walks with support	
11 mos			Plays "peek-a-boo"
12 mos	Pincer grasp; tower of two cubes; handedness develops	Walks alone or holding hand/furniture	Two words (besides "mama," "dada")
15 mos		Should walk by self	Points to what is wanted
18 mos	Cube in box; builds tower of three blocks	Walks forward and back; stoops and recovers; climbs steps	Six words
2 yrs	Tower of eight cubes	Runs; climbs	Combines two to three words
2.5 yrs			Says name; asks questions; says "I"; points to body parts
3 yrs	Copies circle; knows left and right	Throws, catches, kicks ball; pedals tricycle; stands on one foot	Talks constantly; nursery rhymes; knows name; speaks in sentences; follows two commands

Age	Fine motor	Gross motor	Social/verbal
4 yrs	Copies square	Hops	Tells a story; uses syntax; writes name
5 yrs	Writes name	Skips	Begins to read
6 yrs			Reads and writes

C. **School and behavior: standardized tests**
   1. *Infants:* Denver Developmental, Bayley Scales, and Infant Development
   2. *Pre-school:* Gesell, Stanford-Binet, and Bender-Gestalt drawings
   3. *School age:* Wechsler Intelligence Scale (performance intelligence quotient [IQ] and verbal IQ should be within 10 points)
D. *Learning Disorders: achievement score is >20 points lower than IQ*
   1. **Attention deficit disorder:** onset is *before age 7 years; male > female;* duration is >6 months; problems occur in two or more settings; at least *three types of inattentions, three impulsivities, and two hyperactivities* must be present; treatment: behavior modification, methylphenidate, pemoline, imipramine, thioridazine
   2. **Autism:** onset is *before age 3 years; male to female ratio is 4:1;* without clear etiology; failure to develop normal language, lack of imagination, abnormal response to contact, repetitive behavior, and fear of change are key features; treatment: early intervention with behavior modification
   3. **Asperger's syndrome:** features are *flat affect, poor social skills, obsessiveness, fear of change, no clinically significant delays in language or cognition, seems odd and eccentric to other people, may have repetitive patterns*
   4. **Pervasive developmental disorder:** onset is *before age 30 months, with impaired social relationships, anxiety, fear of change, odd mannerisms and speech, and self-mutilation*
   5. *Hearing impairment: in older children results in inattention and poor school performance*
E. **Abnormal development**
   1. Cerebral palsy *(perinatal encephalopathy):* defined as a fixed, *nonprogressive* neurologic deficit of multiple etiologies; incidence: *2:1,000 births;* subtypes: *spastic diplegia* (scissoring legs, tight heel cords, seen in preemies and with hypoxia/ischemia/acidosis/sepsis), *spastic hemiplegia* (usually acquired after birth from trauma or vascular events and one-third have normal IQ), *extrapyramidal cerebral palsy* (basal ganglia lesion results in hypotonia, slow motor development, then chorea/dystonia; usually no mental retardation (MR) or seizures; may be from kernicterus; may occasionally have delayed progression; major seizures are common; those with motor seizures tend to have retardation and poor long-term prognosis; electroencephalography (EEG) may show hypsarrhythmia; psychomotor seizures are common

NB: The study with the highest yield in CP is an MRI. EEG should be obtained only with a history of seizure-like events.

   2. *Macrocephaly:* rapid growth can be normal *in preemies* or after *starvation;* causes include: *familial, gigantism, neurofibromatosis, storage diseases, subdural collections, hydrocephalus* (can be communicating or noncommunicating; congenital secondary to malformations or acquired form mass, meningitis, hemorrhage)
   3. *Microcephaly:* high correlation with MR; causes: genetic or migration problems, infection, vascular, toxic, or nutritional

F. **Genetic syndromes**
   1. **Fragile X syndrome:** site is in the terminal region of the long arm of chromosome X; DNA insertion size correlates with IQ; language, attention, and behavior problems (autistic features) occur; *long face, prominent chin, large ears; females with this have more avoidant and habitual behaviors;* one-third have mild MR; *most common form of inherited MR*

NB: Fragile X is a disorder of trinucleotide repeats.

   2. **Down syndrome:** with an incidence of 1:100; it is responsible for 20% of all cases of severe MR; genetics: *trisomy 21 (increased maternal age), translocation or mosaic abnormality;* small frontal lobes, brain stem, and cerebellum result in low brain weight; hypotonia, round, flat face, up-slanting palpebral fissure, large medial epicanthal fold, large tongue, clinodactyly, simian palmar crease, and septal heart defects are seen; median IQ is 40–50, and Alzheimer's tangles and plaques can develop in middle age

NB: Patients with Down syndrome have a higher risk of atlanto-axial dislocation compared to other children.

   3. **Trisomy 13** *(Patau's syndrome):* has defects of median facial *(cleft palate/lip, micrognathia, arrhinencephaly),* low-set ears/deafness, polydactyly, cardiac defects (patent ductus arteriosus/ventricular septal defect), polycystic kidneys (33%), microcephaly (83%); 2-year survival rate
   4. **5p (Cri du chat) deletion syndrome:** microcephalic *"moon" face;* hypotonia, hypertelorism, and simian crease
   5. **Klinefelter:** XXY (males) gives mild retardation (proportional to the number of extra X chromosomes), delayed language, dyslexia, large breasts/small testes/sparse hair; labs show high follicle-stimulating hormone; EEG can have spike-wave discharge
   6. **XYY:** low average intelligence (extra Ys are less harmful), delayed language, behavior problems, motor incoordination, intention tremor
   7. **Turner syndrome:** appears *similar to Noonan syndrome, with triangular face, webbed neck, posterior ears, and short stature;* 45 chromosomes: XO (80%) or 46 XX (20%); coarctation of the aorta, aortic stenosis, sterile, usually normal IQ, sporadic; Noonan's syndrome: can be XX or XY, may not be sterile, low IQ, sporadic
   8. **Prader-Willi:** *paternal transmission of deletion of 15q11-13* results in neonatal hypotonia, hypogonadism, obesity, short stature, small hands and feet, narrow face with almond-shaped eyes; Angelman's *(happy puppet) syndrome:* maternal transmission results in ataxia, severe retardation, seizures, microbrachycephaly, with onset at 6 months

NB: These two conditions are an example of genetic imprinting, which refers to phenotypic variation depending on the sex of the parent transmitting the disease due to germ-line specific modification of chromosomes and their genetic material.

   9. **Miller-Dieker:** *defect in 17p with agyria and microcephaly;* poor feeding, craniofacial defects, cardiac defects, genital abnormalities
   10. **Cornelia de Lange:** *duplication of 3q* associated with low-pitch cry, bushy eyebrows, hand/feet malformations, marked growth retardation; parkinsonism and dystonia has been reported
   11. **Heller syndrome:** age of onset 1–4 years; male > female; with loss of language and autistic behavior
   12. **Laurence-Moon:** obesity, polydactyly, retinitis pigmentosa, hypogonadism
   13. **Rett's syndrome:** only affects girls; normal until 6–18 months, then show decreased head growth, autistic behavior, writhing/useless hands, ataxia, loss of speech and

other milestones; seizures come late; treatment: naltrexone; X-linked dominant (therefore, lethal in boys)

NB: Mutation causing Rett's syndrome is in the MeCP2 gene.

II. Inherited Metabolic Disease of the Nervous System: the nervous system is the most frequently affected system by genetic abnormality; one-third of all inherited diseases are neurologic
  A. **Modes of inheritance**
    1. *Autosomal dominant:* manifest disease as heterozygotes, but variation in the size of the gene abnormality; may produce *several phenotypes; variable degree of penetrance and expressivity are characteristic;* tendency to *appear long after birth*
    2. *Autosomal recessive:* more *uniform phenotypic expression,* onset soon after birth, usually an *enzyme deficiency*
    3. *X-linked:* mutant gene affects *mainly one sex; Lyon hypothesis:* female will experience same fate as the male if one X chromosome is inactivated in most cells during embryonic development; biochemical abnormality more often a basic protein
    4. *Multifactorial* genetic disease: may present as constitutional disorders with gene abnormalities located on several chromosomes (polygenic); relative contributions of "risk genes" and environmental influences are highly variable
    5. *Mitochondrial* disease: *mitochondrial DNA:* double-stranded circular molecule that encodes protein subunits required; essential feature: inherited maternally; genetic error is most often single point mutation; may also be deletions or duplications that do not conform with maternal inheritance (sporadic, e.g., Kearns-Sayre); some enzymes of respiratory chain are coded by nuclear DNA, which is imported to the mitochondria, resulting in a mendelian pattern of inheritance; of the five complexes that make up the respiratory chain, cytochrome-*c* oxidase (complex IV) is the most often disordered; its deficient function gives rise to lactic acidosis (e.g., Leigh syndrome); complex 1 seen in Leber's optic atrophy
  B. **Suspect hereditary metabolic disease** when presented with the following
    1. A neurologic disorder of similar type in a sibling or close relative
    2. Recurrent nonconvulsive episodes of impaired consciousness
    3. Combination of spastic weakness, cerebellar ataxia, and extrapyramidal disorder
    4. Progression of neurologic disease in weeks, months, or few years
    5. MR in a sibling or close relative
    6. MR in an individual without congenital somatic abnormalities
  C. **Neonatal metabolic diseases:** the *neonate* nervous system functions essentially at a *brain stem-spinal level;* examination should be directed to diencephalic-midbrain, cerebellar-lower brain stem, and spinal functions; control of respiration and body temperature, regulation of thirst, fluid balance appetite (hypothalamus and brain stem); automatisms, sucking, rooting, swallowing, grasping (brain stem-cerebellum); movements and postures of neck, extension of neck, trunk, flexion movement, steppage (reticulospinal, cerebellar, spinal); muscle tone of limbs and trunk; reflex eye movements (tegmental midbrain, pons); state of alertness (diencephalon); reflexes: Moro, placing, etc.; usually manifests as impairment of alertness, hypotonia, disturbance of ocular movements, failure to feed, tremors, clonic jerks, tonic spasms, opisthotonus, chaotic breathing, hypothermia, bradycardia, poor color, seizures
    1. *First hint of trouble: feeding difficulties;* first definite neurologic dysfunction: seizures; divided into three groups: hyperkinetic-hypertonic, apathetic-hypotonic (majority and poorest prognosis), unilateral-hemisyndromic

2. *Three most common hereditary metabolic disorders: phenylketonuria, hyperphenylalaninemia, histidinemia*—does not become clinically manifest in the neonate; clue: history of neonatal disease or unexplained death earlier; history of *rejection of protein foods* (raise suspicion of *hyperammonemia* and *organic aciduria*); distinguish from nonhereditary conditions: hypocalcemia, hypoglycemic reactions (premature, with maternal toxemia, diabetes, adrenal insufficiency), cretinism

3. *Vitamin-responsive aminoacidopathies:* group of diseases that do not respond to dietary restriction of amino acid but to oral supplementation of a specific vitamin

   a. **Pyridoxine dependency:** rare, autosomal recessive; clinical: early onset of convulsions, failure to thrive, hypertonia-hyperkinesia, irritability, jittery baby, hyperacusis—later, psychomotor retardation; lab: increased excretion of xanthurenic acid in response to tryptophan load, decreased levels of pyridoxal-5-phosphate, γ-aminobutyric acid in brain tissue; treatment: 50–100 mg vitamin B_6 and daily doses of 40 mg permit normal development

   b. **Biopterin deficiency:** *lack of tetrahydrobiopterin,* a cofactor of phenylalanine; *increased* concentrations of serum *phenylalanine;* normal phenylalanine hydroxylase (unlike phenylketonuria); lab: measure urine and blood biopterin; clinical: *myoclonic and grand mal seizures,* generalized hypotonia, swallowing difficulty (prominent), developmental delay; treatment: *7.5 mg/kg tetrahydrobiopterin per day with low phenylalanine diet*

   c. **Galactosemia:** autosomal *recessive;* defect in galactose 1-phosphate uridyltransferase; clinical: 1st days of life, *after ingestion of milk,* vomiting, diarrhea, failure to thrive, drowsiness, inattention, hypotonia, hepatosplenomegaly, jaundice, cataracts (due to galactitol in lens); survivors: retarded, visual impairment, cirrhosis; lab: elevated blood galactose, low glucose, galactosuria, deficiency in *galactose 1-phosphate uridyltransferase* in red blood cells, white blood cells, liver cells; treatment: milk substitutes

   d. Hyperglycinemia: two forms

      i. *Ketotic hyperglycinemia (propionic acidemia);* autosomal *recessive;* clinical: vomiting, lethargy, coma, convulsions, hypertonia, respiratory difficulty; onset: neonatal or early infancy; later: retarded, death in a few months; lab: propionic acid, glycine, fatty acids, butanone are elevated in serum; milk protein induces ketosis; also occur in *other organic acidurias: propionic acidemia, β-ketothiolase acidemia, lactic acidemia;* presents in infancy with profound metabolic acidosis, lethargy, vomiting, tachypnea; *methyl malonic acidemia (respond to B_{12}); isovaleric acidemia (striking odor of stale perspiration, respond to restriction of dietary protein); type 2 glutaric acidemia: episodes of acidosis, vomiting, hyperglycinemia;* congenital abnormalities of brain and somatic structures and cardiomyopathy; treatment: *low-protein, carnitine, riboflavin*

      ii. *Nonketotic form: high levels of glycine but no acidosis;* elevated cerebrospinal fluid (CSF) glycine; more devastating than ketotic form; clinical: neonate is *hypotonic, listless, dyspneic, dysconjugate eyes, opisthotonic, myoclonus;* treatment: reduction of protein, sodium benzoate, 120 mg/kg/day

4. *Inherited hyperammonemias:* five disorders of Krebs-Henseleit urea cycle; *all autosomal recessive except type 2 (X-linked);* clinical: severe: asymptomatic at birth, then refuse feedings, vomit, lethargic, lapse into coma; sweating, seizures, rigidity, opisthotonus, respiratory distress; less severe: month later, when protein feeding is increased, failure to thrive, constipation, vomiting, irritability, screaming; *respiratory alkalosis* is constant; liver enlarged; lab: *hyperammonemia* as high as 1500 μg/dL in types 1 and 2

   a. *Carbamoyl phosphate synthetase deficiency*/type 1 hyperammonemia

    b. *Ornithine transcarbamoylase deficiency*/type 2: *sex-linked;* alternating hypertonia and hypotonia, periods of confusion, bizarre behavior; males more severely affected; hyperventilation with alkalosis, retardation, recurrent infections

    c. *Argininosuccinic acid synthetase deficiency*

    d. *Argininosuccinase deficiency:* no signs of metabolic defect during infancy; later, seizures, cerebellar ataxia, excessive dryness and brittleness of hair (trichorrhexis nodosa); treatment: lowering ammonium by hemodialysis, exchange transfusions, and administration of amino and keto acids; sodium benzoate up to 250 mg/day, arginase added to diet (50–150 mg/kg); liver transplantation

    e. *Arginase deficiency*

5. **Maple syrup urine disease and variants:** result of inborn errors of *branched-chain amino acid catabolism;* autosomal *recessive;* clinical: normal at birth, end of 1st week: intermittent hypertonicity, opisthotonus, respiratory irregularities, convulsions, severe ketoacidosis, coma, death; one cause of malignant epileptic syndrome of infancy; milder forms: feeding difficulties, recurrent infections, acidosis, coma, quadriparetic, ataxic; diagnosis: urine smells like maple syrup (due to α-hydroxybutyric acid), positive 2,4-dinitrophenylhydrazine test; increased plasma and urine levels of leucine, isoleucine, valine, and ketoacids; treatment: restrict branched-chain amino acids

6. **Sulfite oxidase deficiency:** extremely rare disorder of *sulfur metabolism;* presents with seizures, spasms, opisthotonus

D. **Hereditary metabolic diseases of early infancy:** hallmark is psychosensorimotor regression; most distinctive members are leukodystrophies and lysosomal storage diseases

1. **Tay-Sachs disease** (GM$_2$ *gangliosidosis, hexosaminidase A deficiency):* autosomal *recessive, mostly Jewish* infants of *eastern European* background; clinical: apparent in 1st weeks and months of life *(always by 4th month);* abnormal *startle* to acoustic stimuli, listless, irritable, delay in psychomotor development, axial hypotonia prominent, later spasticity, visual failure; *cherry-red spot and optic atrophy* in 90%; 2nd year: *seizures, increased head size* with normal ventricles; 3rd year: dementia, decerebration, blindness; death in 3–5 years; EEG: *paroxysmal slow waves with multiple spikes,* basophilic granules in leukocytes, vacuoles in lymphocytes; deficiency in *hexosaminidase A* that cleaves *N*-acetylgalactosamine from gangliosides; large brain, gliosis, enzyme analysis of white blood cells, *normal hexosaminidase B*

2. **Sandhoff disease:** affects *non-Jewish;* deficiency in *both hexosaminidase A and hexosaminidase B;* moderate *hepatosplenomegaly,* coarse granulations in bone marrow histiocytes; same as Tay-Sachs except for additional signs of visceral lipid storage

3. **Infantile Gaucher's disease** (type 2 *neuronopathic form, glucocerebrosidase deficiency):* autosomal *recessive,* no ethnic predominance, before age 6 months; clinical: more rapid than Tay-Sachs, 90% do not survive beyond 1 year; rapid loss of head control, ability to roll over, purposeful movements, bilateral corticospinal signs, persistent retroflexion of the neck and strabismus, enlarged spleen, slightly large liver; CSF normal, EEG nonspecific; lab: *increased serum acid phosphatase* and characteristic *histiocytes (Gaucher's cells)* in marrow smears and liver biopsies; deficiency in *glucocerebrosidase* in leukocytes and hepatocytes; *type 1 Gaucher's disease* is *nonneuropathic, benign;* third type, late childhood and adolescence: slowly progressive mental decline, seizures, ataxia, spastic weakness; *normal lateral gaze (as compared to Niemann-Pick)*

4. **Infantile Niemann-Pick disease:** autosomal *recessive, two-thirds Ashkenazi Jews,* age of onset 3–9 months; clinical: marked *enlargement of liver, spleen, lymph nodes,* infiltration of lungs; loss of spontaneous movements, lack of interest, axial hypotonia, bilateral corticospinal signs, *macular cherry red spot (one-fourth),* seizures (late); lab: *vacuolated*

histiocytes (foam cells) in bone marrow and vacuolated lymphocytes; *deficiency in sphingomyelinase* in leukocytes and fibroblasts and hepatocytes is diagnostic

5. **Infantile, generalized GM$_1$ gangliosidosis** (type 1, *β-galactosidase deficiency, pseudo-Hurler disease*): probably autosomal *recessive*; abnormal at birth with *dysmorphic facial features* (like mucopolysaccharidoses: depressed wide nasal bridge, frontal bossing, hypertelorism, epicanthi, puffy eyelids, long upper lip, low-set ears, macroglossia), impaired awareness, no development after 3–6 months; hypotonia, later hypertonia, spasticity, seizures, variable head size, loss of vision, coarse nystagmus, and strabismus, *cherry-red spot (one-half)*, pseudocontractures, kyphoscoliosis, hepatosplenomegaly; lab: *deficiency of β-galactosidase and accumulation of GM$_1$ ganglioside*

6. **Globoid cell leukodystrophy** (*Krabbe's disease, galactocerebrosidase deficiency*): autosomal recessive, before age 3–6 months; clinical: early, generalized rigidity, loss of head control, dim alertness, vomiting, opisthotonus; later, adduction of the legs, flexion of the arms, clenching of fists, Babinski sign, increased tendon reflexes; most dead by end of 1st year; EEG is nonspecific, CSF protein is elevated; lab: *deficiency in galactocerebrosidase*, accumulation of galactocerebroside; characteristic *globoid cells*; variants: occurring in 2–6-year period, adult years as well

7. **Lipogranulomatosis** (*Farber's disease, ceramidase deficiency*): rare disorder, onset in 1st weeks of life; clinical: *hoarse cry* (due to fixation of laryngeal cartilage), respiratory distress, sensitivity of joints, characteristic *periarticular and subcutaneous swellings and progressive arthropathy*; severe retardation; recurrent infections lead to death in 2 years; *deficiency in ceramidase*, accumulation of ceramide

8. **Sudanophilic leukodystrophies and Pelizaeus-Merzbacher disease:** heterogeneous group of disorders that have a common defective myelination of cerebrum, brain stem, cerebellum, spinal cord, and peripheral nerves
   a. *Pelizaeus-Merzbacher disease:* predominantly *X-linked*, infancy, childhood, adolescence; *defective synthesis of proteolipid protein encoding for one of two myelin basic proteins*; clinical: first signs are abnormal movement of eyes (rapid, irregular, *asymmetric pendular nystagmus*), jerk nystagmus on extreme lateral movements, upbeat nystagmus, hypometric saccades; spastic weakness of limbs, ataxia, optic atrophy, intention tremor, choreiform or athetotic movements of the arms; psychomotor retardation; seizures occasionally; computed tomography (CT)/magnetic resonance imaging (MRI): white matter involvement; one group resembles *Cockayne syndrome: photosensitivity of the skin, dwarfism, cerebellar ataxia, corticospinal tract signs, cataracts, retinitis pigmentosa, deafness*; pathology: islands of preserved myelin impart a *tigroid pattern of degenerated and intact myelin in the cerebrum; this disease and Cockayne: only leukodystrophies with invariable nystagmus*

9. **Spongy degeneration of infancy** (*Canavan-van Bogaert-Bertrand disease*): autosomal *recessive*, onset is early, recognized in 1st 3 months; clinical: lack of development, or psychomotor regression, loss of sight, optic atrophy, lethargy, difficulty sucking, irritability, hypotonia, followed by spasticity, corticospinal signs, *macrocephaly*; no visceral or skeletal abnormality; *blond hair, light complexion*; CSF: normal or slightly elevated protein; increased urinary excretion of N-acetyl-aspartic acid due to *deficiency of aspartoacylase*; MRI: increased T2 signal intensity with normal ventricles, huge brain; must be distinguished from GM$_2$ gangliosidosis, Alexander's disease, Krabbe's disease, nonprogressive megalocephaly

10. **Alexander's disease:** shares certain features with leukodystrophies and gray matter diseases; onset is in infancy, with failure to thrive, psychomotor retardation, and seizures; early and progressive *macrocephaly*; pathology: severe destruction of cerebral

white matter, especially frontal lobes; *Rosenthal fibers:* eosinophilic hyaline bodies around blood vessels, represent glial degeneration products

11. **Alpers disease:** progressive *disease of cerebral gray matter, progressive cerebral poliodystrophy,* diffuse cerebral degeneration in infancy; familial and sporadic forms exists; clinical: loss of smile, sweating attacks, seizures, diffuse myoclonic jerks, followed by incoordination, progressive spasticity, blindness, optic atrophy, growth retardation, microcephaly; occasional hepatic changes, anemia, thrombocytopenia, trichorrhexis; pathology: *walnut brain,* cerebral white matter, and basal ganglia are preserved; occasional spongiform appearance

12. **Congenital lactic acidosis:** very rare disease, death before the 3rd year, acidosis with high anion gap, *high serum lactate, and hyperalaninemia*

13. **Cerebrohepatorenal** (Zellweger) disease: *peroxisomal* disorder, autosomal *recessive;* onset: neonatal to infancy; death within a few months; clinical: motor inactivity, *dysmorphic features* of the skull and face (high forehead, shallow orbits, hypertelorism, high arched palate, retrognathia), poor visual fixation, multifocal seizures, swallowing difficulties, *cataracts,* hepatomegaly, *optic atrophy, cloudy corneas,* stippled, irregular calcification of the patellae and greater trochanter; pathology: dysgenesis of cortex, white matter, renal cysts, hepatic fibrosis, biliary dysgenesis, agenesis of thymus; lab: *increase in very-long-chain fatty acids* in plasma and fibroblasts due to lack of liver peroxisomes

14. **Oculocerebrorenal (Lowe) syndrome:** probably *X-linked recessive;* clinical: bilateral *cataracts, glaucoma, large eyes, megalocornea and buphthalmos, corneal opacities, pendular nystagmus,* hypotonia, corticospinal signs, psychomotor regression; later frontal lobes prominent, eyes shrunken; characteristic *renal tubular acidosis, death by renal failure,* demineralization of bones, typical *rachitic deformities*

15. **Kinky- or steely-hair disease** (*Menkes disease, trichopoliodystrophy*): rare, *sex-linked recessive,* rarely survive beyond 2nd year; birth is premature, poor feeding, hypothermia, seizures, hair is normal at birth, later like steel wool, twisted (pili torti) under microscope; radiology: metaphyseal spurring; angiography: tortuosity and elongation of the cerebral and systemic arteries; due to *deficiency of copper-dependent enzymes* (including cytochrome oxidase) resulting in *failure to absorb copper from gastrointestinal tract, profound copper deficiency*

E. **Inherited metabolic diseases of late infancy and early childhood**

1. *Leukodystrophies:* early-onset spastic paralysis, with or without ataxia, and visual impairment with optic atrophy but normal retina; seizures and intellectual impairment are later events; MRI: white matter involvement (e.g., Krabbe's, metachromatic leukodystrophy, spongy degeneration, Pelizaeus-Merzbacher, Schilder's, sudanophilic, and adrenoleukodystrophy)

2. *Poliodystrophies:* gray matter disease, early-onset seizures, myoclonus, blindness with retinal changes and mental regression; choreoathetosis, ataxia, spastic paralysis occurs later; MRI shows generalized atrophy and ventricular enlargement; e.g., Tay-Sachs, Niemann-Pick, Gaucher's, Alpers, neuroaxonal dystrophy, lipofuscinosis, Leigh

3. *Aminoacidopathies:* 48 inherited aminoacidopathies, one-half with neurologic abnormalities; mostly a lag in psychomotor development

   a. **Phenylketonuria:** most frequent of aminoacidurias; autosomal *recessive;* classic phenylketonuria: psychomotor regression later part of 1st year, by age 5–6 years, IQ <20; hyperactivity, aggressivity, clumsy gait, fine tremors, poor coordination, odd posturing, repetitive digital mannerisms, seizures in 25%; *fair skin, blue-eyed; skin is rough* and dry; *musty body odor;* two-thirds *microcephalic,* fundi normal, no visceral or skeletal abnormality; *increased serum phenylalanine* (>15 mg/dL), with phenylpyruvic acid in blood, CSF and urine is diagnostic: *emerald green color by Guthrie test with ferric chloride* (green-brown for histidinemia; navy blue for maple syrup; purple for propionic and methylmalonic aciduria); deficiency in phenylalanine hydroxylase, localized to *chromosome 12*; treatment: *low-phenylalanine diet*

b. **Hereditary tyrosinemia** *(Richner-Hanhart disease):* one-half with mild to moderate MR; *self-mutilation,* incoordination, language defects are prominent; lacrimation, *photophobia, redness due to corneal herpetiform erosions; palmar and plantar keratosis,* pain; *elevated tyrosine* in blood and urine diagnostic; treatment: *low-tyrosine and low-phenylalanine diet,* retinoids for skin lesions

c. Hartnup's disease: autosomal *recessive;* clinical: intermittent red *scaly rash* over face, neck, hands, legs resembling pellagra; growth failure, developmental delay; emotional lability, confusional-hallucinatory psychosis, episodic cerebellar ataxia, dysarthria, occasionally spasticity, nystagmus, ptosis and diplopia; *attacks are triggered by sunlight, stress, sulfonamide drugs;* due to *transport error of neutral amino acids* across renal tubules, excretion in urine and feces; loss of tryptophan causes *decreased niacin synthesis;* treatment: *nicotinamide, 50–300 mg/day; L-tryptophan ethyl esterase*

4. *Progressive cerebellar ataxia of early childhood*

  a. No biochemical abnormality identified

   i. *Disequilibrium and dyssynergia syndrome of Hagberg and Janner:* early-life onset of relatively pure cerebellar ataxia and psychomotor retardation

   ii. *Cerebellar ataxia with diplegia, hypotonia, and MR (atonic diplegia of Foerster)*

   iii. *Agenesis of the cerebellum:* early cerebellar ataxia and hyperventilation

   iv. Cerebellar ataxia with cataracts and oligophrenia; childhood (mainly) to adulthood *(Marinesco-Sjšgren disease)*

   v. Cerebellar ataxia with retinal degeneration, cerebellar ataxia with cataracts and ophthalmoplegia

   vi. Familial cerebellar ataxia with mydriasis

   vii. Familial cerebellar ataxia with deafness and blindness (retinocochleodentate degeneration)

   viii. Familial cerebellar ataxia with choreoathetosis, corticospinal tract signs, and mental and motor retardation

  b. *Biochemical abnormality identified*

   i. *Refsum's disease (hereditary motor and sensory neuropathy [HMSN] type 4):* autosomal *recessive; deficiency of phytanic acid oxidase* affecting lipid metabolism; onset usually in childhood (1st to 3rd decade) with *cerebellar ataxia, chronic hypertrophic demyelinating neuropathy and retinitis pigmentosa;* other findings: night blindness, deafness, ichthyosis, cardiomyopathy, hepatosplenomegaly, and increased CSF protein; pathology shows *hypertrophic nerves, onion bulb*

   ii. *Abetalipoproteinemia (Bassen-Kornzweig syndrome):* autosomal recessive; clinical: symptoms begin by age 12 years, *fat malabsorption with diarrhea and steatorrhea, acanthocytosis, retinopathy, vitamin A, D, E, and K deficiency, neuropathy with decreased reflexes and sensation, progressive ataxia,* positive Romberg, decreased night vision (retinitis pigmentosa); lab: *acanthocytosis, absent β-lipoproteins,* decreased triglyceride and cholesterol, *low vitamin A, D, E, and K levels;* slowed nerve conduction velocity; pathology: *loss of large myelinated fibers, spinocerebellar and posterior column degeneration;* treatment: dietary restriction of triglycerides, vitamin E supplements

   iii. *Ataxia-telangiectasia (Louis-Bar syndrome):* autosomal *recessive;* onset with walking, *ataxic-dyskinetic, choreoathetosis,* dysarthric speech, jerky eye movements, slow saccades, apraxia of voluntary gaze, optokinetic nystagmus is lost; intellectual decline by age 9–10 years; mild polyneuropathy; lesions: transversely oriented subpapillary venous plexus in the outer part of bulbar conjunctiva, ears, neck, bridge of nose, cheeks in butterfly pattern, and flexor creases of forearms; many with endocrine alterations; progressive, death in 2nd decade due *to pulmonary infection, lymphoma, or glioma;* central nervous system (CNS): cerebellar degeneration, demyelination in posterior columns, spinocerebellar tracts, peripheral nerves, sympathetic ganglia, anterior horn cells; *absence or decrease in immunoglobulin A (IgA), IgE, isotypes ^2IgG and ^4IgG; hypoplasia of thymus*

   iv. *Galactosemia:* autosomal *recessive;* defect in *galactose 1-phosphate uridyltransferase*
   v. *Friedreich's ataxia:* mutation is an *unstable expansion of a GAA repeat in the first intron of the gene X25 on chromosome 9q12-21.1, leading to deficiency of the protein frataxin;* clinical: *progressive gait disturbance, gait ataxia, loss of proprioception in the lower limbs, areflexia, dysarthria and extensor plantar responses* with an age of onset <25 years; other features: hypertrophic cardiomyopathy; diabetes mellitus in fewer than one-half the patients; also with skeletal deformities such as scoliosis and pes cavus; treatment: coenzyme Q10 and vitamin E may improve cardiac and skeletal muscle bioenergetics, idebenone (a coenzyme Q10 analog) may have benefit on cardiomyopathy

5. **NB: Metachromatic leukodystrophy:** another *lysosomal (sphingolipid) storage disease, localized in chromosome 22, absence of aryl sulfatase A,* preventing the conversion of sulfatide to cerebroside; autosomal recessive; manifests between ages 1 and 4 years (variants up to adult life due to variability of gene mutation)
   a. Clinical: progressive impairment of motor function (gait and spasticity) with reduced speech output and mental regression; early, brisk reflexes, but later peripheral nerves become involved, reflexes are lost; later, with visual impairment, squint, nystagmus, intention tremor, dysarthria, dysphagia, drooling, optic atrophy (one-third); seizures are rare, no somatic abnormality; normal head size
   b. CSF protein elevated; widespread demyelination in cerebrum; presence of metachromatic granules in glial cells and macrophages from a biopsy of peripheral nerve; marked increase of sulfatide in urine, absence of aryl sulfatase A in white blood cells, serum, and cultured fibroblasts; treatment: enzyme replacement, bone marrow transplantation (ongoing trial)
   c. Variant: *"multiple sulfatase deficiency"*—due to deficiency in *aryl sulfatase A, B, and C;* clinical: same as metachromatic but, in addition, has skeletal and facial changes
6. **Neuroaxonal dystrophy** *(degeneration):* rare, autosomal *recessive* onset, onset in 2nd year
   a. Clinical: psychomotor retardation, marked hypotonia, brisk reflexes, Babinski sign, *progressive blindness due to optic atrophy* but normal retina; relentlessly progressive, decorticate in 3–8 years; no hepatosplenomegaly, no facial and skeletal abnormality; some of late onset may be indistinguishable from Hallervorden-Spatz
   b. Pathology: *spheroids of swollen axoplasm in posterior columns,* nuclei of Goll and Burdach, and Clarke's column, nigra, subthalamus, brain stem, cortex CT and CSF are normal; no identified biochemical abnormality; EEG shows characteristic *high-amplitude fast rhythms* (16–22 Hz)
7. **Late infantile and early childhood Gaucher's and Niemann-Pick disease (types 3 and 4):** diagnosis of *Gaucher's established with splenomegaly;* variants of *Niemann-Pick: juvenile dystonic lipidosis* (extrapyramidal symptoms and paralysis of vertical eye movements) and *syndrome of the sea-blue histiocytes* (liver, spleen, and bone marrow contain histiocytes with sea-blue granules)

8. **Late infantile-childhood GM$_1$ gangliosidosis:** *type 2 (juvenile) onset* between ages 12 and 24 months, survival 3–10 years
    a. Clinical: first sign is difficulty walking with frequent falls, followed by spastic quadriparesis; with facial dysmorphism resembling Hurler
    b. Lab findings: hypoplasia of thoracolumbar vertebral bodies, hypoplasia of the acetabula; marrow with histiocytes with clear vacuoles or wrinkled cytoplasm; deficiency in β-galactosidase
9. **Neuronal ceroid lipofuscinosis:** *most frequent lysosomal abnormality;* except for a few adult cases, mostly autosomal *recessive;* no biochemical markers
    a. Four types: *Santavuori-Haltia Finnish type* (age 3–18 months, psychomotor regression, ataxia, retinal changes, myoclonus; later: blind, spastic quadriplegia, microcephaly); *Jansky-Bielschowsky early childhood type* (age 2–4 years, survive 4–8 years), first with petit mal or grand mal seizures, myoclonic jerks evoked by proprioceptive and other sensory stimuli; incoordination, deterioration of mental faculties; retinal degeneration), *Vogt-Spielmeyer juvenile type; Kufs adult type*
    b. Pathology: neuronal loss in cortex, *curvilinear storage particles* and osmophilic granules in the neurons, inclusions in nerve twigs
10. *Mucopolysaccharidoses:* storage of lipids in neurons and polysaccharides in connective tissue—result in unique combination of neurologic and skeletal abnormalities; seven clinical subtypes; basic defect prevents degradation of acid mucopolysaccharides (glucosaminoglycans) that can be measured in serum, leukocytes, and fibroblasts; autosomal *recessive (except Hunter, sex-linked)*
11. *Mucolipidoses and sialidoses* (disease of complex carbohydrates): due to α-N-acetylneuraminidase defect; autosomal *recessive;* manifest similar to Hurler but normal mucopolysaccharides in urine
    a. *Mucolipidosis I:* features of *gargoylism,* with slowly progressive MR; cherry-red spots in macula; corneal opacities; ataxia
    b. *Mucolipidosis II:* most common, early-onset psychomotor retardation; abnormal facies, periosteal thickening *(dysostosis multiplex like GM$_1$ and Hurler);* gingival hyperplasia; *hepatosplenomegaly; typical vacuolation of lymphocytes* and Kupffer cells; inclusion cell in bone marrow
    c. *Mucolipidosis III: pseudo-Hurler polydystrophy;* symptoms do not appear until age 2 years, mild; major abnormalities: retardation, *corneal opacities, valvular heart disease*
    d. *Mucolipidosis IV:* "new disease"
    e. *Mannosidosis:* rare, onset 1st 2 years; *Hurler-like facial and skeletal deformities;* MR; *spoke-like opacities of lens;* normal urinary mucopolysaccharides; mannosiduria due to defect in α-mannosidase is diagnostic
    f. *Fucosidosis:* rare, autosomal *recessive;* onset 12–15 months, progressing to spastic quadriplegia in 4–6 years; hepatosplenomegaly, enlarged salivary glands, beaking of vertebral bodies; lack of *lysosomal L-fucosidase,* resulting in accumulation of fucose-rich sphingolipids in skin, conjunctivae, rectal mucosa
    g. *Aspartylglycosaminuria:* autosomal *recessive;* early-onset psychomotor regression; bouts of hyperactivity mixed with apathy; progressive dementia; beaking of vertebral bodies
12. **Cockayne syndrome:** probably autosomal *recessive;* onset late infancy
    a. Clinical: stunting of growth, *photosensitivity* of skin, *microcephaly, retinitis pigmentosa, cataracts, blindness, pendular nystagmus,* delayed psychomotor, weakness, and ataxia

b. Pathology: *small brain*, striatocerebellar calcifications, leukodystrophy like Pelizaeus-Merzbacher, severe cerebellar and cortical atrophy; some with calcification of basal ganglia; normal CSF, no biochemical abnormalities identified

13. **Rett's syndrome:** occurs exclusively in *females*, fatal in homozygous males; 1:10,000 females; normal birth, early postnatal development, normal head circumference, onset at age 6–15 months: loss of voluntary hand movements; later, communication, growth retardation, *stereotypy of hand movements* (wringing, rubbing, tapping), gradual ataxia, rigidity, episodic hyperventilation, seizures; mutation of X-chromosome postulated

14. *Neurologic signs specific for metabolic disorders*

Acousticomotor obligatory startle	Tay-Sachs
Abolished tendon reflexes but with Babinski	Krabbe's disease
	Leigh disease
	Metachromatic leukodystrophy
	Adrenomyeloneuropathy
	Vitamin B_{12} deficiency
Peculiar eye movements, pendular nystagmus	Pelizaeus-Merzbacher
	Leigh disease
	Lesch-Nyhan syndrome
Marked rigidity, opisthotonus, tonic spasms	Krabbe's disease
	Gaucher's disease
	Alpers disease
Intractable seizures, multifocal myoclonus	Alpers disease
Intermittent hyperventilation	Leigh disease
	Congenital lactic acidosis
Involvement of peripheral nerve (weakness, hypotonia, areflexia, slow conduction) plus CNS	Metachromatic leukodystrophy Krabbe's disease
	Neuroaxonal dystrophy
	Leigh disease (rare)
Extrapyramidal signs	Niemann-Pick (rigidity, abnormal postures)
	Juvenile dystonic lipidosis (dystonia, choreoathetosis)
	Rett's (abnormal hand movements and dystonic rigidity)
	Ataxia-telangiectasia (athetosis)
	Sanfilippo
	Type 1 glutaric acidemia

15. *Ocular abnormalities of diagnostic value*

Rapid pendular nystagmus	Pelizaeus-Merzbacher
	Krabbe's disease
Cherry-red spot	Tay-Sachs
	Sandhoff
	Niemann-Pick (occasionally)
	Lipofuscinosis
	GM_1 (one-half of cases) and GM_2 gangliosidosis
	Refsum's
	Mucolipidosis II
	Sialidosis
	Multiple sulfatase deficiency
Corneal opacification	Lowe's syndrome
	GM_1 gangliosidosis
	Mucopolysaccharidoses
	Mucolipidosis
	Tyrosinemia
	Aspartylglycosaminuria (rare)
Cataracts	Galactosemia
	Lowe's (oculocerebral)
	Zellweger
	Congenital rubella
	Marinesco-Sjšgren
	Fabry's disease
	Mannosidosis
	Cerebrotendinous xanthomatosis
	Cockayne syndrome
Retinal degeneration with pigmentary deposits	Jansky-Bielschowsky
	GM_1 gangliosidosis
	Sea-blue histiocytes
Optic atrophy and blindness	Metachromatic leukodystrophy
	Neuroaxonal dystrophy
	Leber's (X-linked; lateral geniculate affected)
	Behr's (autosomal recessive, cortical and cerebellar involvement)
Vertical eye impairment	Niemann-Pick

	Juvenile dystonic lipidosis
	Sea-blue histiocytes
Jerky eye movements	Late infantile Gaucher's
Telangiectasia and optic apraxia	Ataxia-telangiectasia
	Niemann-Pick
Glaucoma	Lowe's
	Zellweger
	Sturge-Weber
Lens dislocation	Homocystinuria
	Marfan's syndrome
Red eyes	Ataxia-telangiectasia
Retinitis pigmentosa	Refsum's
	Bassen-Kornzweig
	Kearns-Sayre
	Spielmeyer-Vogt
	Cockayne syndrome

16. *Other medical findings of diagnostic value*

Gingival hypertrophy	Mucolipidoses
	Mannosidosis
Deafness	Mucopolysaccharidoses
	Mannosidosis
	Cockayne
Skin abnormalities	Cockayne (photosensitivity)
	Fabry's and fucosidosis (papular nevi)
	Ataxia-telangiectasia (telangiectasia of ears, conjunctiva, etc.)
	Sjögren-Larsen (ichthyosis)
	Hunter (plaque-like lesions)
Dwarfism, spine deformities, arthropathies	Mucopolysaccharidoses
	Cockayne
Colorless friable hair	Menkes kinky hair syndrome
Multiple arthropathies and raucous dysphonia	Farber's disease
Dysmorphic features	GM_1 gangliosidosis
	Lowe's
	Zellweger
	Mucopolysaccharidosis
	Mucolipidosis

	Aspartylglycosaminuria
	Mannosidosis
	Fucosidosis (some)
	Multisulfatase deficiency
Hepatosplenomegaly	Gaucher's
	Niemann-Pick
	Sandhoff
	All mucopolysaccharidoses
	Mucolipidoses
	Fucosidosis
	GM_1 gangliosidosis
Macrocephaly without hydrocephalus	Canavan
	Tay-Sachs
	Alexander's
Beaking of vertebral bodies	GM_1 gangliosidosis
	All mucopolysaccharidoses
	Mucolipidoses
	Mannosidosis
	Fucosidosis
	Aspartylglycosaminuria
	Multiple sulfatase deficiency
Stroke/Stroke-like episodes	MELAS
	Homocystinuria
	Propionic acidemia
	Methylmalonic acidemia
	Isovaleric acidemia
	Glutaric acidemia type I
	Urea cycle disorders
	Congenital disorders of glycosylation
	Menkes' syndrome
	Fabry's disease
Reye-like syndrome	Fatty acid disorders
	Urea cycle disorders
	Organic acidemia
Cardiomyopathy	VLCAD deficiency
	LCHAD deficiency
	Carnitine transporter deficiency

	Infantile CPT2 deficiency
	Glycogen storage disease II (Pompe's disease)
	GSD III (Cori's disease)
	Mitochondrial disorders
Rhabdomylysis/ myoglobinuria	GSD V (McArdle's disease)
	Adult CPT2 deficiency
	VLCAD deficiency
	LCHAD deficiency
	Carnitine transporter deficiency
	Mitochondrial disorders
Progressive myoclonic epilepsies	MERRF
	Unvericht-Lundborg disease (Baltic myoclonus)
	Neuronal ceroid lipofuscinosis
	Lafora's disease
	Sialidosis type I
Psychiatric changes	Wilson's disease
	Neuronal ceroid lipofuscinosis
	X-linked adrenoleukodystrophy
	Metachromatic leukodystrophy
	Late-onset GM_2 gangliosidosis
	Porphyria
	Lesch-Nyhan syndrome
	Urea cycle disorders
	Mucopolysaccharidosis II and III (Sanfilippo's and Hunter's syndrome)

F. **Inherited metabolic encephalopathies of late childhood and adolescence:** grouped according to mode of clinical presentation

1. *Progressive cerebellar ataxia:* occurs in late childhood; essentially nonmetabolic, postinfectious encephalomyelitis, postanoxic, postmeningitic, posthyperthermic states, drug intoxications; pure cerebellar forms: postinfectious cerebellitis, cerebellar tumors

   a. *Bassen-Kornzweig acanthocytosis (abetalipoproteinemia):* extremely rare, autosomal recessive, symptoms between 6 and 12 years; clinical: weakness of the limbs with areflexia, ataxia of sensory type (tabetic); later, cerebellar component; steatorrhea often precedes weakness; retinal degeneration, kyphoscoliosis, pes cavus, Babinski signs; lab: spiky or thorny red blood cells *(acanthocytes),* low erythrocyte sedimentation rate, low low-density lipoproteins; pathology: *foamy, vacuolated epithelial cells* in intestinal mucosa; demyelination in sural nerve biopsies, depletion of Purkinje and granule cells in cerebellum, etc.; basic mechanism: inability to synthesize the proteins of cell membranes; treatment: low-fat diet, high doses of vitamins A and E

b. *Familial hypobetalipoproteinemia:* resembles *abetalipoproteinemia with hypercholesterolemia, acanthocytosis, retinitis pigmentosa, pallidal atrophy (HARP syndrome);* autosomal *dominant;* fat droplets in intestinal mucosa (malabsorption); treatment: low fat, high vitamin E

c. *Hereditary paroxysmal cerebellar ataxia;* periodic ataxia; autosomal *dominant; chromosome 19p;* onset childhood or early adult, disabling episodic ataxia, nystagmus, dysarthria, lasting few minutes to hours; asymptomatic or mild nystagmus between attacks; treatment: *acetazolamide, 250 mg tid*

d. Other causes: *Unverricht-Lundborg (Baltic) disease, Cockayne syndrome, Marinesco-Sjögren disease, cerebrotendinous xanthomatosis, Prader-Willi*

2. *Myoclonus and epilepsy*

a. *Myoclonic epilepsy of infants:* widespread, continuous myoclonus except during sleep; male and female; age of onset 9–20 months; myoclonus of all muscles, rapid irregular conjugate movement *(dancing eyes of opsoclonic type);* all lab tests are normal; treatment: adrenocorticotropic hormone and dexamethasone (1.5–4.0 mg/day); *other causes* of opsoclonus-myoclonus: *neuroblastoma, bronchogenic and other occult carcinomas, neural crest tumors, viral infections, hypoxic injury*

b. *Familial progressive myoclonus:* five major categories

   i. **Lafora body polymyoclonus with epilepsy:** autosomal *recessive;* large *basophilic cytoplasmic bodies* in dentate, thalamus, and brain stem; onset late childhood with *seizure* or *myoclonic jerks,* initiated by startle, tactile stimulus, excitement, or motor activities; speech marred, cerebellar *ataxia,* occasional deafness; often do not survive 25th birthday; no abnormalities in blood, urine, or CSF; antiepileptic drugs control seizures but not basic process

   ii. **Polyglycosan body disease:** *glycosamine bodies* found in CNS and peripheral nervous system; diagnosis: bodies in axons of peripheral nerves or liver; includes *dementia, chorea, amyotrophy*

   iii. **Juvenile cerebroretinal degeneration (ceroid lipofuscinosis):** one of the most variable forms; severe myoclonus, seizures, visual loss; yellow-gray maculae; course: visual impairment—generalized seizures, myoclonus—intellectual deterioration—dementia—death in 10–15 years; diagnosis: in *sweat glands; Kufs type:* 15–25 years, no visual impairment, slower

   iv. **Cherry-red spot myoclonus syndrome:** relatively new class, storage of sialidated glycopeptides in tissues due to *neuraminidase deficiency;* clinical: *cherry-red spot, episodic pain* in hands, legs, and feet during hot weather, later followed by *polymyoclonus, cerebellar ataxia;* lab: urinary *excretion of sialidated oligosaccharides, sialidase deficiency in fibroblasts*

   v. Dentatorubral cerebellar atrophy with polymyoclonus (dyssynergia cerebellaris myoclonica, Ramsay-Hunt): onset is late childhood, both sexes; progressive ataxia with action myoclonus, seizures infrequent, intellect preserved

   vi. *Other causes: childhood or juvenile GM$_2$ gangliosidosis, late Gaucher's disease with polymyoclonus*

3. *Extrapyramidal syndrome of parkinsonian type*

a. **Hepatolenticular degeneration (Wilson's disease, Westphal-Strümpell pseudosclerosis):** *Kayser-Fleischer ring* golden-brown in *Descemet's layer* of cornea (pathognomonic); impairment of ceruloplasmin synthesis, with *excessive copper deposition* in tissues; reduced rate of copper incorporation to ceruloplasmin and a reduction in biliary excretion of copper; autosomal *recessive; esterase D locus on chromosome 13;* onset 2nd to 3rd decade

i. Clinical: all instances, first expression is acute or chronic hepatitis—multilobar cirrhosis, splenomegaly (asymptomatic or attacks of jaundice, thrombocytopenia or bleeding); first neurologic manifestations: tremor, slowness, dysarthria, dysphagia, hoarseness, occasional chorea and dystonia; mouth hangs open in early stage of the disease; classic syndrome: dysphagia, drooling, rigidity, slowness, flexed postures, mouth agape giving *"vacuous smile,"* virtual anarthria, *wing-beating tremor,* slow saccadic movements; cerebellar ataxia and intention tremor are variable

ii. Lab: *low serum ceruloplasmin (<20 mg/dL); low serum copper (3–10 μM/L; normal, 11–24) and increased urinary copper excretion (>100 μg/24 hours);* early in the course: most reliable—*high copper in liver biopsy;* most with aminoaciduria secondary to renal tubular abnormalities; CT: large lateral and 3rd ventricles, cerebellar, cerebral, brain stem atrophy, hypodense lenticular, red, and dentate

iii. Neuropathology: frank cavitation of lenticular nuclei or neuronal cell loss in chronic cases; striking hyperplasia of *Alzheimer's type 2 astrocytes* in cortex, basal ganglia, brain stem nuclei cerebellum

iv. Treatment: *reduce dietary copper* to <1 mg/day (copper rich: liver, mushrooms, cocoa, chocolate, nuts, shellfish); copper chelating agent *D-penicillamine* (1–2 g/day) in divided doses; pyridoxine should be added to prevent anemia (25 mg/day); temporary reduction or prednisone for 20% chance of penicillamine reaction (rash, arthralgia, fever, leukopenia); *triethylene tetramine* (trientine) for severe reactions (lupus-like or nephrotic syndromes) or *zinc,* 100–150 mg daily in three to four divided doses; appropriate drug should be continued for life; *tetrathiomolybdate* is often better tolerated; *liver transplantation* is curative for the underlying metabolic defect (indication for severe liver damage or intractable neurologic deterioration); screen relatives and start treatment before neurologic symptoms

b. Hallervorden-Spatz disease: pigmentary degeneration of the globus pallidus, substantia nigra, and red nucleus; autosomal *recessive,* onset late childhood, early adolescence; progresses slowly over 10 or more years

i. Clinical: corticospinal (spasticity, hyperreflexia) and extrapyramidal (rigidity, dystonia, choreoathetosis); intellect deterioration

ii. No known biochemical test; *iron deposits in basal ganglia;* high uptake of radioactive iron in basal ganglia; CT with hypodense zones in lenticular nuclei resembling Wilson's, sulfite oxidase, glutaric acidemia, Leigh; MRI in T2 pallidum appears intensely black with a small white area in medial part ("eye of the tiger" sign)

iii. Neuropathology: intense brown pigmentation of globus pallidus, substantia nigra, red nucleus; also unique are *swollen axon fragments like neuroaxonal dystrophy;* no known treatment

c. Other differential diagnoses to be considered

i. *Chediak-Higashi disease:* massive granulation of leukocytes in blood and marrow with partial albinism; polyneuropathy is most prominent

ii. *Huntington's disease,* juvenile type

iii. *Juvenile parkinsonism*

iv. *Status dysmyelinatus of Vogt and Vogt:* obscure disease in which all myelinated fibers and nerve cells in the lenticular nuclei disappear

v. *Late Lafora body disease*

vi. *Leigh disease* (rarely)

vii. *Dentatorubropallidoluysian degeneration*

4. *Dystonia, chorea, and athetosis*
   a. **Lesch-Nyhan syndrome:** rare *X-linked; uricemia* in association with *spasticity and choreoathetosis* in early childhood with *self-mutilation;* normal at birth up to 6–9 months, self-mutilation (mainly lips) occurs early; spasticity, athetosis, tremor later; MR moderately severe; *gouty tophi* appear on ears, risk for *gouty nephropathy;* lab: serum uric acid 7–10 mg/dL; deficiency in *hypoxanthine-guanine-phosphoribosyl transferase, which lies on X chromosome* by DNA analysis; treatment: allopurinol (xanthine oxidase inhibitor) but no effect on CNS; transitory success with 5-hydroxytryptophan with L-dopa; fluphenazine/haloperidol for self-mutilation; behavior modification
   b. **Fahr syndrome:** *calcification of vessels* in basal ganglia and cerebellum, choreoathetosis and rigidity prominent; some mentally retarded; may be *sporadic, autosomal recessive, or dominant*
   c. *Hypoparathyroidism* (idiopathic or acquired) and *pseudohypoparathyroidism:* rare familial with skeletal and developmental abnormalities; decrease in serum ionized calcium induces tetany, seizures, choreoathetosis (probably due to calcification of the basal ganglia)
   d. *Other causes: ceroid lipofuscinosis of Kufs type, GM$_1$ gangliosidosis, late-onset metachromatic leukodystrophy, Niemann-Pick, Hallervorden-Spatz, Wilson's, glutaric aciduria type 1, kernicterus, Crigler-Najjar form of hereditary hyperbilirubinemia, torsion dystonia, Segawa disease* (familial dopa-responsive dystonia; autosomal recessive); *paroxysmal and kinesogenic form of familial choreoathetosis; phenytoin toxicity in cerebral palsy*
5. *Leukodystrophies and other focal cerebral symptoms*
   a. **Adrenoleukodystrophy (sudanophilic leukodystrophy with bronzing of skin and adrenal atrophy):** *X-linked recessive;* impairment of *peroxisomal oxidation of very-long-chain fatty acids,* accumulation in brain and adrenals, encoded by *gene in X28;* onset between 4 and 8 years, *usually only males;* episodic vomiting, decline in scholastic performance, change in personality, circulatory collapse, ataxia, tremor, cortical blindness; late: bilateral hemiplegia, pseudobulbar paralysis, blindness, deafness
      i. *Adrenomyeloneuropathy:* progressive spastic paraparesis with mild polyneuropathy
      ii. Lab: low serum sodium, chloride, high potassium, reduced corticosteroid excretion, low serum cortisol, CSF protein may be elevated; definitive: *high levels of very-long-chain fatty acids* in plasma, erythrocytes, or fibroblasts; pathology: *massive degeneration of myelin* in cerebrum, brain stem, optic nerves, spinal cord
      iii. Treatment: adrenal replacement, avoid long-chain fatty acid
   b. **Familial orthochromic leukodystrophy:** diffuse symmetric, cerebral, cerebellar, and spinal degeneration without visceral lesions; autosomal recessive
   c. **Cerebral sclerosis of Scholz:** begins in childhood, white matter disease, characterized by cerebral blindness, deafness, aphasia, spastic quadriparesis, occasional choreoathetosis
   d. **Polycystic white matter degeneration:** probably autosomal *recessive*
   e. **Cerebrotendinous xanthomatosis:** probably autosomal *recessive;* rare, usually begins in childhood; *cataracts, xanthochromia* of tendon sheaths and lungs; early neurologic findings: difficulty learning, poor retentive memory, visual-spatial perception, later dementia, ataxic-spastic gait, dysarthria, dysphagia, polyneuropathy; neuropathology: *crystalline cholesterol in brain stem and cerebrum,* with symmetric demyelination; basic *defect: synthesis of primary bile acids,* leading to increased hepatic production of *cholesterol and cholestanol then accumulate in brain* and tendons; treatment: *chenodeoxycholic acid, 750 mg daily*

6. *Strokes*
   a. **Homocystinuria:** autosomal *recessive* trait, *simulates Marfan's; cystathionine synthetase deficiency;* tall, slender, great *limb length,* scoliosis, *arachnodactyly (long spidery fingers and toes),* thin muscles, knock knees, highly arched feet, kyphosis; sparse blond brittle hair, malar flush, livedo reticularis, *dislocation of lens; only neurologic abnormality is mild MR (normal in Marfan's syndrome);* thickening and fibrosis of coronary, cerebral, and renal arteries—later; ?abnormality of platelets favoring clot formation; lab: homocysteine elevated in blood, CSF, urine; treatment: *low-methionine diet, large doses of pyridoxine* (50–500 mg)
      i. May also be secondary to *5,10 methylenetetrahydrofolate reductase deficiency* (due to coincidental folic acid deficiency or phenytoin), causing multiple cerebrovascular lesions, dementia, epilepsy, and polyneuropathy
   b. **Fabry's disease:** also known as *angiokeratoma corporis diffusum; X-linked recessive*—complete form in men, incomplete in women; primary deficit: α-*galactosidase A,* results in accumulation of *ceramide trihexoside* in endothelial, perithelial, and smooth muscle of blood vessels and nerve cells of hypothalamus, substantia nigra, brain stem, dorsal root ganglia, et cetera; intermittent lancinating pains and dysesthesias of the extremities; provoked by fever, hot weather, exercise; later, *diffuse vascular damage*—hypertension, renal damage, cardiomegaly, myocardial infarction, strokes; angiokeratomas most prominent periumbilically
   c. **Sulfite oxidase deficiency:** child ~4.5 y/o, retarded since birth, becomes hemiplegic; may have seizures, aphasia, *upward subluxation of lens;* increased level of *sulfite and thiosulfite, S-sulfocysteine* in blood; treatment: ?low-sulfur amino acid diet
   d. Less common causes: *protein C deficiency, Tangier disease, familial hypercholesterolemia, MELAS (mitochondrial myopathy, encephalomyopathy, lactic acidosis, and stroke-like episodes)*
7. *Disorders with personality and behavioral changes*
   a. *Wilson's disease*
   b. *Hallervorden-Spatz pigmentary degeneration*
   c. *Lafora body myoclonic epilepsy*
   d. *Late-onset neuronal ceroid lipofuscinosis (Kufs form)*
   e. *Juvenile and adult Gaucher's (type 3)*
   f. *Some mucopolysaccharidoses*
   g. *Adolescent Schilder's*
   h. *Metachromatic leukodystrophy*
   i. *Adult GM_2 gangliosidosis*
   j. *Mucolipidosis I*
   k. *Non-Wilsonian copper disorder with dementia, spasticity, and paralysis of vertical eye movement*
8. *Mitochondrial disorders:* huge diversity in clinical presentation and age of onset; many, but not all, show elevations of lactate or lactate-pyruvate ratio in blood and CSF, most prominent after exercise, infection, or alcohol ingestion
   a. *Mitochondrial myopathies:* in mildest form may cause only benign proximal weakness, more severe in arms; severe form, fatal infantile myopathy with lactic acidosis; located on 3250 position of mitochondrial genome; muscle tissue with numerous ragged red fibers and absent cytochrome oxidase activity
   b. *Progressive external ophthalmoplegia and Kearns-Sayre syndrome:* progressive ptosis, ophthalmoplegia, no diplopia despite dysconjugate gaze (progressive external ophthalmoplegia); retinitis pigmentosa, ataxia, heart block, elevated CSF protein, sensorineural deafness, seizures, pyramidal signs (Kearns-Sayre syndrome)

   c. Subacute necrotizing encephalomyopathy (Leigh disease): familial or sporadic with wide range of clinical manifestations; onset subacute or abrupt precipitated by fever or surgery; in infants: hypotonia, poor suck, seizures, myoclonic jerks; 2nd-year onset: ataxia, dysarthria, intellectual regression, tonic spasms, episodes of hyperventilation during infections, with periods of apnea, gasping; may be episodic or progressive; pathology: symmetric foci of spongionecrosis, demyelination, gliosis of thalamus, brain stem, spinal cord, and basal ganglia; muscle is histologically normal; *NARP (neuropathy, ataxia, retinitis pigmentosa) syndrome; due to substitution of one amino acid in position 8993, creating error in adenosinetriphosphatase-6 of complex V*

   d. *Congenital lactic acidosis and recurrent ketoacidosis:* consider in types of organic acidemia of unproved genetic etiology; important findings: *acidosis, high lactate, hyperalaninemia; diagnosis by finding fibers in muscle* or by enzyme activity

   e. **Myoclonic epilepsy with ragged red fiber myopathy:** myoclonus in the young most typical feature; seizures are often photosensitive; ataxia worsens progressively eclipsing the myoclonus and seizures; coupled with other mitochondrial features: *deafness, mental decline, optic atrophy, ophthalmoplegia,* cervical lipomas, short stature, neuropathy; familial with maternal inheritance; quantitative burden of mutant DNA related to time of onset and severity; *80% due to point mutation in locus 8344 (lysine tRNA mtDNA mutation)*

   f. **MELAS:** characteristic feature: clinical pattern of focal seizures, which herald a stroke, unique radiologic pattern of cortex and immediate subcortical matter involvement. CT may show numerous low-density regions without clinical correlates; *most with ragged red fibers* but rarely with weakness; 80% mutation at the 3243 site (leucine tRNA mtDNA mutation)

   g. *Leber's hereditary optic neuropathy:* acute: optic nerve hyperemia, vascular tortuosity; chronic: optic atrophy; uncommonly with cardiac conduction abnormalities; painless, initially asymmetric, progresses over weeks to months

III. Neuromuscular Disorders

  A. *Neuropathies*

    1. **HMSN type 1:** *Charcot-Marie-Tooth, peroneal muscular atrophy;* all types generally have insidious clinical onset and *slow progression* from adolescence; rarely, they can present in infancy; *pes cavus and hammer toes* often cause initial complaints; *segmental demyelination and remyelination* occur, resulting in distal muscle atrophy and weakness and tremor and ataxia in some (39%); autosomal *dominant;* genetic subtypes: Ia *(chromosome 17p11) with a duplication or point mutation, Ib (chromosome 1q), Ic (?chromosome 1q),* and *IX-1 (X-linked form with normal conduction but with axonal neuropathy);* in older patients, nerve biopsy shows a hypertrophic *onion bulb* appearance; may have elevated CSF protein; life expectancy is normal

NB: Peroneal muscular atrophy gives the appearance of "champagne bottle legs."

    2. **HMSN type 2a:** autosomal *dominant;* map to *chromosome 1; axonal neuropathy;* milder course compared to type 1; *HMSN type 2b: childhood onset; autosomal recessive*

    3. **HMSN type 3** *(Dejerine Sottas):* autosomal *recessive;* presents at birth; may be a homozygous form due to a *sporadic point mutation;* hypotonia and slow motor development are common in the 1st year; sensory ataxia develops; clubfoot and scoliosis are seen; usually with elevated CSF protein

    4. **HMSN type 4** *(Refsum's):* autosomal *recessive deficiency of phytanic acid oxidase* affects lipid metabolism; onset is 1st to 3rd decade with cerebellar *ataxia, chronic hypertonic neuropathy, and retinitis pigmentosa;* other findings: *night blindness, deafness, ichthyosis,*

cardiac myopathy, hepatosplenomegaly, and increased CSF protein; dietary restriction of phytanic acid (avoiding nuts, spinach, and coffee) is beneficial, as phytanic acid is not produced endogenously; infant and adult forms are seen

5. **Hereditary neuropathy with liability to pressure palsies** *(tomaculous neuropathy):* 10% have *deletion of 17p11.2-13; PMP-22 protein*

NB: Same chromosomal area as Charcot-Marie-Tooth, but in Charcot-Marie-Tooth it is a duplication of the region, whereas in hereditary neuropathy with liability to pressure palsies it is a deletion of the same region.

6. Other neuropathies: *Riley-Day (familial dysautonomia with hyperpyrexia, skin color changes, mild retardation, neuropathy, dysphagia, and postural hypotension); metachromatic leukodystrophy; familiar amyloid*

7. *Polyneuropathies with possible onset in infancy*

Axonal	Familial dysautonomia
	HMSN type 2
	Idiopathic with encephalopathy
	Infantile neuronal degeneration
	Subacute necrotizing encephalopathy (Leigh disease)
Demyelinating	Guillain-Barré syndrome
	Chronic inflammatory demyelinating polyneuropathy
	Congenital hypomyelinating neuropathy
	Globoid cell leukodystrophy
	HMSN type 1
	HMSN type 3
	Metachromatic leukodystrophy

B. *Anterior horn cell/muscle disorders*

1. **Infantile spinal muscular atrophy:** three types, all related to *chromosome 5;* frequency of carriers is 1:60; prenatal screening available

   a. *Werdnig-Hoffman: infantile form; autosomal recessive;* presents at birth with proximal hypotonia and respiratory insufficiency; reduced fetal movement, hypotonia, areflexia, quivering tongue; progressive feeding difficulty and death can occur by age 6 months; muscle biopsy is also diagnostic

   b. *Kugelberg-Welander: chronic form; autosomal recessive or sporadic;* presents after 3 months with pelvic girdle weakness and runs a variable course; mean survival is 30 years

   c. Third form affects primarily the neck and respiratory muscles; presenting with head droop; survival to age 3 years

2. **Neurogenic arthrogryposis:** *sporadic* disease; affects fetus, causing *contractures* by the time of birth; electromyography (EMG) is normal but shows a neuropathic process

3. **Fazio-Londe:** onset in early childhood; *progressive bulbar paralysis, with anterior horn cell involvement*

4. *Glycogen storage diseases:* autosomal *recessive*

   a. **Type 2 (Pompe's):** *deficient acid maltase activity (1,4 glycosidase)* results in glycogen deposition in the anterior horn cells; infantile form presents as *floppy infant with congestive* *heart failure, macroglossia, hepatomegaly; muscle biopsy shows periodic acid–Schiff-positive deposits and vacuolation*

b. **Type 3 (Forbes-Cori):** *debrancher enzyme (1,6 glucosidase) deficiency* associated with hypotonia, hypoglycemia, hepato/cardiomegaly; prognosis is variable; skeletal and cardiac muscles affected

c. **Type 5 (McArdle's):** results from *inactive myophosphorylase;* childhood and adult forms seen; exercise induces painful cramps; *ischemic exercise test shows no lactate production;* biopsy shows periodic acid–Schiff-positive subsarcolemmal blebs or crescents

d. **Tarui's (type 7):** *phosphofructokinase deficiency* results in cramping and fatigue

NB: McArdle's disease and Tarui's disease do not produce lactate in the exercise ischemic test.

e. *Nonmyopathic types:* **type 1** *(von Gierke; deficient glucose-6-phosphate causes neonatal seizures);* **type 4** *(Anderson's; deficiency of 1,4 debrancher enzyme* results in failure to thrive); **type 6** *(Hers'; liver phosphorylase deficiency* results in growth retardation)

5. *Muscular dystrophies*

a. **Paramyotonia congenita:** autosomal *dominant;* defect on *chromosome 17q23.1* affects voltage-gated *Na+ channels;* cause myotonia on exposure to cold; electrolytes are normal; compare to: **myotonia congenita** *(Thomsen's disease)*—autosomal *dominant on chromosome 7; mutation of the chloride channel;* seen at birth, muscle hypertrophy (mini-Hercules); EMG: myotonic discharges

b. **Duchenne's muscular dystrophy:** the *most common* dystrophy, affects boys by age 5; incidence is 1:3,500; 30% mutation rate; *localized to Xp21;* defects in the gene for *dystrophin* results in variable amounts of this essential muscle structural protein; weakness, *pseudohypertrophy of the calf muscles and tendon shortening* are classic; mild MR and cardiac involvement are also present; treatment: prednisone may improve strength and function; creatine phosphokinase (CPK) is elevated; death usually by age 20 years; biopsy: atrophy and hypertrophy, central nuclei, fiber splitting, necrosis, fibrosis, fatty changes, and hyaline fibers; EMG: myopathic units denervation, fibrillation and sharp waves

c. **Becker's dystrophy:** also *X-linked;* but *milder* defect, slower progression

d. **Limb-girdle dystrophy:** autosomal *recessive (chromosome 15), autosomal dominant (chromosome 5), severe childhood autosomal recessive muscular dystrophy (chromosome 13);* slowly progressive proximal weakness: iliopsoas, quadriceps, hamstrings, deltoids, biceps, triceps; facial and extraocular muscles spared; slightly elevated CPK; EMG: myopathic changes; pathology: fiber size variations; fiber splitting; degeneration/regeneration

e. **Fascioscapulohumeral dystrophy:** autosomal *dominant;* on *chromosome 4;* onset at end of the 1st decade; slowly progressive *weakness of facial musculature (Bell's phenomenon); serratus anterior (winging of the scapula) and biceps;* deltoid and forearm muscles preserved (giving *Popeye appearance*); scapuloperoneal form: on chromosome 5; CPK slightly elevated; EMG and pathology: myopathic changes

f. **Congenital muscular dystrophy:** rare; onset at age 2–3 years

g. **Emery-Dreifuss** *(humeroperoneal):* X-linked *recessive;* weakness over biceps, triceps, distal leg; *contractures early, rigid spine, cardiac conduction block*

h. **Oculopharyngeal dystrophy:** common in French-Canadians or Spanish-Americans; autosomal *dominant;* onset in 5th decade, slowly progressive; ptosis first, pharyngeal weakness later; CPK slightly elevated; pathology: myopathic changes, rimmed vacuoles, and intranuclear tubulofilamentous inclusions

i. **Myotonic dystrophy:** autosomal *dominant; CTG triplet repeat* (>50 copies on *chromosome 19q);* related to defective protein kinase and membrane instability; it is a multisystem disease that usually presents in adults (20–40 y/o), not in children; results in facial weakness (ptosis, *fish mouth*), *hatchet face, some MR, posterior capsule cataracts, cardiac disease, diabetes, testicular or ovarian atrophy;* congenital form is severe at birth but improves in 4–6 weeks; *EMG: spontaneous bursts of high frequency amplitude discharges;* pathology: type 1 fiber hypertrophy and *ring fibers;* congenital myotonic dystrophy in children of mothers with myotonic dystrophy

6. *Myopathies*
    a. **Nemaline:** autosomal *recessive on chromosome 1; occasionally autosomal dominant;* nonprogressive; also high-arched palate, small jaw and thin face; Marfanoid features, cardiomyopathy; CPK is normal; type 1 fiber predominance with Z-line rods
    b. **Central core:** autosomal *recessive on chromosome 19;* floppy baby, motor delay, spine abnormalities, proximal, nonprogressive; CPK is normal; type 1 fibers have *central pallor; on electron microscopy: core lacks mitochondria*
    c. **Myotubular** *(centronuclear): X-linked recessive;* age of onset is 5–30 years; involvement of ocular, facial, and distal muscle; variable progression; CPK is normal or mildly increased; biopsy: central nuclei with halos and type 1 fiber atrophy
    d. **Dermatomyositis:** *female > male; skin lesions: diffuse erythema, maculopapular eruption, heliotrope rash, eczematoid dermatitis of extensor surface joints;* carcinoma in 15% (affects more adults than children); lab: CPK high, aldolase high, IgG and IgA levels may be elevated; myoglobinuria; inflammatory muscle changes; sometimes tissue calcification
    e. **Hypokalemic periodic paralysis:** may be autosomal *dominant or associated with thyrotoxicosis;* age between 10 and 20 years; attacks are frequent and usually severe, lasting for hours to days; trigger: rest, cold, stress; low serum K^+; *calcium channelopathy;* treatment: acetazolamide, K^+ replacement

NB: The mutation in hypokalemic paralysis is in the dihydropyridine receptor. There is vacuolization of the muscle fibers during and immediately after the attacks.

    f. **Hyperkalemic periodic paralysis:** autosomal *dominant;* age between 10 and 20 years; attacks are frequent with moderate severity lasting minutes to hours; triggers: rest, cold, hunger; high serum K^+, occasional myotonia, *Na$^+$ channelopathy;* treatment: acetazolamide, low potassium

NB: In contrast to hypokalemic periodic paralysis, hyperkalemic periodic paralysis may show myotonic discharges in EMG. The mutation is in the voltage-gated sodium channel.

C. *Neuromuscular junction disorders*
    1. **Neonatal (transient) myasthenia:** *transient disorder seen in 15% of infants born to mothers with myasthenia gravis; due to placental transfer of acetylcholine receptor (AChR) antibodies;* symptoms: intrauterine hypotonia; may be born with arthrogryposis; usually evident within 24 hours of life, lasting for 18 days (range, 5 days to 2 months); may need exchange transfusion and/or neostigmine, 0.1 mg intramuscularly before feeding
    2. **Congenital myasthenia:** heterogeneous disorder due to *genetic defects in the presynaptic (mostly autosomal recessive) and postsynaptic (mostly autosomal recessive, some autosomal dominant [slow channel syndrome]) neuromuscular junction;* not associated with antibodies to AChR; symptoms: usually begin in the neonatal period, ocular, bulbar, respiratory weakness, worse with crying or activity; ptosis, ophthalmoplegia, or ophthalmoparesis; diagnosis: positive family history in some, Tensilon® (edrophonium chloride) test negative in most, *AChR is negative,* EMG: decremental response and increased jitter

NB: In contrast to neonatal myasthenia, congenital myasthenia is not an autoimmune disorder.

    3. **Juvenile myasthenia:** *sporadic, autoimmune; due to antibodies to AChR; similar to adult myasthenia gravis;* special characteristics: less often have detectable AChR antibodies, have other autoimmune disorders such as diabetes mellitus/rheumatoidarthritis/asthma/thyroid disease, also have nonautoimmune disease such as epilepsy/neoplasm; thymectomy recommended for moderate to severe cases; *little to no correlation with thymus pathology and response to surgery (77% with hyperplasia, 16% normal, and 3% thymoma)*

IV. Infections

  A. *Perinatal infections (TORCH [toxoplasmosis, other infections, rubella, cytomegalovirus infection, and herpes simplex])*

    1. **Toxoplasmosis:** protozoan comes from *cat feces or uncooked meat;* transmission *is least likely in the 1st trimester; hydrocephalus, chorioretinitis, granulomatous meningoencephalitis, late periventricular and cortical calcification,* seizures, MR, hepatosplenomegaly, thrombocytopenia; diagnosis by enzyme-linked immunosorbent assay; CT for congenital toxoplasmosis: periventricular calcifications; treatment: sulfadiazine, pyrimethamine and folate

    2. **Rubella:** fetus is most susceptible in the 1st trimester; clinical findings: *MR, heart disease, cataracts, deafness, microgyria/-cephaly, seizures, spasticity*

    3. **Cytomegalovirus:** infection occurs transplacentally in the 2nd to 3rd trimester, and reinfection can occur at the time of birth; multifocal necrosis, periventricular calcification, and hydrocephalus are seen; clinical findings: MR, microcephaly, rash, hepatosplenomegaly, jaundice, and chorioretinitis; treatment: acyclovir/ganciclovir

NB: The most common sequela after congenital cytomegalovirus infection is deafness.

    4. **Herpes simplex virus (type 2;** *adult encephalitides are usually type 1*): infection is usually due to exposure at birth and may not be recognized by age 1–3 weeks; there is a high risk (35–50%) with primary (active) maternal infection and lower risk (3–5%) with recurrent maternal infection; predilection is for the temporal lobes, insula, cingulate gyrus; clinically: *cyanosis/respiratory distress, jaundice, fever, microcephaly, periventricular calcification;* treatment: acyclovir or vidarabine; pathology: *Cowdry type A inclusions*

    5. **Congenital syphilis:** etiology: *Treponema pallidum;* meningovascular form may present as hydrocephalus; general paresis can occur by age 10 years; tabes dorsalis is rare in the young

  B. *Other viruses*

    1. **Coxsackie A:** encephalitis, herpangina, rash (usually ages 5–9 years during summer)

    2. **Coxsackie B:** pleurodynia and encephalitis

    3. **Echovirus**: meningitis, morbilliform rash (summer and fall months)

    4. **Human immunodeficiency virus:** CNS signs (motor and cognitive) occur in 50–90% of infected children; 10% develop opportunistic infection; 30% develop bacterial infections; seizures are common, stroke in 10%; mothers treated with zidovudine (AZT) have a lower transmission rate

    5. **Measles:** encephalitis can occur in children <10 y/o with low mortality; pathology: multinucleated giant cells, intranuclear and intracytoplasmic inclusions are present

    6. **Subacute sclerosing panencephalitis:** rare but often *fatal complication of measles (rubeola);* onset occurs at age 5–15 years in children with previous rubeola infection; personality changes, poor school performance, macular changes, progress to myoclonus, ataxia, spasticity, dementia; treatment is with γ-globulin or intrathecal interferon-α;

pathology: *rod cells and Cowdry type A nuclear inclusions,* patchy demyelination and gliosis, CSF increased IgG and measles antibodies, + oligoclonal bands; *EEG: periodic sharp wave complexes (like burst suppression)*

7. **Mumps:** encephalitis presents 2–10 days *after parotitis and orchitis;* note: parotitis and encephalitis can also occur with coxsackie A, cytomegalovirus, Epstein-Barr virus, and lymphocytic choriomeningitis

8. **Poliomyelitis:** etiology: *enterovirus (picornavirus), coxsackie, echovirus;* rare in the United States with widespread use of vaccine; transmission: feco-oral; clinical: *mild flu-like illness in 95% with no CNS involvement;* nonparalytic: flu-like illness, muscle pains, aseptic meningitis; paralytic: rapid limb and bulbar weakness, fasciculations, most patients recover completely, some with residual weakness (atrophied limb); pathology: *neuronophagia; immune response in thalamus, hypothalamus, cranial nerve motor nuclei, anterior horn and cerebellar nuclei, Cowdry B inclusions in the anterior horn cells*

9. **Reye syndrome:** *after varicella or influenza B infection and use of salicylates,* acute encephalopathy develops; results in hypoglycemia, hyperammonemia, increased intracranial pressure, cerebral edema and seizures; treatment: glucose, hyperventilation, fluid restriction, and mannitol; mortality is high unless caught early

C. *Bacterial*
1. Meningitis risk increases with prematurity, maternal infection, complicated delivery; subdural effusion is a common complication of purulent meningitis; etiology: *newborns up to 1 year (Enterobacter coli, group B streptococcus), 6 months to 1 year (Haemophilus influenzae, pneumococcus, meningococcus), post-traumatic (pneumococcus), abscess (staphylococcus, streptococcus, pneumococcus)*

NB: Frontal lobe abscesses are more likely contaminated with streptococcus; in the temporal lobe, it is more likely polymicrobial.

2. **Sydenham's chorea:** initial manifestation: usually disturbance in school function, daydreaming, fidgety, inattentiveness, and increased emotional lability; onset of chorea is rather sudden, *lag time between streptococcal infection and chorea averages 6 months;* serologic evidence is absent in one-third of patients; risk of developing carditis with Sydenham's chorea is 30–50%; *recurrent episodes of chorea are most common at the time of pregnancy in female patients;* lab: *elevated erythrocyte sedimentation rate or C-reactive protein, prolonged PR interval;* treatment for chorea: dopamine receptor blocking agents such as *haloperidol, pimozide, phenothiazines, or amantadine;* for acute rheumatic fever: *penicillin V, 400,000 U (250 mg) tid for 10 days followed by prophylaxis (benzathine penicillin G, 1.2 million U intramuscularly every 3–4 weeks or penicillin V, 250 mg orally bid or sulfisoxazole, 0.5–1.0 g orally qd)*
   a. Differential diagnosis: phenothiazine reactions, tics, Huntington's disease, Wilson's disease, benign paroxysmal choreoathetosis, lupus, polyarteritis and other vasculopathies, hyperparathyroidism, neoplastic lesions of the basal ganglia, and ataxia-telangiectasia
   b. *Jones criteria for acute rheumatic fever:* diagnosis—*two major manifestations or one major and two minor manifestations* plus evidence of streptococcal infection
      i. Major manifestations: *carditis, polyarthritis, chorea, erythema marginatum, subcutaneous nodules*
      ii. Minor manifestations: arthralgia, fever, increased erythrocyte sedimentation rate, increased C-reactive protein, increased PR interval
      iii. Supporting evidence of streptococcus group A infection: throat culture or rapid streptococcus antigen screen, high or rising streptococcus antibody titer

V. Anoxic-Ischemic Injury/Toxins

A. *Perinatal injury:* 90% are prenatal or at delivery; *ulegyria:* shrunken necrotic "mush-rooms" of cortex remaining (sulcal loss is greatest); *hydranencephaly:* membranous tissue in a vascular territory suggests perinatal ischemia; cerebral hemiatrophy: multiple etiologies can result in this unilateral hydrocephalus ex-vacuo; *status marmoratus (état marbré):* marbled pattern of gray matter loss and abnormal myelin overgrowth especially in the basal ganglia and thalamus

B. *Intraventricular hemorrhage:* due to hemodynamic instability or hypoxia in premature infants, occurring at the subependymal germinal matrix (neuroectoderm) where veins are fragile; rupture into the ventricles increases the risk of subsequent hydrocephalus; bleed itself produces little morbidity; development can be gradual and asymmetric, but usually occurs by day 3; bulging of fontanelles and sudden decline are indicators; 44% survive with residual sequelae; subarachnoid hemorrhage due to anoxia is less common than that due to trauma

NB: In the premature infant, intracerebral hemorrhage is more likely at the subependymal germinal matrix, but in the term infant is more likely in the choroid plexus.

C. *Toxins*
1. **Kernicterus:** *(bilirubinemia) is usually from ABO and Rh incompatibility,* especially in the premature, hypoxic, acidotic, or septic newborns; it can affect the pallidum, substantia nigra, cranial nerves III, VIII, and XII selectively or be diffuse, staining neurons yellow
2. **Fetal alcohol syndrome:** growth delay, small face, MR, abnormal cortical lamination, small cerebrum and brain stem; alcohol is also associated with stillbirth, prematurity, and low birth weight
3. **Thallium:** axonal neuropathy, vomiting, diarrhea, headache, and confusion
4. **NB: Lead:** irritability, motor regression and encephalopathy; testing shows *positive urine coproporphyrin III and basophilic stippling of red blood cells;* treatment: oral chelation with dimercaptosuccinic acid; lead paint may have been used in homes until 1973
5. **Arsenic:** *Mees' lines* are seen in the nail bed
6. **Mercury (organic):** in utero exposure at Minamata resulted in severe MR, cerebral > cerebellar atrophy
7. **Botulism:** spores can be found in honey; results in hypotonia, mydriasis, and apnea

VI. Neurophakomatosis

A. **NB: Neurofibromatosis type 1 (NF1):** autosomal *dominant; chromosome band 17q11.2;* spontaneous mutations occur in approximately 50% of patients; the most common genetic disorder of the nervous system: 1 in 3,000 people; chromosome 17 encodes the tumor suppressor *neurofibromin;* the loss of neurofibromin, may contribute to tumor progression
1. *National Institutes of Health criteria for NF1*
   a. *Café au lait macules: six or more*
   b. *Two or more neurofibromas or one plexiform neurofibroma (neurofibromas often multiple, nonpainful, intermingled with nerves, and can become malignant)*
   c. *Axillary or inguinal freckling*
   d. *Optic glioma*
   e. *Lisch nodules (iris hamartomas)*
   f. *Dysplasia or thinning of long bone cortex*
   g. *First-degree relative with NF1*

2. Neurologic complications of NF1: *optic gliomas are the most common*, occur in approximately 15% of patients; other associated CNS neoplasms are *astrocytomas, vestibular schwannomas (acoustic neuroma), and, less often, ependymomas and meningiomas;* hydrocephalus, seizures, learning disabilities; bilateral optic nerve gliomas; congenital *glaucoma; pheochromocytoma (0.1–5.7%) or renal artery stenosis;* growth hormone deficiency, short stature, and precocious puberty have been reported in patients with NF1

B. **Neurofibromatosis type 2 (NF2)** *(central type): autosomal dominant; chromosome 22q11-13.1; this gene codes for schwannomin/merlin proteins,* which may affect tumor suppressor activity at the cell membrane level; spontaneous mutations exists in 50–70% of patients; NF2 is *less common* than NF1, occurring in 1 in 35,000; paucity of cutaneous lesions
   1. *Diagnostic criteria for NF2*
      a. *Bilateral vestibular schwannomas (visualized with CT scan or MRI)*
      b. *A first-degree relative with the disease plus a unilateral vestibular schwannoma before 30 y/o*
      c. *Any two of the following: neurofibroma, meningioma, glioma, schwannoma, or juvenile posterior subcapsular opacity*
   2. Complications of NF2: ocular manifestations include *juvenile posterior subcapsular lenticular opacity, retinal hamartomas, optic disc glioma, and optic nerve meningioma; intracranial and spinal meningiomas, astrocytomas, and ependymomas;* subcutaneous schwannomas are superficial-raised papules with overlying pigment and hair

C. **Tuberous sclerosis (TS):** autosomal *dominant;* two gene loci have been identified: *chromosome 9q34, which codes for a protein (termed* hamartin) and is a probable tumor suppressor gene, and *chromosome 16q13.3, which codes for an amino acid protein (termed* tuberin): triad of MR, epilepsy, and adenoma sebaceum is characteristic
   1. Neurologic complications of TS
      a. *Infantile spasms* (EEG may show *hypsarrhythmia*): generalized tonic-clonic, complex partial, and myoclonic seizures are the most common forms; of children with infantile spasms, 10% have TS
      b. *Cortical tubers:* potato-like nodules of glial proliferation occurring in the cortex, ganglia, or ventricle walls; often calcified
      c. Other CNS findings include *subependymal hamartomas, paraventricular calcifications, or "candle gutterings," and giant cell astrocytomas*
   2. Cutaneous presentation of TS
      a. Congenital *ash-leaf hypopigmented macules:* in 87% of patients
      b. *Confetti macules:* 1–3 mm, hypopigmented, on the pretibial area
      c. *Shagreen patch* (subepidermal fibrous patches): 1–10 cm, flat, flesh-colored plaque, most often in the lumbosacral region; orange-peel appearance
      d. *Facial angiofibromas* (adenoma sebaceum): diagnostic of TS, usually appear in children aged 4–10 years
      e. Koenen tumors: on nail plates *(ungual fibroma)* appear at puberty
   3. Other complications of TS: retinal hamartomas (phacomata); gingival fibromas; renal cysts; phalangeal cysts and periosteal thickening; lung cysts, pulmonary lymphangiomyomatosis; rhabdomyomas occur in 50% of patients; angiomyolipomas; *renal failure* the most common cause of death

NB: Giant cell astrocytomas are nonmalignant and treatable but may cause obstruction of the foramen of Monroe.

D. **Sturge-Weber syndrome:** *trigeminocranial angiomatosis with cerebral calcification; not an inherited disorder* but with higher prevalence among relatives; congenital facial *port-wine* *stains and leptomeningeal angiomatosis;* present clinically as epilepsy, MR, and hemiplegia; complications: ocular complications in 30–60% of patients; *glaucoma* can begin at age 2 years; the most common ocular manifestation is diffuse choroidal angioma; parenchymal calcifications (*train tracks* on radiographs by age 2 years) are classic

E. **Ataxia-telangiectasia** *(Louis-Bar syndrome):* autosomal *recessive; chromosome 11q22-23;* 1 in 80,000 live births; characterized by progressive cerebellar *ataxia, oculocutaneous telangiectasia, abnormalities in cellular and humoral immunity, and recurrent viral and bacterial infections*

   1. Neurologic manifestations: cerebellar ataxia at 2 y/o, nystagmus; chorea, athetosis, dystonia, oculomotor apraxia, impassive facies; decreased deep tendon reflexes, and distal muscular atrophy; intelligence progressively deteriorates; polyneuropathy
   2. Other manifestations: immunodeficiency (thymic hypoplasia); patients *lack helper T cells, but suppressor T cells are normal; IgA is absent in 75% of patients, IgE in 85%, IgG is low;* α-*fetoprotein and carcinoembryonic antigen are elevated;* ovarian agenesis, testicular hypoplasia, and insulin-resistant diabetes; malignant neoplasms in 10–15% of patients; most common are lymphoreticular neoplasm and leukemia; death by 2nd decade from neoplasia or infection
   3. Cutaneous manifestations: telangiectasias develop at age 3–6 years: first on the bulbar conjunctiva (red eyes) and ears and later on the flexor surface of the arms, eyelids, malar area of the face, and upper chest; granulomas, café au lait macules, graying hair, and progeria can occur

F. **Incontinentia pigmenti:** *X-linked dominant disorder; lethal to male* patients; few affected males have been documented, and most had Klinefelter syndrome (47,XXY); *skin lesions arranged in a linear pattern (begin as linear bullous lesions and progress to hyperkeratosis and hyperpigmentation with linear streaks and whorls),* slate-grey pigmentation, alopecia, ocular defects, dental, and neurologic abnormalities; >700 cases have been reported; pathology: atrophy, microgyria, focal necrosis in white matter; lab: eosinophilia

   1. Complications: characterized by seizures, MR, and generalized spasticity, cortical blindness in 15–30% of patients; the findings include cerebral ischemia, cerebral edema, brain atrophy, and gyral dysplasia
   2. Ocular manifestations include *strabismus, cataracts, retinal detachments, optic atrophy, and vitreous hemorrhage*

G. **Osler-Weber-Rendu disease** *(hereditary hemorrhagic telangiectasia; familiar telangiectasia):* autosomal *dominant; chromosome 9q33-q34 (endoglin gene);* 1 in 100,000 births; neurologic complications include vascular lesions, including telangiectasias, arteriovenous malformations, and aneurysms of the brain and/or spinal cord, cerebellar ataxia, varying degrees of MR, and possible hearing loss; multiple telangiectasias on the face, hands, a white forelock, and depigmented patches with spots of hyperpigmentation, epistaxis

H. **von Hippel-Lindau syndrome** *(hemangioblastoma of the cerebellum): autosomal dominant; chromosome 3; cerebellar hemangioblastomas (obstructive hydrocephalus); retinal hemangioblastomas; renal cell carcinoma; hepatic, pancreatic cysts; polycythemia (increased erythropoietin); pheochromocytomas;* usually presents in adults

I. **Sneddon syndrome:** characterized by *livedo reticularis and multiple strokes* resulting in dementia; antiphospholipid antibodies and anti-β$_2$-glycoprotein antibodies also have been detected in some patients with this disorder; not usually a pediatric disorder but a neurocutaneous syndrome

J. **Chediak-Higashi syndrome:** autosomal *recessive; defective pigmentation and peripheral neuropathy*

VII. Table of differential diagnoses

Chorea	Sydenham's chorea
	Huntington's chorea
	Wilson's disease
	Fahr's disease
	Hallervorden-Spatz
	Ramsay-Hunt (dentatorubral atrophy)
	Neuroaxonal dystrophy
	Lesch-Nyhan
	Pelizaeus-Merzbacher
	Metabolic: hyper-/hypothyroidism or /parathyroidism
	Drug: phenytoin; phenothiazines; lithium; amphetamine; oral contraceptives
	Toxins: mercury, carbon monoxide
Dystonia	Huntington's chorea
	Wilson's disease
	Fahr's disease
	Hallervorden-Spatz
	Ceroid lipofuscinosis
	Sea-blue histiocytosis
	Leigh disease
	GM_1/GM_2 gangliosidosis
	Dystonia musculorum deformans
	Dopamine-responsive dystonia
	Tumors
	Trauma
	Encephalitis
Ataxia, acute	Acute cerebellar ataxia
	Occult neuroblastoma
	Traumatic posterior fossa subdural/epidural
	Fischer variant of Guillain-Barré syndrome
	Basilar migraine (Bickerstaff)
	Metabolic: maple syrup urine disease, Hartnup's, pyruvate decarboxylase deficiency, argininosuccinic aciduria, hypothyroidism
	Acute intermittent familial ataxia
	Childhood multiple sclerosis/Schilder's disease
	Leigh disease

Ataxia, chronic, nonprogressive	Cerebellar hypoplasia
	Arnold-Chiari
	Dandy-Walker
	Cerebral palsy
Ataxia, progressive	Tumors: medulloblastoma, cerebellar astrocytoma
	Malformations: Arnold-Chiari, posterior fossa cyst
	Spinocerebellar ataxias, e.g., Friedreich's ataxia, Roussy-Levy (form of HMSN type 1)
	Ataxia-telangiectasia
	Bassen-Kornzweig
	Refsum's
	Metachromatic leukodystrophy
	Tay-Sachs
	Maple syrup urine disease
Myoclonus	Wilson's disease
	Hallervorden-Spatz
	Lafora body disease
	Ceroid lipofuscinosis
	Ramsay-Hunt (dyssynergia cerebellaris myoclonica)
	Ataxia-telangiectasia
	Subacute sclerosing panencephalitis
	Herpes simplex virus
	Herpes zoster
	Human immunodeficiency virus
	Hypoglycemia
	Hypoxia
	Uremia
	Hepatic failure
	Hyponatremia
	Bismuth toxicity
	Paraneoplastic (opsoclonus-myoclonus)
Floppy infant	*Cerebral lesion:* atonic cerebral palsy, Prader-Willi, Down syndrome, storage/amino acid disorders
	Cord lesion: transection during breech delivery, myelopathy from umbilical artery catheters, spina bifida, dysraphism
	Anterior horn cell: Werdnig-Hoffman, Kugelberger-Welander, Pompe's, poliomyelitis
	Peripheral nerves: metachromatic leukodystrophy, Krabbe's

Neuromuscular junction: botulism, aminoglycosides, hypermagnesemia (from maternal treatment of eclampsia)

Muscle: nemaline, core, myotubular myopathy, congenital muscular dystrophy

Systemic: hypercalcemia, hypothyroidism, renal acidosis, celiac, cystic fibrosis, Marfan, Ehlers-Danlos

Benign: Amyotonia congenita (diagnosis of exclusion)

ADDITIONAL NOTES

Subspecialties

CHAPTER 12

Neurourology

I. Anatomy and Nerve Supply: micturition, an intricate and well-coordinated activity, is *primarily a parasympathetic function;* the sympathetic system is involved in urine storage and bladder capacity (provided by the hypogastric nerves with cell bodies at the T11–L2 segment of the intermediolateral column); volitional control is exerted through the corticospinal pathways and spinal nerves innervating the external sphincter, periurethral muscles, and other abdominal and pelvic muscles; cerebral cortex, basal ganglia, cerebellum, and brain stem pontine detrusor nuclei exert suprasegmental influence over the sacral spinal nuclei.

NB: The parasympathetic nerves at the S2–S4 dorsal roots mediate the urge to urinate.

    A. *1st circuit:* connects the *dorsomedial frontal lobe to the pontine detrusor nucleus* (with additional connections to the basal ganglia); provides *volitional control*

    B. *2nd circuit:* the *spinobulbospinal pathway;* a reflex arc that starts in the sensory nerves of the bladder and projects to the pontine detrusor nucleus and its outflow connections to the spinal sacral motor nuclei that make up the detrusor motor axons; constitutes the parasympathetic innervation; brain stem control over micturition

    C. *3rd circuit:* a spinal segmental reflex arc; afferents from the detrusor muscles that synapse with the cells in the pudendal nucleus to the striated sphincter muscles

    D. *4th circuit:* supraspinal component; afferents running in the dorsal nerve of the penis and the posterior columns to the cortex and efferents through the corticospinal tracts to the sacral motor neurons; also provides voluntary control (like the 1st circuit)

NB: The anterior cingulate gyrus has an inhibitory influence on the micturition reflex.

II. Clinical Evaluation

    A. *History:* patient should be questioned regarding urinary incontinence, pattern of incontinence, changes in urinary habits, frequency and urgency of urination, desire to void, ability to initiate and terminate urination, force of urinary stream, urine volume, and sensations associated with urination

    B. *Examination*

        1. *Frontal lobe lesions and suprasegmental spinal cord lesions:* increased frequency and urgency of urination with reduced bladder capacity; bladder sensation may be preserved in incomplete spinal cord lesions; neurogenic bladder

2. *Lower spinal cord lesions*

Feature	Conus medullaris	Cauda equina
Location	S3–Cocc 1	L3–Cocc 1 roots
Onset	Often sudden and bilateral	Usually gradual and unilateral
Motor	Mild dysfunction; fasciculations may be present	Marked dysfunction; fasciculations are rare
Sensory	Symmetric, bilateral saddle-type distribution; mild pain if present	Asymmetric, unilateral saddle-type distribution; radicular pain may be present
Reflexes	Variable loss of Achilles' tendon reflexes	Variable loss of patellar and Achilles' tendon reflexes
Bladder	Paralytic, atonic bladder with increased capacity, incontinence	Paralytic, atonic bladder with increased capacity, incontinence, variable severity
Rectum	Patulous anus, decreased sphincter tone	Patulous anus, decreased sphincter tone, variable severity

NB: In cauda equina lesions, if the motor nerves are preferentially involved, volitional voiding may be severely compromised, although bladder sensation may be largely preserved (motor paralytic bladder).

   C. **Lab evaluation:** magnetic resonance imaging (MRI) of the spine, and sometimes the brain, may be essential in the workup; bladder neck obstruction must be excluded (especially in motor paralytic type)

     1. *Urine studies:* urinalysis and urine culture; patients often with associated urinary tract infection

     2. *Renal function studies:* blood urea nitrogen, creatinine, creatinine clearance, glomerular filtration rate; to detect renal impairment intravenous pyelography: useful for patient with neurogenic bladder dysfunction

     3. *Urodynamic studies*

       a. *Cystometry:* provides information about the pressure-column relationship on filling (bladder compliance), bladder capacity, volume at first sensation and at urge to void, voiding pressure, and the presence of uninhibited detrusor contractions

NB: Normal adult bladder: can usually be filled with 500 mL of fluid without the pressure rising >10 cm of water; urodynamic findings in various types of neurogenic bladder.

Spastic bladder	Decreased capacity
	Reduced compliance
	Uninhibited detrusor contractions
Atonic bladder	Increased capacity
	Increased compliance
	Low voiding pressure and flow rate
Sphincter dyssynergia	Fluctuating voiding pressure
	Intermittent flow rate

b. *Micturating cystourethrogram:* often combined with cystometry; sphincter dyssynergia, position and opening of the bladder neck, urethral anomaly, stricture and ureteric reflux can be visualized

c. *Cystourethroscopy:* assess the structural integrity of the lower urinary system (urethra, bladder, ureteral orifices); not useful for functional disorders

d. *Retrograde urethrography:* supplement to cystourethrography for delineation of urethral strictures, valves, diverticula, and false passages

4. *Neurophysiologic studies:* sphincter and pelvic floor electromyography (EMG); detecting denervation potentials in selected muscles in lesions of the anterior horn cells; pudendal nerve conduction velocity and terminal latency are abnormal in neuropathic etiologies

III. Common Etiologies

Urinary incontinence with urgency	Alzheimer's disease
	Parkinson's disease
	Myxedema
	Hydrocephalus
	Bilateral frontal lobe lesions
	Parasagittal tumors
	Multiple sclerosis
	Transverse myelitis
	Cervical spondylosis
	Spinal cord injuries
	Spinal cord tumors
	Syphilis
	Sacral agenesis
	Tethered cord syndrome
	Myelomeningocele
	Cystitis (non-neurologic etiology)
Atonic bladder	Acute spinal shock
	Acute transverse myelitis
	Conus medullaris lesions
	Cauda equina lesions
	Peripheral neuropathy
	Diabetes mellitus
	Alcoholic neuropathy
	Heavy metal toxicity
	Guillain-Barré syndrome (GBS)
	Amyloid neuropathy
	Tabes dorsalis

Multiple systems atrophy

Friedreich's ataxia

Pelvic radiation

Acute intoxications, such as alcohol

Plexopathy

IV. Management
A. *Urinary incontinence with urgency*
1. *Bladder training:* timed bladder emptying, intermittent catheterization, biofeedback techniques
2. *Pharmacotherapy:* anticholinergics (propantheline bromide, glycopyrrolate), musculotropics (oxybutynin, flavoxate, dicyclomine), tolterodine, β-adrenergic agonists (terbutaline), tricyclic antidepressants (imipramine)

NB: In patients with detrussor hyperreflexia without outlet obstruction or urinary retention, anticholinergic drugs, including oxybutinin, are the most appropriate treatment. If retention occurs, this should be combined with intermittent self-catheterization.

3. *Surgical:* dorsal root rhizotomy, selective sacral root rhizotomy, peripheral bladder denervation, cystoplasty
B. *Atonic bladder with overflow incontinence*
1. Crede's maneuver or Valsalva's maneuver
2. Intermittent self-catheterization
3. Pharmacotherapy: bethanecol
C. *Detrusor sphincter dyssynergia:* the external urethral sphincter fails to relax when there is constriction of the detrusor muscles during voiding; often with increased residual volume (**NB:** normal accepted residual volume is 100 mL) with low flow and an intermittent pattern of voiding; urodynamic studies (cystometry) are useful in diagnosis

V. Sexual Dysfunction: manifested by diminished libido, impaired penile erection, or failure to ejaculate; psychogenic causes are common (depression and anxiety are the most common causes of organic sexual dysfunction); other causes include vascular, endocrine, and neurologic (somatic, sympathetic, and parasympathetic) abnormalities
A. *Anatomy*
1. *Somatic motor and sensory nerve supply:* pudendal nerve carries motor and sensory fibers that innervate the penis and clitoris; motor fibers arise from the nucleus of Onufrowicz (Onuf's nucleus) at the S2–S4 level; three pudendal nerve branches: inferior rectal nerve (innervates external anal sphincter), perineal nerve (supplies external urethral sphincter; bulbocavernosus muscles; other perineal muscles; skin of the perineum, scrotum, labia), and dorsal sensory nerve of the penis or clitoris
2. *Parasympathetic nerve supply:* cell bodies in the sacral cord; preganglionic fibers travel with roots S2–S4, join inferior hypogastric plexus, innervate erectile penile and clitoral tissues, smooth muscles in the urethra, seminal vesicles and prostate, vagina and uterus
3. *Sympathetic nerve supply:* from the intermediolateral cell column in the lower thoracic and upper lumbar spinal cord; innervates the same structures as do the parasympathetic nerves

B. *Etiologies*

Diminished libido	Chronic ill health
	Addison's disease
	Hypothyroidism
	Excessive estrogen in males
	Chronic hepatic disease
	Drugs: reserpine, propranolol, cimetidine, tricyclic antidepressant, selective serotonin reuptake inhibitor, monoamine oxidase inhibitor, sedatives, and narcotics
	Alcohol
	Depression
	Anxiety
Erectile impotence	Conus medullaris lesions
	Cauda equina lesions
	Spinal cord injury
	Myelopathy
	Multiple sclerosis
	Peripheral neuropathy
	Diabetes
	Amyloid neuropathy
	Sacral plexus lesions
	Multiple systems atrophy
	Pure autonomic failure
	Hyperprolactinemia
	Drugs: antihypertensive, anticholinergics, antipsychotics, antihistamines
	Alcohol
	Syphilis
	Arteriosclerosis
	Excessive venous leakage
	Depression
	Anxiety

C. *Lab evaluation*
1. *Endocrine:* fasting blood sugar, oral glucose tolerance test, liver function tests, thyroid function tests, prolactin levels, testosterone levels
2. *Neurophysiologic tests:* sleep studies, electromyography, somatosensory-evoked potentials (some cases of myelopathy)

3. *Vascular studies:* low doses of vasoactive agents (e.g., papaverine) into the corpora cavernosa (response to vasoactive agents is poor in vascular etiologies); may consider arteriography of the major leg and pelvic muscles

4. *Psychiatric evaluation*

D. **Treatment:** endocrine, metabolic, vascular, and psychogenic etiologies must be treated; others: cavernosal unstriated muscle relaxant injection, penile implants, sacral root stimulation, pharmacologic treatment (i.e., sildenafil, etc.)

ADDITIONAL NOTES

CHAPTER 13

Neuro-ophthalmology

I. Anatomy and Examination

A. *Photoreceptors*
1. *Rods:* use *rhodopsin* pigment; mediate *light perception*
2. *Cones:* use *iodopsin* pigment; mediate *color vision*

B. **Eyelids**
1. *Three muscles control lid position*
   a. *Levator palpebrae superioris*
      i. Main elevator of the upper lid
      ii. Innervated by the superior division of cranial nerve (CN) III
      iii. Right and left levators originate from the caudal central nucleus
   b. *Muller's muscle:* upper and lower eyelids; innervated by sympathetic fibers
   c. *Orbicularis oculi:* closes eyelids; innervated mainly by ipsilateral CN VII

C. **Ocular muscles**
1. *Horizontal eye movement*
   a. Lateral rectus—abducts the eye
   b. Medial rectus—adducts the eye
   c. Superior oblique—depresses the eye
   d. Inferior oblique—elevates eye
2. *Torsional eye movement:* superior muscles produce intorsion (superior oblique muscle) and the inferior eye muscles produce extorsion (inferior oblique muscle)
3. When eye is turned outward, eye depressor is inferior rectus, and when turned inward, is superior oblique

D. *Ocular motor nerves*
1. *Oculomotor nerve (CN III)*
   a. Innervates: superior rectus, inferior rectus, medial rectus, inferior oblique, levator palpebrae superioris, iris sphincter, ciliary muscle (required for focusing on near objects)
   b. Controls all adduction, extorsion, and elevation of the eye; most depression; and contributes to intorsion through the secondary action of the superior rectus
   c. Edinger-Westphal nucleus: rostral part of CN III, supplies the iris sphincter and ciliary muscle
2. *Trochlear nerve (CN IV):* innervates: superior oblique; intorsion, particularly during abduction
3. *Abducens nerve (CN VI):* innervates: lateral rectus muscle; eye abduction

E. *Oculomotor systems*
1. *Vestibulo-ocular response system*
   a. Three semicircular canals
      i. Resting firing rate increased by acceleration/rotation of the head
      ii. Canal function is initiated by head rotation toward it
      iii. Each canal works in tandem with one on the opposite side

        iv. Generate compensatory eye movements in the direction opposite the head motion to keep the eye stable

        v. Project through the vestibular component of CN VIII

    b. *Otoliths*

        i. *Also component of the vestibular system*

        ii. *Saccule and utricle consist of maculae embedded in a gelatinous substance with calcium crystals*

        iii. *Detect linear accelerations of the head*

  2. *Optokinetic response*

    a. Main function is to hold images steady on the retina during sustained head movement

    b. Precise pathways are unknown but likely associated with *pathways for smooth pursuit extending from visual association areas (Brodmann's 18 and 19) to the horizontal pontine gaze center*

    c. Smooth eye movement generated when large portions of the visual scene move across the retina, which usually happens when the head is moving

    d. Generates a *jerk nystagmus with the slow phase in the direction of stripe motion*

    e. Vestibulo-ocular response works together with optokinetic response: vestibulo-ocular response: rapid head rotation >0.5 Hz; optokinetic response: slower rotations

    f. *Pursuit*

        i. *Main function is to hold an object of interest on the fovea*

        ii. *Motion-sensitive regions of the extrastriate cortex, occipitoparietal cortex, and the frontal eye fields*

        iii. Involved in horizontal ipsilateral pursuit

    g. *Saccades*

        i. Main function is to bring objects of interest onto the fovea

        ii. Saccades are quick eye movements that shift gaze from one object to another

        iii. Involve parietal and frontal eye fields

        iv. Mediate saccades toward the opposite side

        v. Superior colliculus involved in triggering saccades

        vi. Parapontine reticular formation generates horizontal saccades

F. **Pupillary anatomy**

  1. *Parasympathetic pathway*

    a. *Muscles innervated*

        i. *Iris sphincter: for pupillary constriction*

        ii. *Ciliary muscle: for accommodation*

    b. *Pupillodilator muscles innervated by C8–T2*

    c. *Edinger-Westphal nucleus*

    d. CN III

        i. Innervation of intraocular muscles is located in the inner aspect of CN III

        ii. Pupillomotor fibers are located on the outside (susceptible to compression)

        iii. Courses within the cavernous sinus, where it bifurcates into an inferior (preganglionic pupillomotor fibers) and superior division

        iv. Within the orbit, the parasympathetic fibers synapse in the ciliary ganglion and postganglionic parasympathetic fibers proceed anteriorly as short ciliary nerves to innervate the iris sphincter and ciliary muscles

        v. Acetylcholine released at both the preganglionic presynaptic terminal within the ciliary ganglion and the postganglionic neuromuscular junction

  2. *Sympathetic pathway*

    a. First-order neurons: originate in the *posterolateral hypothalamus and synapse within the intermediolateral gray matter column* of the lower cervical and upper thoracic spinal cord

b. *Second-order (preganglionic) neurons:* arise *from the ciliospinal center and exit the spinal cord through the ventral roots of C8–T2* to synapse in the superior cervical ganglion

NB: Exit in the lower trunk of the brachial plexus.

    c. *Third-order (postganglionic) neurons: originate* from the superior cervical ganglion and travel as a plexus along the internal carotid artery

NB: These fibers, if lesioned, produce a Horner's syndrome in carotid dissection.

  G. *Retina:* light first enters the innermost layer of the retina through the ganglion cell layer

II. Clinical Assessment
  A. *Localization*
    1. Ocular
      a. Loss of vision in one eye vs. both eyes
      b. Homonymous hemianopia may be misinterpreted by patient as monocular vision loss
    2. Retro-ocular
      a. Hemianopia vs. quadrantanopia
      b. Peripheral visual fields vs. central visual field
    3. Time
      a. Duration: transient vs. permanent
      b. Time of onset (acute, subacute, chronic)
      c. Prior events

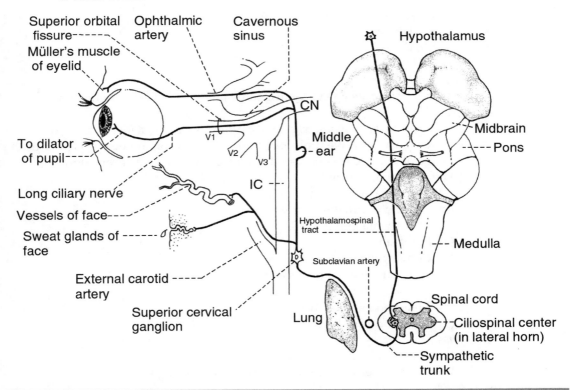

Figure 13-1. The course of the oculosympathetic pathway, where any interruption results in Horner's syndrome. Hypothalamic fibers project to the ipsilateral ciliospinal center of the intermediolateral cell column at T1, which then projects preganglionic sympathetic fibers to the superior cervical ganglion. The superior cervical ganglion projects postganglionic sympathetic fibers through the tympanic cavity, cavernous sinus, and superior orbital fissure. CN, cranial nerve; IC, internal carotid.

4. Associated phenomenology
   a. Positive (hallucinations, scotoma, diplopia, etc.)
   b. Negative (vision loss with darkness; complete vs. partial)
   c. Associated symptomatology (eye pain, headache, focal weakness)
B. *Examination*
   1. General examination of eye
      a. Eyelids
         i. Periorbital edema
         ii. Ptosis
         iii. Blepharospasm
      b. Conjunctiva
         i. Transparent with only a few visible blood vessels
         ii. Tortuous conjunctival vessels—carotid cavernous fistula
         iii. Halo of redness at the limbus—uveitis or acute glaucoma
         iv. Palpebral redness—keratopathy or dry eye syndrome
         v. Diffuse eye injection—viral conjunctivitis
      c. Visual acuity: *Snellen visual acuity test*
         i. *Pseudoisochromatic color plates—assessment of color discrimination*
         ii. Visual field testing: confrontation methods—comparisons between hemifields and quadrants; Goldmann perimetry—standardized visual field testing
      d. *Visual fields*
         i. *Nasal: 50 degrees*
         ii. *Superior: 60 degrees*
         iii. *Inferior: 70 degrees*
         iv. *Temporal: 80 degrees*
      e. Extraocular movement
         i. Supranuclear upgaze palsy: confirmed by an intact Bell's phenomenon
         ii. *Tropias*
            (A) *Both eyes are not aligned, whether the patient is viewing with one eye or both.*
            (B) Patients usually have diplopia (if not, either vision in one eye is poor or the image of one eye is suppressed, which can occur with chronic lesions).
            (C) Differential diagnosis
               (1) CN VI palsy
               (2) Thyroid ophthalmopathy
               (3) Myasthenia gravis (MG)
               (4) Botulism
               (5) Convergence spasm
               (6) Traumatic medial rectus entrapment
               (7) Duane's retraction syndrome
               (8) Childhood strabismus
               (9) Posterior fossa tumors
         iii. *Phorias*
            (A) *Eyes are misaligned when either eye is viewing alone.*
            (B) When both eyes are viewing, the two eyes are aligned.
         iv. *Fixation*
            (A) Opsoclonus: fixation interrupted by repetitive saccades that immediately reverse direction and randomly directed
         v. *Smooth pursuit:* assessed as the patient follows an object; requires attention
         vi. *Saccades*

(A) Hypometria: nonspecific

(B) *Hypermetria: cerebellar disturbance*

(C) Saccadic velocity

vii. *Nystagmus*

    (A) Evaluation

        (1) Waveform

        (2) Direction: horizontal vs. vertical vs. torsional

        (3) Monocular vs. binocular

    (B) *Pendular nystagmus has a sinusoidal oscillation without fast phases*

    (C) *Jerk nystagmus:* has a slow drift of the eyes in one direction alternating rhythmically with a fast movement in the other

    (D) *Latent nystagmus*

        (1) Only when one eye covered

        (2) Fast component away from covered eye

        (3) Decreased visual acuity due to nystagmus

        (4) Usually congenital and often seen in conjunction with esotropia

    (E) *Downbeat nystagmus*

    (F) *Upbeat nystagmus*

    (G) *Seesaw nystagmus*

    (H) *Torsional nystagmus*

    (I) *Rotary nystagmus:* differential diagnosis/etiologies—thalamic lesion

    (J) *Convergence retraction nystagmus*

    (K) *Gaze-evoked nystagmus*

viii. *Ocular myoclonus*

ix. *Ocular bobbing*

x. *Opsoclonus*

f. Pupillary reactivity

  i. Direct vs. indirect

  ii. Swinging flashlight

g. Red reflex

  i. Routine step before the fundus is examined

  ii. Detect corneal opacities, cataracts, vitreous blood, and retinal detachments

h. Ophthalmoscopic examination

  i. Funduscopic examination

    (A) Optic disc: assess for edema, pallor, and cupping

    (B) Vessels

    (C) Macula

    (D) Retina

    (E) Assess for emboli, edema, and hemorrhage

III. Disorders

A. Disorders of the eyelids

1. *Periorbital edema*

  a. Ocular inflammation

  b. Cavernous sinus disease

  c. Thyroid ophthalmopathy

2. *Ptosis*

  a. Originate anywhere from the cortex to the levator aponeurosis

  b. Differential diagnosis

       i. Supranuclear palsy
      ii. CN III palsy
     iii. Horner's syndrome
     iv. Neuropathic
      v. Neuromuscular junction (MG, botulism)
     vi. Myopathic
    vii. Congenital
   viii. Progressive external ophthalmoplegia
     ix. Endocrine (thyroid)
      x. Trauma

3. *Blepharospasm*
   a. Abnormally low upper lid position that results from excessive contraction of the orbicularis oculi
   b. Form of focal dystonia, often with transient resolution during sensory input
   c. Usually transient
   d. Orbicularis oculi resulting in eyelid closure may contract in synchrony with lower facial muscles with aberrant regeneration of CN VII after Bell's palsy
   e. Types and etiologies
      i. Isolated
      ii. Associated with other facial dystonias: Meige's syndrome
      iii. Part of a generalized dystonia
      iv. Occurs with parkinsonian syndromes
      v. Medications (levodopa or the neuroleptics)
      vi. Focal brain stem or basal ganglia lesions
   f. Treatment
      i. Botulinum type A toxin injections of the orbicularis muscles (treatment of choice)
      ii. Medications: anticholinergic agents, baclofen, clonazepam

B. ***Disorders of eye movement***
   1. *Myopathic disorders*
      a. *Congenital myopathy*
         i. Myotubular
         ii. Central core
      b. *Muscular dystrophy*
         i. Myotonic dystrophy
         ii. Oculopharyngeal dystrophy
      c. *Myotonic disorders*
         i. Thomsen's disease
         ii. Paramyotonia congenita
         iii. Hyperkalemic and hypokalemic periodic paralyses
      d. *Mitochondrial myopathy*
         i. Progressive external ophthalmoplegia/Kearns-Sayre syndrome
         ii. *MELAS (Mitochondrial myopathy, Encephalomyopathy, Lactic Acidosis, and Stroke-like episodes)*/myoclonus epilepsy with ragged red fiber
      e. *Metabolic myopathy:* abetalipoproteinemia
      f. *Endocrine myopathy*
         i. *Thyroid (Graves') ophthalmopathy:* characteristic feature is lid retraction; downgaze increases the distance between the cornea and upper lid, transiently resulting in lid lag (von Graefe's sign)
         ii. *Steroid myopathy*

g. *Traumatic myopathy (muscle entrapment)*
h. Infectious
    i. Autoimmune

2. *Neuromuscular disorders*
  a. **MG**
    i. Symptoms more likely as day progresses or with significant motor activity
    ii. Ptosis that increases throughout the day, ptosis that worsens with repeated eye opening or prolonged upgaze, and Cogan's lid twitch
    iii. Lid retraction may also occur
    iv. Diplopia with extraocular muscle involvement
  b. Lambert-Eaton myasthenic syndrome: ocular signs are rare
  c. Amyotrophic lateral sclerosis
  d. *Toxins*
    i. Organophosphate insecticides
    ii. Botulism
    iii. Venom (cobras, kraits, coral snakes, and sea snakes)

3. *Neuropathic disorders*
  a. *Etiologies*
    i. Ischemic (atherosclerotic, diabetes mellitus)
    ii. Hemorrhagic
    iii. Intra-axial tumors
    iv. Compression (tumor, aneurysm)
    v. Trauma
    vi. Acute inflammatory demyelinating polyradiculopathy (Miller-Fisher variant)
      (A) Clinical
        (1) *Ophthalmoplegia: symmetric paresis of upgaze with progressive impairment of horizontal gaze and late involvement or relative sparing of downgaze*
        (2) *Areflexia*
        (3) *Ataxia*
      (B) 2 males:1 female
      (C) Upper respiratory infection or gastrointestinal (*Campylobacter jejuni*) infection preceding the neurologic symptoms
      (D) Autoantibodies to *GQ1b-ganglioside*
    vii. Demyelinating (multiple sclerosis [MS])
    viii. Meningitis (basilar-cryptococcus)
    ix. Increased intracranial pressure
    x. Cavernous sinus
      (A) Compression/metastatic (carcinoma, meningioma)
      (B) Pituitary adenoma
      (C) Chordoma
      (D) Carotid aneurysm
      (E) Inflammation (Tolosa-Hunt)
      (F) Infection (mucormycosis, infiltrating sinus infection)
      (G) Carotid-cavernous fistula
  b. *Oculomotor (CN III) palsy*
    i. Pathophysiology
      (A) Etiologies in adults
        (1) Idiopathic (30–35%)
        (2) Vascular (25%)

          (3) Trauma (15%)

          (4) Tumor (10%)

          (5) Inflammatory/infectious (5–10%)

    ii. Clinical

      (A) Symptoms

          (1) Diplopia: usually oblique in primary position

          (2) Ptosis

          (3) Blurred near vision

      (B) Complete CN III palsy

          (1) Eye in primary position is down and out

          (2) Cannot elevate or adduct

          (3) Full abduction

          (4) Some residual depression accompanied by intorsion

          (5) *Ptosis is severe*

          (6) Accommodation impaired

          (7) Pupil is large and does not constrict to light or on convergence

      (C) *Pupil rule*

          (1) *Ischemic: pupil is spared in 75%*

          (2) *Aneurysm: pupil involved in >90%*

      (D) *Oculomotor synkinesis*

          (1) Anomalous contraction of muscles

          (2) Most common is lid elevation on adduction

  c. *Trochlear (CN IV) palsy*

    i. Pathophysiology

      (A) Etiologies in adults

          (1) Trauma (30%)

          (2) Idiopathic (20–25%)

          (3) Ischemic (15%)

          (4) Congenital (10%)

          (5) Tumor (5–10%)

    ii. Clinical

      (A) Vertical separation largest in downgaze

      (B) Compensatory lateral head tilt away from the side of the lesion to minimize the diplopia

      (C) Extraocular muscles examination: decreased depression of the adducted eye

      (D) Bilateral CN IV = head trauma

      (E) Differential diagnosis of vertical diplopia

          (1) Ocular MG

          (2) Thyroid ophthalmoplegia

          (3) Orbital lesion (i.e., tumor)

          (4) CN III palsy

          (5) CN IV palsy

          (6) Skew deviation

  d. *Abducens (CN VI) palsy*

    i. Pathophysiology

      (A) Etiologies in adults

          (1) Idiopathic (25%)

          (2) Tumor (20%)

          (3) Trauma (15%)

          (4) Ischemia (15%)

ii. Clinical
>   (A) Horizontal diplopia that is uncrossed, meaning that the ipsilateral image belongs to the ipsilateral eye and is more noticeable for distant targets

4. Cavernous sinus syndromes
   a. May also affect CN V-1 or CN V-2
   b. Can produce a Horner's syndrome
   c. Anterior disease may damage the optic nerve
   d. Etiologies
      i. Tumors (70%)
>   (A) Nasopharyngeal carcinoma (most common cause)
>   (B) Pituitary
>   (C) Adenoma
>   (D) Meningioma
>   (E) Craniopharyngioma
>   (F) Chondroma
>   (G) Metastatic (breast, lung, and prostate) carcinoma
      ii. Aneurysms (20%)
      iii. Infection
   e. **Tolosa-Hunt syndrome**
      i. Pathophysiology
>   (A) Accounts for only 3% of cavernous sinus syndromes
>   (B) Pathology: *idiopathic noncaseating granulomatous inflammation in the cavernous sinus*
>   (C) Diagnosis of exclusion
      ii. Clinical
>   (A) Acute painful ophthalmoplegia
>   (B) Progression over days to weeks
>   (C) Most commonly, CNs III and VI involved
>   (D) CN IV and CN V-1 in one-third of cases
>   (E) Optic nerve is affected in 20%
>   (F) CN V-2 sensory loss in 10%
>   (G) Horner's syndrome, CN V-3 sensory loss, and CN VII palsy are unusual
>   (H) May have elevated erythrocyte sedimentation rate and positive systemic lupus erythematosus preparation
>   (I) May have recurring attacks over months to years
      iii. Treatment
>   (A) High dose oral prednisone

5. **Pituitary apoplexy**
   a. Multiple oculomotor palsies
   b. Severe headache
   c. Bilateral vision loss

6. **Wallenberg's lateral medullary syndrome**
   a. *Infarction in posterior-inferior cerebellar artery usually due to ipsilateral vertebral arterial occlusion or possibly MS*
   b. Clinical
      i. *Imbalance*
      ii. *Vertigo*
      iii. *Numbness of the face or limbs*
      iv. *Dysphagia*

      v. *Headache*
     vi. *Vomiting*
    vii. *Horner's syndrome*
   viii. *Decreased pain and temperature sensation of ipsilateral face and contralateral body*
     ix. *Skew deviation with ipsilateral eye hypotropic causing diplopia*
      x. *Primary position horizontal or horizontal-torsional nystagmus*

7. *Internuclear ophthalmoplegia*
  a. *Lesion of the medial longitudinal fasciculus (MLF) blocks information from the contralateral CN VI to the ipsilateral CN III*
  b. *Internuclear ophthalmoplegia named after ipsilateral MLF lesion*
  c. Clinical
    i. Impaired adduction during conjugate gaze away from the side of the MLF lesion
    ii. Nystagmus of the abducting during conjugate version movements
    iii. Slowed adducting saccades with lag in the adducting eye compared with the abducting eye
  d. Etiologies
    i. Brain stem ischemia (usually unilateral)
    ii. MS (usually bilateral)
    iii. Brain stem encephalitis
    iv. Behcet's disease
    v. Cryptococcosis
    vi. Guillain-Barré syndrome

8. *One-and-a-half syndrome*
  a. *Combined damage to*
    i. *MLF plus ipsilateral paramedian pontine reticular formation*
    ii. *MLF and ipsilateral CN VI nucleus*
  b. Clinical
    i. Internuclear ophthalmoplegia on gaze to the contralateral side (the "half")
    ii. Pontine conjugate gaze palsy to the ipsilateral side (the "one")

9. *Mobius syndrome:* heterogeneous group of congenital anomalies consisting of *facial palsies and abnormal horizontal gaze*

C. **Nystagmus**
1. *Pendular nystagmus*
  a. Etiologies
    i. MS (most common)
    ii. Strokes
    iii. Encephalitis
    iv. Brain stem vascular
  b. Pathophysiology unclear
  c. Treatment unclear

2. *Spasmus nutans*
  a. *Disorder of young children, with age at onset usually 6–12 months and resolves by age 3 years*
  b. *Clinical triad (not all three are required)*
    i. *Ocular oscillations*
    ii. *Head nodding*
    iii. *Head turn*
  c. Pathophysiology is uncertain

3. *Seesaw nystagmus*
  a. Pendular

  b. Present in all gaze positions
  c. Etiologies
    i. Tumor
      (A) Pituitary adenoma
      (B) Craniopharyngioma
    ii. Stroke
      (A) Pontomedullary infarct
      (B) Midbrain/thalamic infarct
    iii. Trauma
    iv. Congenital
    v. Vision loss
    vi. Prognosis variable
4. *Jerk nystagmus*
  a. *Downbeat nystagmus*
    i. Clinical
      (A) Associated signs/symptoms
        (1) Ataxia
        (2) Blurred vision
        (3) Oscillopsia
    ii. Etiologies
      (A) Arnold-Chiari syndrome (20–25%)
      (B) Idiopathic (20%)
      (C) Spinocerebellar degeneration (20%)
      (D) Brain stem stroke (10%)
      (E) MS (5–10%)
      (F) Tumor
      (G) Medication (lithium, antiepileptic drugs)/alcohol
      (H) Trauma
  b. *Upbeat nystagmus*
    i. Associated with
      (A) Oscillopsia
      (B) Ataxia
    ii. Etiologies
      (A) Spinocerebellar degeneration (20–25%)
      (B) Brain stem stroke/vascular malformation (20%)
      (C) MS/inflammatory (10–15%)
      (D) Tumor (10%)
      (E) Infection
      (F) Medication/alcohol
      (G) Trauma
  c. *Torsional nystagmus*
    i. Usually attributed to dysfunction of vertical semicircular canal inputs
    ii. Etiologies
      (A) Stroke
      (B) MS
      (C) Vascular malformation
      (D) Arnold-Chiari syndrome
      (E) Tumor
      (F) Encephalitis
      (G) Trauma

5. *Gaze-evoked nystagmus*
   a. Most common nystagmus
   b. Dysfunction of cerebellar flocculus in conjunction with the lateral medulla for horizontal gaze and the midbrain for vertical gaze
   c. Differential diagnosis/etiologies
      i. Medications
         (A) Antiepileptic agents
         (B) Sedative hypnotics
      ii. Bilateral brain stem lesion
      iii. Cerebellar lesion
      iv. MG
6. *Convergence retraction nystagmus*
   a. Jerk retraction movements due to co-contraction of the muscles of extraocular movement on attempted convergence or upgaze
   b. Best seen when testing eyes with a downward moving optokinetic nystagmus tape/drum because this requires upward saccades
   c. Differential diagnosis/etiologies
      i. Differential diagnosis by age
         (A) 10 y/o: pinealoma
         (B) 20 y/o: head trauma
         (C) 30 y/o: brain stem vascular malformation
         (D) 40 y/o: MS
         (E) 50 y/o: basilar stroke
   d. **Parinaud syndrome**
      i. *Dorsal midbrain lesion*
      ii. *Supranuclear upgaze palsy*
      iii. *Lid retraction*
      iv. *Convergence-retraction nystagmus*
7. *Treatment of nystagmus*
   a. Drug therapy relatively ineffective
   b. Botulinum injections (note: normal extraocular movements are also impaired, which is just as debilitating)
   c. Prisms: shift the eyes toward more favorable gaze position
   d. Surgery: immobilize the eye rigidly, which also impairs normal extraocular movements
D. *Opsoclonus*
   1. Pathophysiology: *dentate nucleus lesion*
   2. Clinical
      a. Involuntary bursts of spontaneous saccades in all directions
      b. Classic triad
         i. Opsoclonus
         ii. Myoclonus
         iii. Ataxia (trunk and gait)
   3. Etiologies
      a. Neuroblastoma (childhood)
      b. Infection (young adults)
         i. Enterovirus
         ii. Coxsackie virus B3, B2
         iii. St. Louis encephalitis

        iv. *Rickettsia*

        v. *Salmonella*

        vi. Rubella

        vii. Epstein-Barr virus

        viii. Mumps

    c. Paraneoplastic (older adults)

        i. Breast

        ii. Lung

        iii. Uterine/ovarian

    d. Brain stem stroke

    e. Head trauma

    f. MS

    g. Midbrain tumor

    h. Medications/toxins

E. *Ocular bobbing*

    1. Clinical: rapid downward jerk with slow return to primary gaze

    2. Etiology

        a. Pontine lesion

        b. Subarachnoid hemorrhage

        c. Head trauma

        d. Leigh disease

        e. Cerebellar hemorrhage

F. *Ocular myoclonus* (see Chapter 5: Movement Disorders): lesion associated with Mollaret's triangle

G. *Oculogyric crisis*

    1. Temporary period of frequent spasms of eye deviation, often upward

    2. Lasts seconds to hours

    3. Etiology

        a. Medication

            i. Neuroleptics

            ii. Carbamazepine

            iii. Tetrabenazine

            iv. Lithium toxicity

        b. Brain stem encephalitis

        c. Paraneoplastic

        d. Rett's syndrome

        e. Tourette's syndrome

H. **Disorders of the visual system and pathways**

    1. *Optic disc edema*

        a. Optic disc edema results from stasis of axoplasmic flow at the optic disc with swelling of the axons that cause an elevation of the disc and an increase in the diameter of the disc

        b. Causes of optic disc edema

            i. Papilledema (elevated intracranial pressure)

            ii. Optic neuritis

            iii. Anterior ischemic optic neuropathy (AION)

            iv. Giant cell arteritis

            v. Diabetic papillitis

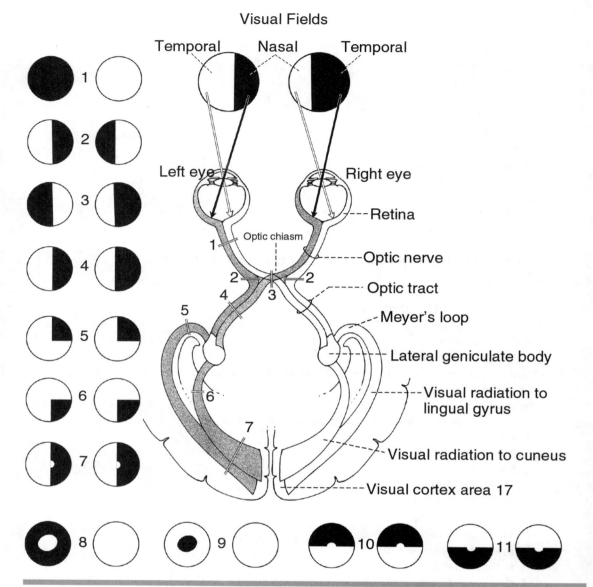

Figure 13-2. The visual pathway from the retina to the cortex illustrating the visual field defects. (1) Ipsilateral blindness. (2) Binasal hemianopia. (3) Bitemporal hemianopia. (4) Right hemianopia. (5) Right upper quadrantanopia. (6) Right lower quadrantanopia. (7) Right hemianopia with macular sparing. (8) Left constricted field as a result of end-stage glaucoma. (9) Left central scotoma seen in optic neuritis. (10) Upper altitudinal hemianopia from destruction of the lingual gyri. (11) Lower altitudinal hemianopia from bilateral destruction of the cunei.

      vi. Orbital or intracranial mass
     vii. Graves' disease
   viii. Infiltration (tumor, lymphoma)
      ix. Retinal vein occlusion
       x. Venous congestion
     xi. Malignant hypertension

xii. Infection

xiii. Uveitis

xiv. Pseudotumor cerebri

2. *Optic neuritis*

a. Describes any condition that causes inflammation of the optic nerve

b. Pain in the involved eye worsened with eye movement followed by monocular vision loss

c. Usually young adults

d. 5 females:1 male

e. Visual acuity is usually affected with central scotoma as the classic finding

f. *Relative afferent pupillary defect may persist even after the visual function improves*

g. *Visual-evoked potential: prolonged P100*

h. Treatment

   i. The Optic Neuritis Treatment Trial

   (A) Three groups

   (1) Placebo tablets

   (2) Moderate-dose oral prednisone

   (3) High-dose intravenous (i.v.) methylprednisolone for 3 days (followed by 11 days' therapy with oral prednisone)

   (B) Results

   (1) Oral steroids: higher rate of recurrence of optic neuritis.

   (2) Abnormal brain magnetic resonance imaging (MRI) more likely to develop MS, but the risk of new events was reduced in those patients who received i.v. methylprednisone

   (3) Patients treated with i.v. steroids improved more quickly, but all patients improved to the same degree within 6 months to 1 year.

3. **AION**

a. Pathophysiology: ischemic infarct of the optic disc due to atherosclerotic disease (nonarteritic AION), or from vasculitis, most commonly giant cell arteritis (arteritic AION)

b. Clinical

   i. **NB:** Sudden *painless* vision loss associated with unilateral optic disc swelling

   ii. *Usually >45 y/o*

   iii. *Arteritic AION*

   (A) Giant cell arteritis

   (1) Inflammation of small- and medium-sized extracranial arteries

   (2) Usually >60 y/o

   (3) 3 females:1 male

   (4) Vision loss most commonly from vasculitic occlusion of the posterior ciliary

   (5) Systemic symptoms include headache, scalp and temple tenderness, myalgias, arthralgias, low-grade fever, anemia, malaise, weight loss, anorexia, or jaw claudication

   (6) Associated with polymyalgia rheumatica

   (7) Inflamed temporal arteries can be palpated as a firm "cord" with a poor pulse

   (8) Labs: elevated erythrocyte sedimentation rate >50 (erythrocyte sedimentation rate may be normal in ~10%); elevated C-reactive protein

   (9) Diagnosis via biopsy at least 2–3 cm long and sectioned serially, because the vasculitis is patchy (skip lesions)

(10) Treatment
  (a) *High-dose i.v. steroids (1 g/day) for patients with vision loss (duration variable) followed by maintenance oral prednisone (sometimes for years)*
  (b) *Patients without acute vision loss can be started immediately on oral prednisone, 60–80 mg/day*

4. *Papilledema*
  a. Associated with bilateral optic disc edema due to elevated intracranial pressure
  b. Secondarily, compression of the venous structures within the nerve head that causes venous engorgement and tortuosity, capillary dilation, and splinter hemorrhage
  c. Etiologies
    i. Intracranial mass lesion
    ii. Pseudotumor cerebri
    iii. Hydrocephalus
    iv. Intracranial hemorrhage
    v. Venous thrombosis/obstruction
    vi. Meningitis

5. *Graves' disease*
  a. Autoimmune disorder
  b. Clinical
    i. Enlargement of the extraocular muscles and oversized rectus muscles compress the optic nerve
    ii. Increase in orbital fat volume
    iii. Proptosis
    iv. Diplopia
    v. Eyelid retraction
    vi. Ocular congestion

6. *Tumors affecting the anterior visual system*
  a. *Optic nerve sheath meningiomas*
    i. *Classic triad*
      (A) Disc pallor
      (B) Optic disc venous collaterals
      (C) Progressive vision loss
    ii. In children, usually bilateral and often associated with neurofibromatosis type 2
    iii. May extend into the optic canal or may originate from the dura within the optic canal
    iv. MRI with contrast and orbital fat suppression shows enhancement of the sheath with optic nerve sparing ("railroad track" on axial images and "bull's eye" on coronal views)
    v. Treatment
      (A) Surgery
      (B) Radiation (most viable)
  b. *Optic nerve gliomas*
    i. Usually present in childhood (75% before 20 y/o)
    ii. Clinical
      (A) Proptosis
      (B) Vision loss
      (C) Strabismus
      (D) Nystagmus
    iii. In children: associated with neurofibromatosis type 1 (15%); usually are pilocytic astrocytomas

iv. In adults: more malignant rapidly lead to blindness and death

7. Inflammatory optic neuropathies

8. Infectious optic neuropathies

9. *Toxic/nutritional optic neuropathies*

   a. Nutritional deficiencies

      i. Pyridoxine

      ii. B$_{12}$

      iii. Folate

      iv. Niacin

      v. Riboflavin

      vi. Thiamine

   b. Toxic

      i. Ethambutol

      ii. Ethanol with tobacco

      iii. Methanol

      iv. Ethylene glycol

      v. Amiodarone

      vi. Isoniazid

      vii. Chloramphenicol

      viii. Chemotherapy

   c. *Toxic amblyopia*

      i. Typically affects heavy drinkers and pipe smokers deficient in B vitamins

      ii. Insidious onset of slowly progressive bilateral visual field impairment associated with loss of color vision

      iii. Ophthalmoscopic examination: splinter hemorrhages or minimal disc edema, but most are normal

10. *Hereditary optic neuropathies*

    a. **Leber's optic neuropathy**

       i. Pathophysiology: maternal *mitochondrial DNA point mutation*

       ii. Clinical

          (A) Optic neuropathy: upper limb, acute, painless optic neuritis

          (B) *Asymptomatic cardiac anomalies including accessory cardiac atrioventricular conduction pathways (Wolff-Parkinson-White and Lown-Ganong-Levine syndromes)*

          (C) Adolescent males

11. Ophthalmoscopic examination: mild hyperemia and swelling of optic discs with irregular dilation of peripapillary capillaries (telangiectasia microangiopathy)

I. *Disorders associated with the optic chiasm*

   1. Clinical: classic pattern is bitemporal visual field defects, but variable

   2. Etiologies

      a. Sella tumors

         i. Pituitary macroadenomas (may have associated endocrine abnormalities): pituitary apoplexy—acute enlargement of a pituitary adenoma due to necrotic hemorrhage or postpartum (Sheehan's syndrome)

         ii. Craniopharyngiomas

         iii. Gliomas

      b. MS

      c. Aneurysm

      d. Trauma

3. *Anterior chiasm lesion (Willebrand's knee)*
   a. *Nasal retinal fibers cross anterior in the chiasm before joining the contralateral temporal fibers*
   b. Signs/symptoms
        i. Ipsilateral monocular central scotoma
       ii. Contralateral upper temporal field cut

NB: This is also known as a junctional scotoma.

J. *Retrochiasmal visual pathways*
   1. Disorders of the optic tract
      a. Etiologies
           i. Tumors
          ii. Aneurysm
   2. *Disorders involving the lateral geniculate nucleus*
      a. **NB:** Lateral geniculate nucleus is somatotopically arranged
           i. *Uncrossed fibers = layers 2, 3, 5*
          ii. *Crossed fibers = layers 1, 2, 6*
      b. Etiologies
           i. Stroke
          ii. Tumors
   3. *Optic radiations:* etiologies: stroke, tumors
   4. *Occipital lobe*
      a. Etiologies
           i. Stroke: thromboembolism from the heart and vertebrobasilar system
          ii. Tumors
      b. Clinical
           i. Produces highly *congruous homonymous visual field defects,* usually without any other accompanying neurologic symptoms
          ii. *Riddoch phenomenon: patient can detect motion in an otherwise blind hemifield (can be associated with any retrochiasmal visual field defect)*
         iii. Bilateral occipital lobe infarctions
              (A) Bilateral blindness
              (B) Normal pupillary response
              (C) No other neurologic signs
          iv. Closed head injury can cause transient cortical blindness (may be difficult to distinguish from functional vision loss)

K. **Disorders of pupillary function**
   1. Topical cholinergic agents that influence pupil size
      a. *Cholinergic agonists that produce miosis*
           i. *Pilocarpine*
          ii. *Carbachol*
         iii. *Methacholine*
          iv. *Physostigmine*
           v. *Organophosphate insecticides*
      b. *Cholinergic antagonists that produce mydriasis*
           i. *Atropine*
          ii. *Scopolamine*
   2. Topical adrenergic agents that influence pupil size

      a. *Adrenergic agonists that produce mydriasis*
         i. *Epinephrine*
        ii. *Phenylephrine*
       iii. *Hydroxyamphetamine*
       iv. *Ephedrine*
        v. *Cocaine*
      b. *Adrenergic antagonists that produce miosis*
         i. *Guanethidine*
        ii. *Reserpine*
       iii. *Thymoxamine*
3. *Afferent pupillary defect (Marcus Gunn pupil)*
      a. Diagnosis via swinging flashlight test
      b. Etiologies
         i. Amblyopia
        ii. Retinopathies
       iii. Maculopathies
       iv. Optic neuropathies
        v. Optic chiasm lesions
       vi. Optic tract lesions
      vii. Midbrain lesion involving the pretectal nucleus or the brachium of the superior colliculus
     viii. Lateral geniculate nucleus
4. *Large and poorly reactive pupil*
      a. Differential diagnosis
         i. Unilateral
           (A) Adie's tonic pupil
           (B) Pharmacologic (anticholinergic agent, jimson weed, adrenergic agonist)
           (C) Trauma/surgery
           (D) Ischemia (carotid artery insufficiency, giant cell arteritis, carotid cavernous fistula)
           (E) Iridocyclitis
           (F) Complication of infection (e.g., herpes zoster)
           (G) CN III palsy
           (H) Tonic pupil associated with peripheral neuropathy or systemic dysautonomia
        ii. Bilateral
           (A) Adie's tonic pupils
           (B) Pharmacologic (anticholinergic agent, jimson weed, adrenergic agonist)
           (C) Parinaud syndrome
           (D) Argyll-Robertson pupils
           (E) CN III palsy
           (F) Carcinomatous meningitis
           (G) Chronic basilar meningitis
           (H) Guillain-Barré syndrome
           (I) Eaton-Lambert syndrome
           (J) Botulism
5. *Argyll-Robertson syndrome*
      a. Clinical
         i. *Miotic irregular pupils*

      ii. *Light-near dissociation*
        (A) Absence of light response associated with normal anterior visual pathway function
        (B) Brisk pupillary constriction to near object
      iii. Normal visual acuity
      iv. Diminished pupillary dilatation, particularly in dark
      v. Usually bilateral
    b. Etiology
      i. Neurosyphilis
      ii. Muscular dystrophy
      iii. MS
      iv. Chronic alcoholism
      v. Sarcoidosis
6. **Horner's syndrome**
    a. Clinical
      i. Miosis
      ii. Ptosis (denervation of Müller's muscle)
      iii. Anhidrosis (ipsilateral facial)
      iv. Transient signs: dilated conjunctival and facial vessels, decreased intraocular pressure, and increased accommodation
    b. Etiologies
      i. Central (1st-order) neuron
        (A) Brain stem (Wallenberg's) or thalamic stroke
        (B) Intra-axial tumor involving the thalamus, brain stem, or cervical spinal cord
        (C) Demyelination or inflammatory process involving the brain stem or cervical spinal cord
        (D) Syringomyelia
        (E) Neck trauma
      ii. Preganglionic (2nd-order) neuron
        (A) Tumors involving the pulmonary apex, mediastinum, cervical paravertebral region, or C8–T2 nerve roots
        (B) Lower brachial plexus injury
        (C) Subclavian or internal jugular vein catheter placement
        (D) Stellate or superior cervical ganglion blocks
        (E) Carotid dissection below the superior cervical ganglion
      iii. Postganglionic (3rd-order) neuron
        (A) Internal carotid artery dissection
        (B) Cluster headache
        (C) Skull base or orbital trauma or tumors
        (D) Intracavernous carotid artery aneurysm
        (E) Carotid endarterectomy
        (F) Herpes zoster ophthalmicus
        (G) Complicated otitis media
    c. **NB:** Diagnostic procedures
      i. **Cocaine 4–10%**
        (A) *Confirms oculosympathetic denervation by blocking presynaptic reuptake of norepinephrine, allowing norepinephrine to accumulate at the iris and produce mydriasis.*
        (B) *If injury occurs anywhere along the oculosympathetic pathway, then the amount of tonically released norepinephrine is reduced and the ability of cocaine to dilate the pupil is impaired.*

ii. **Hydroxyamphetamine 1%**
  (A) *Test 3rd-order neuron*
  (B) Releases stored norepinephrine from the 3rd-order nerve terminal to dilate pupil
iii. Differentiation between pre- and postganglionic Horner's syndrome
  (A) **1% hydroxyamphetamine** → *releases catecholamines from postsynaptic neurons → dilation of the pupil if the lesion is presynaptic*
  (B) **1% phenylephrine** → *dilates supersensitive pupil in postganglionic Horner's syndrome*

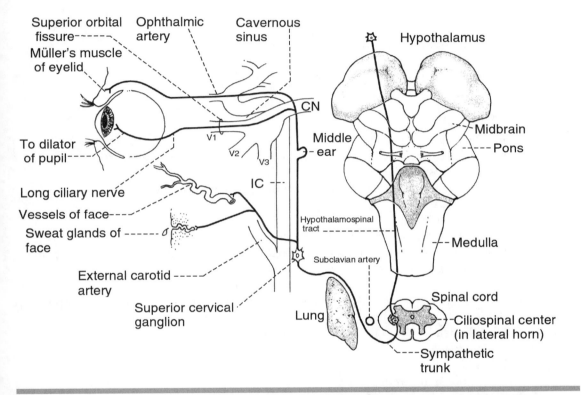

Figure 13-3. The course of the oculosympathetic pathway, where any interruption results in Horner's syndrome. Hypothalamic fibers project to the ipsilateral ciliospinal center of the intermediolateral cell column at T1, which then projects preganglionic sympathetic fibers to the superior cervical ganglion. The superior cervical ganglion projects postganglionic sympathetic fibers through the tympanic cavity, cavernous sinus, and superior orbital fissure. CN, cranial nerve; IC, internal carotid.

7. *Light-near dissociation*
   a. Better pupillary response to near than to light
   b. Differential diagnosis
      i. Severe retinopathy
      ii. Optic neuropathy
      iii. Adie's tonic pupil
      iv. Argyll-Robertson syndrome
      v. Dorsal midbrain syndrome
      vi. Aberrant CN III regeneration

8. *Opiate overdose*
   a. *Bilateral pinpoint pupils*
   b. Also seen in pontine dysfunction
9. *Barbiturate coma: pupils remain reactive*

L. **Other pearls**
1. **Balint's syndrome**
   a. *Paralysis of visual fixation*
   b. *Optic ataxia*
   c. *Simultanagnosia*
2. *External ophthalmoplegia*
   a. Etiologies
      i. MG
      ii. Kearns-Sayre syndrome
      iii. Oculopharyngeal dystrophy
3. **De Morsier's syndrome (Septo-optic dysplasia)**
   a. *Triad*
      i. *Short stature*
      ii. *Nystagmus*
      iii. *Optic disc hypoplasia*
   b. Spectrum of midline anomalies including absent septum pellucidum, agenesis of corpus callosum, dysplasia of anterior 3rd ventricle
   c. 60% have hypopituitarism with decreased growth hormone
4. **Aicardi's syndrome**
   a. *X-linked dominant*
   b. *Only females because lethal in utero for males*
   c. Ophthalmoscopic examination: *chorioretinal atrophy, retinal pigment epithelial changes, large colobomatous disk*
   d. Other ocular features: strabismus, microphthalmos
   e. Associated with infantile spasms, agenesis of corpus callosum, developmental delay
   f. Usually death within first few years of life
5. *Unilateral proptosis*
   a. Etiologies
      i. Intraorbital tumor
      ii. Sphenoid ridge meningioma
      iii. Cavernous sinus/internal carotid artery fistula
      iv. Hyperthyroidism
6. Aberrant regeneration of CN III may cause lid elevation on attempted adduction and infraduction
7. Cerebellar disease can cause
   a. Vertical or horizontal nystagmus
   b. Ocular dysmetria
   c. Impaired saccadic pursuit
8. *Most common visual defect in early compressive lesion of the optic nerve is central scotoma*
9. *Differential diagnosis of central scotoma*
   a. Optic neuritis
   b. Macular degeneration
   c. Ischemic papillitis
   d. Note: not seen in papilledema

10. *Achromatopsia*
    a. *Unable to differentiate colors on Ishihara plates*
    b. Lesion: occipital lobe inferior to calcarine fissure (therefore, also often have superior visual defect)
11. *Devic's disease*
    a. Variant of MS
    b. Bilateral optic neuritis with transverse myelitis
12. *Behçet's disease*
    a. Recurrent painful orogenital ulcers
    b. Uveitis
    c. CN palsies
    d. Seizures
    e. Strokes
    f. Recurrent meningoencephalitis
    g. Joint effusions
    h. Thrombophlebitis

ADDITIONAL NOTES

CHAPTER 14

Neuro-otology

I. Anatomy and Physiology
A. *Hair cell*
1. Transduces mechanic forces associated with sound into nerve action potentials
2. Moderate the spontaneous afferent nerve-firing rate
   a. Bending stereocilia toward the kinocilium depolarizes the hair cell and increases the firing rate.
   b. Bending away from the kinocilium hyperpolarizes the hair cell and decreases the firing rate.
3. *Stereocilia:* protrude from receptor cell and increase stepwise from one side to the other
4. *Kinocilium*
   a. Longest hair cell.
   b. Bending of hair cells toward kinocilium results in an increase in spontaneous firing rate.
   c. Bending of hair cells away from kinocilium results in a decrease in spontaneous firing rate.
B. *Receptor organs*
1. *Vestibular labyrinth*
   a. Hair cells are mounted in the macules and cristae
      i. *Maculae: sensitive to gravitational forces*
      ii. *Cristae*
         (A) *Not affected by gravitational forces*
         (B) *Sensitive to angular head acceleration*
   b. *Cupula: hair-cell cilia in the cristae of the semicircular canals are embedded in this gelatinous material*
   c. *Otoconia: made of calcium carbonate crystals*
   d. *Semicircular canals respond best to frequencies <5 Hz*
2. *Cochlea*
   a. Hair cells mounted on the flexible basilar membrane of the organ of Corti
   b. Tectorial membrane
      i. Covers the organ of Corti
      ii. Relatively rigid structure attached to the wall of the cochlea
      iii. Hair cells vibrate at the frequency of sound, and the hair cells are displaced in relation to the tectorial membrane
   c. *Hair cells in the cochlea are sensitive and vary from 20–20,000 Hz*
C. *Fluids*
1. *Perilymph*
   a. Primarily formed by filtration from blood vessels in the ear
   b. Perilymphatic fluid resembles the extracellular fluids (low potassium and high sodium)

2. *Endolymph*
   a. Produced by secretory cells in the stria vascularis of the cochlea and the dark cells of the vestibular labyrinth
   b. Contains intracellular-like fluids (high potassium and low sodium)

D. *Cranial nerve VIII*
   1. Scarpa's ganglion: afferent bipolar ganglion cells of the vestibular nerve
   2. Superior division
      a. Innervates
         i. Cristae of the anterior and lateral canals
         ii. Macule of the utricle
         iii. Anterosuperior part of the macule of the saccule
   3. Inferior division
      a. Innervates
         i. Crista of the posterior canal
         ii. Saccule
   4. Bipolar cochlear neurons are in the spiral ganglion of the cochlea

II. Examination of Vestibular and Auditory Dysfunction

A. *Vestibular*
   1. Past pointing
   2. Romberg's test
   3. *Doll's eye test (oculocephalic reflex)*
      a. Slowly rotating the head back and forth in the horizontal plane induces compensatory horizontal eye movements that depend on fixation pursuit and the vestibular systems.
      b. Useful bedside verification of vestibular function in the comatose patient.
   4. *Caloric testing*
      a. *Cold calorics*
         i. *Cupula deviates away from utricle, producing nystagmus with fast component directed away from stimulated ear*
         ii. Procedure
            (A) Make sure ears are clear.
            (B) The patient lies in the supine position with his head tilted 30 degrees forward.
            (C) 2–3 cc of ice water induces a burst of nystagmus usually lasting from 1 to 3 minutes.
         iii. Clinical
            (A) Comatose patient: only a slow tonic deviation toward the side of stimulation is observed
            (B) Normal subjects: >20% decrease in nystagmus duration suggests an ipsilateral lesion
      b. *Warm calorics: cupula deviates toward utricle, producing nystagmus with fast component directed toward stimulated ear*
      c. **NB:** Remember COWS: *Cold, Opposite, Warm, Same*
   5. *Dix-Hallpike test*
      a. Induced by a rapid change from the erect sitting to the supine head-hanging left or right position
      b. Specific for the benign paroxysmal positional vertigo
   6. Electronystagmogram: quantifies slow component of nystagmus directed toward side of lesion

B. *Auditory*
1. **Rinne's test**
   a. Compares the patient's hearing by air conduction with that produced by bone conduction
   b. Tuning fork (512 Hz) first held against the mastoid process until the sound fades and then placed 1 inch from the ear
   c. *Normal: can hear the fork approximately twice as long by air conduction as by bone conduction*
   d. *Bone conduction > air conduction = conductive hearing loss*
2. **Weber's test**
   a. Compares the patient's hearing by bone conduction in the two ears
   b. *Tuning fork (512 Hz) placed at the center of the forehead and asked which side is tone best heard*
   c. *Normal: center of the head*
   d. *Unilateral conductive loss: hear sound ipsilateral to lesion*
   e. *Unilateral sensorineural loss: hear sound contralateral to lesion*
3. Audiometry brain stem auditory-evoked responses (see Chapter 10: Clinical Neurophysiology)

III. Vestibular Dysfunction
A. **Clinical**
1. Imbalance of labyrinth system
   a. Vertigo
   b. Nystagmus
   c. Ataxia
2. *Semicircular canal damage*
   a. Slow conjugate ipsilateral deviation of the eyes interrupted by fast corrective movements in the opposite direction (vestibular nystagmus)
   b. If eyes try to fixate, it appears to move away from the side of the lesion
   c. If eyes are closed, then the surrounding seems to spin toward side of lesion
   d. Tends to fall toward side of lesion
3. *Bilateral symmetric vestibular dysfunction*
   a. Secondary to ototoxic drugs
   b. Usually do not develop vertigo or nystagmus because their tonic vestibular activity remains balanced
   c. Complain of unsteadiness and vision distortion
   d. Oscillopsia: unable to fixate on objects because the surroundings are bouncing up and down
4. Infection
   a. Chronic otomastoiditis
   b. Malignant external otitis (*Pseudomonas aeruginosa*)
   c. Labyrinthitis
   d. Vestibular neuritis
   e. Acoustic neuritis
   f. Herpes zoster oticus
5. Vertebrobasilar insufficiency
6. Meniere's syndrome
7. Migraine
8. **Benign paroxysmal positional vertigo**
   a. Brief episodes of vertigo with position change
   b. Top-shelf vertigo is nearly always caused by benign paroxysmal positional vertigo.

　　　c. 50% idiopathic
　　　d. Bedside diagnosis: Dix-Hallpike test

IV. Auditory Dysfunction
　A. **Pathophysiology**
　　1. *Conductive hearing loss:* results from lesions involving the *external or middle ear*
　　2. *Sensorineural hearing loss*
　　　a. Results from lesions of the cochlea or the auditory division of cranial nerve VIII
　　　b. Sound distortion is common
　　3. *Central hearing disorders*
　　　a. Do not have impaired hearing levels for pure tones
　　　b. Understand speech if clear and in a quiet room
　　4. *Tinnitus*
　　　a. Subjective (heard by patient only)
　　　b. Objective (heard by examiner)
　　　c. Differential diagnosis
　　　　i. Objective
　　　　　(A) Abnormally patent eustachian tube
　　　　　(B) Tetanic contractions of soft palate muscles
　　　　　(C) Normal vascular flow
　　　　　(D) Vascular malformation
　　　　ii. Subjective tinnitus
　　　　　(A) Lesions involving the external ear canal, tympanic membrane, ossicles, cochlea, auditory nerve, brain stem, and cortex
　　　　　(B) Lesions of the external or middle ear usually accompanied by conductive hearing loss
　　　　　(C) Lesions of the cochlea or auditory nerve are usually associated with sensorineural hearing loss
　　　　　(D) Meniere's syndrome is low pitched and continuous
　B. **Clinical**
　　1. *Presbycusis*
　　　a. Bilateral hearing loss with advancing age
　　　b. Pathology: *degeneration of sensory cells and nerve fibers at base of the cochlea*
　　2. **Cogan's syndrome**
　　　a. *Autoimmune disorder*
　　　b. *Inner ear involvement*
　　　c. *Interstitial keratitis*
　　3. *Glomus body tumor*
　　　a. *Most common tumor of middle ear*
　　　b. *Conductive hearing loss*
　　　c. *Pulsatile tinnitus*
　　　d. *Rhinorrhea*
　　4. *Acoustic neuromas*
　　　a. Slowly progressive hearing loss
　　　b. Tinnitus
　　　c. Vertigo
　　　d. Abnormal brain stem auditory-evoked responses in >95%

5. Alport's syndrome
   a. *X-linked*
   b. *Sensorineural hearing loss*
   c. *Interstitial nephritis*
6. **Usher's syndrome**
   a. *Autosomal recessive*
   b. *Retinitis pigmentosa*
   c. *Sensorineural hearing loss*
7. *Osteosclerosis*
   a. Immobilizes stapes
   b. Conductive hearing loss
   c. Usually presents between ages 10 and 30 years
   d. Positive family history in >50%
   e. Pathology: absorption of bone and replacement by cellular fibrous connective tissue
   f. Treatment
      i. Sodium fluoride
      ii. Calcium
      iii. Vitamin D
      iv. Stapediolysis
8. *Toxins*
   a. **Aminoglycosides**
      i. Auditory and vestibular toxins
      ii. *Streptomycin and gentamicin are more vestibular toxic*
      iii. *Kanamycin, tobramycin, and amikacin are more auditory toxic*
      iv. *Likely due to hair cell damage*
      v. Hearing loss at higher frequencies and progresses to 60–70 dB loss across all frequencies
   b. **Salicylates**
      i. Hearing loss
      ii. Tinnitus
      iii. Involves all frequencies
      iv. Highly concentrated in perilymph and may interfere with enzymatic activity of hair cells, cochlear nuclei
      v. Symptoms reversible if stop medication
9. *Infection*
   a. Chronic otitis media
   b. 70% of infants of mothers who acquire rubella in 1st trimester have some degree of hearing loss
10. **Ménière's syndrome**
    a. Clinical
       i. *Fluctuating hearing loss at low frequencies (shift >10 dB at two frequencies is pathognomonic)*
       ii. *Tinnitus*
       iii. *Episodic vertigo*
       iv. *Sensation of pressure in the ear*
       v. *Pathology: distention of the entire endolymphatic system*

    b. Etiologies
        i. Idiopathic (most cases)
        ii. Bacterial
        iii. Viral
        iv. Syphilitic labyrinthitis

NB: Sudden sensorineural hearing loss is a cause of sudden hearing loss that is treated with steroids. Pentoxifylline may be helpful.

ADDITIONAL NOTES

CHAPTER 15

Neurorehabilitation

I. Background and General Principles: approximately 500 million people worldwide are disabled in some way; prevalence: 1 in 10 of the world population; three main groups of roughly equal size: developmental, acute, and chronic conditions; four-fifths of disabled live in developing countries; one-third are children.

II. Mechanisms of Functional Recovery
    A. *Artifact theories:* secondary tissue effects, such as inflammation, edema, and vasospasm, may be associated with temporary changes in neurotransmitter pathways and nonspecific inhibition of neural activity *(diaschisis)*; as innervation is regained elsewhere, so does function return to otherwise undamaged structures; examples: spinal shock or the remote effects of a cortical stroke
    B. *Regeneration:* classically regarded as confined to the peripheral nervous system; potential for regeneration within the central nervous system (CNS) may exist; animal experiments with neural trophic factors or transplantation offer an additional method of artificial tissue regeneration
    C. *Anatomic reorganization:* after damage to higher cortical levels of control, certain functions could be taken over by a lower, subcortical level, albeit in a less sophisticated way; rather than strict hierarchical ordering, certain adjacent cortical association areas or even symmetric regions in the contralateral cerebral hemisphere might fulfill equipotential roles, or have the capacity to take over what are termed *vicarious functions*; greatest potential exists in the immature, developing brain
    D. *Behavioral substitution:* a person with a right hemiplegia may recover the ability to write by learning how to use the left hand; also called *functional adaptation*
    E. *Pharmacologic intervention:* examples: amphetamine, physostigmine, nerve growth factor, corticosteroids, 21-aminosteroids, opiate receptor antagonists, free radical scavengers

III. Aims of Rehabilitation
    A. *Ethical issues*
        1. *Respect for autonomy* is paramount: do not ignore the disabled person's responsibility for self-care
        2. *Beneficence:* doing good
        3. *Nonmaleficence:* doing no harm
        4. *Justice:* ethical duty to ensure that disabled patients receive equal high standards of care and equitable distribution of resources
    B. *Management aims*
        1. Prevent complications
        2. Promote intrinsic recovery
        3. Teach adaptive strategies
        4. Facilitate environmental interaction

IV. Management of Specific Neurologic Impairments

A. *Cognitive impairment*
  1. *Reception by sense organs:* arousal and alerting techniques (e.g., verbal, tactile, visual, oral stimulation in a patient in a vegetative state)
  2. *Perception:* training the patient in obeying commands; miming
  3. *Discrimination:* selective attention may be facilitated by performance of matching and selecting tasks
  4. *Organization:* sorting, sequencing, and completion tasks can be practiced
  5. *Memory and retrieval:* psychological techniques (e.g., interactive visual imagery, mental peg systems, etc.); behavioral techniques (e.g., reinforcement with partial cueing); alerting the environment (e.g., checklists, physical cues, etc.); drugs

B. *Language and speech*
  1. *Aphasia*
     a. *Traditional aphasia therapy:* rote learning; selective stimulation
     b. *Cues or deblocking techniques*
     c. *Behavioral modification* using operant conditioning: programmed instructions break tasks down into small steps, initially with the use of cues, which is later slowly faded
     d. *Melodic intonation or rhythm therapy:* based on the belief that musical and tonal abilities are subserved by an intact right hemisphere
  2. *Dysarthria:* improving person's awareness of deficit may allow him or her to compensate for it; specific exercises for one or two weak muscle groups; self-monitoring; use of ice or palatal training appliances
  3. *Dyslexia:* prognosis for acquired dyslexia is generally poor; use of right hemisphere strategies; arrangment of sentences into vertical columns; tactile presentation of material

C. *Aural impairment:* requires full evaluation of communication; visual acuity is relevant to lipreading; hearing aids: cornerstone of therapy, but unable to overcome the common problem of auditory distortions; environmental aids (e.g., amplification devices); sensory substitution aids (for profound or total deafness; e.g., wearing a belt that converts sound into patterns of vibrotactile stimulation); direct nerve stimulation via cochlear implant; communication training

D. *Visual impairment*
  1. *Vision loss:* magnifying devices; psychological and environmental adjustments (e.g., large print books, radio, prerecorded "talking books," white stick, guide dog)
  2. *Visual agnosia:* intensive visual discrimination training can improve agnosia and neglect
  3. *Diplopia:* alternating covering each eye; prisms; surgery; botulinum toxin injection
  4. *Oscillopsia:* resistant to treatment
  5. *Swallowing and nutrition:* need direct observation; videofluoroscopy; etc.
  6. *Dysphagia:* counseling and advice on positioning, exercises, diet modification; ice may reduce bulbar spasticity; treatments: baclofen, preprandial pyridostigmine (for lower motor neuron weakness); appliances; Teflon injection of vocal cords; cricopharyngeal myotomy (controversial)

E. **Motor impairment**
  1. *Weakness:* physical therapy; variable loading with springs, fixed loads with weights, self-loading; suspension devices and hydrotherapy (for very weak muscles)
  2. *Spasticity:* stretching; drugs: benzodiazepines, baclofen, tizanidine, dantrolene (acts directly on muscle, inhibiting excitation-contraction coupling by depressing calcium release from the sarcoplasmic reticulum); botulinum toxin injection; nerve or motor

point blocks; surgery: lengthening or division of soft tissues; rhizotomy, cordectomy (rare); electrical stimulation of dorsal columns

3. *Ataxia:* use of visual, kinesthetic, and conscious voluntary pathways to compensate should be encouraged; repeated practice of exercises of increasing complexity; avoidance of fatigue; redevelopment of self confidence

V. General Prognostic Pearls after a Cerebrovascular Accident

Ambulation	95% of recovery occurs in 11 wks.
	There is generally no increase in the number of patients that can walk after 2 mos.
Arm weakness	Most recovery occurs in 6 wks.
	There is some increase in neurologic capacity up to 3 mos.
	There is some functional improvement after 1 yr.
Sensory recovery	Usually occurs within 2 mos.
Visual field defect	Usually recovery occurs within 2 wks.
	Some at 3 wks.
	No further recovery at 9 wks.
Neglect	Most recovery occurs in 10 days.
	Some up to 3 mos.
Continence	50% of patients recover in 1 wk.
	Some can take up to 6 mos.
Aphasia	Recovery occurs in weeks to months.
	Some recovery can still occur up to 1 yr, especially with comprehension.
Apraxia	Recovery can occur up to 3 yrs.

NB: After a cerebrovascular accident, tone is usually the first finding to improve.

ADDITIONAL NOTES

CHAPTER 16

Neuroendocrinology

I. Hypothalamus

A. *Hormones that affect pituitary function*

1. *Corticotropin-releasing hormone:* mainly from the paraventricular nucleus; stimulates adrenocorticotropic hormone (ACTH); stimulated by stress, exercise; inhibited by glucocorticoids through negative feedback

2. *Thyrotropin-releasing hormone:* a tripeptide secreted mainly from the paraventricular nucleus; stimulates thyroid-stimulating hormone (TSH) and prolactin; decreased by stress, starvation, and by thyroid hormones through negative feedback

3. *Gonadotropin-releasing hormone (GnRH):* secreted mainly from the arcuate nucleus; pulsatile release stimulates follicle-stimulating hormone (FSH) and luteinizing hormone; continuous exposure to GnRH actually decreases luteinizing hormone and FSH through down-regulation; negatively affected by stress, low body weight, weight loss, excessive exercise (which cause hypothalamic amenorrhea); *clinical application:* treatment of precocious puberty of hypothalamic origin makes use of long-acting GnRH agonists (through down-regulation)

4. *Growth hormone (GH)-releasing hormone:* a peptide secreted from the arcuate nucleus; stimulates GH; *clinical application:* recombinant human GH replacement therapy is given for GH deficiency

5. *Somatostatin or somatotropin release inhibiting factor:* a peptide secreted mainly from the periventricular nuclei; also from the gastrointestinal tract; inhibits release of GH; *clinical application:* somatostatin analogues (e.g., octreotide and lanreotide) and GH receptor antagonists (pegvisomant) are used as adjuncts in treatment of acromegaly (GH excess)

6. *Dopamine:* from the arcuate nucleus: inhibits release of prolactin; prolactin inhibitory factor; suppression, not stimulation of prolactin release is the major hypothalamic effect on prolactin; *clinical applications:* destruction of the hypothalamic-pituitary connection (such as transection of the pituitary stalk) produces a decrease in the release of pituitary hormones, except for prolactin, which is increased because dopamine (prolactin *inhibitory* factor) is the major regulator of this pituitary hormone; dopamine agonists such as bromocriptine and cabergoline are used in the treatment of prolactin-producing tumors

B. *Appetite*

1. The hypothalamus has mediators or *receptors* for mediators of food intake
   a. For increased appetite—ghrelin, neuropeptide Y
   b. For satiety or reduced food intake: leptin, cholecystokinin, serotonin (dexfenfluramine, a serotonergic drug, is an appetite suppressant)
2. Areas of the hypothalamus that control eating
   a. *Lateral nuclei = feeding center;* lesions in this area produce adipsia, aphagia
   b. *Ventromedial nuclei = satiety center;* lesions in this area produce hyperphagia

C. *Emotion/behavior:* stimulation of the *septal region* results in feelings of pleasure and sexual gratification; lesions in the caudal hypothalamus produce attacks of rage; impaired GnRH release causes decreased libido; the opioid peptides enkephalin and dynorphin are involved with sexual behavior

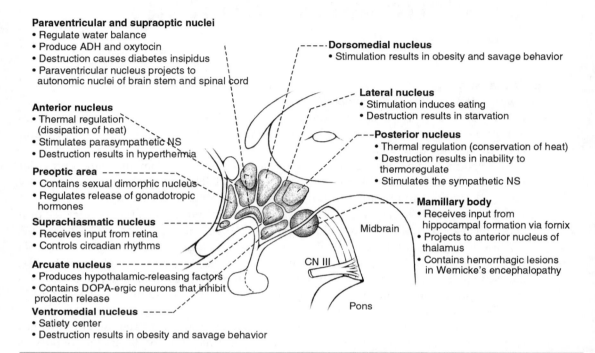

Paraventricular and supraoptic nuclei
• Regulate water balance
• Produce ADH and oxytocin
• Destruction causes diabetes insipidus
• Paraventricular nucleus projects to autonomic nuclei of brain stem and spinal cord

Anterior nucleus
• Thermal regulation (dissipation of heat)
• Stimulates parasympathetic NS
• Destruction results in hyperthermia

Preoptic area
• Contains sexual dimorphic nucleus
• Regulates release of gonadotropic hormones

Suprachiasmatic nucleus
• Receives input from retina
• Controls circadian rhythms

Arcuate nucleus
• Produces hypothalamic-releasing factors
• Contains DOPA-ergic neurons that inhibit prolactin release

Ventromedial nucleus
• Satiety center
• Destruction results in obesity and savage behavior

Dorsomedial nucleus
• Stimulation results in obesity and savage behavior

Lateral nucleus
• Stimulation induces eating
• Destruction results in starvation

Posterior nucleus
• Thermal regulation (conservation of heat)
• Destruction results in inability to thermoregulate
• Stimulates the sympathetic NS

Mamillary body
• Receives input from hippocampal formation via fornix
• Projects to anterior nucleus of thalamus
• Contains hemorrhagic lesions in Wernicke's encephalopathy

Midbrain   CN III   Pons

Figure 16-1. The hypothalamus with its various nuclei and corresponding functions. ADH, antidiuretic hormone; CN, cranial nerve; NS, nervous system.

D. *Temperature*
1. *Pre-optic anterior hypothalamus:* lesions of this area produce *hyperthermia*
2. *Posterior hypothalamus:* lesions of this area produce *hypothermia and poikilothermia*

II. Pituitary
A. *Anterior pituitary (adenohypophysis) hormones*

Pituitary hormone	Excess (adenomas)	Deficiency
ACTH	Cushing's disease	Adrenal insufficiency (glucocorticoid axis)
TSH	Hyperthyroidism	Hypothyroidism
FSH and LH	Usually silent	Infertility, hypogonadism
GH (somatotropin)	Gigantism in children	GH deficiency
	Acromegaly in adults	
Prolactin	Amenorrhea, galactorrhea	Inability to lactate

LH, luteinizing hormone.

1. *Pituitary tumors:* 40–50% are prolactinomas; 20–25% are somatotropinomas; 8–10% are corticotropinomas; 1–2% are thyrotropinomas; 20–25% are clinically nonfunctioning (includes gonadotropinomas)
   a. *Hyperprolactinemia:* produces amenorrhea, galactorrhea, low testosterone levels in males; causes of hyperprolactinemia

Physiologic	Pregnancy
	Sleep
	Nursing
	Stress
	Nipple stimulation
Drugs	Dopamine receptor blockers
	Phenothiazines
	H_2 antagonists
	Estrogens
	α-Methyldopa
CNS lesions	*Prolactinomas*
	Lesions of the hypothalamus or pituitary stalk, granulomatous disease
Others	Liver cirrhosis
	Chronic renal failure
	Primary hypothyroidism (via TRH stimulation)

CNS, central nervous system; TRH, thyrotropin-releasing hormone

   Prolactinomas: *>70% are microadenomas* (<10 mm), the rest are macroadenomas (>10 mm); diagnosis of prolactinomas: prolactin levels, pituitary magnetic resonance imaging (MRI); treatment of choice: dopamine agonists—bromocriptine, cabergoline—for micro- and macroprolactinomas
   b. *Acromegaly:* causes frontal bossing, coarse facial features, increased shoe and ring size, carpal tunnel syndrome, hyperhidrosis; diagnosis: elevated GH and insulin-like growth factor-1; lack of GH suppression after oral glucose tolerance test; pituitary MRI; treatment of choice: transsphenoidal surgery; adjuncts: radiation, dopamine agonists such as bromocriptine (because dopamine attenuates GH secretion in one-third of patients), GH receptor antagonist (pegvisomant), somatostatin analogues (octreotide, lanreotide)
   c. *Cushing's disease:* Cushing's syndrome due to a pituitary adenoma (other causes of Cushing's syndrome are exogenous glucocorticoid intake, adrenal tumors, and ectopic ACTH production); presents with moon facies, buffalo hump, purple striae, diabetes, centripetal obesity; diagnosis: screening by 1 mg overnight dexamethasone suppression test, 48-hour low-dose dexamethasone suppression test, midnight salivary cortisol, or by urinary free cortisol; to differentiate from adrenal or ectopic causes of Cushing's syndrome: high-dose dexamethasone suppression test, 9 a.m. plasma ACTH level, metyrapone test, corticotropin-releasing hormone test; pituitary MRI, inferior petrosal sinus sampling; treatment: transsphenoidal pituitary surgery is the treatment of choice

    d. *Thyrotropinomas:* rare; manifests with hyperthyroidism (symptoms include palpitations, nervousness, weight loss, increased appetite, increased sweatiness), diffuse goiter; diagnosis: TSH levels are normal or high, thyroxine (T_4) and triiodothyronine (T_3) levels are high (as opposed to hyperthyroidism from a thyroid origin such as Graves' disease, in which TSH is low while T_4 and T_3 are high); elevated α subunit levels; pituitary MRI; macroadenoma in 90% of cases; treatment: surgery is the treatment of choice; adjuncts are radiation, somatostatin analogs such as octreotide, or treatment targeted towards the thyroid gland itself, such as antithyroid drugs, radioactive iodine ablation, or thyroidectomy

    e. *Gonadotropinomas:* rare, usually clinically silent

2. *Hypopituitarism:* may be inherited or acquired (e.g., from compression, inflammation, invasion, radiation of the hypothalamus or pituitary); for acquired disorders: prolactin deficiency is rare and occurs only when the entire anterior pituitary is destroyed (e.g., pituitary apoplexy) (remember that tonic inhibition by dopamine is the predominant control of prolactin); of the remaining cells, the corticotrophs and thyrotrophs are usually the last to lose function

    a. *Adrenal insufficiency:* affects the glucocorticoid, not the mineralocorticoid, axis (for adrenal insufficiency originating from the adrenals, both glucocorticoid and mineralocorticoid axes are affected); presents acutely with hypotension, shock; chronic adrenal insufficiency presents with nausea, fatigue; diagnosis: ACTH stimulation test (however, will not differentiate between primary adrenal failure and secondary pituitary failure)—draw baseline cortisol levels, administer synthetic ACTH (e.g., Cortrosyn®), 250 μg intramuscularly or intravenously, then draw cortisol levels again at 30 and 60 minutes; normal if peak cortisol is >20 μg/dL; may give false normal results in acute cases because the adrenal glands may still produce cortisol; in the acute setting, do not need for lab values to come back before instituting glucocorticoid treatment if clinically warranted; in acute stressful situations, hydrocortisone has conventionally been given at a total daily dose of 300 mg intravenously, but lower doses are also effective; maintenance treatment is usually with hydrocortisone, 20 mg in the morning and 10 mg at night, or prednisone, 5 mg in the morning and 2.5 mg at night, or less if tolerated

    b. *Hypothyroidism:* not apparent acutely because the half-life of serum T_4 is approximately 7 days; diagnosis: normal or low TSH, low T_4 and T_3 (as opposed to primary hypothyroidism, in which TSH is high); glucocorticoids should be replaced before thyroid hormone replacement; replacement is with levothyroxine preparations such as Synthroid®

    c. *Hypogonadotropic hypogonadism:* delayed puberty, amenorrhea in females: can be seen in female athletes; low testosterone levels in males (causes sexual dysfunction, decreased libido); treatment of delayed puberty: testosterone for boys, estrogen for girls; luteinizing hormone-releasing hormone or FSH and human chorionic gonadotropin to induce ovulation/fertility; treatment with testosterone replacement in adults: intramuscular or topical preparations; monitoring of prostate-specific antigen levels (link with prostatic cancer though causality not yet proven) and complete blood count (can cause polycythemia); inherited disorders include

      i. **Kallmann's syndrome:** hypogonadotropic hypogonadism, anosmia

      ii. **Laurence-Moon-Biedl:** autosomal recessive, hypogonadotropic hypogonadism, mental retardation, obesity, retinitis pigmentosa, syndactyly

      iii. **Prader-Willi:** hypogonadotropic hypogonadism, hyperphagia, obesity, mental retardation

NB: Condition is produced when chromosomal defect is inherited from the father; if inherited from the mother, the result is Angelman's syndrome.

   d. *GH deficiency:* short stature in children; in adults with pituitary disease, GH is the most frequently deficient of the pituitary hormones; in adults: present with fatigue, increased fat mass, decreased muscle mass, decreased bone density; diagnosis: gold standard is the insulin tolerance test in which GH response to insulin-induced hypoglycemia is measured; treatment: recombinant human GH

B. *Posterior pituitary (neurohypophysis) hormones:* axons from the hypothalamus have direct connections with the posterior lobe of the pituitary

1. *Arginine vasopressin or antidiuretic hormone:* from the supraoptic and paraventricular nuclei

   a. *Hypothalamic diabetes insipidus (DI):* deficiency of arginine vasopressin; causes: head trauma, neurosurgery, tumors such as craniopharyngioma, CNS infections, CNS vascular disease, pituitary apoplexy *(Sheehan's syndrome),* autoimmune disorders, familial DI, idiopathic; presents with polyuria and polydipsia; new-onset enuresis in children; presents with hypernatremia if with deficient thirst mechanism or without access to fluids, otherwise normal serum sodium; dilute urine; differential diagnosis procedure: *dehydration (fluid deprivation) test* to differentiate hypothalamic from nephrogenic DI; treatment of hypothalamic DI: intranasal or oral desmopressin

   b. *Syndrome of inappropriate antidiuretic hormone secretion:* usually a diagnosis of exclusion; hyponatremia with plasma osmolality <275 mOsm/kg H_2O and inappropriate urine osmolality (>100 mOsm/kg H_2O); with normal renal function; with euvolemia; without adrenal insufficiency, hypothyroidism, or diuretics; caused by: CNS infections, tumors and trauma, pulmonary and mediastinal infection and tumors, drugs—phenothiazines, tricyclic antidepressants, desmopressin, oxytocin, salicylates, nonsteroidal anti-inflammatory drugs; diagnosis in difficult cases can be aided by *water loading test* (oral water load of 20 mL per kg body weight in 15–20 minutes, inability to excrete 80–90% of the oral load in 4–5 hours, and inability to suppress the urine osmolality to <100 mOsm/kg H_2O)

2. *Oxytocin:* from the supraoptic and paraventricular nuclei; release during suckling results in myoepithelial cell contraction and milk ejection, as well as myometrial contractions

III. Pineal Gland: secretes melatonin, which is high at night and low during the day; melatonin influences (1) circadian rhythmicity, (2) induction of seasonal responses to changes in day length, and (3) the reproductive axis; melatonin is synthesized from tryptophan; treatment with melatonin has been used for jet lag and to regulate sleep, but controlled clinical trials are lacking

NB: Afferent input to the pineal gland is transmitted from retinal photoreceptors through the suprachiasmatic nucleus and sympathetic nervous system, the supply of which comes from the superior cervical ganglion.

ADDITIONAL NOTES

CHAPTER 17

Neuro-oncology, Transplant Neurology, and Headache Syndromes

I. Central Nervous System (CNS) Tumors

A. *Oncogenes and chromosomal aberrations in the CNS:* oncogenes—genes that are mutated, deleted, or overexpressed during the formation of tumors; *dominant oncogenes*—cause overexpression of growth products in tumors; *recessive oncogenes*—cause loss of function to suppress neoplasia, also called *antioncogenes* or *tumor suppressor genes*

1. *Fibrillary astrocytomas:* loss of the short arm of chromosome 17 in 50% of fibrillary astrocytomas

2. **Li-Fraumeni cancer susceptibility syndrome:** associated with *mutations in p53 tumor suppressor gene* located on the distal short arm of *chromosome 17*; families have dramatically increased incidence of early-onset breast cancer, childhood sarcomas, and brain tumors; 50% likelihood of receiving a diagnosis of cancer by age 30 years

3. *Glioblastoma multiforme (GBM):* loss of chromosome 10 in 80% of GBM cases; gains in chromosome 7; loss of chromosome 22; *loss of tumor suppressor genes P53 in chromosome 17p13.1 and CDKN2 in chromosome 9; amplification of epidermal growth factor receptor*

4. *Retinoblastoma:* sporadic in 60% of cases, autosomal dominant in 40%; emergence of *tumor requires inactivation of retinoblastoma gene (tumor suppressor gene) on chromosome 13q14*; in the familial form, one gene is inactivated in the cell; thus, only one gene needs inactivation to produce the tumor; in the sporadic form, both need inactivation

5. *Pituitary adenoma:* loss of tumor suppressor gene, *MEN 1 on chromosome 11q13*

B. *Neuroepithelial tumors*

1. **Astrocytic tumors**

   a. **Fibrillary (low grade) astrocytoma:** occurs mainly in adults between 30 and 50 y/o; microscopic appearance is very uniform: sparse and fairly regular proliferation of astrocytes without histologic evidence of malignancy, mitotic figures, or vascular endothelial proliferation and without area of necrosis or hemorrhage; malignant change after several years occurs frequently; complete resection/cure often not possible (although may respond to chemotherapy and radiation); *do not enhance on scans*

   b. **Anaplastic astrocytoma:** cellular atypia and mitotic activity, endothelial proliferation is common (but *no necrosis*); poorly responsive to therapy; frequently evolves into GBM

   c. **GBM:** most malignant grade; also the most common malignant primary tumor in adults; chiefly supratentorial; magnetic resonance imaging (MRI): enhancing lesion surrounded by edema (may be indistinguishable from abscess); frequently crosses the corpus callosum *butterfly glioma*

Kernohan Grading System

Grade I	Atypia	Increased cellularity, gliosis	Low-grade astrocytoma
Grade II	Mitosis	Greater cellularity than grade I; pleomorphism	Most anaplastic astrocytoma
Grade III	Endothelial proliferation	Greater cellularity than grade II with vascular proliferation; gemistocytic astrocytes	GBM; accounts for 20–30% of all gliomas; fibrillary type is the most common
Grade IV	Necrosis	Features of grade II plus necrosis with pseudo-palisading	GBM; accounts for 40–50% of all glial tumors

NB: Age is the most important prognostic factor for GBM (younger age is better).

World Health Organization Grading System

Grade I	Pilocytic astrocytoma, subependymal giant cell astrocytoma
Grade II	Fibrillary infiltrating astrocytoma, low-grade astrocytoma
Grade III	Anaplastic astrocytoma
Grade IV	GBM (requires necrosis)

NB: For approximate survival years, remember the rule of nines: astrocytoma—36 months, anaplastic astrocytoma—18 months, glioblastoma—9 months.

    d. **Juvenile pilocytic astrocytoma:** *cerebellar astrocytoma/optic nerve glioma/pontine glioma/hypothalamic glioma;* more common in children and young adults; *location:* commonly in the cerebellum, optic nerve, hypothalamus; generally discrete and well-circumscribed; *pathology:* cystic structures containing mural nodule, hair-like cells with pleomorphic nuclei, contain *Rosenthal fibers* (opaque, homogeneous, eosinophilic structures), microcystic, endothelial proliferation; *MRI:* cystic lesion surrounding some amount of central enhancement (**NB:** low-grade astrocytomas generally do not enhance); course: *indolent;* surgically curable if gross removal is possible

    e. **Subependymal giant cell astrocytoma:** *grade I astrocytoma;* well-demarcated; *location:* lateral ventricles; *associated with tuberous sclerosis;* may produce hydrocephalus; *MRI:* well circumscribed, enhance homogenously; *pathology:* large, round nuclei, few mitoses, few endothelial proliferations; prognosis: good

NB: In tuberous sclerosis, tumor may occur at the foramen of Monro, causing hydrocephalus.

    f. **Pleomorphic xanthoastrocytoma:** common in adolescents and young adults; located in the superficial cortex; frequently in the temporal lobe; thus, often causing seizures; *pathology:* often cystic, large pleomorphic, hyperchromatic nuclei, minimal mitotic activity, no necrosis; most patients live many years

    g. **Desmoplastic cerebral astrocytoma of infancy:** very rare tumor of the first 2 years of life; predilection for the superficial frontoparietal region; *pathology:* desmoplasia (desmoplastic stroma commonly mistaken as fibrillary until abundant glial fibrillary acidic protein [GFAP] confirms glial nature); good prognosis with surgical resection

h. **Gemistocytic astrocytoma:** variant of astrocytoma; contains neoplastic astrocytes with abundant cytoplasm; 80% subsequently transform into GBM

i. **Gliomatosis cerebri:** fairly uncommon; diffuse, neoplastic astrocytic infiltration; hemispheric or bihemispheric

j. **Gliosarcoma:** *collision tumor;* combination of malignant glial and mesenchymal elements; dural and endothelial transformations are theories; prognosis and treatment are similar to GBM

2. *Ependymal tumors*

a. **Ependymoma:** accounts for 6% of gliomas; occur at any age but more common in childhood and adolescence; location: more likely infratentorial, with the most frequent site being the 4th ventricle; in the spinal cord, 60% are located in the lumbosacral segments and filum terminale; *pathology:* gross—reddish nodular and lobulated; microscopic—rudimentary canal and gliovascular (pseudo) rosettes, ciliated cells, but can have *Flexner-Wintersteiner (true) rosettes;* GFAP positive; prognosis has been better, although tumor generally recurs at some point

b. **Anaplastic ependymomas:** usually well circumscribed and benign, however, can be malignant

c. **Myxopapillary ependymomas:** more commonly at the cauda equina or filum terminale; may mimic herniated disc or present with posterior rectal mass; generally benign and well circumscribed; pathology: contain mucinous structures surrounded by ependymal cells

NB: Two particular tumors that occur in the filum terminale are the myxopapillary ependymoma and the paraganglioma of the filum terminale. Myxopapillary ependymoma is positive for GFAP and S-100 protein.

d. **Subependymoma:** usually incidental findings at autopsy in adults; well-circumscribed ventricular lesions; usually asymptomatic (or can cause obstructive hydrocephalus); cluster of nuclei separated by acellular areas; GFAP positive

3. *Choroid plexus tumors*

a. *Choroid plexus papilloma:* account for 2% of intracranial tumors; most frequently in the 1st decade of life; location: 4th ventricle, lateral ventricle (left > right), 3rd ventricle; in children, more commonly supratentorial; in adults, more commonly infratentorial; more common to cause ventricular obstruction than cerebrospinal fluid (CSF) overproduction; *MRI:* well-delineated ventricular lesion with fairly homogeneous enhancement; *pathology:* papillary, calcified, single layer of cuboidal or columnar cells with a fibrovascular core; curable by surgical resection; does not invade the brain (no recurrence)

b. **Choroid plexus carcinoma (ca):** also affects young children; location: 4th ventricle, occipital lobe; pathology: less differentiated, increased mitosis, necrosis, invades the parenchyma, may seed CSF

4. *Oligodendroglial tumors:* **NB:** significant portion are chemosensitive

a. **Oligodendroglioma:** account for approximately 5% of intracranial gliomas; most frequently between ages 30 and 50 years; location: usually cerebral hemispheres, clinical behavior is unpredictable and depends on degree of mitotic rate; pathology: uniform *fried egg cells,* delicate vessels, calcification; mitotic figures are rare, GFAP negative; MRI: diffuse wispy white matter appearance; treatment: radiation and chemosensitive; better prognosis than astrocytic tumors

NB: Mutations in chromosomes 1 and 19 usually have better response to treatment.

  b. **Anaplastic oligodendroglioma:** larger pleomorphic nuclei; with mitotic activity, endothelial proliferation and necrosis
  c. **Mixed oligoastrocytomas:** with oligodendroglial and astrocytic components; low grade or anaplastic; **NB:** glioblastoma with presence of oligodendroglial component may have better prognosis (more responsive to chemotherapy)
5. *Neuronal and mixed neuronal-glial tumors*
  a. **Gangliocytoma:** tumor of mature-appearing neoplastic neurons only
  b. **Ganglioglioma:** mature neoplastic neurons and neoplastic astrocytes; almost always benign; commonly in the temporal lobe of a young adult; may cause long-standing seizure; *pathology:* may appear *cystic with a mural nodule,* microscopic—binucleate, round, GFAP negative, and synaptophysin-positive neoplastic neurons

NB: Synaptophysin is the most specific marker of neuronal differentiation.

  c. **Ganglioneuroblastoma:** mature and immature neurons
  d. **Anaplastic ganglioglioma:** more malignant form of ganglioglioma
  e. **Central neurocytoma:** relatively uncommon intraventricular tumor in the lateral ventricle; discrete, well circumscribed; enhance with contrast administration; *pathology:* microscopically indistinguishable from oligodendroglioma; small, round, bland nuclei, *Homer-Wright rosettes,* no histologic anaplasia (benign), confirmation comes with immunohistochemical demonstration of neural antigens or electron microscopy showing neuronal features
  f. **Dysembryoplastic neuroectodermal tumor:** small islands of mature neurons mimicking oligodendrocytes floating in a *mucin-like substance;* multiple intracortical lesions mainly in the temporal lobe
  g. **Dysplastic infantile ganglioglioma:** highly characteristic supratentorial neuroepithelial neoplasms that occur as large cystic masses in early infancy; most frequently in the frontal and parietal region; *pathology:* marked fibroblastic and desmoplastic component but mature neuroepithelial cells of both glial and neuronal lineage; more primitive cells are also present; very favorable clinical course after successful complete or subtotal resection
  h. **Dysplastic gangliocytoma of the cerebellum (Lhermitte-Duclos):** slowly evolving lesion that forms a mass in the cerebellum, composed of granule, Purkinje, and glial cells; lack of growth potential, therefore, favorable prognosis
  i. **Paraganglioma (chemodectoma):** neural crest derived; location: filum terminale, supra-adrenal, carotid body; *glomus jugulare, glomus vagale;* can produce neurotransmitters; *pathology:* nodules surrounded by reticulin—Zellballen; treatment: surgery or chemo-/radiotherapy
  j. **Olfactory neuroblastoma (esthesioneuroblastoma):** nasal obstruction/epistaxis may be the presenting symptoms; may erode through the cribriform plate; pathology: small blue cell tumor (also a type of primitive neuroectodermal tumor [PNET]); treatment: responsive to chemo-/radiotherapy; fairly good prognosis
6. *Embryonal tumors*
  a. **PNETs:** small blue cell tumors that are named depending on their location; they resemble germinal matrix; >90% are nondifferentiated cells (capable of differentiating along astrocytic, ependymal, oligodendroglial, and neuronal lines); 50% are calcified; 50% are cystic; propensity to spread along CSF; generally sensitive to radiotherapy (**NB:** blastomas are PNET tumors except for hemangioblastoma)
    i. **Medulloblastoma:** the most common intracranial PNET; in children, most commonly located at the cerebellar midline (25% of pediatric brain tumors); 50%

have drop metastasis; 50% 10-year survival with multimodality therapy (surgery, radiation, chemotherapy); *pathology: Homer-Wright rosettes,* carrot-shaped nuclei, mitosis, necrosis; *loss of alleles on chromosome 17p; oncogenes called c-myc and n-myc are known to be amplified in some medulloblastomas*—poor prognostic indicators

NB: Suspect medulloblastoma in child presenting with headaches and ataxia.

    ii. **Pineoblastoma:** PNET of the pineal gland; occurs most commonly in children; *frequent leptomeningeal metastasis (drop metastasis); radiology:* contrast-enhancing pineal region mass; *pathology:* resembles medulloblastomas, may form *fleurettes;* treatment: surgical resection; prognosis: rapid recurrence with wide dissemination

NB: The most common pineal gland tumor is the germinoma.

    iii. **Ependymoblastoma:** usually 1st 5 years of life; location: commonly cerebrum with craniospinal metastasis; radiology: large discrete, contrast-enhancing lesion; pathology: ependymoblastic rosettes in field of undifferentiated cells; treatment: surgical resection ± radiation ± chemotherapy

    iv. **Retinoblastoma:** sporadic in 60% of all cases, *autosomal dominant in 40%; emergence of tumor requires inactivation of Rb gene (tumor suppressor gene) on chromosome 13q14;* in the familial form, one gene is inactivated in the cell; thus, only one gene needs inactivation to produce the tumor; in the sporadic form, both need inactivation; trilateral (rare): bilateral retinoblastomas + pineoblastoma; *pathology: Flexner-Wintersteiner rosettes* with mitosis and necrosis; treatment: enucleation

    v. **Esthesioblastoma:** from the olfactory neuroepithelium

    vi. **Neuroblastoma:** rare in the CNS; most commonly arise in the sympathetic chain (or in adrenal) in childhood; clinical correlate of dancing eyes (opsoclonus) and dancing feet syndrome; *pathology:* small blue cell tumors, *Homer-Wright rosettes*

  b. **Medulloepithelioma:** prototype of embryonal central neuroepithelial tumors; characterized by papillary and tubular pattern of closely aligned pseudostratified cells (that recall the structure of the primitive epithelium of the medullary plate and neuronal tube); marked capacity for divergent differentiation; thus, may comprise focal areas of ependymoblastoma, astrocytoma, neuroblastoma, and gangliocytoma

7. *Pineal parenchymal tumors:* 80% are calcified; **NB:** computed tomography scan is the modality of choice in the evaluation of pineal region tumors owing to the calcification

  a. **Pineocytoma:** occurs primarily in middle to late adulthood; radiology: contrast-enhancing solid mass in the pineal region; pathology: noninvasive, sheets of small cells resembling pineal gland with pineocytomatous rosettes; treatment: surgical resection; prognosis: favorable after resection

  b. **Pineoblastoma:** a PNET; highly malignant

  c. **Mixed or transitional pineal tumors**

8. *Neuroepithelial tumors of uncertain origin*

  a. **Astroblastoma:** circumscribed, usually paraventricular or subcortical gliomas occurring in young persons and characterized by a prominent arrangement of the tumor cells in perivascular pseudorosettes; the better differentiated forms have good prognosis, but tumors may convert to glioblastoma

  b. **Polar spongioblastoma:** extremely rare gliomas of primitive character; often involve the wall of one of the ventricles; most frequently in young persons; pathology: conspicuous palisading arrangement of the tumor cells in rather compact groups; cells are thin and tapering unipolar or bipolar spongioblasts with very delicate neuroglial fibrils

  c. **Gliomatosis cerebri**

C. *Tumors of nerve sheath cells*

1. **Neurilemmoma (schwannomas; neurinoma):** benign tumors arising from Schwann cell; usually *solitary except in neurofibromatosis type 1* in which they are multiple; *in neurofibromatosis type 2, bilateral acoustic schwannomas* can be found; location: most commonly cranial nerve VIII, also other cranial nerves, spinal roots (thoracic segments > cervical, lumbar, cauda equina); pathology: *Antoni type A*—dense fibrillary tissue, narrow elongated bipolar cells with very little cytoplasm and nuclei that are arranged in whorls or palisades; *Antoni type B*—loose reticulated type tissue, round nuclei are randomly arranged in a matrix that appears finely honeycombed; *MRI:* hyperintense on T2; gross total resection usually possible

NB: Schwannomas are strongly positive for S-100 protein.

2. **Neurofibroma:** differ from schwannomas in that they almost always occur within the context of neurofibromatosis type 1, almost always multiple, may undergo malignant transformation in 0.5–1.0% of tumors (neurofibrosarcoma); *plexiform neurofibroma:* cord-like enlargement of nerve twigs; pathology: single cells, axons, myxoid background, parent nerve is usually intermingled with tumor

NB: Tumors occurring in the nerve roots may have a dumbbell appearance.

3. **Malignant peripheral nerve sheath tumor:** includes malignant schwannomas and neurofibroma; most common in neurofibromatosis type 1; aggressive tumors clinically: 12-month survival; usually involves the limb, requiring limb amputation

D. *Tumors of the meninges*

1. **Meningioma:** benign tumors originating from arachnoid cells; account for 13–18% of primary intracranial tumors and 35% of intraspinal tumors (frequently in the thoracic segment in the lateral compartment of the subdural space); most meningiomas have *a partial or complete deletion of chromosome 22;* primarily in adults (20–60 y/o), although it may occur in childhood; female predominance, especially in the spinal epidural space (**NB:** women with breast cancer have a higher incidence of meningioma); *pathology:* gross—spherical, well circumscribed, and firmly attached to the inner surface of the dura; microscopic—*psammoma bodies* (whorls of cells wrapped around each other with a calcified center), xanthomatous changes (presence of fat-filled cells), myxomatous changes (homogeneous stroma separating individual cells), areas of cartilage or bone within the tumor, foci of melanin pigment in the connective tissue trabeculae, rich vascularization; may produce hyperostosis (local osteoblastic proliferation of skull); most are epithelial membrane antigen positive; *radiology:* dural-based tumors cause enhancement of the peripheral rim of the dura surrounding the meningioma producing *the dural tail*

   a. *Histologic types: meningothelial, syncytial, fibroblastic, transitional, psammomatous, angiomatous, microcystic, secretory, clear cell, choroid, lymphoplasmacyte-rich, metaplastic*

   b. *"Aggressive" variants with tendency to bleed or metastasize: hemangiopericytic, papillary or anaplastic meningioma*

   c. *Location:* convexity meningiomas (parasagittal, falx, lateral convexity); basal meningiomas (olfactory groove, lesser wing of the sphenoid, pterion, suprasellar meningiomas); posterior fossa meningiomas, meningiomas of the foramen magnum, as well as intraventricular meningiomas are considerably less common

NB: Meningiomas are strongly positive for epithelial membrane antigen.

NB: Meningioma in the planum sphenoidale that could involve both the olfactory groove and optic canal is a common etiology for Foster-Kennedy syndrome—unilateral anosmia and optic neuropathy with increased ICP (papilledema in the opposite eye).

2. **Lipoma:** hamartomatous rather than neoplastic; midline lesions arising from cellular rests; commonly found in the cauda equina, spinal cord, corpus callosum (**NB:** no adipose tissue normally exists in the CNS except the filum terminale); *pathology:* mature adipose tissue; prognosis: good, usually an incidental finding

3. **Hemangiopericytoma:** identical to the systemic soft tissue tumor; generally intracranial; no gender predilection (unlike meningiomas); intensely vascular with contrast enhancement; *pathology:* hypercellular and lacking whorls or nodules, staghorn vasculature, mitosis and necrosis common; epithelial membrane antigen negative

4. **Melanoma:** a wide variety ranging from a simple increase in normal leptomeningeal pigmentation to highly malignant melanomas; primary melanomas of the nervous system are extremely rare; **NB:** therefore, it is essential to exclude rigorously a small occult primary cutaneous or ocular melanoma.

5. *Others:* **chondrosarcoma, malignant fibrous histiocytoma, fibrous histiocytoma, osteocartilaginous tumors, rhabdomyosarcomas, meningeal sarcomatosis, melanocytoma**

E. *Tumors of uncertain histogenesis*

1. **Hemangioblastoma:** the most common primary cerebellar neoplasm; sporadic or genetic; 20% are associated with von Hippel-Lindau syndrome (hemangioblastoma, retinal angiomatosis, renal cell ca, renal and pancreatic cysts); location: cerebellum > brain stem > spinal cord; pathology: gross—cystic lesion with mural nodule, microscopic—foamy cells in clusters separated by blood-filled channels, surrounding parenchyma contains Rosenthal fibers; gadolinium-enhanced MRI is the best modality for detection

NB: Von Hippel-Lindau syndrome is inherited as an autosomal dominant trait.

NB: The most common cerebellar tumor is metastatic.

F. *Lymphomas and hematopoietic neoplasms*

1. **Malignant lymphoma:** **NB:** most CNS lymphomas *are B cell;* usually non-Hodgkin's (usually a diffuse large cell variety); more common in the immunocompromised population; Epstein-Barr virus may play a role; *ghost tumor:* initially may respond dramatically to steroids and/or radiation but eventually recurs; commonly originate in the basal ganglia or periventricular white matter; may be multifocal; angiocentric or perivascular distribution; radiology: homogeneous contrast enhancement located in the deep brain rather than the gray-white interface; treatment: methotrexate; responds to steroids and radiation but recurs; prognosis: overall survival in human immunodeficiency virus is 3 months or less, in nonhuman immunodeficiency virus is 19 months

NB: The main differential diagnosis for CNS lymphoma in human immunodeficiency virus patients is toxoplasmosis.

2. *Others:* plasmacytoma, granulocytic sarcoma

G. **Germ cell tumors:** most occur within the 1st three decades of life (except pineocytoma); *Parinaud syndrome:* limited upgaze due to compression of the tectal plate; more common in males

1. **Germinoma:** *seminoma;* account for >50% of pineal tumors; two-thirds of tumors are calcified; location: suprasellar (in females), pineal region (in males); two cell populations: large malignant cells and small reactive lymphocytes; placental alkaline-phosphatase positive; responsive to therapy but often seed CSF

2. **Embryonal cell ca:** increased α-fetoprotein; increased β-human chorionic gonadotropin

3. **Yolk sac tumor** *(endodermal sinus tumor):* increased α-fetoprotein

4. **Teratoma:** may arise in utero and present as hemispheric mass; pathology: three germ cell layers are present—ectoderm, mesoderm, and endoderm; benign, but any component may become malignant; location: generally midline (pineal region, sellar, suprasellar, posterior fossa) and sacrococcygeal area; treatment: resection; prognosis: favorable with resection

5. *Others:* teratocarcinoma, mixed germ cell tumors

H. *Cysts and tumor-like lesions*

1. **Rathke cleft cyst:** epithelial cyst in the sella

2. **Epidermoid cyst:** due to slow-growing ectodermal inclusion cysts; secondary to ectoderm trapped at the time of closure of neural tube; cyst lined by keratin producing squamous epithelium; leakage of contents into the CSF produces chemical meningitis; occurs mostly laterally instead of midline; *radiology:* low-density cyst with irregularly enhancing rim, may not enhance with contrast; treatment: surgical excision preferred; prognosis: recurrence with subtotal excision

3. **Dermoid cyst:** mostly present in childhood; hydrocephalus common; pathology: comprising mesoderm and ectoderm lined with stratified squamous epithelium and filled with hair, sebaceous glands, and sweat glands; location: usually midline, related to fontanel, 4th ventricle, spinal cord; treatment: surgical resection; prognosis: recurrence with subtotal excision

4. **Colloid cyst:** account for 2% of intracranial gliomas; mainly in young adults; location: always at the anterior end of the 3rd ventricle, adjacent to the foramen of Monro; *MRI:* increased signal on T1-weighted images (due to the proteinaceous composition of contents); obstructive hydrocephalus is common; therapy: drainage, surgical resection

NB: Patients may present with lightning headaches that improve with positional changes of the head.

5. **Hypothalamic hamartomas:** rare; associated with gelastic seizures and endocrine abnormalities; location: hypothalamus; radiology: small discrete mass near the floor of the 3rd ventricle; *pathology:* well-differentiated but disorganized neuroglial tissue; treatment: surgical resection or ablation, if possible; prognosis: cure is possible if resected

6. *Others:* **nasal glial heterotopia, plasma cell granuloma, neurenteric (enterogenous) cyst, granular cell tumor**

I. *Tumors of the sellar region*

1. **Pituitary adenoma:** 15% of all intracranial neoplasms; women > men; most common neoplasm of the pituitary gland; can present early if they hypersecrete hormones or later owing to compressive effects; microadenoma (<10-mm diameter) tend to be hormone secreting with hyperprolactinemia as the most common hormonal abnormality; may be due to hypersecretion or stalk effect in which the flow of prolactin inhibitory factor (dopamine) is absent; treatment: bromocriptine—may induce tumor fibrosis (which may make pathologic diagnosis difficult); older classification system

a. *Acidophilic:* growth hormone ± prolactin; rare follicle-stimulating hormone or luteinizing hormone; acromegaly

b. *Basophilic:* adrenocorticotropic hormone >> thyroid-stimulating hormone; hyperadrenalism (Cushing's disease)

c. *Chromophobic:* prolactin; null; rarely follicle-stimulating hormone/luteinizing hormone; amenorrhea-galactorrhea; men impotent

d. *Mixed*

2. **Pituitary ca:** adenocarcinoma; rarely primary; usually metastatic (commonly from breast)

3. **Craniopharyngioma:** *Rathke pouch cyst;* origin is uncertain; bimodal age of distribution of childhood and adult life; calcified and cystic; *crankcase oil;* more commonly adenomatous but can be papillary; benign but locally adherent; **NB:** chemical meningitis is a rare complication of craniopharyngioma with seeding of the cyst into the subarachnoid space.

J. *Local extensions from regional tumors*
   1. **Paraganglioma (chemodectoma)/glomus jugulare tumor:** rare; originate from the cells of the jugular body; proliferates in the middle ear and may present in the external meatus, but, in the majority of the cases, the growth reaches the posterior fossa especially in the cerebellopontine angle
   2. **Chordoma:** notochord remnant; approximately 40% of chordomas arise in the clivus; the remainder are distributed unevenly along the vertebral column: cervical, thoracic, lumbar, and sacral (5:1:1:20 respectively); relentlessly locally invasive
   3. *Others:* chondroma, chondrosarcoma, chondrocarcinoma

K. *Metastatic tumors:* 20–40% of all brain tumors; well-defined, round, with surrounding edema; *location:* gray-white junction
   1. *Primary CNS tumors:* can metastasize to extracranial regions (any anaplastic glial tumor, PNET, meningioma), lymph nodes and/or lung (gliomas, meningiomas) or bone (PNET)
   2. *Secondary metastasis to brain:* bronchogenic ca > breast ca > melanoma > hypernephroma
   3. *Hemorrhagic transformation*—melanoma, bronchogenic ca, choriocarcinoma (the only pineal region tumor that may bleed spontaneously; increased β-human chorionic gonadotropin), renal ca, thyroid ca
   4. Metastasis to the skull/dura: prostate, lung, breast, lymphoma
   5. Meningeal carcinomatosis: adenocarcinomas (gastrointestinal, breast, lung)

NB: The most common site of CNS metastasis is the cerebellum.

L. *Common tumor classifications*
   1. Most common tumors by location

Supratentorial tumors	Hemispheric	Sellar region	Pineal region
	Astrocytoma	Pituitary adenoma	Pineocytoma
	GBM	Craniopharyngioma	Pineoblastoma
	Metastasis	Meningioma	Germinoma
	Meningioma	Optic glioma	Astrocytoma
		Germ cell tumor	
		Epidermoid/dermoid	
		Esthesioneuroblastoma	
		Hypothalamic glioma/hamartoma	
Infratentorial tumors	Cerebellar midline	Cerebellar hemisphere	
Pediatric	Medulloblastoma	Juvenile astrocytoma	
	Ependymoma		
	Pontine glioma		
Adult	Medulloblastoma	Hemangioblastoma	

	Schwannoma	Astrocytoma	
	Meningioma	Metastasis	
	Choroid plexus papilloma	Medulloblastoma	
	Metastasis		
Spinal cord tumors	Extradural	Intradural extramedullary	Intramedullary
	Metastasis—prostate	Meningioma	Astrocytoma
	Metastasis—breast	Schwannoma	Ependymoma
	Metastasis—kidney	Neurofibroma	Glioblastoma
	Metastasis—thyroid		
	Metastasis—lung		
	Metastasis—lymphoma		

NB: Children <1 y/o have mainly supratentorial tumors; after 1 year, approximately 70% are infratentorial; only 30% of tumors in adults are infratentorial.

Extra-axial CNS tumors	Meningioma
	Epidermoid cyst
	Dermoid cyst
	Arachnoid cyst
	Rare dural tumors
	Meningeal sarcomas (fibrosarcoma, polymorphic cell sarcoma, primary meningeal sarcomatosis)
	Xanthomatous tumors (fibroxanthoma, xanthosarcoma, primary melanotic tumors: primary melanoma, meningeal melanomatosis)
Intraventricular tumors	Ependymoma: frequency—20%; location: 4th ventricle (in pediatrics) or lateral ventricle (in adults); calcified in 20–40%
	Astrocytoma: frequency—18%; location: frontal horn, 3rd ventricle; calcified in 30%
	Colloid cyst: frequency—12%; location: 3rd ventricle (anterior roof); may be associated with hydrocephalus
	Meningioma: frequency—11%; location: lateral ventricle (atrium)
	Choroid plexus papilloma: frequency—7%; location: lateral ventricle (pediatrics), 4th ventricle (adults)
"Seeding" CNS tumors	Medulloblastoma: >66% have subarachnoid space seeding at the time of first operation
	Glioblastoma
	PNET
	Ependymoma

Pineal region tumors	Pineoblastoma
	Germinoma
	Plexus papilloma
	Germ cell tumors
	Germinoma
	Teratoma
	Embryonal cell tumor
	Choriocarcinoma
	Endodermal sinus tumor/yolk sac tumor
	Pineal cell origin
	Pineocytoma
	Pineoblastoma
	Astrocytoma: second most common
	Meningioma
	Cyst
	Lipoma
Corpus callosum tumors	GBM
	Oligodendroglioma
	Lipoma
Conus/filum terminale	Ependymoma
	Lipoma
	Paraganglioma
	Meningioma
	Drop metastasis
Cystic tumors	Pilocytic astrocytoma
	Hemangioblastoma
	Ganglioglioma
	Pleomorphic xanthoastrocytoma
	GBM

2. *Posterior fossa lesions*

Extra-axial	Foramen magnum	Chordoma (clival)	
		Meningioma (anterior)	
		Neurofibroma (posterior)	
	Cerebello-pontine angle	M	Meningioma[a]
			Metastasis
		E	Epidermoid[a]

			Exophytic brain stem glioma
		A	Acoustic neuroma[a]
			Arachnoid cyst
			Aneurysm
		T	Trigeminal neuroma
		S	Seventh nerve neuroma
Intra-axial	Anterior compartment	Brain stem glioma (25% of pediatric, 3% of adults)	
		Syringobulbia	
		Cavernous malformations	
	Posterior compartment	Metastasis (most common adult tumor)	
		Hemangioblastoma (most common primary adult tumor)	
		Ependymoma (>70% are posterior fossa; peak ages: 5 and 50 y/o; 0% Ca^{2+})	
		Medulloblastoma (most common pediatric tumor; midline in pediatrics; lateral in adults)	
		Choroid plexus papilloma	
		Oligodendroglioma (rare in the posterior fossa; 90% are calcified)	

NB: [a]Meningioma/epidermoid/acoustic neuroma account for 75% of cerebello-pontine angle lesions.

II. Chemotherapy

A. *Nervous system complications of chemotherapy*

Altretamine	Peripheral neuropathy
	Ataxia
	Tremor
	Visual hallucinations
Amsacrine	Seizures
Azacitidine	Muscle pain and weakness
Bleomycin	Raynaud's phenomenon
Busulfan	Seizures
	Venous thrombosis

Carboplatin	Peripheral neuropathy
	Hearing loss
	Transient cortical blindness
Cladribine	Peripheral neuropathy
Cisplatin	Peripheral neuropathy
	Ototoxicity (high frequency is affected; tinnitus)
	Encephalopathy
Cytarabine	Cerebellar dysfunction
	Somnolence
	Encephalopathy
	Personality changes
	Peripheral neuropathy
	Rhabdomyolysis
	Myelopathy
Dacarbazine	Paresthesia
Etoposide	Peripheral neuropathy
5-Fluorouracil	Acute cerebellar syndrome
	Encephalopathy
	Seizures
Fludarabine	Visual disturbances
Interleukin-2	Parkinsonism
	Brachial plexopathy
Isotretinoin	Pseudotumor cerebri
L-Asparaginase	Central vein thrombosis
	Headache
Levamisole	Peripheral neuropathy
Methotrexate	Leukoencephalopathy
	Chemical arachnoiditis (if given intrathecally)
Nitrourease (Carmustine [BCNU])	Encephalopathy
Paclitaxel (Taxol®)	Peripheral neuropathy
Procarbazine	Peripheral neuropathy
	Autonomic neuropathy
	Encephalopathy
	Ataxia
Suramin	Peripheral neuropathy
Tamoxifen	Decreased visual acuity

Teniposide	Peripheral neuropathy
Thiotepa	Myelopathy
Trimexetrate glucoronate	Peripheral neuropathy
Vinblastine	Peripheral neuropathy
	Myalgias
	Cranial neuropathy
	Autonomic neuropathy
Vincristine	Peripheral neuropathy
	Autonomic neuropathy
	Decreased antidiuretic hormone secretion
Vinorelbine	Peripheral neuropathy
	Autonomic neuropathy

B. **Acute encephalopathy:** occurs most often with high doses of L-asparaginase and 5-fluorouracil; clinical picture is characterized by lethargy, confusion, and hallucinations; usually reversible by discontinuation of treatment

C. **Chronic encephalopathy:** described after methotrexate administration in the form of disseminated necrotizing leukoencephalopathy; the onset of clinical symptoms (confusion, drowsiness, irritability, ataxia, tremor, seizures, and dementia) is often insidious and may occur months or years after treatment; pathology: mainly present in the white matter; areas of creamy-white necrosis with petechial hemorrhages and cavitations; loss of myelin, extensive damage to axons with bulb formation and astrocytosis, but absence of an inflammatory cell response

D. **Other complications:** gliosis in the white matter, diffuse cortical atrophy, sclerosis of the cerebellum, neuroaxonal dystrophy, peripheral neuropathy, and spinal myelopathy

III. Radiation Side Effects

A. *Acute reactions:* occur during the course of irradiation; usually minor and cause signs and symptoms of increased intracranial pressure; reaction is dose related

B. *Early delayed reactions:* probably secondary to injury to oligodendrocytes; appear a few weeks to 2–3 months later; usually transient and disappear without treatment; clinically presents with lethargy and somnolence; pathology: when fulminant, multiple small foci of demyelination with perivascular infiltration by lymphocytes and plasma cells

C. *Late delayed reactions:* appear from a few months to many years after irradiation; represent either diffuse damage to the white matter *(leukoencephalopathy)* or a space-occupying gliovascular reaction *(radionecrosis)*; macroscopic appearance of radionecrosis is similar to that of malignant gliomas; histologically: ranges from coagulative necrosis to foci of demyelination, loss of axons, macrophage, lymphocyte and plasma cell infiltration; most important change: fibrinoid necrosis and hyalinization of the walls of blood vessels and proliferation of the endothelium (causing obliterative endarteritis and thrombotic occlusion of small vessels); in the cerebellum: formation of small cysts in the Purkinje cell layer, loss of Purkinje and granule cells, atrophy of folia, demyelination and gliosis; incidence is dose related: <57 Gy (rare), 57–65 Gy (3%), >65 Gy (up to 20%)

IV. Paraneoplastic Syndromes

A. **Recommended diagnostic criteria for *definite* PNS** (from Graus et al. JNNP 2004)

1. A classical syndrome and cancer that develops within 5 years of the diagnosis of the neurological disorder
2. A nonclassical syndrome that resolves or significantly improves after cancer treatment without concomitant immunotherapy, provided that the syndrome is not susceptible to spontaneous remission
3. A nonclassical syndrome with onconeural antibodies and cancer that develops within 5 years of the neurological disorder
4. A neurological syndrome with well characterized onconeural antibodies (anti-Hu, Yo, CV2, Ri, Ma2, or amphiphysin) and no cancer

Brain and cranial nerves	Cerebellar degeneration
	Opsoclonus/myoclonus
	Limbic encephalitis
	Brain stem encephalitis
	Encephalomyelitis
	Optic neuritis
	Retinopathy/photoreceptor degeneration
	Paraneoplastic chorea
Spinal cord and dorsal root ganglia	Necrotizing myelopathy; myelitis (as part of encephalomyelitis)
	Subacute motor neuropathy
	Motor neuron disease
	Myelitis
	Sensory neuronopathy
Peripheral nerves	Subacute or chronic sensorimotor peripheral neuropathy
	Guillain-Barré syndrome
	Mononeuritis multiplex and microvasculitis of the peripheral nerves
	Brachial neuritis
	Autonomic neuropathy
	Peripheral neuropathy with islet cell tumors
	Peripheral neuropathy associated with paraproteinemia
Neuromuscular junction and muscle	Lambert-Eaton myasthenic syndrome
	Myasthenia gravis
	Dermatomyositis, polymyositis
	Acute necrotizing myopathy
	Carcinoid myopathies
	Myotonia
	Cachectic myopathy

B. **Neuromuscular junction and muscle disorders**
1. *Inflammatory myopathies:* frequent form of paraneoplastic syndrome; usually from bronchogenic ca
2. *Lambert-Eaton myasthenic syndrome:* associated most often with small cell bronchial ca (or with other autoimmune disorders, e.g., type 1 diabetes, thyroid disease, pernicious anemia, vitiligo); disrupt the function of neuronal voltage-gated calcium channels, leading to reduction in the release of acetylcholine at the neuromuscular junction; diagnosis: reduced amplitude compound motor action potential with facilitation characterized by a twofold increase in compound motor action potential after rapid stimulation at 20–50 Hz; repetitive stimulation at 2 Hz is associated with a decremental response

NB: Lambert-Eaton myasthenic syndrome is usually caused by blockade of P/Q-type voltage-gated calcium channel, responsible for acetylcholine release. Treated with 3,4-diaminopyridine, which blocks voltage-gated potassium channels (in charge of repolarization of the action potential), thereby increasing the action potential duration.

C. *Motor neuron diseases:* may present with motor neuropathy with loss of anterior horn cells, motor neuropathy with multifocal conduction block; encephalomyelitis syndrome, necrotizing myelopathy; presence of *anti-Hu* antibodies; associated with non-Hodgkin's lymphoma, paraproteinemia, Hodgkin's disease (subacute motor neuronopathy)
D. *Peripheral neuropathy:* very heterogeneous
1. *Paraneoplastic sensory neuronopathy (of Denny Brown):* associated with small cell anaplastic ca; lesions in the dorsal spinal root ganglia associated with degeneration of dorsal columns and wallerian degeneration
2. *Sensory-motor polyneuropathy:* most frequent paraneoplastic neuropathy; seen in almost all types of ca (bronchus, gastric, mammary, uterine, lymphomas); axonal, demyelination, lymphocytic infiltration of small blood vessels
3. *Guillain-Barré* type described in malignancies, including Hodgkin's disease
4. *Stiff-person syndrome:* muscle rigidity and painful spasms; associated with breast cancer and autoantibodies against a 128-kDa neuronal antigen concentrated at synapses and identified as *amphiphysin*

NB: An autoimmune form of this disease is characterized by antibodies against glutamic acid decarboxylase, the enzyme that converts glutamic acid to γ-aminobutyric acid.

E. *Brain and cranial nerves paraneoplastic syndromes*
1. Paraneoplastic necrotizing myelopathy: extremely rare; associated with malignant lymphoma
2. *Subacute cerebellar cortical degeneration:* rare, often in gynecologic ca (ovary, breast, uterus), also in small cell ca, Hodgkin's; massive diffuse disappearance of Purkinje cells with proliferation of Bergman glia and sparing of basket fibers and granular layer; anti-Yo antibodies
3. *Subacute polioencephalomyelitis:* usually in bronchial ca; inflammatory lesions in the gray matter of variable proportion; predilection to mesial temporal cortex *(limbic encephalitis)*, rhombencephalon *(medullary-pontine encephalitis)* and cerebellum, and gray matter of the spinal cord *(poliomyelitis)*; presence of *anti-Hu* antibody; small cell ca, some neuroblastomas and medulloblastomas

4. *Opsoclonus-myoclonus:* high titers of *anti-Ri antibodies;* associated with childhood neuroblastoma; in adults, associated with breast, gynecologic, or small cell lung ca; produces saccadic eye movements in combination with myoclonus involving facial muscles, limbs, or trunk and truncal ataxia

NB: Opsoclonus-myoclonus may also occur after viral infections or medication use.

5. *Retinal degeneration or cancer-associated retinopathy:* associated with small cell lung ca, also in melanoma and cervical ca; pathology; widespread degeneration of the outer retinal layers; *clinical: photosensitivity, ring scotomatous visual field loss, attenuated caliber of retinal arterioles*
6. *Cerebral vascular processes: due to hypercoagulation, nonbacterial thrombotic endocarditis, disseminated intravascular coagulation, venous thrombosis*

V Transplant Neurology
A. **Neurological complications of transplantation**

Treatment	Complication
Anti-CD3	Asceptic meningitis
	Cytokine release
Cyclosporine	Anorexia, nausea and vomiting
	Cholestasis
	Confusion, psychosis, coma
	Hyperglycemia
	Hypertrichosis
	Primary CNS lymphoma
	Seizures
	Thrombosis, TTP, hemolytic uremic syndrome
	Tremor
Cytarabine	Cerebellar toxicity (could be reversible)
	Myelopathy
	Neuropathy
FK-506	Anorexia, nausea, and vomiting
	Confusion, psychosis, coma
	Hyperglycemia
	Hypertrichosis
	Primary CNS lymphoma
	Seizures
	Thrombosis, TTP, hemolytic uremic syndrome
Glucocorticoids	Delirium
	Opportunistic infections
	Psychosis

Treatment	Complication
	Steroid myopathy
Methotrexate	Intrathecal: asceptic meningitis, myelopathy
	Intravenous: CVA, epilepsy

Phenomena	Complication
Graft versus Host disease	Acute transverse myelitis
	Inflammatory myositis
	Malignancy
	Myasthenia gravis

B. **CNS infections in transplant recipients**

Time from transplant	Class	Infection
Early (0–1 month)	Viral	HSV
		Hepatitis B or C
	Bacterial	Wound/catheter infections, pneumonia
	Fungal	Candida
Intermediate (1–6 months)	Viral	HSV
		CMV
		EBV, VZV (shingles), influenza, RSV, adenovirus
	Bacterial	Hepatitis B or C
		Nocardia
		Listeria
	Fungal	Mycobacterium tuberculosis
		Pneumocystis
		Aspergillus
		Cryptococcus
	Parasitic	Endemic fungi
		Strongyloides
		Toxoplasma
		Leishmania
		Trypanosoma cruzi
Late (> 6 months post transplantation)	Viral	CMV retinitis/colitis
		Papillomavirus
		post-transplantation lymphoproliferative disease
	Fungal	Endemic fungi

VI Headache Syndromes

A. **International classification of primary and secondary headaches**

1. *Primary Headaches*

   a. Migraine
      i. Migraine without aura
      ii. Migraine with aura
      iii. Childhood periodic syndromes that are commonly precursors to migraine
      iv. Retinal migraine
      v. Complications of migraine
      vi. Probable migraine

   b. Tension-type headache
      i. Infrequent episodic tension-type headache
      ii Frequent episodic tension-type headache
      iii. Chronic tension-type headache
      iv. Probable tension-type headache

   c. Cluster headache and other trigeminal autonomic cephalgias
      i. Cluster headache
      ii. Paroxysmal headache
      iii SUNCT (short-lasting unilateral neuralgiform headache attacks with conjuncti-
          val injection and tearing)
      iv. Probable trigeminal autonomic cephalgia

   d. Other primary headaches
      i. Primary stabbing headaches
      ii. Primary cough headaches
      iii. Primary exertional headaches
      iv. Primary headache associated with sexual activity
      v. Hypnic headache
      vi. Primary thunderclap headache
      vii. Hemicrania continua
      viii. New daily persistent headaches

2. *Secondary headaches*

   a. Headache attributed to head and/or neck trauma
   b. Headache attributed to cranial or cervical vascular disorder
   c. Headache attributed to nonvascular intracranial disorder
   d. Headache attributed to substance or its abuse
   e. Headache attributed to infection
   f. Headache attributed to disorders of homeostasis
   g. Headache of facial pain attributed to disorder of cranium, neck, eyes, ears, nose,
      sinuses, teeth, mouth, or other facial or cranial structures
   h. Headache attributed to psychiatric disorder

NB: Migraines are more likely to be frontal than unilateral in children. Benign paroxysmal vertigo is a frequent precursor of migraine in children. Ibuprofen is more efficacious than triptans in children.

B. **ICHD-II diagnostic criteria for migraine without aura**

1. At least five attacks fulfilling criteria 2–4
2. Headache attacks lasting 4–72 hours
3. Headache has at least two of the following characteristics
   a. Unilateral location
   b. Pulsating quality

    c. Moderate or severe pain intensity

    d. Aggravation by or causing avoidance of routine physical activity

  4. During headache at least one of the following

    a. Nausea and/or vomiting

    b. Photophobia and phonophobia

NB: Caffeine withdrawal is a common cause of acute severe headache among patients with migraine.

  5. Not attributed to another disorder

C. **ICHD-II diagnostic criteria for migraine with typical aura**

  1. At least two attacks fulfilling criteria 2–4

  2. Aura consisting of >1 of the following but no motor weakness

    a. Fully reversible visual symptoms including positive features (e.g., flickering lights, spots, or lines) and/or negative features (i.e., loss of vision)

    b. Fully reversible sensory symptoms including positive features (i.e., pins and needles) and/or negative symptoms (i.e., numbness)

    c. Fully reversible dyphasic speech disturbance

  3. At least two of the following characteristics

    a. Homonymous visual symptoms and/or unilateral sensory symptoms

    b. At least one aura symptom develops gradually over ≥5 mins, and/or different aura symptoms occur in succession over ≥5 mins

    c. Each symptom lasts ≥5 mins and not longer than 60 mins

  4. Headache fulfilling criteria 2–4 for migraine without aura begins during the aura or follows aura within 60 mins

  5. Not attributed to another disorder

D. **ICDH-II diagnostic criteria for frequent episodic tension-type headache**

  1. At least 10 episodes occurring on 1 or more but less than 15 days per month for at least 3 months and fulfilling criteria 2–4

  2. Headache lasting from 30 minutes to 7 days

  3. Headache has at least two of the following characteristics

    a. Bilateral location

    b. Pressing/tightening (nonpulsating) quality

    c. Mild or moderate intensity

    d. Not aggravated by routine physical activity such as walking or climbing stairs

  4. Both of the following

    a. No nausea or vomiting (anorexia my occur)

    b. No more than one of photophobia or phonophobia

  5. Not attributed to another disorder

E. **ICHD-II diagnostic criteria for cluster headache**

  1. At least five attacks fulfilling criteria 2–4

  2. Severe or very severe unilateral orbital, supraorbital, and/or temporal pain lasting 15–180 minutes if untreated

  3. Headache is accompanied by at least one of the following

    a. Ipsilateral conjunctival injection and/or lacrimation

    b. Ipsilateral nasal congestion and/or rhinorrhea

    c. Ipsilateral eyelid edema

    d. Ipsilateral forehead and facial sweating

    e. Ipsilateral miosis and/or ptosis

    f. A sense of restlessness or agitation

  4. Attacks have a frequency from one every other day to eight per day
  5. Not attributed to another disorder

NB: Cluster headaches may be triggered by vasodilating substances such as nitroglycerin, histamine, and ethanol. It will often respond acutely to oxygen inhalation at a flow rate of 8–10L/min via face mask. DHE is an alternative. Preventive treatments: verapamil, lithium, methysergide.

F. **ICDH-II diagnostic criteria for SUNCT and SUNA** (short-lasting unilateral neuralgiform headache with cranial autonomic features)
   1. *SUNCT*
      a. At least 20 attacks fulfilling criteria b–d
      b. Attacks of unilateral orbital, supraorbital, or temporal stabbing or pulsating pain lasting 5–240 secs
      c. Pain is accompanied by ipsilateral conjunctival injection and lacrimation
      d. Attacks occur with a frequency from 3–200 per day
      e. Not attributed to another disorder
   2. *SUNA*
      a. At least 20 attacks fulfilling criteria b–e
      b. Attacks of unilateral orbital, supraorbital, or temporal stabbing pain lasting 5 secs–10 mins
      c. Pain is accompanied by one of the following
         i. Conjunctival injection and/or tearing
         ii. Nasal congestion and/or rhinorrhea
         iii. Eyelid edema
      d. Attacks occur with a frequency from ≥1 per day for more than half the time
      e. No refractory period follows attacks from trigger areas
      f. Not attributed to another disorder

NB: *Paroxysmal hemicrania* is a disorder, more common in women, characterized by frequent episodes of unilateral, severe, but short-lasting headaches associated with autonomic manifestations. Indomethacin is the treatment of choice.

NB: *Psuedotumor cerebri* has been linked to the use of isotretinoin and other vitamin A-containing compounds (and also Vitamin D). It is much more common in women and is characterized by normal CSF composition, normal ventricles on imaging. Neuro exam is typically normal but 6th–nerve palsies and enlarged blind spots may be seen.

G. **Medications associated with probable medication-overuse headache**
   1. Opioid intake for >10 or more days per month
   2. Analgesic intake for >15 days per month
   3. Use of triptans for >10 days per month
   4. Use of ergotamine for >10 days per month
   5. Combination of analgesic medications, or combination of ergotamine, triptans, analgesics, or opioids >10 days per month
H. **Activity-induced headaches**

Primary cough headache	Occurs with coughing or in conjunction with other Valsalva maneuvers
	Sharp, stabbing, or splitting pain
	Usually bilateral, sudden onset, short duration

	Most have underlying cause (i.e., Chiari I malformation, aneurysm, etc.)
Primary exertional headache	Occurs with exercise or other forms of exertion
	Usually bilateral, pulsating, or throbbing
	Lasts for mins to days
	Young onset (early 20s)
Headache associated with sexual activity	Subclassified further into: *preorgasmic* (dull, aching pain that increases in severity during orgasm) or *orgasmic* (maximal and severe during orgasm)
	Lasts less than 3 hours

I. Symptomatic and preventive therapies for migraine

Recommendation	Preventive treatment	Symptomatic treatment
First line	Amitriptyline	All triptan medications (naratriptan, rizatriptan, sumatriptan, zolmitriptan)
	Divalproex sodium	DHE IV +/–antiemetic
	Propranolol	ASA + caffeine
	Topiramate	ASA/Ibuprofen/Naproxen/ Butorphanol IN
		Prochlorperazine IV
Second line	Atenolol/metoprolol/nadolol	Acetaminophen + caffeine
	Verapamil	Butalbital, ASA, caffeine + codeine
	ASA/Naproxen	Chlorpromazine
	Ketoprofen	Metoclopromide IV
	Fluoxetine	Isometheptene
	Gabapentin	Proclorperzine IM, PR
		Ketorolac IM
		Lidocaine IN
		Meperidine IM, IV
		Methadone IM
Third line	Bupropion	Butalbital, ASA + caffeine
	Imipramine	Metoclopromide IM, PR
	Mirtazepine	Ergotamine + caffeine PO
	Nortriptyline	Ergotamine PO
	Paroxetine/Sertraline/ Venlafaxine	
	Cyproheptadine (especially in children)	
	Indomethacin	

ADDITIONAL NOTES

Basic Neurosciences

CHAPTER 18

Neurochemistry/Pharmacology

I. Neurotransmitters (NTs) and Receptors
A. Miscellaneous
1. *Three major categories of NTs*
   a. **Amino acids**
      i. *Glutamate*
      ii. *γ-Aminobutyric acid (GABA)*
      iii. *Aspartic acid*
      iv. *Glycine*
   b. **Peptides**
      i. *Vasopressin*
      ii. *Somatostatin*
      iii. *Neurotensin*
   c. **Monoamines**
      i. *Norepinephrine (NE)*
      ii. *Dopamine (DA)*
      iii. *Serotonin (5-hydroxytryptamine [5-HT])*
      iv. *Acetylcholine (ACh)*
2. Monoamine NTs are nearly always (with a few exceptions) inhibitory
3. *ACh is the major NT in the peripheral nervous system (the only other peripheral NT being NE)*
4. *Major NTs of the brain are glutamate and GABA*
5. Peptides perform specialized functions in the hypothalamus and other regions
6. *Peripheral nervous system has only two NTs*
   a. *ACh*
   b. *NE*
7. *Excitatory NTs*
   a. *Glutamate*
   b. *Aspartate*
   c. *Cystic acid*
   d. *Homocystic acid*
8. *Inhibitory NTs*
   a. *GABA*
   b. *Glycine*

    c. *Taurine*

    d. *β-Alanine*

  9. *Excitatory/inhibitory pairs*

    a. *Glutamate (+): GABA (–) in the brain*

    b. *Aspartate (+): glycine (–) in the ventral spinal cord*

B. **ACh**

  1. Miscellaneous

    a. First NT discovered

    b. The major NT in the peripheral nervous system

      i. *Provides direct innervation of skeletal muscles*

      ii. *Provides innervation of smooth muscles of the parasympathetic nervous system*

    c. *Major locations* of ACh

      i. *Autonomic ganglia*

      ii. *Parasympathetic postganglionic synapses*

      iii. *Neuromuscular junction (NMJ)*

      iv. *Renshaw cells of spinal cord*

    d. Roles of ACh

      i. *Thermal receptors*

      ii. *Chemoreceptors*

      iii. *Taste*

      iv. *Pain perception (possibly)*

    e. Primarily (but not always) an *excitatory* NT

    f. *Main effect of ACh on pyramidal cells is via muscarinic receptor-mediated depletion of K^+ currents, which results in hyperexcitability*

    g. Most dietary choline comes from phosphatidyl choline found in the membranes of plants and animals

    h. Phosphatidyl choline is converted to choline, which is then transported across the blood-brain barrier

    i. Acetylcoenzyme A and choline are independently synthesized in the neuronal cell body and independently transported along the axon to the synapse in which they are conjugated into ACh

  2. Synthesis: *Rate limiting: supply of choline*

  3. Release

    a. Voltage-gated calcium channel is open as the action potential (AP) reaches the terminal button of the presynaptic neuron, producing influx of calcium ions that allows exocytosis of presynaptic vesicles containing ACh into the synaptic cleft.

    b. The activation of postsynaptic ACh receptors results in an influx of Na^+ into the cell and an efflux of K^+, which depolarizes the postsynaptic neuron, propagating a new AP.

  4. Receptors

    a. *Muscarinic receptors*

      i. *Subtypes*

        (A) *M1, 3, 5: activate phosphatidylinositide hydroxylase*

        (B) *M2, 4: inhibit adenyl cyclase*

      ii. *Agonists*

        (A) Bethanecol

        (B) Carbachol

        (C) Pilocarpine

        (D) Methacholine

        (E) Muscarine (from *Amanita* mushroom)

iii. *Antagonists*
   (A) Atropine
   (B) Scopolamine
   (C) Artane
 b. *Nicotinic receptors*
   i. *Antagonists (nondepolarizing)*
      (A) Tubocurare
      (B) Atracurium
      (C) α-Neurotoxin of sea snakes
      (D) Procainamide
      (E) Aminoglycoside antibiotics
   ii. *Antagonists (depolarizing)*
      (A) Succinylcholine
   iii. *Receptor inactivation*
      (A) Myasthenia gravis
   iv. *ACh release augmentation*
      (A) Black widow spider latrotoxin
   v. *ACh release blockade*
      (A) Botulism
      (B) Eaton-Lambert syndrome
      (C) Tick paralysis
      (D) β-Neurotoxin of sea snakes
 c. Specific locations of muscarinic and nicotinic receptors
   i. Both nicotinic and muscarinic
      (A) *Central nervous system (CNS) (muscarinic > nicotinic receptor concentrations)*
      (B) *All sympathetic and parasympathetic preganglionic synapses*
   ii. *Muscarinic only*
      (A) *All postganglionic parasympathetic terminals*
      (B) *Postganglionic sympathetic sweat glands*
   iii. *Nicotinic only*
      (A) *NMJ*
      (B) *Adrenal medulla*
   iv. In brain: muscarinic > nicotinic
5. Inactivation
 a. Metabolism
   i. Within synaptic cleft by acetylcholinesterase
   ii. Acetylcholinesterase found at nerve endings is anchored to the plasma membrane through a glycolipid
6. *Cholinergic agonists*

Agonists	Source	Mode of action
Nicotine	Alkaloid prevalent in the tobacco plant	Activates nicotinic class of ACh receptors, locks the channel open
Muscarine	Alkaloid produced by *Amanita muscaria* mushrooms	Activates muscarinic class of ACh receptors
α-*Latrotoxin*	Protein produced by the black widow spider	Induces massive ACh release, possibly by acting as a Ca^{2+} ionophore

7. *Cholinergic antagonists*

Antagonists	Source	Mode of action
Atropine/ scopolamine	Alkaloid produced by the deadly nightshade, *Atropa belladonna*	Blocks ACh actions only at muscarinic receptors
Botulinum toxin	Eight proteins produced by *Clostridium botulinum*	Inhibits the release of ACh
β-*Bungarotoxin*	Protein produced by *Bungarus* genus of snakes	Prevents ACh receptor channel opening
d-Tubocurarine	Active ingredient of curare	Prevents ACh receptor channel opening at motor end plate

8. *Specific agonists/antagonists action*
    a. *Presynaptic NMJ release blockade*
        i. Botulinum toxin: block presynaptic vesicle mobility
        ii. Lambert-Eaton syndrome: block presynaptic Ca^{2+} channels
        iii. Sea snake venom
    b. *Postsynaptic NMJ receptor blockade*
        i. Myasthenia gravis: ACh receptor antibody
        ii. Succinylcholine: depolarizing blockade
        iii. Curare: nondepolarizing blockade
        iv. α-Bungarotoxin: irreversible ACh receptor blockade
9. *Anticholinesterases*
    a. *Reversible*
        i. Neostigmine
        ii. Pyridostigmine
        iii. Physostigmine
        iv. Tacrine
    b. *Irreversible*
        i. With irreversible anticholinesterases, receptors can be regenerated with pralidoxime (peripherally) and atropine (centrally)
        ii. Agents
            (A) Organophosphates
            (B) Carbamates
            (C) Nerve gas
10. *Conditions/medications that increase ACh concentration*
    a. Acetylcholinesterase inhibitors
        i Pyridostigmine
        ii Physostigmine
        iii Edrophonium
        iv Tacrine
        v Donepezil
        vi Organophosphates
        vii Black widow venom
        viii β-Bungarotoxin
C. **Catecholamines**
    1. Miscellaneous
        a. *Principal catecholamines*

      i. *NE*

     ii. *Epinephrine*

   iii. *DA*

  b. Synthesis

  c. Tyrosine (TYR) transported to catecholamine-secreting neurons in which it is converted into DA, NE, and epinephrine

  d. Direct innervation of the sympathetic nervous system (except for sweat glands) due to NE

  e. *β-Noradrenergic receptors inhibit feeding, whereas α receptors stimulate feeding*

NB: Postganglionic sympathetic neurons to sweat glands use ACh as NT.

2. **DA**

  a. Miscellaneous

      i. 3–4× more dopaminergic cells in the CNS than adrenergic cells

     ii. DA made in the substantia nigra: *neurons in the pars compacta of the substantia nigra account for 80% of DA in the brain; neuromelanin is a DA polymer that makes the substantia nigra appear dark*

   iii. Highest concentration of DA: striatum (caudate and putamen)—although made in the substantia nigra, is transported to the striatum from the substantia nigra in vesicles

   iv. Two primary DA-receptor types found in striatum: D1 (stimulatory) and D2 (inhibitory)

    v. D2 receptors are found predominantly on dopaminergic neurons functioning primarily as autoreceptors to inhibit DA synthesis and release

   vi. *Four main dopaminergic tracts*

     (A) The *nigrostriatal tract* accounts for most of the brain's DA

     (B) The *tuberoinfundibular tract* controls release of prolactin via D2 receptors

     (C) *The mesolimbic tract*

     (D) *The mesocortical tract*

   vii. Parkinson's disease develops when striatal DA is depleted by >80% (<20% of original concentration remaining)

	Schizophrenia	Parkinson's disease	Huntington's disease
DA transporter	Normal	Decreased (midbrain DA also decreased)	—
D1 receptor	Normal	Increased	Decreased
D2 receptor	Increased in caudate and putamen	Increased	Decreased
Linkage between D1 and D2	Decreased	Normal with treatment	Decreased

  b. *Synthesis*

      i. *Rate-limiting step: TYR hydroxylase conversion to L-dopa*

     ii. DA is feedback inhibitor

   iii. TYR

      (A) Not an essential amino acid because it can be synthesized in the liver from phenylalanine

      (B) Cannot be synthesized in the brain

      (C) Must enter the brain by the large neutral amino acid transporter, which transports TYR, phenylalanine, tryptophan, methionine, and the branch-chained amino acids

    iv. L-TYR converted to L-dopa within the brain

    v. DA is synthesized in the cytoplasm

  c. Receptors

    i. The receptor that determines whether the transmitter is excitatory or inhibitory

    ii. *D1 receptor (subtypes D1 and D5)*

      (A) *Postsynaptic receptors*

        (1) *Excitatory*

        (2) *Stimulates cyclic adenosine monophosphate (cAMP)*

      (B) D1 receptor: ↑adenylate cyclase

      (C) D1-receptor activation is required for full postsynaptic expression of D2 effects

    iii. *D2 receptor (subtypes D2, D3, and D4)*

      (A) *Presynaptic receptor: inhibitory (high affinity)*

      (B) *Postsynaptic receptor*

        (1) *Inhibitory (low affinity)*

        (2) *Genetic polymorphisms exist for the D4 receptor that may provide basis for genetic-based schizophrenia*

    iv. *Tardive dyskinesia may be due to supersensitivity of DA receptors that have been chronically clocked (i.e., psychotropic agents)*

    v. Tuberoinfundibular DA system: regulated by prolactin

  d. Inactivation

    i. Reuptake

      (A) Presynaptic intraneuronal monoamine oxidase (MAO) converts DA → 3, 4-dihydroxyphenylacetic acid (DOPAC)

      (B) Extraneuronal MAO and catechol-O-methyltransferase convert DA → homovanillic acid; CNS DA metabolite: homovanillic acid

3. **NE**

  a. Miscellaneous

    i. Neuropeptide Y: co-localized with NE in sympathetic nerve terminals, innervating blood vessels

    ii. *Most concentrated in CNS within locus ceruleus of the pons followed by lateral tegmental area*

    iii. Electrical stimulation of the locus ceruleus produces arousal

    iv. Benzodiazepines decrease firing in the locus ceruleus, which reduces release of NE to rest of brain, causing relaxation and sedation

    v. *Antidepressant effect of MAO inhibitors (MAOIs) is more related to NE than to DA*

  b. Synthesis

    i. *Rate-limiting step*

      (A) *TYR hydroxylase*

      (B) NE is feedback inhibitor

    ii. NE is synthesized in the storage vesicles

    iii. TYR hydroxylase is inhibited by α-methyl-p-TYR

  c. Release and vesicle storage

      i. Calcium influx with depolarization
     ii. Amphetamines increase release
    iii. Inhibition of transport
        (A) Reserpine
        (B) Tetrabenazine
    iv. NE is displaced from vesicles by
        (A) Amphetamine
        (B) Ephedrine

d. *Receptors*
      i. *α-1*
        (A) *Postsynaptic*
        (B) *Most sensitive to epinephrine*
        (C) *Blocked by prazosin and clonidine*
     ii. *α-2*
        (A) *Presynaptic*
        (B) *Inhibits adenyl cyclase via G-protein effects*
        (C) *Inhibited by yohimbine and clonidine*

e. Inactivation
      i. Metabolism
        (A) Catechol-O-methyltransferase in synaptic cleft
        (B) Reuptake
            (1) Primary mode of NE termination
            (2) *Reuptake inhibited by*
                (a) *Cocaine*
                (b) *Tricyclic antidepressants (TCAs) (desipramine)*
                (c) *Tetracyclic antidepressant (maprotiline)*
                (d) *Selective serotonin reuptake inhibitors (SSRIs)*

f. Other medication effects
      i. *Lithium*
        (A) *Decrease NE release*
        (B) *Increase NE reuptake*

4. **Epinephrine**
a. Miscellaneous
      i. *Epinephrine is found with NE in*
        (A) *Lateral tegmental system*
        (B) *Dorsal medulla*
        (C) *Dorsal motor nucleus*
        (D) *Locus ceruleus*
b. Synthesis: epinephrine synthesis occurs only in adrenal medulla via phenyletha-nolamine N-methyltransferase

5. Medications
a. *Catecholamine agonists/antagonists*
      i. *Neuroleptics*
        (A) *Based on D2 and D4 receptor antagonism in the mesolimbic and mesocortical pathways*
        (B) *Antagonism of nigrostriatal pathways produces extrapyramidal side effects*
        (C) Antagonism in the chemoreceptor trigger zone produces antiemetic effect
        (D) *Older neuroleptics mainly block D2 receptor but can block multiple DA receptors*
        (E) D2 affinity correlates to efficacy
        (F) *Clozapine*

             (1) *Newer neuroleptic that is more selective for the D1 and D4 receptors; also binds to:* 5-HT$_2$ receptor, α_1-Adrenergic receptor, muscarinic receptor, histamine (histamine$_1$) receptor

             (2) DA neurons in ventral tegmentum develop depolarization inactivation, but neurons in the substantia nigra do not have this effect (i.e., minimal parkinsonism)

       ii. *Amphetamines*

          (A) *Increase release of DA and NE centrally and peripherally*

          (B) *Decrease reuptake of DA*

      iii. *MAOIs: decrease metabolism of DA*

      iv. *Cocaine: block reuptake of DA and NE*

       v. *TCAs: block reuptake of DA*

      vi. *Reserpine and tetrabenazine: prevent vesicle storage of DA, epinephrine, and 5-HT, both centrally and peripherally*

     vii. *Selegiline and rasagiline: MAO$_B$ inhibitor increasing DA stores*

D. 5-HT

   1. Miscellaneous

     a. An *indolamine*

     b. Most prominent effects on cardiovascular system, with additional effects in the respiratory system and the intestines

     c. *Vasoconstriction is a classic response to the administration of 5-HT*

     d. Only 1–2% of 5-HT in the body is in the brain; widely distributed in platelets, mast cells, etc.; greatest concentration of 5-HT (90%) is found in the enterochromaffin cells of the gastrointestinal tract

     e. *High concentration in CNS found in*

       i. *Raphe nuclei that project to the limbic system*

      ii. *Pons/upper brain stem*

     iii. *Area postrema*

     iv. *Caudal locus ceruleus*

      v. *Interpeduncular nucleus*

     vi. *Facial (cranial nerve VII) nucleus*

     f. *Raphe nuclei*

       i. *5-HT neurons are located in the CNS*

      ii. Projects caudally mainly to the medulla and spinal cord for the regulation of pain

     iii. Projects rostrally to the limbic structures and the cerebral cortex

     iv. Stimulation produces similar effects as lysergic acid diethylamine (LSD)

     g. *5-HT and NE regulate arousal*

     h. *Low 5-HT associated with anxiety and impulsive behavior*

       i. *5-HT syndrome*

       i. *SSRI + MAOI*

      ii. *Clinical: restlessness, tremor, myoclonus, hyperreflexia, diarrhea, diaphoresis, confusion, and possible death*

     iii. *Must wait 2–3 weeks after stopping MAOI before initiating SSRI*

     iv. *Wait 5 weeks after stopping SSRI before initiating MAOI*

   2. *Synthesis*

     a. *Rate-limiting step: tryptophan hydroxylase*

     b. 5-HT in the brain is independently synthesized from tryptophan transported across the blood-brain barrier

3. Receptors

Receptor	Linked to/associations	Agonist	Antagonist
5-HT$_{1a}$	G-protein→inhibit adenyl cyclase	Buspirone	None
5-HT$_{1b/1d}$, both act as autoreceptors	G-protein→inhibit adenyl cyclase	Sumatriptan (5-HT$_{1d}$)	None
5-HT$_{1c}$	Linked to G-protein→ to increase DAG and IP$_3$	LSD α-Methyl-5-HT	Ritanserin Pizotifen Clozapine
5-HT$_2$	Linked to G-protein → to increase DAG and IP$_3$	LSD α-Methyl-5-HT	Ritanserin Pizotifen Clozapine
5-HT$_3$	Ion channel	2-α-5-HT	Metoclopramide Ondansetron (potent) Cocaine (weak)

DAG, dimeric acidic glycoprotein.

a. Most receptors are coupled to G proteins that affect the activities of adenylate cyclase or phospholipase C
b. *5-HT$_1$ receptor function*
    i. *Thermoregulation*
    ii. *Sexual behavior*
    iii. *Hypotension*
c. *5-HT$_2$ receptor function*
    i. *Vascular contraction*
    ii. *Platelet aggregation*
d. *5-HT$_3$ receptor function: ion channels*
4. Inactivation
a. Metabolism
b. Reuptake
    i. Primary mode of inactivation
    ii. Mechanism similar to NE
c. 5-HT also converted to melatonin (only in pineal gland)
5. Agonists/antagonists
a. Storage
    i. Disrupted by reserpine and tetrabenazine
        (A) *Reserpine (an extract of the Rauwolfia plant) prevents the transport of all the monoamines and ACh into storage vesicles in the presynaptic membrane, allowing MAO metabolism to occur.*
b. Release
    i. *Increased release of 5-HT*
        (A) *Amphetamine*
        (B) *Fenfluramine*

      ii. *Increased release and block reuptake of 5-HT*
         (A) *Clomipramine*
         (B) *Amitriptyline*
   c. Reuptake
      i. *Blocked by*
         (A) *TCAs: inhibit NE and 5-HT reuptake by presynaptic nerve terminals*
         (B) *SSRIs (fluoxetine, sertraline): selectively prevent the reuptake of 5-HT*
         (C) *Clomipramine: although a TCA, it is an SSRI*
   d. *LSD*
      i. Acts most strongly on the 5-HT$_2$ receptors (and some effect on NE receptors).
      ii. Small doses potentiate 5-HT activity.
      iii. High doses inhibit 5-HT activity, leading to psychedelic action.
   e. *5-HT agonists*
      i. *Sumatriptan: potent 5-HT$_2$ agonist*
      ii. *Methylsergide*
      iii. *Cyproheptadine*
   f. *5-HT antagonist: clozapine*

E. Glutamate
   1. Miscellaneous
      a. *Excitatory* NT
      b. Glutamate is NT of corticostriate fibers
      c. *Most common NT in the brain*
      d. *High concentration in dorsal spinal cord and dentate nucleus*
      e. Aspartic acid and glutamate have the capacity for neuronal damage via excitotoxicity
   2. *Receptors*
      a. *N-methyl-D-aspartate*
         i. Only known receptor that is regulated both by a ligand (glutamate) and by voltage
         ii. *Mainly activate Ca^{2+} channels*
         iii. *N-methyl-D-aspartate receptor locations*
            (A) *Cortex*
            (B) *Hippocampal neurons, particularly the CA1 region*
            (C) *Amygdala*
            (D) *Basal ganglia*
         iv. *Five binding sites alter channel opening*
            (A) *Glutamate (increase)*
            (B) *Glycine (increase)*
            (C) *Polyamine (increase): binds the hallucinogenic substance phencyclidine*
            (D) *Magnesium (decrease)*
            (E) *Zinc (decrease)*
         v. *Glycine binding is required for activation*
         vi. *Voltage-dependent blockers*
            (A) *Phencyclidine*
            (B) *Ketamine*
            (C) *Magnesium*
         vii. *Voltage-independent blocker: zinc*
         viii. Associated with long-term potentiation, which is integral for learning and memory
      b. *AMPA*
         i. Mainly activate *sodium channel*
         ii. Major source of excitatory postsynaptic potentials (EPSPs)

        iii. Receptor affinity: AMPA > glutamate > kainate

        iv. *GluR3 receptor: implicated in Rasmussen's encephalitis*

    c. *Kainate*

        i. Receptor affinity: kainate > glutamate > AMP

        ii. No specific antagonists

        iii. Derived commercially from seaweed

    d. 1-amino-1,3-cyclopentone dicarboxylic acid (ACPD): G-coupled formation of IP_3

    e. L-AP4

        i. G-coupled formation of AMP

        ii. Inhibitory autoreceptor

  3. Inactivation

  4. Other

    a. *Caffeine:* increases alertness and possibly produces anxiety by blocking adenosine receptors that normally inhibit glutamate release

    b. *Mercury poisoning:* damage to astrocytes prevents resorption of glutamate, resulting in excitotoxicity

    c. *Lamotrigine* inhibits release of excitatory NTs glutamate and aspartate

F. **GABA**

  1. Miscellaneous

    a. *Inhibitory NT: inhibitor of presynaptic transmission in the CNS and retina*

    b. *30–40% of all synapses (second only to glutamate as a major brain NT)*

    c. *Most highly concentrated in the basal ganglia (with projections to the thalamus); also concentrated in the hypothalamus,* periaqueductal gray, *and hippocampus*

  2. Synthesis: *glutamate decarboxylase decreased in striatum of Huntington's disease*

NB: Antibodies targeting glutamate decarboxylase represent the autoimmune form of stiff-person syndrome.

  3. *Receptors*

    a. *Connected to a chloride ion channel, allowing chloride to enter the cell and increasing the threshold for depolarization*

    b. *GABA-A*

        i. Fast inhibitory postsynaptic potentials (IPSPs)

        ii. Increase chloride conductance

        iii. Five binding sites

            (A) *Benzodiazepine: increase chloride conductance of presynaptic neurons*

            (B) *Barbiturate: prolong duration of chloride channel opening*

            (C) Steroid site

            (D) Picrotoxin site

            (E) GABA site

        iv. CNS locations

            (A) *Cerebellum: highest concentration in granule cell layer*

            (B) *Cortex*

            (C) *Hippocampus*

            (D) *Basal ganglia*

        v. GABA-A receptor binds

            (A) GABA

            (B) Benzodiazepine

            (C) β-Carbolines

            (D) Picrotoxin-like convulsant drugs: noncompetitive antagonist

    (E) Bicuculline: competitive antagonist
    (F) Barbiturates
  c. *GABA-B*
    i. *Slow IPSPs*
    ii. *Increased K⁺ conductance via K⁺ channels*
    iii. *Coupled to G-protein that uses adenyl cyclase as a second messenger*
    iv. *Agonist: baclofen*
    v. *Antagonist: phaclofen*
    vi. CNS locations
      (A) Cerebellum
      (B) Cord
4. Inactivation
  a. Reuptake
  b. Enzyme metabolism
5. Agonists/antagonists
  a. *Inhibitors of GABA transaminase*
    i. *Valproic acid*
    ii. *Vigabatrin*
6. Other
  a. *Benzodiazepines*
    i. Increase the frequency of chloride channel opening
    ii. Enhance the effect of GABA on GABA-A receptors
  b. *Caffeine:* neutralize the effects of benzodiazepines by inhibiting GABA release
  c. *Barbiturates:* prolong the duration of opening

G. **MAO**

1. Miscellaneous
  a. *Antidepressant effect of MAOIs is more related to NE than DA*
  b. MAO_A
    i. *MAO_A inhibitors have proven to be better antidepressants because MAO_A metabolizes NE and 5-HT; therefore, inhibition increases NE and 5-HT levels.*
    ii. *MAO_A-inhibiting drugs given for depression have critically elevated blood pressure in patients eating tyramine-containing foods (e.g., cheese).*
  c. MAO_B
    i. Alcohol also selectively inhibits MAO_B.
    ii. MAO_B is the most common form in the striatum.
    iii. *MAO_B metabolizes the neurotoxin 1-methyl-4-phenyl-1,2,3,6-tetrahydropyridine (MPTP).*
    iv. *selegiline, rasagiline: specific MAO_B inhibitor.*
  d. Mitochondrial MAO degrades intraneuronal DA, NE, and 5-HT that is not protected within storage vesicles
  e. **Hypertensive crisis**
    i. *MAO in the gastrointestinal system usually prevents entrance of large amounts of ingested tyramine (or other pressor amines)*
    ii. If MAOI is used, then ingested tyramine can be absorbed and produce sympathetic response
    iii. Clinical: sudden occipital or temporoparietal headache, sweating, fever, stiff neck, photophobia (can be mistaken for meningitis)
    iv. *Foods to avoid with MAOIs*
      (A) *Aged cheese*

NB: Cottage cheese, ricotta, and cream cheese are safe.

      (B) *Smoked or pickled meats, fish, or poultry*

      (C) *Caviar*

      (D) *Nonfresh meat*

      (E) *Liver*

      (F) *Nondistilled alcohol*

      (G) *Broad beans (fava, Italian green, Chinese pea pods)*

      (H) *Banana peel*

      (I) *Sausage*

      (J) *Corned beef*

      (K) *Sauerkraut*

   v. *Medications/drugs to avoid with MAOIs*

      (A) *Amphetamines*

      (B) *Cocaine*

      (C) *Anorectics/dietary agents*

      (D) *Catecholamines*

      (E) *Sympathomimetic precursors (DA, levodopa)*

      (F) *Sympathomimetic (ephedrine, phenylephrine, phenylpropanolamine, pseudoephedrine)*

      (G) *Meperidine*

   vi. Treatment of hypertensive crisis: *phentolamine, 5 mg intravenously, or nifedipine, 10 mg sublingually*

  2. Location

    a. Outer surface of presynaptic mitochondria

    b. Postsynaptic cell membrane

  3. Inhibitors

    a. MAO_A: *Clorgyline*

    b. MAO_B: *Selegiline, Pargyline, Rasagiline*

    c. *Nonspecific MAOIs: Phenelzine, Isocarboxazid, Tranylcypromine*

H. Glycine

  1. Miscellaneous

    a. *Inhibitory NT of cord for inhibitory interneurons (Renshaw cells), which inhibit anterior motor neurons of the spinal cord*

    b. Glycine binds to a receptor that makes the postsynaptic membrane more permeable to Cl^- ion, which hyperpolarizes the membrane, making it less likely to depolarize (inhibitory NT)

    c. *Opposite function of aspartate in the spinal cord*

    d. Anoxia results in loss of inhibitory neurons and decreased glycine

  2. Synthesis

  3. Inactivation: deactivated in the synapse by active transport back into the presynaptic membrane

  4. Agonists/antagonists

    a. *Antagonist*

      i. *Strychnine*

        (A) *Antagonist*

        (B) *Noncompetitively blocks glycine > GABA receptors by inhibiting opening of the chloride channel, which subsequently results in hyperexcitability*

      ii. *Tetanus toxin: blocks release of glycine and GABA*

    b. *Agonist: glycine > β-alanine > taurine >> alanine/serine*

I. **Aspartate**
1. Miscellaneous
   a. *Primarily localized to the ventral spinal cord*
   b. *Opens an ion channel*
   c. *Excitatory NT,* which increases the likelihood of depolarization in the postsynaptic membrane
   d. Opposite function of glycine in the spinal cord
   e. Aspartate (+) and glycine (–) form an excitatory/inhibitory pair in the ventral spinal cord
   f. Nonessential amino acid found particularly in sugar
2. Inactivation: reabsorption into the presynaptic membrane

J. **Histamine**
1. Miscellaneous
   a. Histamine acts as an NT and is found *in mast cells (but histamine of mast cells is not an NT)*
   b. Highest concentration within hypothalamus
2. Synthesis
3. Receptors
   a. Histamine$_1$ receptor
   b. Histamine$_2$ receptor
   c. Histamine$_3$ receptor: functions in autoregulation
4. Agonists/antagonists
   a. Histamine$_1$-receptor antagonists
      i. Diphenhydramine
      ii. Chlorpheniramine
      iii. Promethazine
   b. Histamine$_2$-receptor antagonists: cimetidine
   c. α-Fluoromethylhistidine: selective inhibitor of histamine decarboxylase

K. **Neuropeptides**
1. Miscellaneous
   a. *Most common NTs in the hypothalamus*
   b. Very potent compared to other NTs
   c. May modulate postsynaptic effects of NTs by prolonging effect via second messengers
   d. *Neuropeptides coexist with other NTs*

NT	Neuropeptide
GABA	Somatostatin
	Cholecystokinin
Ach	Vasoinhibitory peptide (VIP)
	Substance P
NE	Somatostatin
	Enkephalin
	Neuropeptide Y
DA	Cholecystokinin

NT	Neuropeptide
	Neurotensin
Epinephrine	Neuropeptide Y
	Neurotensin
5-HT	Substance P
	Enkephalin
Vasopressin	Cholecystokinin
	Dynorphin
Oxytocin	Enkephalin

2. Synthesis: ribosomal synthesis
3. Inactivation: extracellular action is terminated via hydrolysis by proteases and diffusion; not inactivated by reuptake
4. Subtypes
   a. *Enkephalins*
      i. *Enkephalin receptor*
         (A) Opiates and enkephalins bind to the receptor
         (B) Highest concentration found in the sensory, limbic system, hypothalamic, amygdala, and periaqueductal gray
         (C) Located on presynaptic synapses
      ii. *Opiates and enkephalins inhibit the firing of locus ceruleus neurons*
L. **Opioids**
   1. *Receptors*

	μ Receptor	δ Receptor	κ Receptor
Agonist	β endorphin[a]	Leu-enkephalin[a]	Dynorphins[a]
	Morphine	Met-enkephalin	
Antagonist	Naloxone	Naloxone (weak)	Naloxone (very weak)
	Naltrexone		
Function	Analgesia	Cardiac affects	Salt and water resorption
			Analgesia

[a]Most potent.

   a. κ Receptor differs from μ and δ receptors because cannot reverse morphine withdrawal
M. **Substance P**
   1. Release
      a. Ca^{2+} dependent
      b. Inhibited by morphine
   2. Agonists/antagonists
      a. *Capsaicin: depletes substance P (analgesic effect)*

N. *Quick reference for NTs*

NT	Synthesized from	Site of synthesis
ACh	Choline	CNS, parasympathetic nerves
5-HT	Tryptophan	CNS, chromaffin cells of gut, enteric cells
GABA	Glutamate	CNS
Glutamate	—	CNS
Aspartate	—	CNS
Glycine	—	Spinal cord
Histamine	Histidine	Hypothalamus
Adenosine	ATP	CNS, peripheral nerves
Adenosine triphosphate	—	Sympathetic, sensory, and enteric nerves
Nitric oxide	Arginine	CNS, gastrointestinal

O. *Other*
   1. Quisqualate-type receptor is coupled to phospholipase C
   2. CNS sites of high neurochemical concentrations
      a. NE: locus ceruleus
      b. 5-HT: median and dorsal raphe
      c. DA: substantia nigra
      d. GABA: cerebellum
      e. Cholinergic: substantia innominata and nucleus basalis of Meynert
      f. Histamine: hypothalamus
   3. Calmodulin: prominent calcium-binding protein in the CNS
   4. Ascending pathways mediating arousal

II. Neurochemistry
A. *Electrolyte concentrations*

Ion	Intracellular concentration (mEq/L)	Extracellular concentration (mEq/L)
Na^+	15	140
K^+	135	4
Ca^{2+}	2×10^{-4}	4
Mg^{2+}	40	2
Cl^-	4	120
HCO_3^-	10	24

B. **Basic neurophysiology**
   1. *AP generation*
      a. Definition: a self-propagating regenerative change in membrane potential
      b. An AP only develops if the depolarization reaches the threshold determined by the voltage-dependent properties of the sodium channels; sodium channels are also time dependent, staying open for only a limited period
      c. *Ion fluxes and membrane potentials*

      i. Most of the charge movement in biological tissue is attributed to passive properties of the membrane or changes in ion conductance

     ii. Important cations: K^+, Na^+, Ca^{2+}

   iii. Important anions: Cl^-, proteins

  d. *Three phases*

      i. *Resting membrane potential*

        (A) *Potential = –70 mV*

        (B) Due to difference in permeability of ions and sodium-potassium pump forcing K^+ in and Na^+ out

        (C) Resting membrane potential is based on outward K^+ current through passive leakage channels

        (D) If resting membrane potential is diminished and threshold is surpassed and the AP is generated

     ii. *Depolarization*

        (A) *Potential = +40 mV*

        (B) Dependent on sodium permeability

           (1) Voltage-gated opening of sodium channels

              (a) Sodium permeability increases as membrane potential decreases from the resting membrane potential (–70 mV) toward 0.

              (b) When the membrane potential reaches approximately –55 mV, sodium channels open dramatically.

              (c) The transient increase in sodium permeability allows results in membrane potential of +40 mV.

              (d) Voltage-dependent potassium channels will also open in conjunction with sodium channels.

   iii. *Repolarization:* closure of voltage-gated sodium channels re-establishes potassium as the determining ion of the membrane potential

  e. Myelinated are faster than unmyelinated nerves

      i. *Myelin decreases membrane capacitance and conductance and the time constant.*

     ii. Increases the space constant of the segment of axon between the nodes of Ranvier.

   iii. Velocity is proportional to axon radius.

2. *NMJ*

  a. Presynaptic components

      i. Motor neuron

     ii. Axon

   iii. Terminal bouton

        (A) *Synaptic vesicles: contain 5,000–10,000 molecules (1 quanta) of ACh*

        (B) *Release based on voltage-gated calcium channels*

  b. Synaptic cleft: 200–500 μm

  c. Postsynaptic components

      i. Motor end plate

     ii. ACh receptors

   iii. Voltage-gated sodium channels

3. Synaptic transmission

  a. *AP is based on sodium inward current and potassium outward current through voltage-dependent channels.*

  b. *When AP reaches presynaptic region, causes release of NT.*

  c. NTs bind to postsynaptic receptors, opening postsynaptic membrane channels.

  d. Depending on the ionic currents flowing through the transmitter (ligand)-operated channels, two types of postsynaptic potentials are generated.

 i. *EPSPs*

   (A) Occur when sodium inward current prevails

   (B) Increase the probability that AP will be propagated

 ii. *IPSPs*

   (A) Occur when potassium outward current or chloride inward current prevail

   (B) Cause hyperpolarization of the postsynaptic membrane, making it more difficult to reach the threshold potential

e. Summation

   i. EPSPs and IPSPs interact to determine whether AP is propagated postsynaptically.

   ii. *Temporal summation: EPSPs/IPSPs sequentially summate at a monosynaptic site.*

   iii. *Spatial summation: EPSPs/IPSPs simultaneously evoke an end-plate potential polysynaptically.*

f. Depolarization of the nerve terminal results in opening of all ionic channels, including those for calcium; calcium entry causes release of NT from the presynaptic terminal, which binds to postsynaptic receptor sites.

g. Chemical transmission is the main mode of neuronal communication and can be excitatory or inhibitory (if postsynaptic binding opens sodium channels and/or calcium channels → EPSP; if opens potassium channels and/or Cl channels → IPSP); most common excitatory NT is glutamate, common inhibitory NTs are GABA and glycine.

C. *Membrane channel dysfunction*

 1. *Sodium channel*

   a. *Sodium channel inhibitors*

     i. *Tetrodotoxin (puffer fish)*

     ii. *Saxitoxin (dinoflagellate, shellfish)*

   b. *Sodium channel potentiators*

     i. *Batrachotoxin (arrow poisoning)*

     ii. *Grayanotoxin (Amazon amphibians)*

   c. *Sodium channel closure inhibitors*

     i. *Scorpion toxin*

     ii. *Sea anemone toxin*

   d. *Mutational disorders*

     i. *Failure of sodium channel to inactivate*

     ii. *Disorders*

       (A) *Hyperkalemic periodic paralysis*

       (B) *Paramyotonia congenita*

 2. *Potassium channel*

   a. *Antagonists*

     i. *Tetraethyl ammonium chloride: voltage-gated potassium channels*

     ii. *4-Aminopyridine: antagonizes fast voltage-gated potassium channels*

NB: May be used in the treatment of Lambert-Eaton myasthenic syndrome.

   b. *Mutational disorders: hypokalemic periodic paralysis*

 3. *Calcium channel disorders*

   a. *Absence seizures: thalamic calcium channels*

   b. *Hypokalemic periodic paralysis*

ADDITIONAL NOTES

CHAPTER 19

Neurogenetics

I. **Genes and Amino Acids:** the major function of DNA is to specify the sequence of amino acids in proteins synthesized within the cell; a given protein is the final expression of a given gene; genes consist of *exons,* sequences of DNA that find expression in protein amino acid sequence, and *introns,* intervening sequences between exons that are not expressed in the final protein amino acid sequence.

  A. **Transcription:** DNA is transcribed into *heteronuclear RNA, which contains both introns and exons;* the heteronuclear RNA is edited so that introns are excised and adjacent exons are fused (spliced) together to give a *final RNA product—the messenger RNA (mRNA)*

  B. **Translations:** mRNA is translated into protein on the cytoplasmic ribosomes; *transfer RNA complexed with amino acids bind to mRNA on the ribosome with complementation of three nucleotides on the mRNA, specifying which transfer RNA will bind;* the linear sequence of nucleotides on mRNA is translated into the primary sequence of the synthesized protein

  C. *Classes of mutations*

Mutation	Mutation type	Leads to
Single DNA base change	Missense	Abnormal protein
	Nonsense	No or truncated protein
	Premature stop codon	No or truncated protein
mRNA processing	Splicing mutation	Abnormal protein
Codon insertion or deletion	Frame shift	Abnormal protein
	Codon insertion	Abnormal protein
	Codon deletion	Abnormal protein
Gene fusion	Fusion mRNA	Chimera protein
Triplet repeat amplification	Polyglutamate runs abnormal methylation	Abnormal protein
Mitochondrial	Deletions	No protein
	Transfer RNA deletions	Many proteins not made

  D. *Patterns of inheritance*
    1. *Autosomal dominant (AD):* one damaged allele is sufficient to produce disease; *50% of offspring of an affected individual have the defective allele and, therefore, have the disease;* the degree of expression (penetrance) of the defect is variable according to the specific disease
    2. *Autosomal recessive (AR):* both alleles must be damaged for the disease to be manifest; many of the classic inborn errors of metabolism; *25% of the offspring of two carriers are affected;* carriers are usually asymptomatic

3. *X-linked recessive:* alleles on the sex chromosomes are abnormal; the Y-chromosome does not contain the full complement of alleles to match the X-chromosome; if the male offspring receives a defective unmatched allele from his carrier mother, he will be affected; 50% of the male offspring receive the defective X-chromosome and 50% receive the mother's normal X-chromosome, then *50% of male progeny are affected*

4. *Mitochondrial:* mitochondria are semiautonomous owing to the presence of 10–12 circular genomes within each mitochondria coding for an independent protein synthetic apparatus; *at fertilization, the ovum contributes all of the mitochondria,* and the sperm contributes none; *mitochondrial inheritance is exclusively maternal;* also, during development, the mitochondria do not segregate randomly, accounting for genetic variability from tissue to tissue (heteroplasmy)

II. Oncogenes and Chromosomal Aberrations in the Central Nervous System (CNS) Tumors: *oncogenes*—genes that are mutated, deleted, or overexpressed during the formation of tumors; *dominant oncogenes*—cause overexpression of growth products in tumors; *recessive oncogenes*—cause loss of function to suppress neoplasia, also called *antioncogenes* or *tumor suppressor genes*

A. **Fibrillary astrocytomas:** loss of the short arm of *chromosome 17* in 50% of fibrillary astrocytomas

B. **Li-Fraumeni cancer susceptibility syndrome:** associated with mutations in p53 tumor suppressor gene located on the distal short arm of *chromosome 17*; families have dramatically increased incidence of early-onset breast cancer, childhood sarcomas, and brain tumors; 50% likelihood of receiving a diagnosis of cancer by age 30 years

C. **Glioblastoma multiforme:** *loss of chromosome 10* in 80% of glioblastoma multiforme cases; *gains in chromosome 7; loss of chromosome 22;* loss of *p53* tumor suppressor genes *in chromosome 17p13.1 and CDKN2 in chromosome 9;* amplification of *epidermal growth factor receptor*

D. **Retinoblastoma:** sporadic in 60% of cases, AD in 40%; emergence of tumor *requires inactivation of Rb gene (tumor suppressor gene) on chromosome 13q14*; in the familial form, one gene is inactivated in the cell; thus, only one gene needs inactivation to produce the tumor; in the sporadic form, both need inactivation

E. **Pituitary adenoma:** loss of tumor suppressor gene, multiple endocrine neoplasia 1 on chromosome 11q13

III. Dementia

Disease	Inheritance	Chromosome	Gene/protein
Alzheimer's	AD	21q11-22	Amyloid precursor protein
Alzheimer's	AD	14q24.3	Presenilin-1
Alzheimer's	AD	1	Presenilin-2
Alzheimer's	Risk factor only	19q	Apolipoprotein E4
Familial prion disorders	AD	20p	Prion protein
Creutzfeldt-Jakob, Gerstmann-Sträussler syndrome, fatal familial insomnia			
Fragile X	AD	Xq27.3	FMR
Cerebral amyloid angiopathy	—	20	—

IV. Movement Disorders

A. *Parkinson's disease/parkinsonism*

Locus/Disease	Chromosome	Gene mutation	Inheritance
Park 1	4q21-23	α Synuclein	AD
Park 2	6q25.2-27	Parkin	AR
Park 3	2p13	—	AD
Park 4	4p14-16.3	Alpha-synuclein triplications and duplications	AD
Park 5	4	Ubiquitin carboxy-terminal hydrolase L1	AD
Park 6	1p35-36	PINK1	AR
Park 7	1p36	DJ-1	AR
Park 8	12cen	LRRK-2	AD
Park 9	1q36	ATP13A2	AR
Park 10	1p32	?	?AD
Park 11	2q34	?	?AD
Frontotemporal dementia with parkinsonism	17q21-23	τ	?AD
Familial multisystem degeneration with parkinsonism	mtDNA11778	Mitochondrial mutation	Maternally transmitted

B. *Trinucleotide-repeat diseases*

Disease	Inheritance	Repeats	Chromosome	Protein
Huntington's	AD	CAG	4p16	Huntingtin
Fragile X	AD	CGG	X	FMR-1
Myotonic dystrophy	AD	CTG	19	Myotonin
Spinocerebellar ataxia type 1 (SCA 1)	AD	CAG	6p23	Ataxin-1
SCA 2	AD	CAG	12q24	Ataxin-2
SCA 3 (Machado-Joseph)	AD	CAG	14q32	Ataxin-3
SCA 6	AD	CAG	19p13	Voltage-dependent calcium channel
SCA 7	AD	CAG	13p12	Ataxin-7
SCA 12	AD	CAG	5q31-33	Regulatory subunit of protein phosphatase (PP2A)
SCA 17	AD	CAG	6q27	TATA–binding protein

Disease	Inheritance	Repeats	Chromosome	Protein
Spinobulbar muscular atrophy (Kennedy's)	X-linked recessive	CAG	Xq13	Androgen receptor
Dentatorubropallidoluysian atrophy	AD	CAG	12p13	Atrophin-1
Friedreich's ataxia	AR	GAA	9q13-21.1	Frataxin

C. Dystonia

Dystonia type	Gene	Inheritance	Chromosome	Gene product/ mutation
Early-onset generalized torsion dystonia	DYT 1	AD	9q34	GAG deletion in the DYT1 gene—loss of one glutamic acid residue in Torsin A
AR torsion dystonia	DYT 2	AR	Unknown	Unknown
X-linked dystonia parkinsonism (lubag)	DYT 3	X-linked	Xq13.1	Unknown
Non-DYT1 torsion dystonia	DYT 4	AD	Unknown	Unknown
Dopa responsive dystonia and parkinsonism (Segawa syndrome)	DYT 5	AD	14q22.1-22.2	GTP cyclohydrolase I gene
Adolescent and early-adult torsion dystonia of mixed phenotype	DYT 6	AD	8p21-22	Unknown
Late-onset focal dystonia	DYT 7	AD	18p	Unknown
Paroxysmal nonkinesigenic dyskinesia	DYT 8	AD	2q	Unknown
Paroxysmal choreoathetosis with episodic ataxia and spasticity	DYT 9	AD	1p21-13.3	Unknown
Paroxysmal kinesigenic dyskinesia	DYT 10	AD	16p11.2-12.1	Unknown
Myoclonus dystonia	DYT 11	AD	7q21-31	Mutation in ε-sarcoglycan
Rapid-onset dystonia parkinsonism	DYT 12	AD	19q	Unknown
Early- and late-onset cervical cranial dystonia	DYT 13	AD	1p36.13	Unknown

D. AR ataxias with known gene loci

Disease	Chromosome	Gene
Friedreich's ataxia	9q13-21.1	X25/frataxin
Ataxia telangiectasia	11q22-23	ATM

Disease	Chromosome	Gene
Ataxia with isolated vitamin E deficiency	8q	α TTP
AR ataxia of Charlevoix-Saguenay	13q11	SACS
Ataxia with oculomotor apraxia	9p13	Aprataxin
Ataxia, neuropathy, high α-fetoprotein	9q33-34	Unknown
Infantile onset olivopontocerebellar atrophy	10q24	Unknown
Ataxia, deafness, optic atrophy	6p21-23	Unknown
Unverricht-Lundborg	21q	Cystatin B

E. *AD ataxias*

Disease	Chromosome	Gene	Mutation
SCA 1	6p23	Ataxin-1	CAG expansion
SCA 2	12q23-24.1	Ataxin-2	CAG expansion
SCA 3/Machado-Josephs disease	14q21	Ataxin-3	CAG expansion
SCA 4	16q24	—	—
SCA 5	11p11-q11	—	—
SCA 6	19p	CACNA1	CAG expansion
SCA 7	3p21.2-12	Ataxin-7	CAG expansion
SCA 8	13q21	—	CAG expansion
SCA 10	22q13	—	—
SCA 11	15q14-21.3	—	ATTCT expansion
SCA 12	5q31-33	PP2R2B	CAG expansion
SCA 13	10q13.3-13.4	—	—
SCA 14	19q13.4	—	—
SCA 16	8q23-24.1	—	—
SCA 17	6p21	TBP	CAG expansion
Dentatorubral-pallidoluysion atrophy	12p	Atrophin	CAG expansion
Episodic ataxia 1	12p13	KCNA 1	Point mutations in ion channels (K)
Episodic ataxia 2	19p13	CACNA 1	Point mutations in ion channels (Ca)

V. Neuromuscular Disorders

Disease	Protein	Chromosome
Spinal muscular atrophy 1 (Werdnig-Hoffman)	SMN, NAIP, BTFII	5
Familial amyotrophic lateral sclerosis	Superoxide dismutase	21q22.1-22.2

Disease	Protein	Chromosome
AR amyotrophic lateral sclerosis	—	2q33-35
Charcot-Marie-Tooth 1A	PMP 22	17p11.2
Charcot-Marie-Tooth 1B	P_0 myelin	1q21.2-23
Tomaculous neuropathy/hereditary neuropathy with liability to pressure palsy	PMP 22	17p11.2
Charcot-Marie-Tooth 2	—	1p35-36
Charcot-Marie-Tooth 3	—	8q13-21
Charcot-Marie-Tooth X	Connexin 32	Xq13
Familial amyloidotic peripheral neuropathy	Transthyretin	18q11.2
Familial dysautonomia	—	9q31-33
Becker's/Duchenne's dystrophy	Dystrophin	Xp21.2
Myotonic dystrophy	Myotonin	19
Nemaline myopathy (AD)	—	1q21-q23
Familial hyperthermia	Ryanodine receptor	19q12-13.2
Central core	—	19p13.1-13.2
Myotubular myopathy	—	Xq28
Fukuyama congenital dystrophy	—	9q31-33
Severe childhood muscular dystrophy	—	17 (AR)
Infantile spinal muscular atrophy (Werdnig-Hoffman)	—	5q11.2-13.3
Juvenile spinal muscular atrophy (Kugelberg-Welander)	—	5q11.2
Spinobulbar muscular atrophy (Kennedy's)	—	Xq21.3
Fascioscapulohumeral dystrophy	—	4q35
Limb-girdle dystrophy	—	15q (AR); 2p (AR); 5 (AD)
Emery-Dreifuss muscular dystrophy	—	Xq28
Distal myopathy	—	14q11
Kearns-Sayre syndrome	—	Mitochondrial deletion
Progressive external ophthalmoplegia	—	Mitochondrial deletion
Myoclonic epilepsy with ragged red fibers	—	mtDNA 3344, 3356
Hyperkalemic periodic paralysis	Sodium channelopathy	17q22-24
Paramyotonia congenita	—	—
Hypokalemic periodic paralysis	Calcium channelopathy	1q31
Thomsen's myotonia congenita	Chloride channelopathy	7q35

Disease	Protein	Chromosome
McArdle's	—	11q13
Acute intermittent porphyria	—	11q23.2
Familial spastic paraplegia	—	2p21-24; 8 (AR); 14q (AD); 15q (AD); Xq13-22 and Xq28 (X-linked)
Hyperekplexia (startle)	Glycine receptor	5q

VI. Stroke/Narcolepsy/Seizures/CNS Tumors

Disease	Protein	Chromosome
NB: Cerebral autosomal dominant arteriopathy with subcortical infarcts and leukoencephalopathy (CADASIL)	NOTCH3	19
Homocystinuria	—	21q22.3
Cystatin C/Icelandic cerebral amyloid angiopathy	—	20p11.22-11.21
Mitochondrial encephalomyopathy with lactic acidosis and stroke-like episodes	—	mtDNA 3243, 3271
Narcolepsy	—	6p21.3
Benign neonatal seizures	—	20q
Juvenile myoclonic epilepsy	—	6p21
Myoclonic epilepsy (Unverricht-Lundborg)	—	22q22.3
Glioblastoma multiforme	p53	10p12-q23.2
	CDKN2	17p13.1
	—	9p21
Retinoblastoma	RB1	13q14
Pituitary adenoma	Multiple endocrine neoplasia 1	11q13
Familial meningioma	Merlin	22q12.3

VII. Genetic Syndromes Associated with Brain Tumors (from Kesari and Wen 2004)

Syndrome	Inheritance	Gene/Protein	Associated Tumors
Neurofibromatosis type 1	AD	NF/neurofibromin (chromosome 17)	Schwannomas, astrocytomas, optic nerve gliomas, meningiomas, neurofibromas, neurofibrosarcomas
Neurofibromatosis type 2	AD	NF2/merlin (chromosome 22)	Bilateral vestibular schwannomas, astrocytomas, multiple meningiomas, ependymomas

Syndrome	Inheritance	Gene/Protein	Associated Tumors
von Hippel-Lindau disease	AD	VHL/VHL tumor suppressor (chromosome 3)	Hemangioblastomas, pancreatic cysts, retinal angiomas, renal cell carcinomas, pheochromocytomas
Li-Fraumeni syndrome	AD	TP53/p53 (chromosome 17)	Gliomas, sarcomas, breast CA, leukemias
Turcot's syndrome	AD	APC/adenomatous polyposis coli (chromosome 5)	Gliomas, medulloblastomas, adenomatous colon polyps, adenocarcinoma
Basal cell nevus (Gorlins's syndrome)	AD	PTCH/patched (Chromosome 5)	Basal cell carcinoma, medulloblastomas

VIII. Known Channelopathies with Neurologic Manifestations

Disease	Gene	Ion channel
Hypokalemic periodic paralysis	SCN4A	Sodium channel
Paramyotonia congenita	SCN4A	Sodium channel
Potassium-aggravated myotonia	SCN4A	Sodium channel
Myotonia congenita	CLCN1	Chloride channel
Hypokalemic periodic paralysis type 1	CACNLA3	Calcium channel
Andersen-Tawil syndrome	KCNJ2	Potassium channel
Congenital myasthenic syndrome	CHRNA, CHRNB, CHRNE	Acetylcholine receptor
Other myasthenic syndromes	CHRNA, CHRNB, CHRNE	Acetylcholine receptor
Episodic ataxia type 1 (with myokymia)	KCNA1	Potassium channel
Episodic ataxia type 2 (with nystagmus)	CACNA1A	Calcium channel
NB: Familial hemiplegic migraine	CACNA1A and ATP1A2	Calcium channel
SCA 6	CACNA1A	Calcium channel
Hereditary hyperekplexia	GLRA1	Glycine receptor

IX. Pediatric Neurology
A. *Phakomatoses*

Disease	Protein	Chromosome
Neurofibromatosis 1	Neurofibromin	17q11.2
Neurofibromatosis 2	Merlin	22q11-13.1
von Hippel-Lindau	VHL (elongation factor)	3p26-25
Tuberous sclerosis	TSC1 (hamartin)	9q34.1-34.2
	TBS2 (tuberin)	16
Ataxia telangiectasia	—	11q22-q23

Disease	Protein	Chromosome
Sturge-Weber	—	3 (AR); usually sporadic
Incontinentia pigmenti	—	X

B. *Metabolic disorders/developmental disorders*

Disease	Inheritance	Enzyme deficiency	Chromosome
Ceroid lipofuscinosis—Santavuori's	AR	—	1p32
Gaucher's	AR	β-galactosidase	1q21
Carnitine palmitoyltransferase deficiency	AR	—	1p32-12
Bassen-Kornzweig	AR	—	2p24
Cerebrotendinous xanthomatosis	AR	—	2q
GM$_1$ galactosidase	AR	—	3p21-14.2
Morquio syndrome	AR	Galactose-6-sulfate sulfatase (type A) β-galactosidase (type B)	3
Phenylketonuria	AR	—	4q16.1; 12q24.1
Sandhoff	AR	Hexosaminidase A and B	5q13
Tay-Sachs	AR	Hexosaminidase A	5q; 15 q22-25.1
Lafora's	AR	—	6
Zellweger syndrome	AR	—	7q11.3
Holoprosencephaly	AD	—	7q36 (AD); 13, 18 (sporadic)
Argininosuccinic acid deficiency	AR	Argininosuccinase	9
Galactosemia	AR	Galactose-1-phosphate uridyl transferase	9p13
Lactate dehydrogenase deficiency	AR	Lactate dehydrogenase	11p15.4
Niemann-Pick	AR	Sphingomyelinase	11p15 (types A and B); 18p (type C)
McArdle's	AR; rarely AD	Myophosphorylase	11q13
Pyruvate carboxylase deficiency (Leigh)	—	Pyruvate carboxylase	11q
Lipofuscinosis, late infantile	AR	—	12q21-32
Wilson's	AR	—	13p14.2-21

Disease	Inheritance	Enzyme deficiency	Chromosome
Krabbe's leukodystrophy	AR	Galactocerebrosidase	14q24.3-32
Prader-Willi/Angelman's syndrome	Sporadic	—	15q11-12
Juvenile lipofuscinosis (Batten)	AD	—	16p12
Bardet-Biedl (mental retardation, retinitis pigmentosa, polydactyly)	AR	—	16q
Pompe's	AR	1,4 glycosidase	17q23
Lissencephaly (Miller-Dieker)	—	G proteins	17p13.3
Canavan leukodystrophy	AR	Aspartoacylase	17p13
Sjšgren-Larsson syndrome	AR	—	17q
Maple syrup urine	AR	Branched chain acylcoenzyme A dehydrogenase	19p13.1-q13.2
Sialidosis	AR	Oligosaccharide sialidase	20 (type 1) 10 (type 2)
Unverricht-Lundborg	AR	—	21q23.2
Metachromatic leukodystrophy	AR	Arylsulfatase A	22q13.31
Hurler-Scheie	AR	α-L-iduronidase	22
Hunter's	X-recessive	Iduronate-2-sulfate sulfatase	X
Ornithine transcarbamoylase deficiency	X-recessive	Ornithine transcarbamoylase	Xp21.1
Fabry's	X-recessive	α-Galactosidase A	X q21-22
Menkes	X-recessive	Copper dependent enzymes (including cytochrome oxidase)	Xp11.4-11.23
Lesch-Nyhan	X-recessive	Hypoxanthine-guanine-phosphoribosyl transferase	Xq26
Pelizaeus-Merzbacher	X-recessive	—	X
Adrenoleukodystrophy	X-recessive	adenosine triphosphate-binding cassette transporter	Xq28
Kallmann's anosmia-hypogonadism	X-recessive	—	Xp22.3
Ataxia/sideroblastic anemia	X-recessive	—	Xq13
Aicardi syndrome	X-dominant	—	X

Disease	Inheritance	Enzyme deficiency	Chromosome
Incontinentia pigmenti	X-dominant	—	X
Rett syndrome	X-dominant	—	X
Leber hereditary optic atrophy	Mitochondrial	—	Deletion
Neuropathy, ataxia, retinitis pigmentosa syndrome	Mitochondrial	—	Substitution of one amino acid in position 8993

C. *Mitochondrial disorders*

Complex I	Nicotinamide adenine dinucleotide-coenzyme Q reductase	Congenital lactic acidosis, hypotonia, seizures, and apnea
		Exercise intolerance and myalgia
		Kearns-Sayre syndrome
		Mitochondrial encephalomyopathy with lactic acidosis and stroke-like episodes
		Progressive infantile poliodystrophy
		Subacute necrotizing encephalomyelopathy (Leigh disease)
Complex II	Succinate-coenzyme Q reductase	?Encephalomyopathy
Complex III	Coenzyme QH_2-cytochrome-*c* reductase	Cardiomyopathy
		Kearns-Sayre syndrome
		Myopathy and exercise intolerance with or without progressive external ophthalmoplegia
Complex IV	Cytochrome-*c* oxidase	Fatal neonatal hypotonia
		Menkes syndrome
		Myoclonic epilepsy with ragged red fibers
		Progressive infantile poliodystrophy
		Subacute necrotizing encephalomyelopathy (Leigh disease)
Complex V	Adenosine triphosphate synthase	Congenital myopathy
		Neuropathy, retinopathy, ataxia, and dementia
		Retinitis pigmentosa, ataxia, neuropathy, and dementia

ADDITIONAL NOTES

CHAPTER 20

Neurohistology, Embryology, and Developmental Disorders

I. Neurohistology

A. *Neurons:* classified by the number of processes
1. *Pseudounipolar:* located in the spinal dorsal root ganglia and sensory ganglia of the cranial nerves V, VII, IX, X
2. *Bipolar:* found in the cochlear and vestibular ganglia of cranial nerve VIII, in the olfactory nerve, and in the retina
3. *Multipolar:* the largest population of nerve cells in the nervous system; includes the motor neurons, neurons of the autonomic nervous system, interneurons, pyramidal cells of the cerebral cortex, and Purkinje cells of the cerebellar cortex

B. *Nissl substance:* consists of rosettes of polysomes and rough endoplasmic reticulum; therefore, it has a role in protein synthesis; found in the nerve cell body (perikaryon) and dendrites and not in the axon hillock or axon

C. *Axonal transport:* mediates the intracellular distribution of secretory proteins, organelles, and cytoskeletal elements; inhibited by colchicine, which depolarizes microtubules
1. *Fast anterograde axonal transport:* responsible for transporting all newly synthesized membrane organelles (vesicles) and precursors of neurotransmitters; occurs at *a rate of 200–400 mm per day;* mediated by neurotubules and kinesin; neurotubule dependent
2. *Slow anterograde transport:* responsible for transporting fibrillar cytoskeletal and protoplasmic elements; occurs at a rate of 1–5 mm per day
3. *Fast retrograde transport:* returns used materials from the axon terminal to the cell body for degradation and recycling at a rate of 100–200 mm per day; transports nerve growth factor, neurotropic viruses, and toxins (e.g., herpes simplex, rabies, poliovirus, and tetanus toxin); mediated by neurotubules and dynein

D. *Wallerian degeneration:* anterograde degeneration characterized by the disappearance of axons and myelin sheaths and the secondary proliferation of Schwann cells; occurs in the central nervous system (CNS) and peripheral nervous system (PNS)

E. *Chromatolysis:* the result of retrograde degeneration in the neurons of the CNS and PNS; there is loss of Nissl substance after axotomy

NB: Axonal sprout grows at the rate of 3 mm per day in the PNS.

F. *Glial cells:* non-neural cells of the nervous system
1. *Macroglia:* consists of astrocytes and oligodendrocytes
   a. *Astrocytes:* project foot processes that envelop the basement membrane of capillaries, neurons, and synapses; form the external and internal glial-limiting membranes of the CNS; play a role in the metabolism of certain neurotransmitters (e.g., γ-aminobutyric acid, serotonin, glutamate); buffer the potassium concentration of the extracellular space; form glial scars in damaged areas of the brain; contain glial fibrillary acidic protein, a marker for astrocytes; contain glutamine synthetase

    b. *Oligodendrocytes:* myelin-forming cells of the CNS; *one oligodendrocyte can myelinate up to 30 axons*

2. *Microglia:* arise from monocytes and function as the scavenger cells (phagocytes) of the CNS

3. *Ependymal cells:* ciliated cells that line the central canal and ventricles of the brain; also line the luminal surface of the choroid plexus; produce the cerebrospinal fluid

4. *Tanycytes:* modified ependymal cells that contract capillaries and neurons; mediate cellular transport between the ventricles and the neuropil; project to hypothalamic nuclei that regulate the release of gonadotropic hormone from the adenohypophysis

5. *Schwann cells:* derived from the neural crest; myelin-forming cells of the PNS; *one Schwann cell can myelinate only one internode;* separated from each other by the nodes of Ranvier

G. **Blood–brain barrier:** consists of the right junctions of nonfenestrated endothelial cells; some authorities include the astrocytic foot processes; while the *blood-cerebrospinal fluid barrier* consists of the tight junctions between the cuboidal epithelial cells of the choroid plexus, it is permeable to some circulating peptides (e.g., insulin) and plasma proteins (e.g., prealbumin)

NB: Areas of the brain that contain no blood-brain barrier include the subfornical organ, area postrema, and neurohypophysis.

H. *Classification of nerve fibers*

Fiber	Diameter (µm)	Conduction velocity (m/sec)	Function
Sensory axons			
Ia (A)	12–20	70–120	Proprioception, muscle spindles
Ib (A)	12–20	70–120	Proprioception, Golgi tendon organs
II (A)	5–12	30–70	Touch, pressure, and vibration
III (A)	2–5	12–30	Touch, pressure, fast pain, and temperature
IV (C)	0.5–1.0	0.5–2.0	Slow pain and temperature (unmyelinated fibers)
Motor axons			
α (A)	12–20	15–120	Innervate the extrafusal muscle fibers
γ (A)	2–10	10–45	Innervate the intrafusal muscle fibers
Preganglionic autonomic fibers (B)	<3	3–15	Myelinated preganglionic autonomic fibers
Postganglionic autonomic fibers (C)	1	2	Unmyelinated postganglionic autonomic fibers

I. *Cutaneous receptors*

1. *Free nerve endings:* nociceptors (pain) and thermoreceptors (cold and heat)

2. *Encapsulated endings:* touch receptors (Meissner's corpuscles) and pressure and vibration receptors (pacinian corpuscles)

3. *Merkel disks:* unencapsulated light-touch receptors

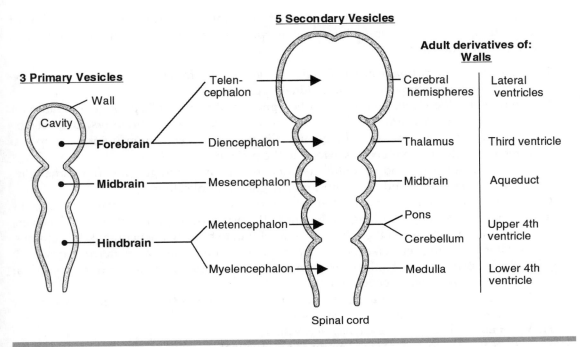

Figure 20-1. Embryologic derivatives of walls and cavities.

II. Embryology
A. NB: Divisions

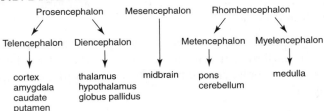

NB: Telencephalon produces the striatum except for the globus pallidus, which is from the diencephalon.

B. **Sulcus limitans:** marks boundary between basal and alar plates
1. *Alar plate* forms: posterior horn, gray matter, cerebellum, inferior olive, quadrigeminal plate, red nucleus, sensory brain stem nuclei
2. *Basal plate* forms: anterior horn, gray matter, motor nuclei of the cranial nerves
C. **Cells *derived from neural crest*:** *chromaffin cells, preganglionic sympathetic neurons, dorsal root ganglia cells, skin melanocytes, adrenal medulla, cranial nerve sensory ganglia, autonomic ganglia, cells of pia/arachnoid, Schwann cells, odontoblasts* (which elaborate predentin)

NB: The olfactory epithelium is from the ectoderm.

D. *Neural tube formation*
1. Closure of neural tube: *begins at the region of 4th somite* and proceeds in cranial and caudal directions; fusion begins on day 22
2. *Anterior neuropore: closes on day 25*
3. *Posterior neuropore: closes on day 27*

NB: α-Fetoprotein is found in the amniotic fluid and maternal serum; it is an indicator of neural tube defects (e.g., spina bifida, anencephaly); it is reduced in mothers of fetuses with Down syndrome.

 E. ***Secondary neurulation*** *(caudal neural tube formation):* forms days 28–32; forms the sacral/coccygeal segments, filum terminale, ventriculus terminalis

 F. ***Neuronal proliferation:*** *radial glia*—earliest glia in embryonic CNS, provides guidance for neuron migration from ventricular region to cortex, may be *precursors to astrocytes/ oligodendrocytes* but persist as Bergmann glia in mature cerebellum (which are special cerebellar cells whose processes extend to the pial surface)

  1. *Phase 1:* between 2 and 4 months; neuronal proliferation and generation of radial glia

  2. *Phase 2:* between 5 and 12 months; mostly glial multiplication

 G. ***Neuronal migration:*** radial cells send foot processes from the ventricular surface to the pial surface, forming a limiting membrane at the pial surface; proliferate units of the ventricular zone migrate via the radial glia scaffolding to become the neuronal cell columns; the later migrating cells take a more superficial position (inside out pattern); types

  1. *Radial:* primary mechanism for formation of the cortex and deep nuclei, cerebellar Purkinje cells, and cerebellar nuclei

  2. *Tangential:* originates in the germinal zones of the rhombic lip and migrate to form the external and internal granular layers

 H. ***Myelination:*** begins in the *4th month of gestation*

  1. *PNS:* myelinates before CNS; motor fibers myelinate before sensory; myelination in the PNS is accomplished by the *Schwann cells*

  2. *CNS:* sensory areas myelinate before motor, association cortices myelinate last; *most rapid myelination is between birth and age 2 years;* myelination in the cerebral association cortex continues into the 3rd decade; myelination in the CNS is accomplished *by oligodendrocytes* (which are not found in the retina)

NB: The lateral corticospinal tract does not fully myelinate until age 2 years (correlating to development of motor skills); the earliest structures to be myelinated at 14 weeks include medial longitudinal fasciculus/dorsal roots/cranial nerves (except II, VIII, and sensory V); myelination continues until age 12 years.

 I. **Positional changes in the spinal cord**

  1. *Newborn:* the conus medullaris *ends at L3*

  2. *Adult:* the conus medullaris *ends at L1*

 J. ***Optic nerve and chiasma:*** *derived from the diencephalon;* the optic nerve fibers occupy the choroid fissure; failure of this fissure to close results in *coloboma iridis*

 K. ***Pituitary gland:*** derived from two embryologic substrata

  1. *Adenohypophysis:* derived from the ectodermal diverticulum of the primitive mouth cavity (stomodeum), which is also called *Rathke pouch; remnants of Rathke pouch may give rise to a craniopharyngioma*

  2. *Neurohypophysis:* develops from a ventral evagination of the hypothalamus (neuroectoderm of the neural tube)

III. Developmental Disorders

 A. *Disorders of primary neurulation*

  1. **Anencephaly:** *meroanencephaly; failure of anterior neuropore closure* (less than day 24); as a result, the brain does not develop; frequency: 1:1,000; risk in subsequent pregnancies is 5–7%; 75% are stillborn; affects the forebrain and variable portions of the brain stem

   a. *Holoacrania:* up to the foramen magnum

   b. *Meroacrania:* slightly higher than the foramen magnum

2. Encephalocele: restricted to anterior neuropore defects; 75% are occipital, 50% have hydrocephalus

3. **Spina bifida:** results from failure of the posterior neuropore to form; the defect usually occurs in the *sacrolumbar region*

    a. *Spina bifida occulta:* skin-covered defect; rarely associated with a neurologic deficit; frequency: 10%; associated with diastematomyelia, lipomeningocele, tethered cord, filum terminale, intraspinal dermoid, epidermoid cyst

    b. *Spina bifida aperta:* associated with a neurologic deficit in 90%; 85% with spinal dysraphism

        i. **Meningocele:** herniation of cerebrospinal fluid-filled sac without neural elements

        ii. **Myelomeningocele:** herniated neural elements covered by meningeal sac; 80% are lumbar; 90% have hydrocephalus if lumbar is involved; symptoms include motor, sensory, and sphincter dysfunction

        iii. **Myeloschisis:** neural elements at surface completely uncovered; associated with iniencephaly (malformed skull base); most babies are stillborn

        iv. **Myelocystocele:** herniation of meninges and cord with dilated central canal

4. **Arnold-Chiari malformation**

    a. *Chiari I:* typical characteristics include

        i. Kinked cervical cord

        ii. Brain stem elongation

        iii. Cerebellar tonsillar dysmorphic tissue displaced downward (radiologically, cerebellar tonsils are >5 mm below foramen magnum)

        iv. Beaked mesencephalic tectum

        v. Atretic aqueduct

        vi. Small cerebellum with small posterior fossa and large foramen magnum

    b. *Chiari II:* similar to Chiari I *plus lumbar spinal fusion defect;* almost 100% with myelomeningocele; 96% with cortex malformation (heterotopia, polymicrogyria); with hydrocephalus (due to 4th ventricle obstruction); with tectum deformity; frequency: 1:1,000

    c. *Chiari III:* Chiari II *plus occipital encephalocele or myelocerebellomeningocele* (due to cervical spina bifida with cerebellum herniating through the foramen magnum); with downbeat nystagmus or periodic alternating nystagmus, cranial nerve dysfunction, altered respiratory control, abnormal extraocular movements

    d. *Chiari IV: with cerebellar hypoplasia*

5. **Meckel's syndrome:** associated with *maternal hyperthermia/fever on days 20–26;* characterized by encephalocele, microcephaly, micro-ophthalmia, cleft lip, polydactyly, polycystic kidneys, ambiguous genitalia

NB: Chromosomal abnormalities associated with neural tube defects: trisomy 13 and 18; other causes of neural tube defects: teratogens (thalidomide, valproate, phenytoin), single mutant gene (Meckel's syndrome), multifactorial.

  B. *Disorders of secondary neurulation: occult dysraphic states;* 100% have abnormal conus and filum; 90% with vertebral abnormalities; 80% have overlying dermal lesions (dimple, hair tuft, lipoma, hemangioma), although with an intact dermal layer over lesions; 4% with siblings with a disorder of primary neurulation

    1. **Caudal regression syndrome:** 20% are infants of diabetic mothers; characterized by dysraphic sacrum and coccyx with atrophic muscle and bone; symptoms: delayed sphincter control and walking, back and leg pain, scoliosis, pes cavus, leg asymmetry

    2. **Myelocystocele:** cystic central canal

   3. **Diastematomyelia:** bifid cord
   4. **Meningocele:** rare; no associated hydrocephalus
   5. **Lipomeningocele**
   6. **Subcutaneous lipomas/teratoma**
   7. **Dermal sinus**
  C. *Disorders of porencephalic development*
   1. **Aprosencephaly:** absent telencephalon and diencephalon
   2. **Atelencephaly:** absent telencephalon (diencephalon present); characterized by intact skull and skin, cyclopia with absent eyes, abnormal limbs, and abnormal genitalia
   3. **Holoprosencephaly:** single-lobed cerebrum and only one ventricle; 100% associated with anosmia; facial defects include *ethmocephaly* (hypertelorism with proboscis between eyes), *cebocephaly* (single nostril), *cyclopia* (single eye with or without proboscis), *cleft lip;* associated with hypoplastic optic nerves; corpus callosum may be absent; associated chromosomal abnormality: *trisomy 13 (Patau syndrome)* or ring 13; also the most severe manifestation of **fetal alcohol syndrome** (i.e., the most common cause of mental retardation and is associated *with microcephaly and congenital heart disease*); 2% are infants of diabetic mothers; 6% recurrence rate
    a. *Alobar:* characterized by facial anomalies, hypotelorism, microphthalmia, micrognathia
    b. *Semilobar:* facial anomalies are less severe and less common; septum pellucidum and corpus callosum are absent; the falx and interhemispheric fissure are partially developed posteriorly
    c. *Lobar:* shallow, incomplete interhemispheric fissure anteriorly; septum pellucidum is absent; facial anomalies are uncommon
   4. **Agenesis of corpus callosum:** associated with
    a. *Holoprosencephaly*
    b. *Absent septum pellucidum*
    c. *Schizencephaly and other migrational disorders*
    d. *Chiari type 2*
    e. *Septo-optic dysplasia:* absent or hypoplastic septum pellucidum, hypoplastic optic nerves, schizencephaly in approximately 50% but normal-sized ventricles, pituitary axis dysfunction (50% with diabetes insipidus)
    f. **Aicardi syndrome:** *X-linked dominant* condition with agenesis of the corpus callosum, neuronal migrational defects and chorioretinal lacunes
    g. **Dandy-Walker malformation:** failure of foramen of Magendie development; cystic dilation of 4th ventricle and cerebellar vermis agenesis with enlarged posterior fossa; elevation of the inion; agenesis of the corpus callosum; 70% with migrational disorders; associated with cardiac abnormalities and urinary tract infections; frequency: 1:25,000; may result from riboflavin inhibitors, posterior fossa trauma, or viral infection
  D. *Disorders of proliferation*
   1. **Microcephaly:** decreased size of proliferative units
   2. **Radial microbrain:** decreased number of proliferative units
   3. **Macrencephaly:** well formed but large brain
   4. **Hemimegalencephaly**
  E. *Neuronal migrational disorders*
   1. **Schizencephaly:** clefts between ventricles and subarachnoid space; no gliosis; associated with heterotopias in the cleft wall
   2. **Porencephaly:** variable communication between ventricle and subarachnoid space + gliosis; usually due to ischemia later in gestation

3. **Lissencephaly:** few or no gyri (smooth surface); **Miller-Dieker syndrome** (lissencephaly, 90% with *chromosome 17 deletion;* characterized by microcephaly, seizures, hypotonia, craniofacial defects, cardiac defects, genital abnormalities)
4. **Pachygyria:** few broad, thick gyri
5. **Polymicrogyria:** too many small gyri (like a wrinkled chestnut); seen in Zellweger syndrome (cerebrohepatorenal syndrome): autosomal recessive peroxisomal disorder linked to *chromosome 13,* characterized by increased low-chain fatty acids, polymicrogyria, heterotopias, seizures, hepatomegaly, renal cysts
6. **Heterotopias:** rests of neurons in the white matter secondary to arrested radial migration; associated with seizures; may be periventricular, laminar (in the deep white matter) or band-like (between the cortex and the ventricular surface)

F. *Disorders of myelination*
   1. Aminoaciduria/organic acidurias
      a. Ketotic hyperglycinemia
      b. Nonketotic hyperglycinemia
      c. Phenylketonuria
      d. Maple syrup urine disease
      e. Homocystinuria
   2. Hypothyroidism
   3. Malnutrition
   4. Periventricular leukomalacia
   5. Prematurity

G. *Congenital hydrocephalus:* frequency: 1:1,000; common etiologies are
   1. Aqueductal stenosis: 33%
   2. Chiari types 2 and 3: 28%
   3. Communicating hydrocephalus: 22%
   4. Dandy-Walker malformation: 7%
   5. Others: tumors, vein of Galen, X-linked aqueductal stenosis

NB: The most common cause of congenital hydrocephalus is aqueductal stenosis.

H. **Walker-Warburg syndrome:** associated with congenital muscular dystrophy, cerebellar malformation, retinal malformation, and macrocephaly
I. **Hydranencephaly:** results from bilateral hemisphere infarction secondary to occlusion of the carotid arteries; hemispheres are replaced with hugely dilated ventricles
J. *Differential diagnosis of skull and spine disorders*

Platybasia (flattened skull base)	Osteomalacia
	Rickets
	Hyperparathyroidism
	Fibrous dysplasia
	Paget's disease
	Arnold-Chiari malformation
Craniosynostosis: premature closure of the sutures (normally closes at approximately 30 mos); 4 males:1 female; sagittal suture is most commonly affected	Primary Secondary Hematologic (sickle-cell anemia, thalassemia)
Scaphocephaly = dolichocephaly: premature closure of sagittal suture causing a long skull	Metabolic (rickets, hypercalcemia, hyperthyroidism, hypervitamin D)

Brachycephaly = turricephaly: premature closure of coronal/lambdoid sutures causing a short and tall skull

Plagiocephaly: premature closure of coronal and lambdoid sutures

Trigonocephaly: metopic suture
Oxycephaly: premature closure of coronal, sagittal, and lambdoid sutures; causing a cloverleaf skull (kleeblattschädel)

Wormian bones: intrasutural ossification; normal up to 6 mos old

Bone dysplasia (hypo-PO_4, achondroplasia, metaphyseal dysplasia, mongolism, Hurler disease, skull hyperostosis)
Syndromes (Crouzon, Apert, Carpenter, Treacher-Collins, cloverleaf skull, arrhinencephaly)
Microcephaly
After ventriculoperitoneal shunt

P: Pyknodysostosis

O: Osteogenesis imperfecta

R: Rickets that are healing

K: Kinky hair syndrome

C: Cleidocranial dysplasia

H: Hypothyroidism

O: Olopalatodigital syndrome

P: Primary acro-osteolysis

S: Down syndrome

Increased focal skull thickness

H: Hyperostosis frontalis

I: Idiopathic

P: Paget's disease

F: Fibrous dysplasia

A: Anemia

M: Metastasis

Absent greater sphenoid wing

M: Meningioma

F: Fibrous dysplasia

O: Optic glioma

R: Relapsing hematoma

M: Metastasis

A: Aneurysm

R: Retinoblastoma

I: Idiopathic

N: Neurofibromatosis

E: Eosinophilic granuloma

ADDITIONAL NOTES

CHAPTER 21

Clinical Neuroanatomy

I. Spinal Reflexes and Muscle Tone

A. *Monosynaptic reflex* **response:** *mediated by two neurons, one afferent and one efferent (e.g., deep tendon reflexes; polysynaptic reflex):* involves several neurons, termed *interneurons* or *internuncial cells,* in addition to afferent and efferent neurons

B. *Muscle spindles:* receptor organs that provide the afferent component of many spinal stretch responses; encapsulated structures, 3–4 mm in length; consists of 2–12 thin muscle fibers of modified striated muscle; because they are enclosed in a fusiform spindle, they are termed *intrafusal muscle fibers* (to contrast them with large extrafusal fibers); they are *connected to the muscle's tendons in parallel with the extrafusal fibers;* the sensory function of the intrafusal fibers is *to inform the nervous system of the length and rate of change in length of the extrafusal fibers;* supplied by types of spindles

1. *Nuclear bag fiber:* longer, larger fiber containing large nuclei closely packed in a central bag
2. *Nuclear chain fiber:* shorter, thinner, and contains a single row of central nuclei
3. Bag_2: intermediate in structure between bag and chain fibers

NB: Both bag and chain fibers are innervated by γ motor neurons, which terminate in two types of endings—plates (occur chiefly on nuclear bag fibers) and trails (occur mostly on nuclear chain fibers, but found on bag fibers as well); muscle spindles are supplied by group 1a and group 2 nerve fibers.

C. *Motor neurons:* muscle contraction in response to a stimulus involves activation of the α, β, and γ motor neurons of lamina IX

1. *α Motor neurons: largest of the anterior horn cells;* may be stimulated monosynaptically by group 1a primary and 2 secondary afferents, corticospinal tract fibers, lateral vestibulospinal tract fibers, reticulospinal and raphe spinal tract fibers; however, the vast majority are stimulated through interneurons in the spinal cord gray matter; they *activate the large extrafusal skeletal muscle fibers and interneurons in the ventral horn (Renshaw cells*—which are capable of inhibiting α motor neurons, producing a negative feedback response)
2. *γ Motor neurons: fusimotor neurons; innervate the intrafusal muscle fibers only, thus do not produce extrafusal muscle contraction;* smaller, not excited monosynaptically by segmental inputs, not involved in inhibitory feedback by Renshaw cells; discharges spontaneously at high frequencies
    a. *Dynamic γ motor neurons:* affects the afferent responses to phasic stretch more than static stretch; terminate in plate endings on nuclear bag fibers
    b. *Static γ motor neurons:* increase spindle response to static stretch; terminate in trail endings on bag and chain fibers
3. *β Motor neurons:* have axons intermediate in diameter between α and β motor neurons; *innervate extrafusal and intrafusal muscle fibers*

D. *Stretch reflex:* the basic neural mechanism for maintaining tone in muscles (e.g., tapping the patellar tendon stretches the extrafusal fibers of the quadriceps femoris group)—because the intrafusal fibers are arranged in parallel with the extrafusal fibers, the muscle spindles will also be stretched—which then stimulates the sensory nerve endings in spindles (particularly group 1a)—group 1a monosynaptically stimulates the α motor neurons that supply the quadriceps muscle and polysynaptically inhibits the antagonist muscle group (the hamstring muscles)—thus, the quadriceps suddenly contract and the hamstring relaxes, causing the leg to extend the knee

E. *Golgi tendon organs:* encapsulated structures attached in series with the large, collagenous fibers of tendons at the insertions of muscles and along the fascial covering of muscles; *group 1b afferents terminate* in small bundles within the capsule; when muscle contraction occurs, shortening of the contractile part of the muscle results in lengthening of the noncontractile region where the tendon organs are located—resulting in vigorous firing of the Golgi tendon organs—their afferents project to the spinal cord, where they polysynaptically inhibit the α motor neurons innervating the agonist muscle and facilitate motor neurons of the antagonist muscle; central action of the Golgi tendon organs are responsible for the "clasp knife" phenomenon in spasticity

II. Peripheral Nerves

A. *Brachial plexus:* originates from the *anterior rami of spinal nerves C5–T1;* variations are common

1. *Muscles of the shoulder girdle innervated by nerves* that originate *proximal to the formation of the brachial plexus;* these muscles are important to evaluate clinically and by nerve conduction study/electromyography (EMG) when trying to determine if the lesion is at the level of the plexus or roots

   a. **Serratus anterior**: innervated by the long thoracic nerve (C5–C7)

   b. **Rhomboids**: innervated by the dorsal scapular nerve (C5)

2. *Trunks of the brachial plexus*

   a. *Upper trunk:* C5, C6; branches include

   i. **Suprascapular nerve**: innervates the supraspinatus and infraspinatus muscles

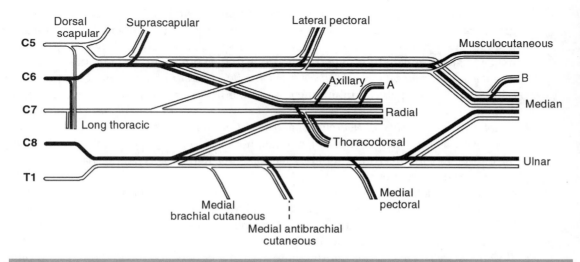

Figure 21-1. Schematic diagram of the brachial plexus. A, branch to extensor carpi radialis longus and brachioradialis; B, branch to flexor carpi radialis and pronator teres.

NB: The suprascapular nerve is susceptible to compression in the suprascapular notch.

       ii. **Nerve to the subclavius muscle**: innervates the subclavius
    b. *Middle trunk:* C7
    c. *Lower trunk:* C8, T1
  3. *Cords of the brachial plexus*
    a. *Lateral cord:* formed by the anterior divisions of the upper and middle trunks (C5–C7); branches include
       i. *Part of the median nerve:* supplies pronator teres, flexor carpi radialis

NB: The sensory supply to the median nerve derives from the lateral cord.

       ii. *Musculocutaneous nerve:* supplies the biceps, brachialis, and coracobrachialis
      iii. *Lateral antebrachial cutaneous nerve:* skin of the lateral forearm
      iv. *Branch to the pectoral nerve:* supplies the pectoralis major
    b. *Medial cord:* formed by the anterior division of the lower trunk (C8, T1)
       i. *Part of the median nerve:* supplies the flexor digitorum sublimes, one-half of the flexor digitorum profundus, pronator quadratus, flexor pollicis longus, and 1st and 2nd lumbricals, abductor pollicis brevis, opponens pollicis, and one-half of flexor pollicis

NB: Martin-Gruber anastomosis occurs in 15–30% of the population, consisting of a communicating branch from the median nerve to the ulnar nerve in the forearm to supply the first dorsal interosseous, adductor polices, and abductor digiti minimi.

       ii. *Ulnar nerve:* supplies one-half of the flexor digitorum profundus, flexor carpi ulnaris, 3rd and 4th lumbricals, interossei, adductor pollicis, abductor digiti minimi, opponens digiti minimi, and one-half flexor pollicis brevis
      iii. *Medial antebrachial cutaneous nerve:* supplies the skin to the medial forearm

NB: This nerve is a branch of the medial cord and would be expected to be injured in the neurogenic thoracic outlet syndrome, and would be spared in an ulnar nerve mononeuropathy at the elbow.

      iv. *Branch to pectoral nerve:* supplies the pectoralis major and minor muscles
    c. *Posterior cord:* formed by the posterior division of the upper, middle, and lower trunks (C5–T1); branches include
       i. *Subscapular nerve:* supplies the subscapularis and teres major
      ii. *Thoracodorsal nerve:* supplies latissimus dorsi
      iii. *Axillary nerve:* supplies the deltoid and teres major
      iv. *Radial nerve:* supplies the triceps, brachioradialis, extensor carpi radialis longus, extensor carpi radialis brevis, anconeus, supinator, extensor digitorum communis, extensor carpi ulnaris, abductor pollicis longus, extensor pollicis longus, extensor pollicis brevis, and extensor indicis proprius muscles
      v. *Posterior antebrachial cutaneous nerve*
  4. *Anatomic lesions of the brachial plexus*

NB: Lesions in the brachial plexus will spare the paraspinals at the corresponding levels.

    a. *Trunk lesions*
       i. *Upper trunk lesion:* **Erb-Duchenne paralysis**; nerves involved: *suprascapular nerve* (paralysis of the shoulder adductors/external rotators), C5, C6 portions of *the lateral cord and posterior cord* (paralysis of forearm flexors, elbow flexors, external

rotators of the forearm), *lateral antebrachial cutaneous nerve;* clinical presentation: arm is adducted, internally rotated and extended *(porter tip position)* with sparing of the intrinsics, absent biceps/brachioradialis reflexes, absent sensation over the lateral forearm

    ii. *Lower trunk lesions:* **Klumpke's paralysis**—involves the C8, T1 portion of the *medial cord; paralysis of the finger flexors and intrinsics; paresis of triceps and extensor digitorum communis* (C8, T1 portion of the posterior cord); the arm is mildly flexed at the elbow and wrist, with a *"useless" hand;* may be accompanied by Horner's syndrome

    iii. *Middle trunk lesions:* rarely in isolation

  b. *Cord lesions*

    i. *Lateral cord:* weakness in the elbow and wrist flexors; sensory loss over the lateral forearm

    ii. *Medial cord:* weakness in the hand intrinsics and partial weakness in long finger flexors; sensory loss over medial forearm

    iii. *Posterior cord:* weakness in shoulder abduction and elbow/wrist/finger extensors; sensory loss over posterior aspect of the arm and hand

NB: Idiopathic brachial plexopathy (Parsonage Turner syndrome)—most common among young, healthy males; 25% preceded by a viral syndrome; symptoms include pain, weakness, paresthesias; elevated cerebrospinal fluid protein in 10%; two-thirds begin to improve by 1 month and two-thirds recover by 1 year

  5. *Muscles innervated by the brachial plexus*

Muscle	Nerve	Spinal segment	Action/test
Trapezius	Spinal accessory	C3, C4	Have the patient elevate shoulder against resistance.
Rhomboids	Dorsal scapular	C4, C5	With the patient's hand behind the back, order to press against you while you press on the palm.
Serratus anterior	Long thoracic	C5–C7	Have the patient push against a wall.
Pectoralis major	Lateral and medial pectoral	C6–C8	Have the patient adduct the upper arm against resistance.
Supraspinatus	Suprascapular	C5, C6	With the arm close to the body, have the patient abduct the upper arm against resistance.
Infraspinatus	Suprascapular	C5, C6	Have the patient externally rotate the upper arm at the shoulder against resistance.
NB: Latissimus dorsi	Thoracodorsal	C6–C8	With the upper arm up at shoulder level, have the patient adduct against resistance.
Teres major	Subscapular	C5–C7	Have the patient adduct the elevated upper arm against resistance.
Biceps	Musculocutaneous	C5, C6	Have the patient flex supinated forearm against resistance.

Muscle	Nerve	Spinal segment	Action/test
Deltoid	Axillary	C5, C6	Have the patient abduct the upper arm against resistance while elevated to the level of the shoulder.
Triceps	Radial	C6–C8	Have the patient extend the forearm at the elbow against resistance.
Brachioradialis	Radial	C5, C6	Have the patient flex the forearm against resistance with the forearm midway between pronation and supination.
Extensor carpi radialis	Radial	C5, C6	Have the patient extend and abduct the hand at the wrist against resistance.
Supinator	Radial	C6, C7	Have the patient supinate the forearm against resistance with the forearm extended at the elbow.
Extensor carpi ulnaris	Posterior interosseous	C7, C8	Have the patient extend and adduct the hand at the wrist against resistance.
Extensor digitorum	Posterior interosseous	C7, C8	Have the patient maintain extension of fingers at the metacarpophalangeal joints against resistance.
Abductor pollicis longus	Posterior interosseous	C7, C8	Have the patient abduct the thumb at the carpometacarpal joint in a plane at right angles to the palm.
Extensor pollicis longus	Posterior interosseous	C7, C8	Have the patient extend the thumb at the interphalangeal joint against resistance.
Extensor pollicis brevis	Posterior interosseous	C7, C8	Have the patient extend the thumb at the metacarpophalangeal joint against resistance.
Pronator teres	Median	C6, C7	Have the patient pronate the forearm against resistance.
Flexor carpi radialis	Median	C6, C7	Have the patient flex the hand at the wrist against resistance.
Flexor digitorum superficialis	Median	C7–T1	Have the patient flex the finger at the proximal interphalangeal joint against resistance.
Flexor digitorum profundus I, II	Anterior interosseous	C7, C8	Have the patient flex the distal phalanx of the index finger against resistance.
Flexor pollicis longus	Anterior interosseous	C7, C8	Have the patient flex the distal phalanx of the thumb against resistance.
Abductor pollicis brevis	Median	C8, T1	Have the patient abduct the thumb at right angles to the palm against resistance.

Muscle	Nerve	Spinal segment	Action/test
Opponens pollicis	Median	C8, T1	Have the patient touch the base of the little finger with the thumb against resistance.
1st lumbrical-interosseous	Median and ulnar	C8, T1	Have the patient extend the finger at the proximal interphalangeal joint against resistance.
Flexor carpi ulnaris	Ulnar	C7–T1	Have the patient flex and adduct the hand at the wrist against resistance.
Flexor digitorum profundus III, IV	Ulnar	C7, C8	Have the patient flex the distal interphalangeal joint against resistance.
Adductor digiti minimi	Ulnar	C8, T1	Have the patient adduct the little finger against resistance.
Flexor digiti minimi	Ulnar	C8, T1	Have the patient flex the little finger at the metacarpophalangeal joint against resistance.
1st dorsal interosseous	Ulnar	C8, T1	Have the patient abduct the index finger against resistance.
2nd palmar interosseous	Ulnar	C8, T1	Have the patient adduct the index finger against resistance.
Adductor pollicis	Ulnar	C8, T1	Have the patient adduct the thumb at right angles to the palm against resistance.

B. *Median nerve:* derived from the lateral cord (C5, C6) and medial cord (C8, T1) of the brachial plexus; passes between the two heads of the pronator teres muscle
   1. *Innervates: pronator teres, flexor carpi radialis, flexor digitorum sublimis, and palmaris longus muscles*
   2. *Anterior interosseous innervation—flexor digitorum profundus, flexor pollicis longus, pronator quadratus*
   3. *Branches to palmar cutaneous nerve*—which supplies the skin of the proximal median palm; passes through the carpal tunnel to innervate: abductor pollicis brevis, opponens pollicis, one-half of flexor pollicis brevis, skin of the distal median palm and 1st through 3rd digits, and one-half of the 4th digit
   4. *Clinical syndromes*
      a. **Carpal tunnel syndrome**: *symptoms:* pain, tingling, or burning in thumb, 1st two fingers, most prominent at night, aggravated by activities involving repetitive wrist action; *clinical findings:* thenar muscle weakness, sensory deficit, *Phalen's sign, Tinel's sign* (to percussion at wrist flexor crease); *EMG/nerve conduction study (NCS):* relative slowing of the conduction between the palm and wrist as compared to the adjacent ulnar nerve may be the most sensitive method of detecting carpal tunnel syndrome, the motor conduction and compound motor action potential amplitude are normal in the majority unless severe disease

NB: Median nerve sensory nerve action potential is the most sensitive study for the detection of carpal tunnel syndrome. Motor studies are recorded over the abducens pollicis brevis.

     b. **Anterior interosseous nerve syndrome**: *symptoms:* spontaneous onset or associated with vigorous exercise, pain over proximal flexor surface of the forearm but can be painless, weakness is a common complaint; *clinical:* tenderness over proximal flexor surface of the forearm, weakness of the flexor pollicis longus is most common, no weakness of the thenar muscles, no sensory deficit; etiology: accessory head of the flexor pollicis longus, fibrous origin or tendinous origin of the flexor digitorum sublimes to the long finger; *EMG:* abnormalities in the flexor pollicis longus, 1st and 2nd flexor digitorum profundus, and pronator quadratus sparing all other muscles, especially thenar groups

NB: Approximately one-half of the cases of Martin-Gruber anastomosis arise from the anterior interosseous nerve.

NB: Martin-Gruber anastomosis is detected by an increased amplitude of compound motor action potential with stimulation at the elbow when compared with stimulation at the wrist.

     c. **Pronator syndrome**: *symptoms:* pain in the flexor muscles of the proximal forearm, paresthesias of the hand, symptoms worse with forceful pronation, weakness of grip is not a common complaint; *clinical:* tenderness over pronator teres, Tinel's sign over site of entrapment, weakness is often slight, sensory deficit over the cutaneous distribution of the median nerve including the thenar eminence; etiology: hypertrophy of the pronator teres, fibrous band from the ulnar head of the pronator teres to the "sublimis bridge," ligament from medial epicondyle to the radius; *EMG/NCS:* sparing of the pronator teres, abnormalities of other median innervated forearm muscles plus the thenar muscles, slowing of the conduction through proximal forearm distal latencies

     d. **Humeral supracondylar spur syndrome (ligament of Struthers)**: presents clinically like a pronator syndrome; aggravated by forearm supination and elbow extension, which may obliterate the radial pulse, the spur may be palpable, EMG abnormalities of all median nerve-innervated muscles, including pronator teres; supracondylar conduction abnormalities may be demonstrated

  C. ***Ulnar nerve:*** derived directly from the lower trunk and medial cord (C8, T1) of the brachial plexus; in the midarm, it becomes superficial and reaches the grove behind the median epicondyle; it passes between the two heads of the flexor carpi ulnaris (cubital tunnel); runs down the medial forearm innervating the flexor carpi ulnaris and the ulnar half of the flexor digitorum profundus

    1. Before entry into the Guyon's canal, gives off two small branches: *dorsal cutaneous* (supplies the dorsal ulnar aspect of the hand) and *palmar cutaneous* (supplies the skin of the ulnar palm)

    2. *Within Guyon's canal*, gives off two branches: *superficial branch* to the skin over the distal ulnar palm and 5th digit and one-half of 4th digit, and *deep branch* to innervate adductor digiti minimi, opponens digiti minimi, flexor digitorum minimi, 3rd and 4th lumbricals, all interossei, one-half flexor pollicis brevis, adductor pollicis

NB: The ulnar nerve does not supply sensory innervation proximal to the wrist.

    3. *Clinical syndromes*

     a. *Compression at the elbow:* site of compression: adjacent to posterior aspect of medial epicondyle of the humerus is most common (due to trauma), *cubital tunnel syndrome* (due to entrapment between the two heads of the flexor carpi ulnaris), *arcade of Struthers syndrome* (due to entrapment as the nerve passes through the medial intermuscular septum); *clinical:* gradual onset of pain along the ulnar side of the forearm and/or hand, numbness in the ring and little fingers, atrophy and weakness of ulnar innervated intrinsic hand muscles, weakness of 4th and 5th flexor digitorum profundus, flexor carpi ulnaris is seldom weak (except entrapment at the arcade of Struthers), hypesthesia and hypalgesia over cutaneous distribution of the ulnar nerve in most cases, nerve in the ulnar grove may enlarge and dislocate; *EMG/NCS:* abnormally large motor unit potentials and decreased number of motor unit potentials are common, positive waves and fibrillation also seen frequently, findings are much more prominent in the hand than the forearm (except in the Arcade of Struthers syndrome), conduction delay is the earliest finding

    b. **Distal ulnar nerve compression syndrome**: *symptoms:* gradual or sudden onset, aching pain along the ulnar side of hand, sensory symptoms may be absent in type 2; *etiology:* fibrous scaring after fracture or soft tissue injury, ganglion, hemorrhage (hemophilia), lipoma, other tumors, ulnar artery disease

       i. *Type 1:* atrophy and weakness of all ulnar innervated intrinsic muscles of the hand, sensory loss in the ulnar cutaneous distribution sparing the dorsum of the hand; EMG/NCS: confined to the ulnar innervated intrinsic muscles, motor conduction delay from wrist to hypothenar muscles, sensory conduction delay from the digit to the wrist

      ii. *Type 2:* atrophy and weakness of all ulnar innervated intrinsic muscles or all but the hypothenar group, no sensory deficit; EMG/NCS: may spare hypothenar muscles on EMG, may have no conduction delay to hypothenar muscles, conduction delay to the 1st dorsal interosseous, no conduction delay from the digit to the wrist

      iii. *Type 3:* sensory loss in the ulnar cutaneous distribution sparing the dorsum of the hand, no motor deficit; EMG/NCS: no EMG abnormality (except possibly palmaris brevis), no conduction delay of hypothenar muscles or 1st dorsal interosseous, with sensory conduction delay from digit to wrist

D. *Radial nerve:* derived from the posterior cord (C5–C8) of the brachial plexus; courses down on medial side of the humerus; winds obliquely around the humerus in the spiral groove and branches to deltoid (axillary nerve) and triceps; passes between the head of the triceps, passes into the forearm and branches to brachioradialis, the extensor carpi radialis brevis, and longus muscles

  1. Divides into

    a. *Posterior interosseous nerve:* deep motor branch, major terminal portion of the nerve, passes through the supinator muscle via arcade of Frohse, innervates extensor groups of forearm and wrist

    b. *Superficial radial nerve:* superficial sensory branch

  2. **Posterior interosseous syndrome**: *symptoms:* usually painless, progression most often gradual, begins with a fingerdrop and then progresses from one finger to another, incomplete wristdrop develops later; *clinical:* no weakness proximal to elbow, weakness of muscles of the extensor surface of forearm (except brachioradialis, extensor carpi radialis, and supinator), no sensory deficit; etiology: tumors (usually lipomas), bursitis or synovitis, chronic trauma; *EMG/NCS:* EMG sparing brachioradialis, extensor carpi radialis, and supinator, delayed latency from elbow to extensor indicis

E. *Musculocutaneous nerve:* derived from the lateral cord (C5–C7) of the brachial plexus; pierces coracobrachialis then passes between biceps and brachioradialis and supplies these muscles; continues as the lateral cutaneous nerve of the forearm

1. **Coracobrachialis syndrome**: *symptoms:* painless weakness of elbow flexion, onset related to strenuous exercise or associated with general anesthesia, recovery is spontaneous and usually complete; *clinical:* weakness is limited to the biceps and brachialis, sensory deficit in the distribution of the lateral cutaneous nerve; *EMG/NCS:* abnormalities noted in biceps and brachialis, but coracobrachialis spared, conduction block can be detected proximal to axilla

F. *Lumbar plexus:* produced by the union of the ventral rami of the 1st three lumbar nerves and the greater part of the 4th, with contribution from the subcostal nerve; lies anterior to the vertebral transverse processes, embedded in the posterior part of the psoas major

  1. *1st lumbar nerve:* receives fibers from the subcostal nerve and divides into
     a. *Upper branch:* splits into iliohypogastric and ilioinguinal (supplying the skin over the root of the penis, adjoining part of the femoral triangle, and upper part of the scrotum) nerves
     b. *Lower branch:* joins a twig from the 2nd lumbar nerve and becomes the *genitofemoral nerve* (divides further into genital—supplying the cremaster muscle and the skin of the scrotum, and femoral—supplying the skin over the upper part of the femoral triangle, branches); all three nerve branches run parallel to the lower intercostal nerves and supply the transverse and oblique abdominal muscles
  2. Large part of the *2nd lumbar* and the entire *3rd* (and the offshoot from the 4th lumbar nerve): split into *ventral (anterior) division and dorsal (posterior) division,* which unite to constitute
     a. Femoral nerve
     b. Obturator nerve
  3. The lower part of the ventral ramus of the 4th lumbar joins the ventral ramus of the 5th to form the *lumbosacral trunk*

G. *Sacral plexus:* formed by the lumbosacral trunk and the ventral rami of the 1st three sacral nerves and the upper part of the 4th sacral ramus; a flattened band that gives rise to many branches before its largest part passes below the piriformis muscle to form the sciatic nerve

NB: The sciatic nerve is divided into peroneal division and tibial division.

H. *Coccygeal plexus:* the lower part of the ventral ramus of the 4th and 5th sacral nerves and the coccygeal nerves form the small coccygeal plexus; it consists of two loops on the pelvic surface of the coccygeus and levator ani muscles; anococcygeal nerve: supplies the skin between the anus and coccyx

I. *Muscle innervated by the lumbar plexus*

Muscles	Nerve	Spinal segment	Action/test
Iliopsoas	Femoral, L1–L3 spinal nerve branches	L1–L3	Have the patient flex the thigh against resistance with the leg flexed at the knee and hip.
Quadriceps femoris	Femoral	L2–L4	Have the patient extend the leg against resistance with the limb flexed at the hip and knee.
Adductors	Obturator	L2–L4	Have the patient adduct the limb against resistance while lying on back with leg extended at the knee.

Muscles	Nerve	Spinal segment	Action/test
Gluteus medius and minimus	Superior gluteal	L4–S1	Have the patient lie on his back and internally rotate the thigh against resistance with the limb flexed at the hip and knee; or, while the leg is extended, have the patient abduct the limb against resistance.
Gluteus maximus	Inferior gluteal	L5–S2	While the patient lies on his back with the leg extended at the knee, extend the limb at the hip against resistance; or while the patient lies on his face, have him elevate the leg against resistance.
Hamstring: semitendinosus, semimembranosus, biceps	Sciatic	L5–S2	While the patient lies on his back with the limb flexed at the hip and knee, have him flex the leg at the knee against resistance.
Gastrocnemius	Tibial	S1, S2	With the leg extended, have the patient plantar flex the foot against resistance.
Soleus	Tibial	S1, S2	With the limb flexed at the hip and knee, have the patient flex the foot against resistance.
Tibialis posterior	Tibial	L4, L5	Have the patient invert the foot against resistance.
Flexor digitorum longus; flexor hallucis longus	Tibial	L5–S2	Have the patient flex the toes against resistance.
Small muscles of the foot	Medial and lateral plantar	S1, S2	Have the patient cup the sole of the foot.
Tibialis anterior	Deep peroneal	L4, L5	Have the patient dorsiflex the foot against resistance.
Extensor digitorum longus	Deep peroneal	L5, S1	Have the patient dorsiflex the toes against resistance.
Extensor hallucis longus	Deep peroneal	L5, S1	Have the patient dorsiflex the distal phalanx of the big toe against resistance.
Extensor digitorum brevis	Deep peroneal	L5, S1	Have the patient dorsiflex the proximal phalanges of the toes against resistance.
Peroneus longus and brevis	Superficial peroneal	L5, S1	Have the patient evert the foot against resistance.

NB: The small head of the biceps femoris is the only muscle supplied by the peroneal division of the sciatic nerve proximal to the knee.

J. *Clinical syndromes of nerves in the lower limb*
1. *Lateral femoral cutaneous nerve:* arises from the lumbar plexus by fusion of the dorsal division of the ventral rami of L2 and L3; **meralgia paresthetica**: burning, numbness, tingling sensation over the anterolateral thigh; usually most intense in the distal half of the thigh, aggravated by standing, walking, relieved by sitting; etiology: intrapelvic—diverticulitis, uterine fibroid; extrapelvic at the anterior superior iliac spine—pressure by belts, girdles, backpacks; stretch by obesity, pregnancy, physical maneuvers (e.g., getting on bicycles)
2. *Femoral nerve:* arises from the lumbar plexus within the psoas muscle, formed by the posterior division of the ventral rami of L2–L4
   a. *Intrapelvic compression:* symptoms: pain in the inguinal region partially relieved by flexion and external rotation of the hip, dysesthesia over the anterior thigh and anteromedial leg; clinical: weakness of hip flexion and knee extension, impaired quadriceps reflex, sensory deficit in the cutaneous distribution of the femoral nerve, pain with hip extension; etiology: iliacus hematoma, tumor, extension of disease from the hip joint

NB: Psoas abscess may cause compression of the lumbar plexus, as well as hematoma in hemophiliac patients.

   b. *Compression in the inguinal region:* symptoms: similar to intrapelvic compression; clinical: same as intrapelvic compression except that there is no weakness of hip flexion; etiology: femoral lymphadenopathy, lithotomy position
3. *Saphenous nerve:* compression at the knee symptoms: history of prolonged external compression over the anteromedial aspect of the knee, numbness limited to the cutaneous distribution of the saphenous nerve; clinical: *no weakness or reflex changes;* etiology: horseback riding, pressure during sleep

NB: Saphenous nerve neuropathy causes exquisite pain in the distribution of the saphenous nerve.

4. *Obturator nerve:* symptoms: pain in the groin and along the medial aspect of the thigh, numb patch over the medial aspect of the thigh, worse with adduction and extension of the hip; clinical: *weakness of hip adduction,* impaired adductor reflex, patch of numbness over the medial aspect of the thigh; etiology: high retroperitoneal hemorrhage, surgical procedures (intra-and extrapelvic), tumor
5. *Superior gluteal nerve:* symptoms: pain in the upper gluteal region, limping gait; clinical: no sensory deficit or reflex changes, weakness of gluteus medius and tensor fascia lata; etiology: involvement at the sciatic notch (in conjunction with the sciatic nerve), post-traumatic entrapment
6. *Inferior gluteal nerve:* symptoms: pain in the posterior gluteal region, limping gait; clinical: no sensory or reflex changes, weakness of gluteus maximus; etiology: involvement at the sciatic notch, neoplasm
7. *Sciatic nerve:* originates from the ventral rami of L4–S3, leaves the pelvis through the sciatic notch; two trunks: *lateral trunk (forms the common peroneal nerve) and medial trunk (forms the tibial nerve)*
   a. *Intrapelvic involvement:* symptoms: pain in the posterior aspect of the thigh and leg, extending into the foot, numbness/paresthesia may be present along the sciatic cutaneous distribution, nocturnal pain prominent in tumor patients, may be associated with low back pain; etiology: tumors, intrapelvic surgical procedures, pyriformis syndrome

b. *Compromise at the notch:* symptoms: similar to intrapelvic involvement; clinical: findings predominate in the peroneal division, may present as a peroneal nerve injury, glutei and hamstrings may or may not be involved; etiology: injection palsy, compression during coma, tumor

c. *Focal involvement in the thigh:* symptoms: similar to intrapelvic and sciatic thigh lesions; etiology: tumors, entrapment by the myofascial band

8. *Peroneal nerve:* continuation of the lateral trunk of the sciatic nerve; separates from the sciatic nerve in the upper popliteal fossa, passes behind the fibular head, pierces the superficial head of peroneus longus muscle to reach the anterior compartment of the leg; *divides into: superficial and deep branch; in the popliteal fossa, gives rise to two sensory nerves: sural nerve and superficial peroneal nerve*

a. **Crossed-leg palsy:** involves the *common peroneal nerve* at the head of the fibula, or occasionally the deep or superficial branches individually near their origin; symptoms: footdrop, unstable ankle, paresthesias over anterolateral leg and dorsum of the foot; clinical: weakness of dorsiflexors and evertors of the foot, sensory deficit over the anterolateral leg and dorsum of the foot; etiology; external pressure over the head of the fibula (crossed legs, bed positioning, etc.), internal pressure (squatting), predisposing factors—dieting, peripheral neuropathy

NB: An L5 lesion will spare the evertors of the foot.

b. **Anterior compartment syndrome**: clinical: tenderness to palpation over the anterior compartment, pain with passive plantar flexion of the foot and flexion of the toes, weakness of the anterior compartment muscles (tibialis anterior, extensor hallucis longus, extensor digitorum longus), sensory deficit over the cutaneous distribution of the deep peroneal nerve; etiology: increased anterior compartment pressure due to bleeding, increased capillary permeability (trauma, postischemia), increased capillary pressure (exercise, venous obstruction)

NB: An area of sensory loss between the big and the 2nd toe may be the initial finding of an L5 lesion.

c. **Lateral compartment syndrome**: symptoms are the same as for the anterior compartment syndrome except that the pain is localized over the lateral aspect of the leg; pain with passive inversion of the foot, weakness of the peronei, sensory deficit over the cutaneous distribution of the superficial peroneal nerve

d. **Anterior tarsal tunnel syndrome**: symptoms: pain in the ankle and dorsum of the foot, dysesthesia in the distribution of the deep peroneal nerve, nocturnal exacerbation, walking provides partial relief; clinical: weakness of extensor digitorum brevis only, no reflex changes, hypesthesia in the cutaneous distribution of the deep peroneal nerve; etiology: edema, swelling due to ankle injuries, tight boots

NB: An accessory deep peroneal nerve may exist and innervate the extensor digitorum brevis, passing behind the lateral malleolus. It will manifest in NCS as a smaller compound motor action potential with stimulation of the deep peroneal nerve in the ankle when compared to stimulation at the knee.

9. *Tibial nerve:* continuation of the medial trunk of the sciatic nerve; from the ventral rami of L5–S2; innervates the posterior calf muscles; *branches into medial plantar nerve and lateral plantar nerve*

a. **Deep posterior compartment syndrome**: tenderness over the distal posteromedial leg; pain with passive foot dorsiflexion and toe extension; weakness of plantar flexion, inversion of the foot and flexion of the toes; plantar hypesthesia

b. **Tarsal tunnel syndrome**: symptoms: burning pain and paresthesias in toes and soles of the foot, aggravated by ambulation, nocturnal exacerbations; clinical: tenderness to palpation over the flexor retinaculum, sensory deficit over the distribution of the tibial nerve; etiology: compression within the flexor retinaculum at the ankle

10. *Digital nerve:* **Morton's neuroma**—metatarsal pain and pain in the toes, *typically the 3rd and 4th*, numbness in one or two toes; clinical: hypesthesia of apposing surfaces of two toes, palpation of the nerve across the deep transverse metatarsal ligament with passive hyperextension of the toes causes acute tenderness; etiology: fixed hyperextended M-P joint secondary to trauma or rheumatoid arthritis, high-heeled shoes, work-related stooping, interphalangeal fracture, barefoot running on a hard surface, shortened heel cord

III. Spinal Cord: an elongated, cylindrical mass of nerve tissue occupying the upper two-thirds of the adult spinal canal within the vertebral column; normally 42–45 cm long; *conus medullaris:* the conical distal end of the spinal cord; *filum terminale:* extends from the tip of the conus and attaches to the distal dural sac, it consists of pia and glial fibers and often contains a vein

A. *Segments and divisions:* divided into 30 segments—8 cervical, 12 thoracic, 5 lumbar, 5 sacral, and a few small coccygeal segments; cross sections show: a deep *anterior median fissure* (commonly contains a fold of pia and blood vessels; its floor is the anterior/ventral white commissure) and a shallow *posterior median sulcus;* the dorsal nerve roots are attached to the spinal cord along the *posterolateral sulcus;* the ventral nerve roots exit the spinal cord in the *anterolateral sulcus*

B. *Gray matter*

1. *Columns:* a cross section of the spinal cord shows an H-shaped internal mass of gray matter surrounded by white matter; made up of two symmetric portions joined across the midline by a transverse connection (commissure) of gray matter that contains the minute central canal or its remnants

   a. *Ventral (anterior) gray column:* contains the cells of origin of the fibers of the ventral roots

   b. *Intermediolateral gray column:* position of the gray matter between the dorsal and ventral gray columns; a prominent lateral triangular projection in the thoracic and upper lumbar regions but not in the midsacral regions; contains the preganglionic cells of the autonomic nervous system

   c. *The dorsal gray column:* reaches almost to the posterolateral sulcus; Lissauer's tract: dorsolateral fasciculus, compact bundle of small fibers as part of the pain pathway

2. *Laminas:* a cross section of the gray matter shows a number of laminas (layer of nerve cells), termed *Rexed laminas* after the neuroanatomist who described them

   a. *Lamina I:* thin marginal layer, contains neurons that respond to noxious stimuli and send axons to the contralateral spinothalamic tract

   b. *Lamina II:* substantia gelatinosa; small neurons, some respond to noxious stimuli; substance P is the neuropeptide involved in pathways mediating sensitivity to pain, which is found in high concentration in laminae I and II

   c. *Laminae III and IV:* nucleus proprius; main input is from fibers that convey position and light touch sense

   d. *Lamina V:* this layer contains cells that respond to both noxious and visceral afferent stimuli

   e. *Lamina VI:* the deepest layer of the dorsal horn and contains neurons that respond to the mechanical signals from joints and skin

   f. *Lamina VII:* a large zone that contains the cells of the dorsal nucleus of Clarke medially, as well as a large portion of the ventral gray column; Clarke's column contains cells that give rise to the posterior cerebellar tract; also contains the intermediolateral nucleus

g. *Laminae VIII and IX:* represent motor neuron groups in the medial and lateral portions of the ventral gray column; the medial portion contains the lower motor neurons (LMNs) that innervate the axial musculature; the lateral motor neuron column contains LMNs for the distal muscles of the arm and leg; in general, motor neurons for flexor muscles are located more centrally, whereas motor neurons for extensor muscles are located more peripherally

h. *Lamina X:* represents the small neurons around the central canal or its remnants

C. *White matter*

1. *Columns:* each lateral half of the spinal cord has white columns (funiculi)—dorsal (posterior), lateral, ventral (anterior); the dorsal column lies between the posterior median sulcus and the posterolateral sulcus (in the cervical region, it is divided into fasciculus gracilis and fasciculus cuneatus); the lateral column lies between the posterolateral sulcus and the anterolateral sulcus; the ventral column lies between the anterolateral sulcus and the anterior median fissure

2. *Tracts*

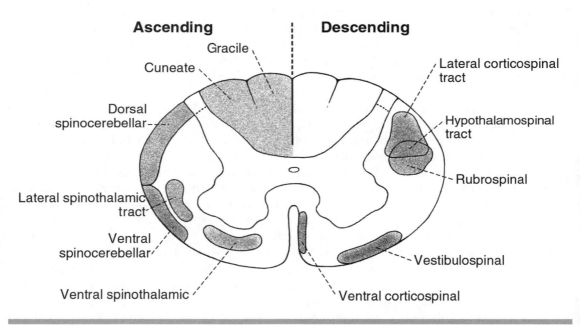

Figure 21-2. Cross section of the spinal cord highlighting the major ascending and descending tracts.

a. *Descending tracts in the spinal cord*

Tract	Origin	Termination	Location	Function
Pyramidal/ corticospinal	Motor and premotor cortex	Contralateral anterior horn cells (after crossing the pyramidal decussation at the medulla)	Lateral column	Fine motor function (distal musculature)

Tract	Origin	Termination	Location	Function
Anterior (ventral) corticospinal	Motor and premotor cortex	Descends uncrossed in the spinal cord then later decussates via anterior white commissure to the contralateral anterior horn neurons (interneurons and LMNs)	Anterior column	Gross and postural motor function (proximal and axial)
Lateral vestibulospinal	Lateral vestibular nucleus	Descend uncrossed to the anterior horn interneurons and motor neurons (for extensors)	Ventral column	Postural reflexes
Medial vestibulospinal	Medial vestibular nucleus	Descends crossed and uncrossed to the anterior horn interneurons and motor neurons	Ventral column	Postural reflexes
Rubrospinal	Red nucleus	Immediately crosses and terminates in contralateral ventral horn interneurons	Lateral column	Motor function
Medial reticulospinal	Pontine reticular formation	Descends uncrossed fibers to the ventral horn	Ventral column	Motor function (excitation of flexor and proximal trunk and axial motor neurons)
Lateral reticulospinal	Medullary reticular formation	Descends crossed and uncrossed to most of the ventral horn and the basal portion of the dorsal horn	Lateral column	Modulation of sensory transmission and spinal reflexes; excitation and inhibition of axial (neck and back) motor neurons
Descending autonomic	Hypothalamus, brain stem	Poorly defined fiber system projecting to the preganglionic autonomic fibers	Lateral columns	Modulation of autonomic functions
Tectospinal	Superior colliculus of the midbrain	Contralateral ventral horn interneurons	Ventral column	Reflex head turning
Medial longitudinal fasciculus (MLF)	Vestibular nuclei	Only up to the cervical gray	Ventral column	Coordination of head and eye movements

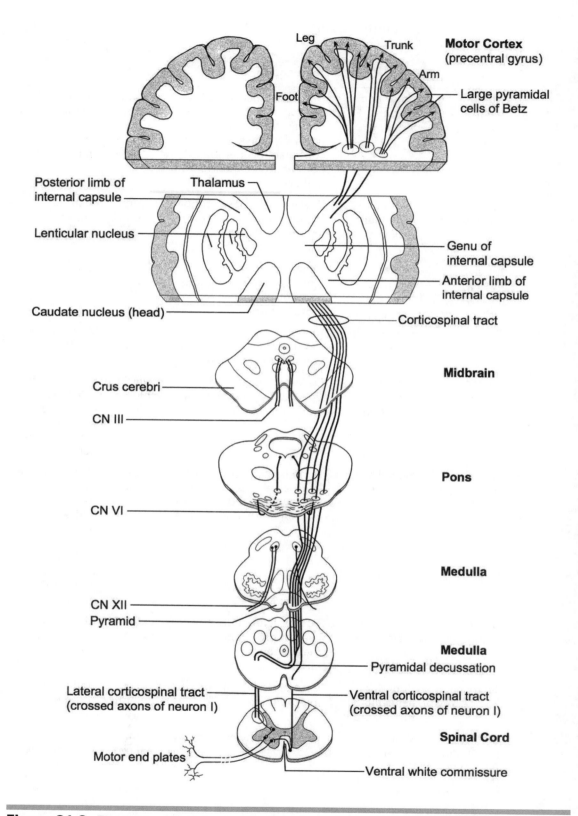

Figure 21-3. The route of the lateral corticospinal tract in the spinal cord from the motor and premotor cortex down to the contralateral anterior horn cells after crossing the pyramidal decussation at the medulla.

b. *Ascending tracts of the spinal cord*

Tract	Origin	Termination	Location	Function
Dorsal column system	Skin, joints, tendons	Dorsal column nuclei; 2nd-order neurons project to the contralateral thalamus (crossing at the lemniscal decussation in medulla)	Dorsal column	(Conscious) proprioception, fine touch, two-point discrimination
Spino-thalamic	Skin	Dorsal horn; 2nd- order neurons project to the contralateral thalamus (cross in the spinal cord close to the level of entry)	Ventrolateral column	Sharp pain, temperature, crude touch
Dorsal spinocere-bellar	Muscle spindles, Golgi tendon organs, touch and pressure receptors	Cerebellar paleocortex (via ipsilateral inferior cerebellar peduncle)	Lateral column	(Unconscious) proprioception-stereognosis
Ventral spinocere-bellar	Muscle spindles, Golgi tendon organs, touch and pressure receptors	Cerebellar paleocortex (via contralateral and some ipsilateral superior cerebellar peduncle)	Lateral column	(Unconscious) proprioception-stereognosis
Spino-reticular	Deep somatic structures	Ipsilateral reticular formation of the brain stem	Polysynaptic, diffuse in the ventrolateral column	Deep and chronic pain

NB: The dorsal and ventral spinocerebellar tracts are the most lateral tracts in the spinal cord and are most likely to be affected first from an extrinsic lateral insult.

D. *Spinal cord syndromes*
   1. *Small central lesion* (e.g., *syringomyelia*): affects the decussating fibers of the spinothalamic tract from both sides without affecting other ascending or descending fibers, producing dissociated sensory abnormalities with loss of pain and temperature sensibility in appropriate dermatomes but with preserved vibration and position sense
   2. *Large central lesion*: in addition to the pain and temperature pathways, portions of the adjacent tracts, gray matter, or both, are affected, producing LMN weakness in the segments involved, together with upper motor neuron (UMN) dysfunction, and occasionally with joint position and vibration sense loss below the lesion

NB: Central cord syndrome at the cervical levels produces LMN findings in the upper extremities, UMN findings in the lower extremities, and a disturbance of pain and temperature sensation noticeable in the upper extremities.

   3. *Dorsal column lesion* (e.g., *tabes dorsalis*): proprioception and vibratory sensation are involved, with other functions remaining normal

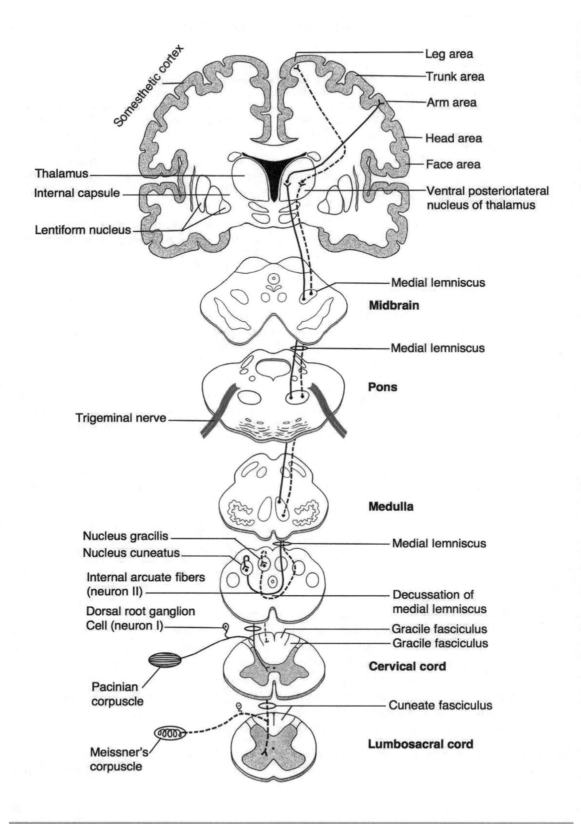

Figure 21-4. The route of the dorsal column system from the dorsal column nuclei to the contralateral thalamus to its termination in the sensory cortex.

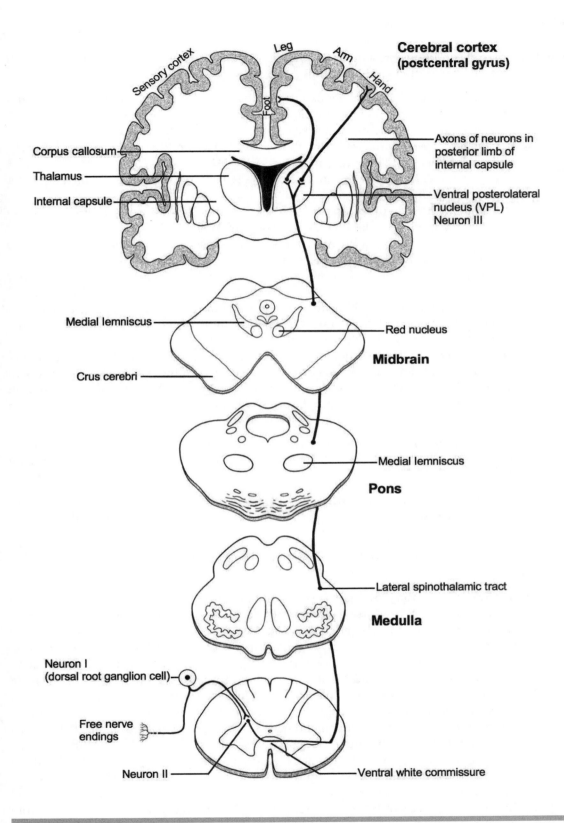

Figure 21-5. The route of the lateral spinothalamic tract from the nucleus in the dorsal horn through the contralateral thalamus to its termination in the sensory cortex.

NB: Examples of conditions presenting findings from dorsal column lesions include latent *Treponema pallidum* infection and vitamin B$_{12}$ deficienc

4. **Brown-Sequard syndrome**: hemisection of the spinal cord as a result of bullet or stab wound, syrinx, tumor, hematomyelia, etc.; signs:
   a. Ipsilateral LMN paralysis in the segment of the lesion (damage of the LMNs)
   b. Ipsilateral UMN paralysis below the level of the lesion (due to damage of the corticospinal tract)
   c. Ipsilateral cutaneous anesthesia in the segment of the lesion (damage of yet uncrossed afferent fibers)
   d. Ipsilateral loss of proprioceptive, vibratory, and two-point discrimination sense below the level of the lesions (damage of dorsal columns)
   e. Contralateral loss of pain and temperature sense below the lesion (damage of spinothalamic tracts that have already crossed)
5. **Posterolateral sclerosis** *(subacute combined degeneration or Friedreich's ataxia): deficiency of vitamin B$_{12}$ (cyanocobalamin) results in degeneration of dorsal and lateral columns;* loss of position sense, two-point discrimination and vibratory sensation; ataxic gait (damage to the spinocerebellar tracts), muscle weakness, hyperactive reflexes, spasticity of the extremities, and positive Babinski sign
6. **Spinal shock**: acute transection of or severe injury to the spinal cord from sudden loss of stimulation from higher levels or from overdose of spinal anesthetic; all body segments below the level of the injury become paralyzed and have no sensation; all reflexes (including autonomic) are suppressed; usually transient; may disappear in 3–6 weeks followed by a period of increased reflex response

NB: Autonomic dysreflexia may occur in patients with lesions at T5, T6, and above. Symptoms include diaphoresis, hypertension, tachycardia, etc. If not treated promptly, death may result.

7. *Combined UMN and LMN disease* (e.g., *amyotrophic lateral sclerosis*): damage to the corticospinal tracts with pyramidal signs and by damage to the LMNs with UMN signs; no sensory deficits

NB: The familial form of amyotrophic lateral sclerosis is secondary to a mutation of superoxide dismutase.

8. **Ventral spinal artery occlusion**: causes infarction of the anterior two-thirds of the spinal cord but spares dorsal columns and horns; damage to the following structures: lateral corticospinal tracts (bilateral spastic paresis with pyramidal signs below the lesion), lateral spinothalamic tracts (bilateral loss of pain and temperature sensation below the lesion), hypothalamospinal tract (at T2 and above, results in bilateral Horner's syndrome), ventral (anterior) horns (results in bilateral flaccid paralysis of the innervated muscles), corticospinal tracts to the sacral parasympathetic centers at S2–S4 (results in bilateral damage and loss of voluntary bladder and bowel control)
9. **Cauda equina syndrome**: for spinal roots L3 through coccygeal; results usually from a nerve root tumor (ependymomas, dermoid tumor, or from a lipomas of the terminal cord); clinical: severe radicular unilateral pain, sensory distribution in unilateral saddle-shaped area, unilateral muscle atrophy and absent quadriceps (L3) and ankle jerks (S1), incontinence and sexual functions are not marked, onset is often gradual and unilateral
10. **Conus medullaris syndrome**: for segments S3 through coccygeal; usually results from an intramedullary tumor, such as ependymomas; clinical: pain usually bilateral but not

severe, sensory distribution in bilateral saddle-shaped area, muscle changes are not marked, quadriceps and ankle reflexes are normal, incontinence and sexual functions are severely impaired, onset is often sudden and bilateral

NB: The collateral blood supply at the T5–T7 level of the SC is relatively tenuous making this area most susceptible to ischemia.

IV. Brain Stem, Cranial Nerves (CNs), and Special Systems: The brain stem includes the medulla, pons, and midbrain; extends from the pyramidal decussation to the posterior commissure; receives blood supply from the vertebrobasilar system; contains CNs III–XII, except the spinal part of XI.

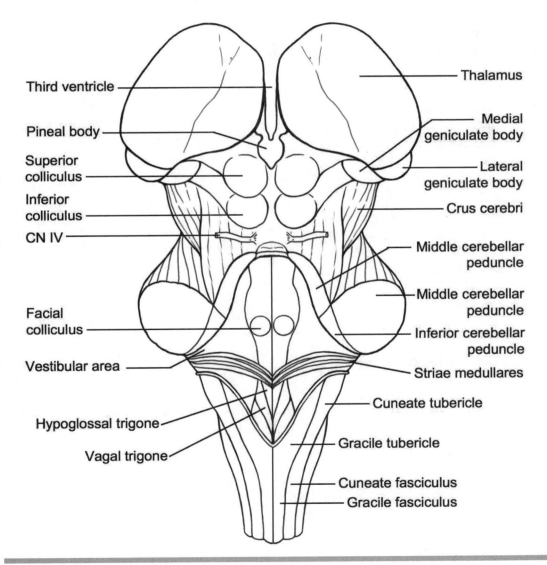

Figure 21-6(A). The dorsal view of the brain stem.

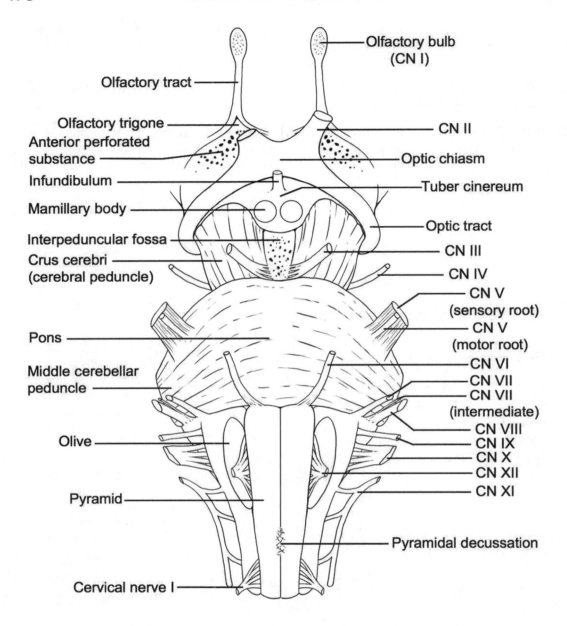

Figure 21-6(B). The ventral view of the brain stem.

A. *Trigeminal system:* provides sensory innervation to the face, oral cavity, and supratentorial dura (general somatic afferent [GSA] fibers); also innervates the muscles of mastication (special visceral efferent [SVE] fibers)

NB: A lesion in the facial nerve will not affect the muscles of mastication.

1. *Trigeminal ganglion: semilunar or gasserian;* contains pseudounipolar ganglion cells; three divisions:

a. *Ophthalmic nerve (V1):* lies in the wall of the cavernous sinus; enters *through the superior orbital fissure;* also mediates the afferent limb of the corneal reflex

b. *Maxillary nerve (V2):* lies in the wall of the cavernous sinus; exits the skull *through the foramen rotundum*

c. *Mandibular nerve (V3):* exits the skull *through the foramen ovale*

NB: V3 does not go through the cavernous sinus. It will be spared in a cavernous sinus thrombosis.

d. *Motor (SVE) component of CN V:* accompanies the mandibular nerve *through the foramen ovale;* innervates the muscles of mastication, mylohyoid, anterior belly of digastric, tensors tympani, and veli palatini; innervates the muscles of the jaw, the lateral and medial pterygoids

2. *Trigeminothalamic pathways*

   a. *Ventral trigeminothalamic tract:* mediates pain and temperature sensation from the face and oral cavity

      i. *First-order neurons:* located in the *trigeminal ganglion;* gives rise to axons that descend in the spinal trigeminal tract and synapse with second-order neurons in the spinal trigeminal nucleus

      ii. *Second-order neurons:* located in the *spinal trigeminal nucleus;* gives rise to the decussating axons that terminate in the contralateral ventral posteromedial (VPM) nucleus of the thalamus

      iii. *Third-order neurons:* located in the *VPM nucleus* of the thalamus; project through the posterior limb of the internal capsule to the face area of the somatosensory cortex (Brodmann's areas 3, 1, 2)

   b. *Dorsal trigeminothalamic tract:* mediates tactile discrimination and pressure sensation from the face and oral cavity; receives input from Meissner's and Pacini's corpuscles

      i. *First-order neurons:* located in the *trigeminal ganglion;* synapse in the principal sensory nucleus of CN V

      ii. *Second-order neurons:* located in the *principal sensory nucleus of CN V;* project to the ipsilateral VPM nucleus of the thalamus

      iii. *Third-order neurons:* located in the *VPM nucleus* of the thalamus; project through the posterior limb of the internal capsule to Brodmann's areas 3, 1, 2

3. *Trigeminal reflexes*

   a. *Corneal reflex:* consensual disynaptic reflex

   b. *Jaw-jerk reflex:* monosynaptic myotatic reflex

   c. *Tearing (lacrimal) reflex*

   d. *Oculocardiac reflex:* pressure of the globe results in bradycardia

4. *Cavernous sinus:* contains the following structures—*internal carotid artery (siphon), CN III, IV, V1, V2, and VI, postganglionic sympathetic fibers* (en route to the orbit)

B. **Auditory system:** an exteroceptive special somatic afferent (SSA) system that can *detect sound frequencies from 20 to 20,000 Hz;* derived from the otic vesicle, which is a derivative of the otic placode, a thickening of the surface ectoderm

1. *Auditory pathway:*

   a. *Hair cells of the organ of Corti:* innervated by the peripheral processes of bipolar cells of the spiral ganglion; stimulated by vibrations of the basilar membrane

      i. *Inner hair cells:* chief sensory elements; synapse with the dendrites of myelinated neurons whose axons comprise 90% of the cochlear nerve

      ii. *Outer hair cells:* synapse with the dendrites of unmyelinated neurons whose axons comprise 10% of the cochlear nerve; they reduce the threshold of the inner hair cells

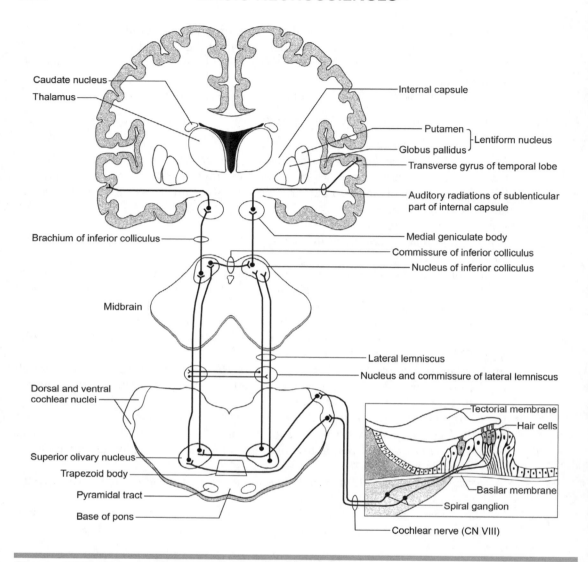

Figure 21-7. The auditory system from the cochlear nucleus—superior olivary nucleus—lateral lemniscus—inferior colliculus—medial geniculate body—to the primary auditory cortex.

b. *Bipolar cells of the spiral (cochlear) ganglion:* project peripherally to the hair cells of the organ of Corti; project centrally as the cochlear nerve to the cochlear nuclei
c. *Cochlear nerve (CN VIII):* extends from the spiral ganglion to the cerebellopontine angle, where it enters the brain stem
d. *Cochlear nuclei:* receive input from the cochlear nerve and project to the contralateral superior olivary nucleus and lateral lemniscus
e. *Superior olivary nucleus:* projects to the lateral lemniscus; plays a role in sound localization; **NB:** the trapezoid body, located in the pons, contains decussating fibers from the ventral cochlear nuclei
f. *Lateral lemniscus:* receives input from the contralateral cochlear nuclei and superior olivary nuclei
g. *Nucleus of the inferior colliculus:* receives input from the lateral lemniscus and projects through the brachium of the inferior colliculus to the medial geniculate body

h. *Medial geniculate body:* projects through the internal capsule as the auditory radiation to the primary auditory cortex (transverse temporal gyri of Heschl-Brodmann's areas 41, 42)

2. *Tuning fork tests*
   a. *Weber's test:* place a vibrating tuning fork on the vertex of the skull; the patient should hear equally on both sides
      i. Unilateral conduction deafness: hears the vibration more loudly in the affected ear
      ii. Unilateral partial nerve deafness: hears the vibration more loudly in the normal ear
   b. *Rinne test:* compares air and bone conduction; place a vibrating tuning fork on the mastoid until the vibration is no longer heard, then hold the tuning fork in front of the ear; the patient should hear the vibration in air after bone conduction is gone
      i. *Unilateral conduction deafness:* patient does not hear the vibration in air after bone conduction is gone
      ii. *Unilateral partial nerve deafness:* patient hears the vibration in the air after bone conduction is gone

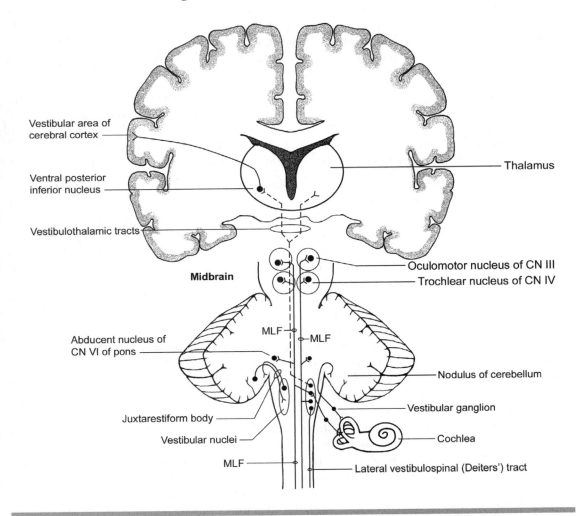

Figure 21-8. The vestibular system from the semicircular ducts, utricle, and saccule and cerebellar projections to the vestibular nuclei to its various projections to the cerebellum, CN III, IV and VI, spinal cord, and ventral posteroinferior and posterolateral nuclei of the thalamus.

C. **Vestibular system:** also derived from the otic vesicle; maintains posture and equilibrium and coordinates head and eye movements

    1. The *labyrinth*

       a. *Three semicircular ducts (superior, lateral, and posterior)* lie within the three semicircular canals; ducts *respond to angular acceleration and deceleration* of the head; contain hair cells in the crista ampullaris; hair cells respond to endolymph flow

       b. *Utricle and saccule:* respond to the position of the head with respect to *linear acceleration and pull of gravity;* also contain hair cells whose cilia are embedded in the otolithic membrane

    2. *Vestibular pathways*

       a. *Hair cells of the semicircular ducts, saccule, and utricle are innervated by the peripheral processes of bipolar cells* of the vestibular ganglion

       b. *Vestibular ganglion:* located on the fundus of the internal auditory meatus; project their central processes as the vestibular nerve to the vestibular nuclei and to the flocculonodular lobe of the cerebellum

       c. *Vestibular nuclei:* receive input from semicircular ducts, saccule, utricle, flocculonodular lobe of the cerebellum; projects to flocculonodular lobe of the cerebellum, CN III, IV, VI (through MLF), spinal cord (through the lateral vestibule spinal tract) and ventral posteroinferior and posterolateral nuclei of the thalamus (which project to the postcentral gyrus)

NB: Cold water irrigation of the external auditory meatus (stimulation of the horizontal ducts) results in nystagmus to the opposite side; in unconscious patients, no nystagmus is observed; with intact brain stem, deviation of the eyes to the side of the cold irrigation is seen; with bilateral MLF transection, deviation of the abducting eye to the side of the cold irrigation is observed; with lower brain stem damage to the vestibular nuclei, no deviation of the eyes.

D. *Visual system:* served by the optic nerve (SSA nerve)

    1. *Visual pathway:* human retina contains *two types of photoreceptors: rods (mediate light perception, provide low visual acuity, used chiefly in nocturnal vision, contain rhodopsin pigment) and cones (mediate color vision, provide high visual acuity, contain iodopsin pigment);* the *fovea centralis* within the macula is a specialized region in the retina adapted for high *visual acuity and contains only cones;* the pathway includes the following structures:

       a. *Ganglion cells* of the retina: form the optic nerve (CN II); project from the nasal hemiretina to the contralateral lateral geniculate body and from the temporal hemiretina to the ipsilateral geniculate body

       b. *Optic nerve:* projects from the lamina cribrosa of the scleral canal, through the optic canal, to the optic chiasm; transection causes ipsilateral blindness, with no direct pupillary light reflex; **NB:** a section of the optic nerve at the optic chiasm transects all fibers from the ipsilateral retina as well as fibers from the contralateral inferior nasal quadrant that loop into the optic nerve (fibers of von Willebrand's knee)—a lesion, therefore, causes ipsilateral blindness plus contralateral upper temporal quadrant defect (junction scotoma)

       c. *Optic chiasm:* contains the decussating fibers from the two nasal hemiretinas and noncrossing fibers from the two temporal hemiretinas and projects to the suprachiasmatic nucleus of the hypothalamus; midsagittal transection or pressure (e.g., pituitary tumor) causes bitemporal hemianopia; bilateral lateral compression (e.g., calcified internal carotid artery) causes binasal hemianopia

d. *Optic tract:* contains fibers from the ipsilateral temporal hemiretina and contralateral nasal hemiretina; projects to the ipsilateral lateral geniculate body, pretectal nuclei, and superior colliculus; transection causes hemianopia

e. *Lateral geniculate body:* Six-layer nucleus; *layers 1, 4, and 6 receive crossed fibers; layers 2, 3, and 5 receive uncrossed fibers;* projects through the geniculocalcarine tract to layer IV of Brodmann's area 17

f. *Geniculocalcarine tract (optic radiation):* projects through two divisions to the visual cortex

    i. *Upper division:* projects to the upper bank of the calcarine sulcus, the *cuneus;* contains input from the superior retinal quadrants, representing inferior visual field quadrants; transection causes contralateral lower quadrantanopia; lesions that involve both cunei *cause a lower altitudinal hemianopia (altitudinopia)*

    ii. *Lower division:* loops from the lateral geniculate body anteriorly (Meyer's loop), then posteriorly, to terminate in the lower bank of the calcarine sulcus, the *lingual gyrus;* contains input from the inferior retinal quadrants representing the superior visual field quadrants; transection causes contralateral upper quadrantanopia ("pie in the sky"); transection of both lingual gyri *causes an upper altitudinal hemianopia*

g. *Visual cortex (Brodmann's area 17)* is located on the banks of the calcarine fissure: cuneus (upper bank) and lingual gyrus (lower bank); lesions cause contralateral hemianopia with macular sparing

2. *Pupillary light reflex pathway:* has an *afferent limb (CN II) and efferent limb (CN III);* the ganglion cells of the retina project bilaterally to the pretectal nuclei—which projects crossed and uncrossed fibers to the *Edinger-Westphal nucleus,* which gives rise to the preganglionic parasympathetic fibers; these fibers exit the midbrain with CN III and synapse with postganglionic parasympathetic neurons of the ciliary ganglion, which innervates the sphincter muscle of the iris

3. *Pupillary dilatation pathway:* mediated by the *sympathetic division* of the autonomic nervous system; interruption at any level causes *Horner's syndrome* (miosis, anhydrosis, ptosis); includes the following structures: hypothalamic neurons of the paraventricular nucleus project directly to the ciliospinal center (T1–T2) of the intermediolateral cell column of the spinal cord, which projects preganglionic sympathetic fibers through the sympathetic trunk to the superior cervical ganglion, which projects postganglionic sympathetic fibers through the perivascular plexus of the carotid system to the dilator muscle of the iris

NB: The pupil in Horner's syndrome is reactive to light.

    a. **Argyll-Robertson pupil**: pupillary light-near dissociation—the absence of a miotic reaction to light, both direct and consensual, with the preservation of a miotic reaction to near stimulus (accommodation-convergence); occurs in syphilis and diabetes

NB: This pupil is typically small, irregular, and fixed to light.

    b. **Relative afferent (Marcus Gunn) pupil**: results from lesion of the optic nerve, the afferent limb of the pupillary light reflex; diagnosis can be made with the swinging flashlight test

NB: When the affected eye is stimulated, the reaction is slower, incomplete, and it may start dilating while still illuminated.

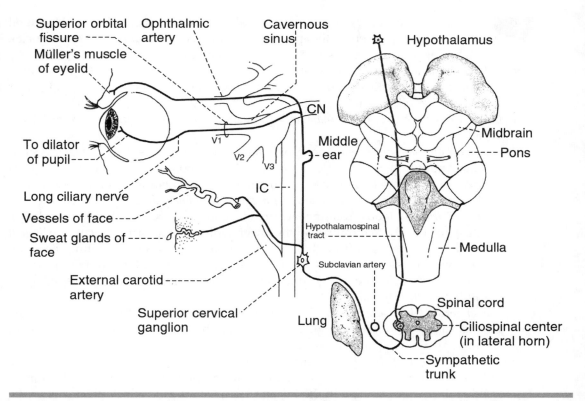

Figure 21-9. The course of the oculosympathetic pathway, where any interruption of this pathway results in Horner's syndrome. Hypothalamic fibers project to the ipsilateral ciliospinal center of the intermediolateral cell column at T1, which then projects preganglionic sympathetic fibers to the superior cervical ganglion. The superior cervical ganglion projects postganglionic sympathetic fibers through the tympanic cavity, cavernous sinus, and superior orbital fissure. CN, cranial nerve; IC, internal carotid.

    c. **Adie's pupil**: a large tonic pupil that reacts slowly to light but shows a more definite response to accommodation (light-near dissociation); frequently seen in females with absent knee or ankle jerks and impaired sweating

NB: Adie's pupil is caused by degeneration of the nerve cells in the ciliary ganglion.

    4. *Near reflex and accommodation pathway:* the cortical visual pathway projects from the primary visual cortex (Brodmann's area 17) to the visual association cortex (Brodmann's area 19), which projects through the corticotectal tract to the superior colliculus and pretectal nucleus, which project to the oculomotor complex of the midbrain; the oculomotor complex includes the following structures:
      a. *Rostral-Edinger-Westphal nucleus:* mediates pupillary constriction through the ciliary ganglion
      b. *Caudal-Edinger-Westphal nucleus:* mediates contraction of the ciliary muscle to increase the refractive power of the lens
      c. *Medial rectus subnucleus of CN III:* mediates convergence
    5. *Cortical and subcortical centers for ocular motility*

a. *Frontal eye field:* located on the posterior part of the middle frontal gyrus (Brodmann's area 8); regulates voluntary (saccadic) eye movements; stimulation causes contralateral deviation of the eyes (i.e., away from the lesion), and destruction causes transient ipsilateral conjugate deviation of the eyes (i.e., toward the lesion)

NB: This means that in a patient with a vascular lesion, the eyes deviate to the side of the lesion, whereas a patient seizing has deviation of the eyes opposite the lesion.

b. *Occipital eye fields:* located in Brodmann's areas 18 and 19; controls involuntary (smooth) pursuit and tracking movements; stimulation causes contralateral conjugate deviation of the eyes

c. *Subcortical center for lateral gaze:* located in the abducens nucleus of the pons (?paramedian pontine reticular formation)

    i. **MLF syndrome or internuclear ophthalmoplegia**: damage to the MLF between the abducens and oculomotor nuclei, causes medial rectus palsy in the adducting eye on the attempted lateral conjugate gaze and monocular horizontal nystagmus in the adducting eye (convergence is normal)

    ii. **One-and-a-half syndrome**: bilateral lesions of the MLF and unilateral lesion of the abducens nucleus; on attempted lateral gaze, the only muscle that functions is the intact lateral rectus

d. *Subcortical center for vertical gaze:* located in the midbrain at the level of the posterior commissure; called the *rostral interstitial nucleus* of the MLF; associated with **Parinaud syndrome** (*paralysis of upward gaze and convergence*)

NB: Parinaud syndrome can result from a pineal gland tumor.

E. **Functional components of the CNs**
1. *General afferent fibers:* have their cells of origin in the cranial and spinal dorsal root ganglia
   a. *GSA fibers:* carry exteroceptive (pain, temperature, and touch) and proprioceptive impulses from sensory endings in the *body wall, tendons, and joints*
   b. *General visceral afferent (GVA) fibers:* carry sensory impulses from the *visceral structures* (hollow organs and glands) within the thoracic, abdominal, and pelvic cavities
2. *Special afferent fibers:* found only in certain CNs
   a. *SSA nerves carry sensory impulses from the special sense organs in the *eye and ear* (vision, hearing, and equilibrium)
   b. *Special visceral afferent (SVA) fibers:* carry information from the *olfactory and gustatory receptors;* designated as visceral because of the functional association with the digestive tract
3. *General efferent fibers:* arise in cells in the spinal cord, brain stem, and autonomic ganglia; innervate all musculature of the body except the branchiomeric muscles
   a. *General somatic efferent (GSE) fibers:* convey motor impulses to *somatic skeletal muscles;* in the head, the somatic musculature is that of the tongue and the extraocular muscles
   b. *General visceral efferent (GVE) fibers:* autonomic axons that innervate *smooth and cardiac muscle fibers and regulate glandular secretion;* sympathetic or parasympathetic
4. *Special efferent fibers:* innervate the skeletal musculature of *branchiomeric origin;* SVE fibers: innervate striated muscles of the jaw, facial expression, pharynx, and larynx; they are not part of the autonomic nervous system

CN	General afferent	Special afferent	General efferent	Special efferent
I		*SVA:* olfactory nerve; consists of unmyelinated axons of bipolar neurons		
II		*SSA:* optic nerve; not a true nerve, rather an evaginated fiber tract of the diencephalon		
III			*GSE:* oculomotor nucleus—innervates ipsilateral inferior rectus, inferior oblique, medial rectus, contralateral superior rectus, and bilateral levators (most medial subnuclei)	
			GVE: Edinger-Westphal nucleus—constricts the pupil and participates in light accommodation reflex	
IV			*GSE:* trochlear nucleus—innervates the superior oblique of the contralateral eye	
V	*GSA:* trigeminal ganglion—sensory innervation of the face, dura of the anterior and middle cranial fossae; *mesencephalic nucleus*—proprioceptive fibers from the muscles of mastication and muscles innervated by the mandibular nerve			*SVE:* motor nucleus of V—innervates muscles of mastication

CN	General afferent	Special afferent	General efferent	Special efferent
VI			*GSE:* abducens nucleus—innervates the lateral rectus	
VII	*GSA:* geniculate ganglion—conveys pain and temperature from the external auditory meatus and skin of the ear region *GVA:* geniculate ganglion—innervates the soft palate and adjacent pharynx	*SVA:* geniculate ganglion—innervates taste buds of the anterior two-thirds of the tongue by way of the chorda tympani and lingual nerves; terminates in the nucleus solitarius	*GVE:* superior salivatory nucleus—preganglionic parasympathetic neurons that innervate the lacrimal, submandibular, sublingual glands	*SVE:* facial nucleus—loops around the abducens nucleus, exits the brain stem, and enters the internal auditory meatus, traverses facial canal and exits through the stylomastoid foramen; innervates muscles of facial expression, stylohyoid muscle, posterior belly of digastric and stapedius muscle
VIII		*SSA: spiral ganglion*—bipolar cells receive stimuli from hair cells in cochlear duct and terminate in dorsal and ventral cochlear nuclei; *vestibular ganglion*—bipolar cells receive stimuli from hair cells in the maculae and cristae and terminate in four vestibular nuclei		
IX	*GSA:* superior ganglion of IX—conveys pain and temperature from the external auditory meatus of the ear	*SVA:* inferior ganglion—carries gustatory sensation from the posterior third of the tongue	*GVE:* inferior salivatory nucleus—preganglionic parasympathetic fibers that innervate the parotid gland	*SVE:* nucleus ambiguus of the medulla—innervates the stylopharyngeus muscle

CN	General afferent	Special afferent	General efferent	Special efferent
	GVA: inferior petrosal ganglion—carries general sensory input from posterior 3rd of the tongue, upper pharynx, tonsils, tympanic cavity, auditory tube and terminate in nucleus solitarius; also innervates the carotid sinus (baroreceptors) and carotid body (chemoreceptors)			
X	*GSA:* superior (jugular) ganglion—conveys pain and temperature from the skin in the ear region and terminates in the spinal nucleus of V *GVA:* inferior (nodose) ganglion—conveys general sensations from the pharynx, larynx, thoracic and abdominal viscera and terminates in nucleus solitarius	*SVA:* inferior ganglion—receives gustatory sensation from epiglottal taste buds and ends in the nucleus solitarius	*GVE:* dorsal motor nucleus of X—preganglionic parasympathetic fibers, innervates the viscera of the neck and thoracic (heart) and abdominal cavities as far as the left colic flexure	*SVE:* nucleus ambiguus—provides efferent limb of the gag reflex, innervates the pharyngeal arch muscles of larynx, pharynx, striated muscles of the upper esophagus, uvula, levator palatini, and palatoglossus muscles

CN	General afferent	Special afferent	General efferent	Special efferent
XI				*SVE:* cranial division—arises from the nucleus ambiguus and innervates the intrinsic muscles of the larynx, exits through the jugular foramen; spinal division—ventral horn of C1–C6 and innervates sternocleidomastoid and trapezius
XII			*GSE:* hypoglossal nucleus—mediates tongue movement, exits skull through the hypoglossal canal	

V. Cerebellum: Three primary functions: maintenance of posture, maintenance of muscle tone, and coordination of voluntary motor activity.

A. *Cerebellar peduncles*
1. *Superior cerebellar peduncle:* brachium conjunctivum
   a. *Afferent tract:* ventral spinocerebellar portion of the rostral spinocerebellar tract, and trigeminocerebellar projections
   b. *Efferent tract:* dentatothalamic tract—terminates in the ventral lateral nucleus of the thalamus; also rubral and reticular projections arise from the dentate and interposed nuclei

NB: Lesion in this tract results in palatal tremor.

2. *Middle cerebellar peduncle:* brachium pontis
   a. Afferent tract: pontocerebellar fibers—crossed fibers from the pontine nuclei that project to the neocerebellum
3. *Inferior cerebellar peduncle:* restiform body
   a. *Afferent tracts*
      i. Dorsal spinocerebellar
      ii. Cuneocerebellar
      iii. Olivocerebellar (from the contralateral olivary nucleus)
      iv. Others: fibers from the vestibular nerve and nuclei, reticulocerebellar fibers, some fibers from the rostral spinocerebellar

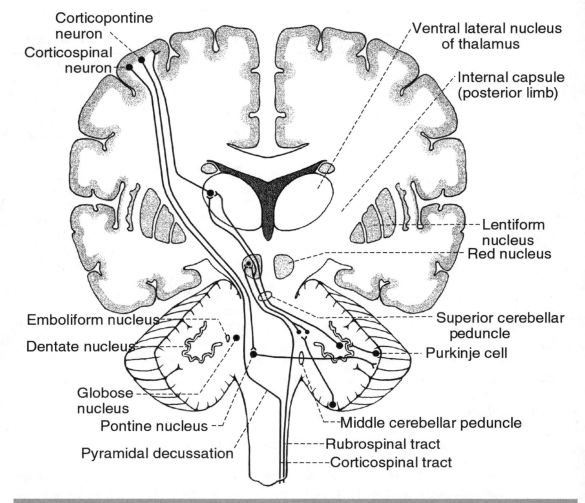

Figure 21-10. Coronal section of the brain and brain stem showing the cerebellar tracts, nuclei, and connections.

B. *Cerebellar cortex, neurons, and fibers*
  1. *Cortex:* has three layers
     a. *Molecular layer:* outer layer underlying the pia; contains stellate cells, basket cells, and dentritic arbor of the Purkinje cells
     b. *Purkinje cell layer:* lies between the molecular and granule cell layers
     c. *Granule layer:* inner layer overlying the white matter; contains granule cells, Golgi cells, and cerebellar glomeruli (which consists of a mossy fiber rosette, granule cell dendrites, and a Golgi cell axon)
  2. *Neurons and fibers of the cerebellum*
     a. *Purkinje cells:* convey the *only output* from the cerebellar cortex; project inhibitory output (γ-aminobutyric acid [*GABA*]) to the cerebellar and vestibular nuclei;

excited by parallel and climbing fibers and inhibited by GABA-ergic basket and stellate cells

b. *Granule cells: excite (by way of glutamate)* Purkinje, basket, stellate, and Golgi cells through parallel fibers; excited by mossy fibers and inhibited by Golgi cells

c. *Parallel fibers:* axons of granule cells; extend into the molecular layer

d. *Mossy fibers:* the afferent excitatory fibers of the spinocerebellar, pontocerebellar, and vestibulocerebellar tracts; terminate as mossy fiber rosettes on granule cell dendrites; excite granule cells

e. *Climbing fibers:* the *afferent excitatory (by way of aspartate)* fibers of the olivocerebellar tract; arise from the contralateral inferior olivary nucleus and terminate on neurons of the cerebellar nuclei and dendrites of Purkinje cells

NB: The major cerebellar pathway: Purkinje cells of the cerebellar cortex project to the dentate nucleus (also emboliform, globose, and fastigial nuclei)—dentate nucleus gives rise to the dentatothalamic tract, which projects (through the superior cerebellar peduncle) to the contralateral ventral lateral thalamus, which projects to the ipsilateral primary motor cortex (Brodmann's area 4), which projects ipsilaterally as the corticopontine tract to the pons; the pontine nuclei then project as the pontocerebellar tract (through the middle cerebellar peduncle) to the contralateral cerebellar cortex, where they terminate as mossy fibers.

VI. Thalamus, Hypothalamus, and Basal Ganglia

A. *Thalamus:* the largest division of the diencephalon; *divided into three unequal parts by the internal medullary lamina;* the centromedian nucleus and other intralaminar nuclei are enclosed within the internal medullary lamina in the center of the thalamus

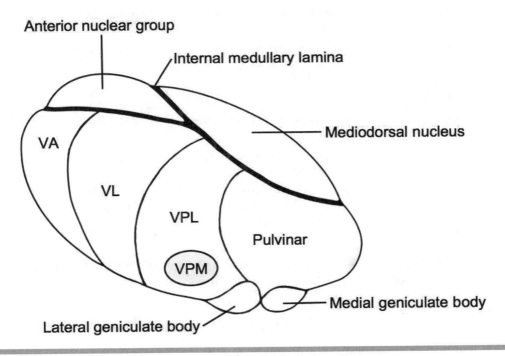

Figure 21-11. Schematic diagram of the thalamus and its various nuclei.

1. **NB**: *Major thalamic nuclei and their connections*

Nuclei	Input	Projection
Anterior	Mamillary nucleus of the hypothalamus	Cingulate gyrus
Dorsomedial	Prefrontal cortex (parvocellular part)	Prefrontal cortex (parvocellular)
	Amygdala, substantia nigra, orbital portion of the frontal lobe (magnocellular)	Many interconnections with other thalamic nuclei
Centromedian	Globus pallidus	Striatum (caudate and putamen) and to the entire neocortex
Pulvinar	Connects reciprocally with large association areas of the parietal, temporal, and occipital lobes; receives input from the superior colliculus, retina, cerebellum, and other thalamic nuclei	Connects reciprocally with large association areas of the parietal, temporal, and occipital lobes
Ventral tier		
Ventral anterior	Globus pallidus and substantia nigra	Prefrontal, orbital, and premotor cortex
NB: Ventral lateral	Cerebellum, globus pallidus, substantia nigra	Motor and supplementary motor cortex
Ventral posterior		
Ventroposterolateral	Spinothalamic tracts and medial lemniscus	Sensory cortex
Ventroposteromedial	Trigeminothalamic tracts, nucleus solitarius (via central tegmental tract)	Sensory cortex
Metathalamus		
Lateral geniculate body	Retinal input (via optic tract)	Visual cortex
Medial geniculate body	Auditory input (brachium of the inferior colliculus)	Primary auditory cortex
Reticular nucleus	Excitatory collateral input from corticothalamic and thalamocortical fibers	Inhibitory fibers to the thalamic nuclei

NB: The dorsomedial nucleus is the most implicated in the amnestic confabulation in Korsakoff's syndrome as it receives input from limbic structures and projects diffusely to the frontal cortex.

NB: Sleep spindles are generated in the reticular nucleus of the thalamus.

NB: Pulvinar is associated with visual attention.

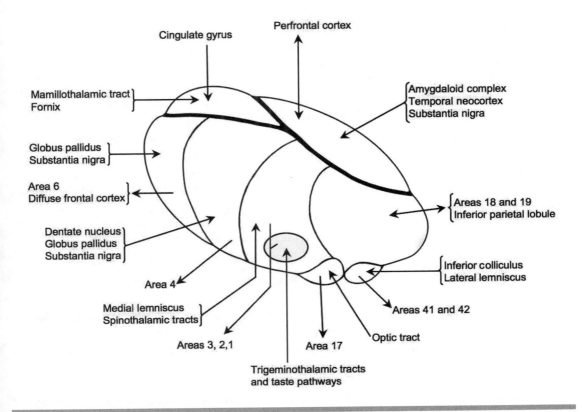

Figure 21-12. The projections of the major thalamic nuclei.

NB: Lesions in the anterior group are more likely to manifest with amnesia, confabulation, anomia, and preserved visual function. Lesions in the paramedian area can manifest with decreased consciousness followed by vertical gaze paresis, disinhibition, and occasionally amnesia.

   2. *Blood supply:* Three arteries
     a. Posterior communicating artery
     b. Posterior cerebral artery
     c. Anterior choroidal artery (to the lateral geniculate body)
   3. *Epithalamus:* the most dorsal division of the diencephalon
     a. *Pineal body:* the dorsal diverticulum of the diencephalon; cone-shaped structure that overlies the tectum; no neurons are present
     b. *Habenular nuclei:* located in the dorsal margin of the base of the pineal body; afferent fibers (via habenulopeduncular tract and stria medullaris): from septal area, lateral hypothalamus, brain stem, interpeduncular nuclei, raphe nuclei, ventral tegmental area; efferent fibers (via habenulopeduncular tract) terminate in the interpeduncular nucleus
     c. *Habenular commissure:* consists of stria medullaris fibers crossing over to the contralateral habenular nuclei
     d. *Posterior commissure:* located ventral to the base of the pineal body; carries decussating fibers of superior colliculi and pretectum (visual reflex fibers)

B. *Hypothalamus:* subserves three systems: autonomic, endocrine, and limbic
   1. *Hypothalamic nuclei and their functions*

Nucleus	Function
Medial preoptic	Regulates the release of gonadotropic hormones from the adenohypophysis; contains sexually dimorphic nucleus, which depends on testosterone levels for development
Suprachiasmatic	Receives direct input from the retina; role in regulation of circadian rhythms
Anterior	Role in temperature regulation; stimulates the parasympathetic nervous system; destruction results in hyperthermia
Paraventricular	Synthesizes the antidiuretic hormone, oxytocin, and corticotropin-releasing hormone; regulates water conservation; destruction results in diabetes insipidus
Supraoptic	Synthesizes antidiuretic hormone and oxytocin
Dorsomedial	In animals, savage behavior results when this nucleus is stimulated
Ventromedial	Satiety center; when stimulated, inhibits the urge to eat; destruction results in hyperphagia
Arcuate (infundibular)	Gives rise to tuberohypophysial tract; contains neurons that produce dopamine ([DA] i.e., prolactin-inhibiting factor)
Mamillary	Receives input from the hippocampal formation through the postcommissural fornix; projects to the anterior nucleus of the thalamus through the mamillothalamic tract; associated with Wernicke's encephalopathy and alcoholism
Posterior hypothalamic	Role in heat conservation and production of heat; lesions result in poikilothermia (inability to thermoregulate)
Lateral hypothalamic	Induces eating when stimulated; lesions cause anorexia and starvation

NB: The paraventricular nucleus provides the bulk of the direct innervation of the preganglionic sympathetic neurons.

NB: The posterior lateral hypothalamus contains the hypocretin/orexin neurons that have a function in preventing abrupt transitions from wakefulness to sleep. They project to cholinergic and monoaminergic neurons in brain stem and ventrolateral preoptic neurons. Narcolepsy results from impaired activity of these neurons.

   2. *Circuit of Papez: hippocampal formation—to the mamillary body (and septal area) through the fornix—to the anterior thalamic nucleus (through the mamillothalamic tract)—to the cingulate gyrus (passing through the anterior limb of the internal capsule)—to the entorhinal cortex (through the cingulum)—back to the hippocampal formation (through the perforant pathway)*

NB: During transcallosal surgery to remove a colloid cyst in the 3rd ventricle, the fornix can be damaged which interrupts Papez's circuit and results in loss of the ability to form new memories.

NB: *Akinetic mutism* may result from lesions in the anterior cingulate gyrus or a disconnection of the limbic connections projecting from the anterior cingulate through subcortical circuits.

    3. *Other limbic connections*
        a. *Stria terminalis:* from the amygdala—follows curvature to the tail of the caudate nucleus—to the septal nuclei and anterior hypothalamus
        b. *Stria medullaris:* from septal nuclei and anterior hypothalamus—to habenular nucleus
        c. *Mamillotegmental tract:* mamillary bodies—raphe nuclei of the midbrain reticular formation
        d. *Medial forebrain bundle:* septal area and amygdala—to the raphe nuclei of the midbrain reticular formation
  C. ***Basal ganglia:*** function is to control and regulate activities of the motor and premotor cortical areas so that voluntary movements can be performed smoothly; consists of five subcortical nuclei
    1. *Caudate:* derived from the telencephalon; three parts: head, body, and tail (ending near the amygdala); along with the putamen, is the major input nuclei of the basal ganglia (i.e., receives most of the input from the cerebral cortex); caudate + putamen = striatum; major neurotransmitter: GABA (inhibitory)

NB: The recurrent artery of Heubner, a branch of the anterior cerebral artery, supplies the anteromedial part of the head of the caudate nucleus, adjacent parts of the internal capsul and putamen, and parts of the septal nuclei.

    2. *Putamen:* derived from the telencephalon; means "shell"; putamen + globus pallidus = lentiform nucleus
    3. *Globus pallidus:* derived from the diencephalon; histologically resembles substantia nigra pars reticulata (SNr) and, along with it, serves as the major output nuclei of the basal ganglia; two divisions: globus pallidus interna (GPi) and externa (GPe); neurotransmitter: major GABA (inhibitory)

NB: The caudate and the putamen serve as the primary input nuclei for the basal ganglia while the globus pallidus, which projects to the ventral anterior nucleus of the thalamus, is the primary output nucleus.

    4. *Substantia nigra:* derived from the diencephalon; means "black substance"; lies in the midbrain and composed of two zones: SNr (pale, GABA-ergic) and substantia nigra pars compacta ([SNc] dark, composed of dopaminergic neurons)
    5. *Subthalamic nucleus:* derived from the diencephalon; involved in the indirect pathway; major neurotransmitter: *glutamate (excitatory)*

NB: The subthalamic nucleus receives inhibitory input from the external part of the globus pallidus and sends excitatory input to the GPi.

NB: The claustrum and amygdala are now part of the limbic system instead of the basal ganglia. The amygdala is associated with emotional memory.

    6. *Basal ganglia connections*
        a. *Direct pathway*
            i. In the *normal state*, DA levels are relatively constant; this produces an output (neurotransmitter release/GABA) from the striatum that is inhibitory in nature (and can be thought of as braking signal to the GPi and SNr); these two populations of neurons (GPi and SNr) also produce an output to the thalamus that is also inhibitory (GABA); so, in effect, the greater the inhibitory signal is to the GPi and SNr, the smaller the inhibitory signal is to the thalamus (braking the brake); the output from

the thalamus (to the motor areas of the brain) is excitatory (so by increasing the braking signal from the striatum to the GPi and SNr, the braking signal to the thalamus is diminished and the excitatory output from the thalamus is increased)

ii. *With Parkinson's disease (PD),* there is a progressive loss of the DA cells (in the SNc); with the diminished DA signal, the output from the striatum (remember, it is inhibitory or a brake signal) is diminished and, in turn, will release the GPi and SNr from inhibition, allowing a larger inhibitory or braking signal to be sent to the thalamus (so by unbraking a brake, the thalamus sends a smaller excitatory signal, which is consistent with the bradykinesia seen in PD)

NB: GABA is inhibitory, and glutamate is excitatory.

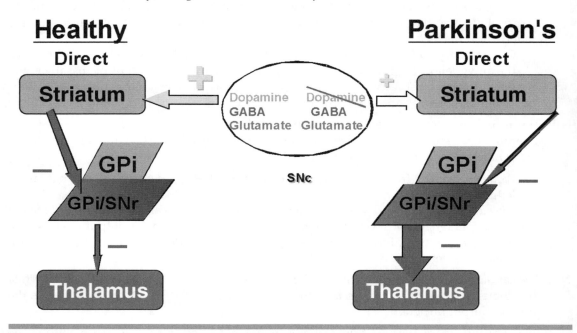

Figure 21-13. Schematic diagram of the direct pathway of the basal ganglia.

b. *Indirect pathway:* DA stimulates the DA receptors in the striatum (as discussed for the *direct pathway*); this courses through a series of inhibitory and excitatory nuclei (GPe, subthalamic nucleus, GPi/SNr) and results in the final inhibitory signal to the thalamus; *output of the globus pallidus = GABA (inhibitory), subthalamic nucleus = glutamate (excitatory)*

NB: The GPe is part of the indirect pathway (not the direct pathway!) that projects inhibitory fibers to the subthalamic nucleus.

VII. Cerebral Cortex: thin gray covering of both hemispheres of the brain; two types: neocortex (90%) and allocortex (10%); motor cortex is the thickest (4.5 mm), and the visual cortex is the thinnest (1.5 mm).

    A. **Layers of the neocortex:** *layers II and IV are mainly afferent; layers V and VI are mainly efferent*

       1. *Layer I:* molecular layer
       2. *Layer II:* external granular layer
       3. *Layer III:* external pyramidal layer; gives rise to association and commissural fibers
       4. *Layer IV:* internal granular layer; receives thalamocortical fibers from the thalamic nuclei of the ventral tier and also input from the lateral geniculate body

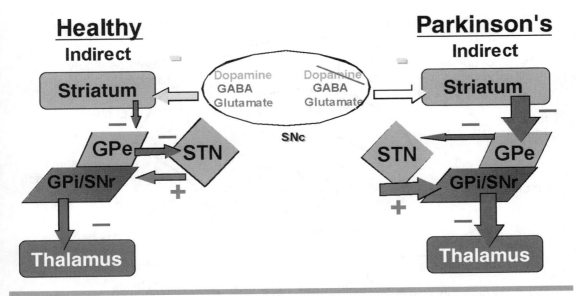

Figure 21-14. Schematic diagram of the indirect pathway of the basal ganglia.

5. *Layer V:* internal pyramidal layer; gives rise to corticobulbar, corticospinal, and corticostriatal fibers; contains giant pyramidal cells of Betz (found only in the motor cortex)
6. *Layer VI:* multiform layer; major source of corticothalamic fibers; gives rise to projection, commissural, and association fibers

B. *Functional areas*

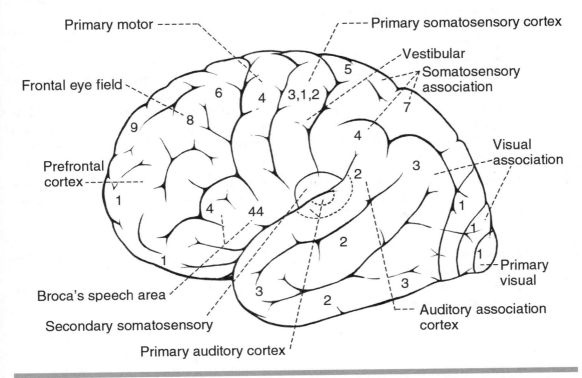

Figure 21-15. Gross lateral view of the brain illustrating the functional (Brodmann's) areas.

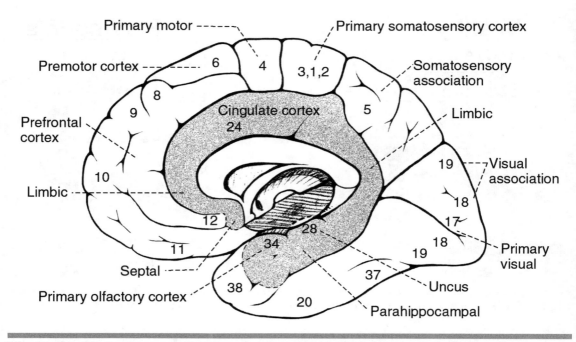

Figure 21-16. Medial surface of the brain hemisphere highlighting the functional (Brodmann's) areas.

1. *Frontal lobe*
   a. *Motor cortex (Brodmann's area 4) and premotor cortex (Brodmann's area 6):* destruction causes contralateral spastic paresis
   b. *Frontal eye field (Brodmann's area 8):* destruction causes deviation of the eyes to the ipsilateral side
   c. *Broca's speech area (Brodmann's areas 44 and 45):* located in the posterior part of the inferior frontal gyrus in the dominant hemisphere; destruction results in expressive, nonfluent aphasia
   d. *Prefrontal cortex (Brodmann's areas 9–12, 46, 47):* destruction of the anterior two-thirds results in deficits in concentration, orientation, abstracting ability, judgment, and problem solving ability; destruction of the orbital (frontal) lobe results in inappropriate social behavior

NB: Medial frontal cortex lesions may result in akinetic mutism, whereas orbitofrontal cortex lesions may result in impulsive and antisocial behavior. Left dorsolateral frontal lesions may produce depression.

2. *Parietal lobe*
   a. *Sensory cortex (Brodmann's areas 3, 1, 2):* destruction results in contralateral hemihypesthesia and astereognosis
   b. *Superior parietal lobule (Brodmann's areas 5 and 7):* destruction results in contralateral astereognosis and sensory neglect

NB: Asomatognosia is a form of neglect in which patients deny ownership of their limbs. It frequently accompanies anosognosia. The lesion is located in the nondominant supramarginal gyrus.

     c. *Inferior parietal lobule of the dominant hemisphere:* damage results in Gerstmann's syndrome: right-to-left confusion, finger agnosia, dysgraphia and dyslexia, dyscalculia, contralateral hemianopia, or lower quadrantanopia

     d. *Inferior parietal lobule of the nondominant hemisphere:* destruction results in topographic memory loss, anosognosia, construction apraxia, dressing apraxia, contralateral sensory neglect, contralateral hemianopia, or lower quadrantanopia

  3. *Temporal lobe*

     a. *Primary auditory cortex (Brodmann's areas 41 and 42):* unilateral destruction results in slight hearing loss; bilateral loss results in cortical deafness

     b. *Wernicke's speech area in the dominant area (Brodmann's area 22):* found in the posterior part of the superior temporal gyrus; destruction results in receptive, fluent aphasia

     c. *Olfactory bulb, tract, and primary cortex (Brodmann's area 34):* destruction results in ipsilateral anosmia, irritative lesion of the uncus results in olfactory and gustatory hallucinations

     d. *Hippocampal cortex (archicortex):* bilateral lesions result in the inability to consolidate short-term memory into long-term memory

     e. *Anterior temporal lobe (including amygdaloid nucleus):* bilateral damage results in Klüver-Bucy syndrome—visual agnosia, hyperphagia, docility, hypersexuality

     f. *Inferomedial occipitotemporal cortex:* bilateral lesions result in the inability to recognize once-familiar faces (prosopagnosia)

  4. *Occipital lobe*

     a. Bilateral lesions: cortical blindness (Anton's syndrome)

NB: Individuals with Anton's syndrome have cortical blindness, often with denial or unawareness of the blindness.

     b. Unilateral lesions: contralateral hemianopia or quadrantanopia

  5. *Corpus callosum*

     a. *Anterior corpus callosum lesions:* may result in akinetic mutism or tactile anomia

     b. *Posterior corpus callosum (splenium) lesion:* may result in alexia without agraphia

NB: Left posterior cerebral artery syndrome presents alexia without agraphia. The lesion is in the splenium of the corpus callosum.

NB: Surface dyslexia is characterized by impairment in linking the visual form system with the phonological output lexicon. Patients are therefore unable to access the visual word images to link to proper pronunciation and will need to rely on "print-to-sound-conversion" and have difficulty reading words that do not sound the way they are spelled.

     c. *Split-brain syndrome:* a disconnection syndrome that results from transection of the corpus callosum (e.g., in a patient with alexia in the left visual field, the verbal symbols seen on the right visual cortex have no access to the language centers of the left hemisphere)

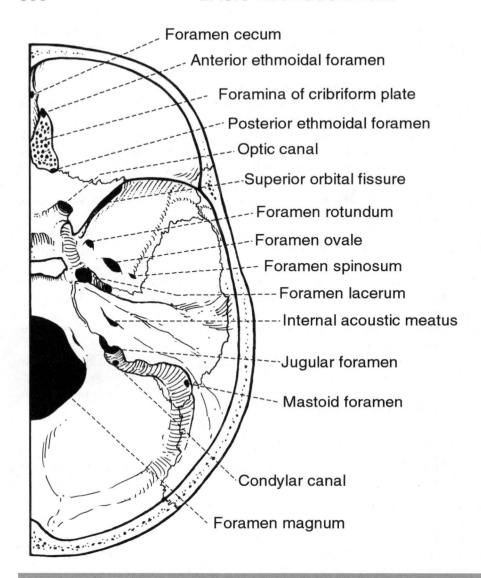

Figure 21-17. Basal view of the skull highlighting the foramina.

VIII. Skull, Arterial Supply, and Venous Drainage

A. Foramina of the skull

Foramen	Structures
Foramen cecum	Vein to superior sagittal sinus
Anterior ethmoidal foramen	Anterior ethmoidal artery, vein, and nerve
Foramina of cribriform plate	Olfactory nerve bundles
Posterior ethmoidal foramen	Posterior ethmoidal artery, vein, and nerve
Optic canal	CN II
	Ophthalmic artery
Superior orbital fissure	CN III
	CN IV
	Ophthalmic nerve
	CN VI
	Superior ophthalmic vein
Foramen rotundum	Maxillary nerve
Foramen ovale	Mandibular nerve
	Accessory meningeal artery
	Lesser petrosal nerve (occasionally)
Foramen spinosum	Middle meningeal artery and vein
	Meningeal branch of the mandibular nerve
Foramen of Vesalius (inconstant)	Small emissary vein
Foramen lacerum	Internal carotid artery
	Internal carotid nerve plexus
Hiatus of canal of lesser petrosal nerve	Lesser petrosal nerve
Hiatus of canal of greater petrosal nerve	Greater petrosal nerve
Internal acoustic meatus	CN VII
	CN VIII
	Labyrinthine artery
Vestibular aqueduct	Endolymphatic duct
Mastoid foramen	Emissary vein
	Branch of occipital artery
Jugular foramen	Inferior petrosal sinus
	CN IX
	CN X
	CN XI
	Sigmoid sinus

Foramen	Structures
	Posterior meningeal artery
Condylar canal (inconstant)	Emissary vein
	Meningeal branch of the ascending pharyngeal artery
Hypoglossal canal	CN XII
Foramen magnum	Medulla oblongata
	Meninges
	Vertebral arteries
	Spinal roots of CN XI

B. **Venous drainage**

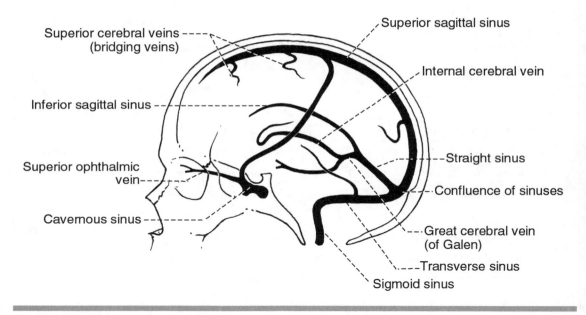

Figure 21-18. The venous system.

C. **Arterial supply**

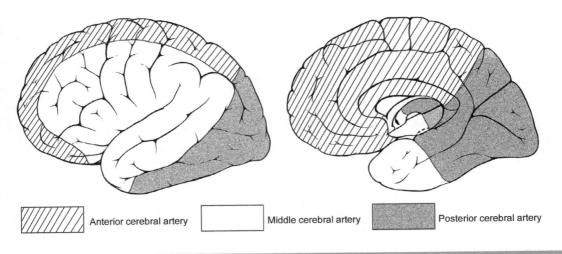

Anterior cerebral artery   Middle cerebral artery   Posterior cerebral artery

Figure 21-19. Sagittal view and section of the brain showing the major arterial supplies.

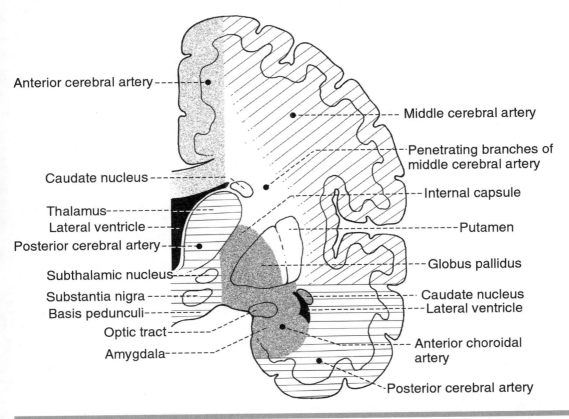

Anterior cerebral artery

Middle cerebral artery

Penetrating branches of middle cerebral artery

Caudate nucleus

Internal capsule

Thalamus

Lateral ventricle

Putamen

Posterior cerebral artery

Subthalamic nucleus

Globus pallidus

Substantia nigra

Caudate nucleus

Basis pedunculi

Lateral ventricle

Optic tract

Amygdala

Anterior choroidal artery

Posterior cerebral artery

Figure 21-20. Coronal section of the brain at the level of the internal capsule and thalamus showing the arterial supply.

ADDITIONAL NOTES

Psychiatry, Neurobehavior, and Neuropsychology

CHAPTER 22

Adult Psychiatry

I. Psychochemistry

A. **Neurotransmitters**

1. **Dopamine** (DA)

   a. Dopaminergic pathways

Pathway	Source (cell type)	Tract	Destination
Nigrostriatal	Substantia nigra pars compacta (SNc), midbrain (A8/9)	Medial forebrain bundle	Striatum (D1, D2), amygdala (D1)
Mesolimbic and mesocortical	Ventral tegmentum (A10)	Medial forebrain bundle	Nucleus accumbens (D1, D2, D3), prefrontal cortex, hippocampus, cingulum
Tuberoinfundibular	Hypothalamus (A12)		Portal vessels → pituitary (D2)
Incertohypothalamic	A11/13–15 (hypothalamus)		Hypothalamus

   b. *Synthesis*

     i. Tyrosine—[*tyrosine hydroxylase*] → L-dopa—[dopa decarboxylase] → DA

     ii. Tyrosine hydroxylase is the rate-limiting enzyme

   c. *Catabolism*

     i. DA is broken down by *monoamine oxidase types A and B (MAO$_{A, B}$)* and *catechol-O-methyl-transferase*

     ii. End products are *homovanillic acid* and *3,4-dihydroxyphenylacetic acid*

   d. *Receptor "families" and their distributions*

     i. D1 family: characteristics—postsynaptic, excitatory; locations: D1—*striatum, accumbens*, olfactory tubercle, cortex, amygdala; D5—hippocampus, dentate gyrus, thalamus (parafascicular), cortex

     ii. D2 family: characteristics—postsynaptic and presynaptic, inhibitory; locations: D2—striatum, accumbens, olfactory tubercle, lateral septum, SNc, ventral tegmentum, olfactory bulb, zona incerta; D3—olfactory tubercle, accumbens; D4—*cortex* (prefrontal and temporal), dentate gyrus, hippocampus

    iii. Psychiatric significance: DA's normal functions include movement, perception, motivation, reward, aggression; DA *excess* or *hypersensitivity* is associated with *positive symptoms* of *schizophrenia* (mesolimbic tract), and *tardive dyskinesia (TD)* (nigrostriatal tract); DA *deficiency* or *blockade* is associated with: *extrapyramidal syndromes* ([EPSs] striatum, nucleus accumbens), *hyperprolactinemia* (tuberoin-fundibular), *negative symptoms of schizophrenia*, depression

2. **Serotonin** (5-hydroxytryptamine [5-HT]): 5-HT is produced in the dorsal and median *raphe nuclei*—periaqueductal gray matter of midbrain and pons, B_{1-9} type cells; raphe neurons project through the *medial forebrain bundle* to hippocampus, hypothalamus, frontal cortex, striatum, and thalamus; receptors are also located on platelets (increase cohesion), sexual organs, and in the gastrointestinal (GI) tract (increase peristalsis)

    a. Synthesis: tryptophan—[*tryptophan hydroxylase*] → 5-hydroxytryptophan—[5-HTPdecarboxylase] → 5-HT

    b. Catabolism: 5-HT—[MAO_A] → 5-hydroxyindoleacetic acid

    c. Psychiatric significance

      i. Normal functions of 5-HT include mood and sleep regulation, appetite, impulse control

      ii. Stimulation of 5-HT_1 receptors is associated with *antidepressant* activity

      iii. Stimulation of $5HT_{1D}$ autoreceptors associated with *migraine* treatment ("triptans")

      iv. Stimulation of 5-HT_2 and 5-HT_3 receptors is associated with *psychosis*

      v. Blockade of 5-HT_3 receptors associated with *antiemetics* (ondansetron)

      vi. Decreased levels of 5-hydroxyindoleacetic acid are found in cerebrospinal fluid of violent and suicidal subjects

      vii. Peripheral 5-HT receptors cause antidepressants side effects (GI distress, sexual dysfunction)

NB: Low levels of CSF 5-HIAA has been reported among patients who have attempted suicide via violent means and in alcoholics with impulsive violent behavior. Norepinephrine and COMT have also been implicated.

3. **Norepinephrine** (NE): produced by cells in *locus ceruleus*; widely distributed targets (cortex, limbic system, thalamus, hypothalamus, reticular formation, dorsal raphe, cerebellum, brain stem, spinal cord)

    a. Synthesis

      i. Tyrosine—[*tyrosine hydroxylase*] → L-dopa (rate-limiting step)

      ii. L-Dopa—[*dopa decarboxylase*] → DA—[*dopamine β-hydroxylase*] → L-NE

    b. *Catabolism* is by MAO_A and *catechol-O-methyl-transferase* to 3-methoxy-4-hydroxy-phenylglycol

    c. Psychiatric significance

      i. Normal functions include focused attention, stress response, aggression.

      ii. NE reuptake inhibition is associated with treatment of *depression* and *attention-deficit/hyperactivity disorder.*

      iii. *Peripheral* blockade leads to *orthostatic hypotension* (common side effect of psychiatric drugs).

4. **Other neurotransmitters**

    a. γ-Aminobutyric acid (GABA): GABA is a widely distributed *inhibitory* amino acid neurotransmitter; synthesis: glutamate—[*glutamate decarboxylase*] → GABA; GABA agonists are prescribed for *anxiety, ethanol (EtOH) withdrawal, seizures,* catatonia, and akathisia

    b. Acetylcholine (ACh)

        i. *Synthesis:* Choline + acetyl coenzyme A—[*choline acetyltransferase*] → ACh

        ii. *Catabolism:* ACh—[*acetylcholinesterase*] → choline + acetate

        iii. Psychiatric significance: ACh is heavily involved in cognition and motor function, degeneration of ACh-ergic neurons is associated with cognitive deficits in Alzheimer's and other degenerative dementias, acetylcholinesterase *inhibitors* are prescribed to treat Alzheimer's disease, anticholinergics should be avoided in the elderly and demented

NB: Alzheimer's disease presents a decrease of choline acetyltransferase in the basalis nucleus of Meynert.

        iv. Central ACh receptor blockade: used to treat EPSs caused by antipsychotics; used to treat parkinsonism; may cause disturbed cognition (particularly in elderly)

        v. Peripheral ACh receptor blockade is responsible for side effects of many psychiatric medications; decreased visceral activity: dry mouth, constipation, urinary retention; parasympathetic: blurred vision, tachycardia

NB: ACh, vital to encoding new memories, is one of the many neurotransmitters deficient in Alzheimer's disease. Medications including tricyclic antidepressants (TCAs), antihistamines, and anti-emetics with strong anticholinergic properties can worsen memory and cause confusion.

    c. Glutamate: excitatory amino acid neurotransmitter; **NB:** normal activity associated with memory (*N-methyl-D-aspartate* [NMDA] receptor); antagonism associated with psychosis; **NB:** hyperactivity associated with excitotoxicity

    d. Histamine (H): excitatory monoamine neurotransmitter; blockade causes drowsiness, weight gain, cognitive slowing

  B. **Antidepressants:** *all antidepressants increase monoamine-dependent neurotransmission,* most commonly in serotonergic systems; *reuptake inhibition* at the synapse increases monoamine activity; *newer agents are generally more selective and less dangerous in overdose*

    1. **Tricyclic antidepressants** (TCAs); *major indications:* depression, migraine prophylaxis, neuropathic pain, anxiety disorders

      a. Tertiary amines

        i. 5-HT > NE reuptake inhibition

        ii. More antihistaminic and anticholinergic activity than the secondary amines

        iii. Examples: amitriptyline (Elavil®), clomipramine (Anafranil®), imipramine (Tofranil®), doxepin (Sinequan®)

NB: More sedating than other secondary amine classes.

      b. Secondary amines

        i. Secondary amine TCAs are derived from metabolism of tertiary amines

        ii. Amitriptyline → nortriptyline

        iii. Imipramine → desipramine

        iv. NE >> 5-HT reuptake inhibition

        v. Examples: nortriptyline (Pamelor®), desipramine (Norpramin®), protriptyline (Vivactil®)

    c. Tetracyclic: these are the only TCAs with some antipsychotic activity; examples: amoxapine (Asendin®), maprotiline (Ludiomil®)

    d. Common *side effects of TCAs*
      i. Potentially lethal in overdose
      ii. Anticholinergic side effects include dry mouth, constipation, blurred vision, urinary retention, delirium, memory impairment
      iii. Antiadrenergic (α_1) activity causes orthostatic hypotension
      iv. Anti-H_1 activity causes sedation and weight gain
      v. Cardiac toxicity in overdose (*Q-T prolongation* → torsades de pointes)

2. **MAO inhibitors** (MAOIs): examples: phenelzine (Nardil®), tranylcypromine (Parnate®); *work through irreversible inhibition* of $MAO_{A, B}$; resynthesis of the enzymes takes 2 weeks

    a. Major uses: depression, migraine prophylaxis, borderline personality disorder, anxiety disorders

    b. Side effects: potentially lethal in overdose; *hypertensive crisis:* sudden headache, hypertension, flushing, neck stiffness; associated with ingestion of large amounts of *tyramine-rich food* (aged cheese/meat, cured meats, some alcoholic beverages, sauerkraut, may be caused by MAOI overdose, treat with nifedipine (10 mg orally) or phentolamine; *orthostatic hypotension*, sedation, headache, sexual dysfunction, decreased sleep, fatigue; *serotonin syndrome*
      i. Signs/symptoms: rest tremor, myoclonus, hypertonicity, hyperthermia, hallucinations
      ii. Results from combining serotonergic drugs; combinations including an MAOI are the most dangerous.
      iii. **NB:** *Avoid other serotonergic, adrenergic, or dopaminergic drugs for 2 weeks before or after ingestion of an MAOI.*

3. **Serotonin-specific reuptake inhibitors** (SSRIs)

    a. Uses: depressive disorders, anxiety disorders, premenstrual dysphoric disorder

    b. Examples:

Fluoxetine (Prozac®)	Paroxetine (Paxil®)
Sertraline (Zoloft®)	Fluvoxamine (Luvox®)
Citalopram (Celexa®)	Escitalopram (Lexapro®)

    c. *Distinguishing characteristics:* in most respects, the SSRIs are relatively interchangeable; most differences are pharmacokinetic
      i. Fluoxetine: **NB:** parent drug has a long half-life ($t_{1/2}$) (5 days) and a long-lived active metabolite (norfluoxetine, $t_{1/2}$ = 10 days); requires 3- to 4-week washout period before initiation of MAOI; cytochrome P3A4 inhibitor
      ii. Paroxetine: **NB:** *most anticholinergic; very short $t_{1/2}$ can cause severe withdrawal syndrome; cytochrome P2D6 inhibitor*
      iii. Fluvoxamine: initially marketed for obsessive-compulsive disorder; cytochrome 1A2 inhibitor
      iv. Sertraline: can sometimes inhibit warfarin (Coumadin®) metabolism
      v. Citalopram: the most serotonin-specific
      vi. Escitalopram: the L-isomer of citalopram; has fewer side effects

    d. Major side effects of SSRIs
      i. Common, reversible side effects include nausea, diarrhea, sexual dysfunction, headache, anxiety.
      ii. **NB:** Mania can be induced in patients even without prior history of bipolar disorder.

iii. Start at low initial dose and titrate slowly to minimize side effects.

iv. Pregnancy class C (uncertain safety, no adverse effects in studies).

NB: Paroxetine is the most potent SSRI; citalopram is the most selective; fluoxetine is the longest lasting.

NB: Sertraline is also a potent blocker of the DA transporter.

NB: Serotonin syndrome results from medications that enhance serotonin transmission (via decreased breakdown or increased production). Combinations of MAOIs and SSRIs, TCA, or dextromethorphan should be avoided. Serotonin syndrome can be differentiated from NMS by the presence of shivering and myoclonus.

4. **Other antidepressants**
   a. **NB:** Venlafaxine (Effexor®)
      i. Works through 5-HT reuptake, but also inhibits NE reuptake at higher doses
      ii. Side effects: *mild hypertension* (5–10 mm Hg in 5–10% of patients); withdrawal syndrome (myalgias, restlessness, poor energy); other side effects similar to the SSRI
   b. Bupropion (Wellbutrin®, Zyban®); increases NE activity; also increases DA activity at very high doses; *no sexual dysfunction*; side effects: **NB:** *lowers seizure threshold,* avoid in patients with seizure risk factors, increased seizure risk in patients with eating disorders, increased risk with single doses >300 mg or total daily dose >450 mg; can cause *irritability* and *anxiety*; also used as a smoking cessation aid (Zyban); approved for treatment of attention deficit disorder
   c. Mirtazapine (Remeron®); *enhances 5-HT and NE transmission:* postsynaptic 5-HT$_{1A}$ agonist, presynaptic 5-HT$_2$ and 5-HT$_3$ antagonist, presynaptic α$_2$ antagonist; *no sexual dysfunction;* anti-H$_1$ side effects *(weight gain, drowsiness)*
   d. Nefazodone (Serzone®): enhances 5-HT and NE neurotransmission: 5-HT reuptake inhibition, presynaptic 5-HT$_2$ antagonism, synaptic NE reuptake inhibition (?); *minimal sexual dysfunction; can cause hepatic dysfunction* and is sedating
   e. **Trazodone** (Desyrel): mostly serotonergic: 5-HT reuptake inhibition, presynaptic 5-HT$_2$ antagonist, postsynaptic 5-HT agonist at high doses (?); side effects: **NB:** priapism, drowsiness, sexual dysfunction
   f. **Electroconvulsive therapy** (ECT)
      i. Indications: *medication resistant depression (80% efficacy), Parkinson's disease (PD),* mania, acute psychosis
      ii. Procedure involves delivery of a small current to the brain, under anesthesia, to induce a generalized seizure
      iii. Mechanism of action unknown: massive monoamine release?; "resetting" of frontal subcortical systems?
      iv. Side effects: *major side effect is temporary anterograde and retrograde amnesia;* other side effects include risks of anesthesia (cardiac arrest, allergic reaction); modern anesthetics and paralytic agents have virtually eliminated risk of broken bones, tongue biting, and broken teeth from the seizure; effect is temporary, usually requires multiple treatments
C. **Repetitive transcranial magnetic stimulation:** application of magnetic field to frontal part of brain, presumably inducing current and neurotransmitter release; may have efficacy in treatment-resistant depression; parameters not fully established
D. **Antimanic and mood-stabilizing agents**

1. Uses in psychiatry
   a. Treatment of mania; the antipsychotics risperidone and quetiapine can treat acute mania; acute mania and mania prophylaxis:

Lithium (Eskalith®)	Valproate (Depakote®)
Carbamazepine (Tegretol®)	Olanzapine (Zyprexa®)
Lamotrigine (Lamictal®)	

   b. Are used in treatment of *impulse control disorders, agitation, and aggression*
   c. Some can also treat bipolar depression (lithium, lamotrigine)
2. Lithium *(therapeutic levels 0.6–1.2)*
   a. Theories about mechanism of action include effects on second messenger systems, serotonergic neurotransmission, and neuronal ion channels
   b. Acute side effects: *tremor, ataxia,* acne, weight gain, polyuria, hypokalemia
   c. Chronic side effects: hypothyroidism, psoriasis, weight gain
   d. **NB:** Toxicity: symptoms: *delirium, tremor, ataxia,* diarrhea, seizure, Q-T prolongation, *renal failure;* risk of toxicity increases with *dehydration, nonsteroidal anti-inflammatory drugs, phenytoin;* dialyze for level >3.0
3. Antimanic antiepileptics (carbamazepine, valproate, lamotrigine)
4. Antimanic antipsychotics (olanzapine, quetiapine, risperidone)
E. *Review of pharmacology of antipsychotics*
   1. **Uses in neurology**
      a. PD-related psychosis: *use atypicals only; clozapine* and *quetiapine* have lowest risk of worsening parkinsonism; less D2 blockade; substantial anti-ACh activity
      b. Dementia/sundowning: *atypicals preferred;* avoid agents with strong anticholinergic or antihistaminic properties; use low nighttime doses to reduce treatment-emergent side effects
      c. **NB:** Tic disorders (including Tourette's): high-potency antipsychotic *(pimozide or haloperidol)*
   2. Uses in psychiatry
      a. Psychotic disorders (schizophrenia, schizoaffective disorder)
      b. Mood disorders (psychotic depression, mania)
   3. **"Typical" antipsychotics** (neuroleptics) work mainly through *D2 blockade*
      a. *Low-potency neuroleptics* (typical daily dose >100 mg)
         i. Significant anti-ACh, anti-NE, and anti-H$_1$ activity
         ii. Examples: chlorpromazine (Thorazine®), thioridazine (Mellaril®)
         iii. **NB:** The antiemetics prochlorperazine (Compazine®), promethazine (Phenergan®), and metoclopramide (Reglan®) have similar pharmacology and side effects
      b. *High-potency neuroleptics* (typical daily dose <50 mg)
         i. Higher anti-DA to anti-ACh ratio—increased risk of EPSs
         ii. Low antiadrenergic and anti-H$_1$ activity
         iii. Examples: haloperidol (Haldol®), thiothixene (Navane®), fluphenazine (Prolixin®)
   4. **"Atypical" antipsychotics**
      a. Defined by 5-HT$_2$ > DA blockade and D4 > D2 blockade; **NB:** much *lower incidence of EPS and TD* than typical agents; increased efficacy for *negative symptoms of schizophrenia and cognition*
         i. Clozapine (Clozaril®): most effective antipsychotic; **NB:** clozapine causes no EPS; *safely treats PD-related psychosis; approved for treatment of TD; side effects:* **NB:** idiosyncratic *agranulocytosis* (~1% incidence), weekly complete blood count for 6 months,

then biweekly complete blood count for duration of treatment, hold or discontinue clozapine if white blood count or neutrophil count declines, **NB:** *lowers seizure threshold* (0.7–1.0% per 100 mg daily dose), severe anti-ACh and anti-H_1 side effects—sialorrhea (excessive salivation)

    ii. Olanzapine (Zyprexa®): *massive weight gain* and moderate sedation because of anti-ACh effects; the only atypical antipsychotic approved for prophylaxis against mania

   iii. Quetiapine (Seroquel®): mostly blocks 5-HT_2 receptors; minimal DA blockade at usual doses; **NB:** useful in patients with *PD*; anti-H_1 activity causes weight gain and sedation; α_1 blockade causes orthostatic hypotension

   iv. Risperidone (Risperdal®): the highest D2/5-HT_2 blockade ratio of the atypicals; dose-related EPS at >6 mg/day; *hyperprolactinemia*—caused by tuberoinfundibular DA blockade (DA suppresses prolactin release), decreased libido, gynecomastia, sexual dysfunction; orthostatic hypotension because of α_1 blockade

    v. Ziprasidone (Geodon®): powerful 5-HT_2 and DA receptor antagonist; no weight gain; newest atypical; high D2 affinity suggests EPS may prove to be a problem; significant α_1 blockade—may cause hypotension; prolongation of QT interval (clinically insignificant)

   vi. Aripiprazole (Abilify®): new form of antipsychotic—partial agonist; extremely high affinity at D2 and 5-HT_{2A} receptor

5. Quick reference chart: atypical antipsychotic receptor affinities

Drug	D2	5-HT_2	a_1	ACh	H_1
Clozapine	+	+++	++	++++	++
Risperidone	+++	+++	++++	–	–
Olanzapine	+	+	+	++	+++
Quetiapine	+/–	++	++	+/–	++++
Ziprasidone	++++	++++	++++	+/–	–

+, weak affinity; ++, moderate affinity; +++, strong affinity; ++++, very strong affinity.

6. lasting intramuscular depot formulations
   a. Haloperidol decanoate (3–4 weeks)
   b. Fluphenazine decanoate (2 weeks)
   c. Risperidone (Risperdal Consta®) (2 weeks)

7. **NB:** EPS—"3 hours, 3 days, 3 weeks"; likelihood of EPS usually correlates with degree of DA blockade
   a. Acute dystonia (usually occurs within 3 hours): usually occurs with *parenteral high-potency* medications; young men, particularly of African descent are at higher risk; usually involves midline musculature, oculogyrus, opisthotonus, torticollis, retrocollis; treat with intramuscular/intravenous *diphenhydramine* (Benadryl®) or *benztropine* (Cogentin®)
   b. Akathisia (within 3 days): "inner restlessness"; *most common* EPS; patients fidget, get up and walk around, unable to sit quietly; treat with *propranolol* (Inderal®), benzodiazepine, or anticholinergic
   c. Parkinsonism (approximately 3 weeks): occurs with *high-potency typicals* and *risperidone (usually >6 mg/day)*; features that distinguish EPS from idiopathic PD: EPS

parkinsonism is usually symmetric, EPS parkinsonism usually has subacute onset, tremor is typically less prominent than rigidity and bradykinesia; treatment: reduce antipsychotic dose, add anticholinergic, switch to a "more atypical" drug (i.e., lower $D2/5\text{-}HT_2$ blockade ratio)

8. **TD**: incidence 3–5% per year of treatment with DA-blocking agent; caused by chronic DA blockade, resulting in striatal D2 receptor hypersensitivity; elderly, female patients and those with underlying central nervous system (CNS) disease are at greater risk for developing TD; syndrome consists of choreoathetoid movements that *can occur anywhere in the body*, with the face (buccolingual) being the most commonly affected region; treatment: *decrease dose of antipsychotic*—may cause worsening initially because DA receptors are left unblocked; *switch to atypical antipsychotic*; clozapine does not cause EPS and *is indicated for treatment of TD*; mixed success with benzodiazepines, anticholinergics, gabapentin, and vitamin E

9. **Neuroleptic malignant syndrome**: incidence <1%
   a. Results from *decreased dopaminergic neurotransmission*
      i. Usually results from addition of DA receptor blocker (i.e., antipsychotic)
      ii. Can happen with removal of DA receptor stimulator (i.e., anti-PD medications)
   b. Causes of increased risk of neuroleptic malignant syndrome: affective disorder, concomitant lithium use, sudden decrease of DA agonist or increase of DA antagonist
   c. Symptoms/signs: earliest sign is mental status change (confusion, irritability); physical signs: *rigidity, fever, autonomic instability*, tremor, diaphoresis; labs: ↑*creatine phosphokinase* (usually >1,000), ↑white blood count, myoglobinuria
   d. Treatment: *discontinue antipsychotic; supportive care in the intensive care unit, especially cooling and hydration;* bromocriptine (DA agonist), dantrolene (muscle relaxant); ECT in refractory cases; patients usually tolerate rechallenge with antipsychotic

NB: Paroxysmal autonomic instability with dystonia (PAID) is a common symptom cluster similar to NMS and commonly appears following severe traumatic or hypoxic brain injury. Treatment consists of beta-adrenergic blockers, opiod analgesia, DA agonists and benzodiazepines. DA antagonists can precipitate PAID-like symptoms. Anticholinergics and SSRIs are largerly ineffective.

F. **Anxiolytics and hypnotics**
   1. *Benzodiazepines*
      a. General properties
         i. All facilitate $GABA_A$ receptor (ligand-gated chloride channel) by binding to its benzodiazepine site.
         ii. Actions include *muscle relaxation, sedation, and amnesia.*
      b. *Indications and uses*
         i. Primary sleep disorders (rapid eye movement [REM] behavior disorder, restless limbs)
         ii. Anxiety disorders (panic disorder, generalized anxiety, phobias, social anxiety disorder)
         iii. Sedation (for agitated patients or medical procedures)
         iv. Muscle spasticity
         v. Alcohol, benzodiazepine, or barbiturate withdrawal
         vi. Epilepsy
      c. Should be used for a brief, well-defined duration
      d. *Tolerance and/or dependence* can develop with all—more likely with rapidly absorbed and short-acting ($t_{1/2}$<20 hours) compounds

e. *Contraindicated in patients with substance use disorders;* can impair memory and cognitive and motor performance
f. Duration of clinical activity is usually significantly shorter than $t_{1/2}$
g. *Quick reference chart: benzodiazepines*

Drug	Brand	Equiva-lent (mg)	Absorption	$t_{1/2}$[a] (hrs)	Dosing (mg/day)	Active metabolites	Special features
Midazolam	Versed®	1.25	Intravenous	2	1–5	Yes	Anesthetic, significant amnesia
Triazolam	Halcion®	0.1	Rapid	2	0.25–0.5	No	—
Alprazolam	Xanax®	0.25	Medium	10	0.5–4	Yes	Has anti-depressant activity
Clon-azepam	Klonopin®	0.5	Rapid	30	0.5–10	No	Effective against mania
Lorazepam	Ativan®	1	Medium	12	2–8	No[b]	—
Temazepam	Restoril®	5	Medium	10	15–30	No[b]	Typically used for insomnia
Diazepam	Valium®	5	Rapid	100	5–45	Yes	Metabolized to oxazepam
Chlordiazepoxide	Librium®	10	Medium	100	10–100	Yes	Use with caution in hepatic disease
Oxazepam	Serax®	15	Slow	9	20–100	No[b]	—

[a]*Benzodiazepines with $t_{1/2} < 20$ hours are considered short acting.*
[b]*Conjugated metabolites are eliminated in the urine—safer for use in patients with liver disease.*

2. Barbiturates: no longer commonly used in psychiatry, but still used as anticonvulsants
   a. Risks: generally similar to those of benzodiazepines; *can cause respiratory depression and severe hypercarbia/hypoxia; can induce hepatic enzymes,* causing rapid elimination of other medications
   b. Modern uses of barbiturates
      i. Amobarbital (Amytal®): used for drug-assisted interviews
      ii. Phenobarbital (Luminal®)
      iii. Seizure prophylaxis
      iv. Medication of choice for barbiturate withdrawal

      v. Methohexital (Brevital®): an ultra-short acting parenteral barbiturate; the *most popular anesthetic for ECT* and other brief surgical procedures

     vi. Pentobarbital (Nembutal®): used to control status epilepticus

3. Zolpidem (Ambien®) and zaleplon (Sonata®): short-acting *nonbenzodiazepine* compounds that interact with the benzodiazepine binding site; approved for the treatment of insomnia; *cannot be used to treat benzodiazepine withdrawal or muscle spasm;* zolpidem: longer acting

4. Buspirone (BuSpar®): 5-HT$_{1A}$ receptor agonist; requires weeks to obtain therapeutic effect (similar to antidepressants); *no dependence, abuse potential, or withdrawal side effects; not effective for benzodiazepine or barbiturate withdrawal*

G. **Medications for treatment of substance related disorders**

1. Flumazenil (Mazicon®, Romazicon®): *benzodiazepine receptor antagonist;* used to reverse benzodiazepine toxicity; *may precipitate seizures or severe anxiety* in patients who are epileptic, benzodiazepine-dependent, or have ingested a large quantity of benzodiazepines; t$_{½}$<15 minutes; dose in 0.2–0.5 mg increments, to max dose of 3 mg/hour

2. Opioid abuse treatments

   a. Naloxone (Narcan®): parenteral opioid antagonist; used to reverse effects of opioid toxicity

   b. Naltrexone (ReVia®): *competitive antagonist* at opioid receptors; used to maintain drug-free state in patients treated for opioid dependence

   c. Methadone (Dolophine®, Methadose®): once-daily opioid agonist; used to replace more illegal, injected, or more addictive opioids; patient remains narcotic-dependent but under a physician's care

   d. Disulfiram (Antabuse®): used for patients being treated for EtOH dependence; requires high level of motivation and compliance; EtOH—[*EtOH dehydrogenase*] → acetaldehyde—[*aldehyde dehydrogenase*] → acetic acid; disulfiram inhibits aldehyde dehydrogenase, causing accumulation of acetaldehyde; causes multiple unpleasant effects—nausea, headache, diaphoresis, vomiting, tachycardia, vertigo; can cause severe reactions to EtOH in food (desserts, sauces), medicine (cough suppressant), or topical products (aftershave, perfume); can cause death and is contraindicated in patients with pulmonary or cardiac illness; *long t$_{½}$ necessitates 2-week washout of disulfiram before EtOH is used again*

H. **β-blockers:** effective for social anxiety, medication-induced tremors, and akathisia; used to treat agitation and aggression; *propranolol (Inderal®) and metoprolol (Lopressor®) have better CNS penetration because they are more lipophilic;* pindolol has been used to augment antidepressants

I. **Psychosurgery:** frontal lobotomy, used in the past, is no longer an acceptable therapeutic option; capsulotomy for treatment of obsessive-compulsive disorder (OCD); stereotactic radioablation of small portions of the internal capsule in the region of the caudate; microelectrode deep brain stimulation of the same area is being studied

II. Psychiatric Illnesses: the *Diagnostic and Statistical Manual of Mental Disorders* (currently in its 4th edition) strictly defines psychiatric disorders; for practical purposes, less rigid criteria are often employed with real patients; in general, all diagnoses (except personality disorders) can be made only if there is a change from prior functioning, significant impairment or distress in the patient, and the behavior has no other reasonable cause (medications, medical illness, bereavement, etc.)

A. **Mood disorders**

1. **Mood states**

a. *Major depressive episode: at least 2 weeks* of symptoms representing a *change from prior functioning;* five or more of the following symptoms (**NB:** *SIGECAPS*):
  i. Depressed mood
  ii. Alteration in **S**leep patterns (hypersomnia or insomnia)
  iii. Diminished **I**nterest or pleasure (anhedonia)
  iv. Excessive **G**uilt or feelings of worthlessness
  v. Decreased **E**nergy or fatigue nearly every day
  vi. Impaired **C**oncentration or unusual indecisiveness
  vii. Change in **A**ppetite or weight (±5%)
  viii. Unusual **P**sychomotor activity (agitation or retardation)
  ix. Thoughts of **S**uicide or death; one of the symptoms must be depressed mood or anhedonia; depressive symptoms can result from many medications (β blockers), or *medical illnesses* (hypothyroidism, B_{12} deficiency, cancer, lupus, *stroke* (30%), myocardial infarction (30%)

b. *Manic episode: at least 1 week* of symptoms (or need for hospitalization) representing a change from prior functioning; elevated, expansive, or irritable mood; at least three of the following symptoms (**NB:** *DIGFAST*), four if mood is predominantly irritable:
  i. **D**istractibility
  ii. **I**nsomnia without tiredness
  iii. **G**randiose ideas or behavior (exaggerated sense of importance)
  iv. **F**light of ideas (constant shifting between connected concepts)
  v. **A**gitation or increased activity
  vi. **S**peech excessive and/or pressured (pressure: internal drive to talk)
  vii. **T**houghtless or reckless behavior; must cause marked social and/or occupational impairment

c. **Hypomanic episode**
  i. Requires only *4 days* of manic symptoms.
  ii. Symptoms must be observable by others but not severe enough to cause marked impairment.
  iii. *Cannot be severe enough to cause hospitalization and/or psychosis.*

d. **Mixed episode**
  i. Meets criteria for both major depressive and manic episodes almost every day for at least a week.
  ii. Symptoms must cause marked impairment.
  iii. Mania, hypomania, or mixed episodes may be induced by *antidepressants, corticosteroids, stimulants,* and *right-sided cerebral damage.*

2. **Mood disorder diagnoses**
  a. *Major depressive disorder: one or more major depressive episodes*
    i. Epidemiology: 15% lifetime prevalence; twice as common in females
    ii. Risk factors: *genetics* (having a 1st-degree relative with mood disorder confers risk); other psychiatric illness (personality disorders, anxiety disorders); neurologic illnesses (Parkinson's, 40–50%; multiple sclerosis, 50%; epilepsy, 40–50%); pregnancy
    iii. Neuropsychiatric research findings: associated with decreased frontal metabolism on positron emission tomography scanning; associated with left frontal brain injury; decreased 5-hydroxyindoleacetic acid in cerebrospinal fluid of suicidal patients
    iv. *Suicide risk factors:* genetics (family history of suicide); medical (intoxication, chronic medical illness); gender (successful suicide is 3× more common in males,

suicide attempts are 4× more common in females); psychiatric: prior suicide attempt, psychosis, substance use disorder; advanced age (peak rates occur in men >45 y/o, and in women >55 y/o, high rate of completion in patients >65 y/o, but remember that suicide is the second-leading cause of death for adolescent males [accidents are the first])

NB: Greater than 50% of epileptics have one or more episodes of significant depression during the course of the disorder and the suicide rate is greater than the general population.

   v. *Treatment:* antidepressants—*avoid tricyclics in the elderly, pregnant, or cardiac compromised; beware of bupropion in patients with seizure disorders;* augmenting agents include lithium and thyroid hormone; *ECT for:* pregnant women; psychotic, medication-resistant, or imminently life-threatening depression; psychotherapy is effective alone but more effective in conjunction with medications; antipsychotics such as aripiprazole are now used as adjunctive treatment for major depressive disorder

b. **Dysthymic disorder**
   i. At least two depressive symptoms, but no major depressive episode
   ii. Symptoms have been present on most days for *at least 2 years*
c. **Bereavement** (not a disorder, but should be distinguished from depression): depressive symptoms *within 2 months* of a loved one's death; symptoms *not associated* with normal bereavement
   i. Hallucinations not related to the deceased
   ii. Excessive guilt unrelated to the death
   iii. Morbid preoccupation with one's worthlessness
   iv. Marked functional impairment
   v. Persistent wish for death
   vi. Marked psychomotor retardation

NB: *Primary melancholia* is characterized by a profound and unremitting autonomous mood change with unnatural sadness, apprehension, or dysphoria, and a pervasive loss of pleasure. At least three of these items must be present for the diagnosis: anorexia, insomnia with early morning awakening, quality of mood distinct from ordinary sadness, diurnal mood swings (worse in the morning), psychomotor retardation or agitation, and feelings of guilt.

d. **Bipolar disorder**
   i. Epidemiology: 2% prevalence; usually presents in 2nd or 3rd decade; approximately 50% of patients have a family history of mood disorder
   ii. Bipolar I vs. bipolar II disorder: any history of a full manic episode → bipolar I; psychosis or hospitalization during elevated mood → bipolar I; mixed episode → bipolar I; hypomanic episodes and major depressive episodes only → bipolar II
   iii. Variants: rapid-cycling—four mood episodes within 1 year; cyclothymia—alternation between hypomanic episodes and episodes of depressive symptoms that do not meet criteria for a major depressive episode
   iv. Treatment: treat manic symptoms with antimanic agent (see section I.D); lithium and valproic acid are 1st-line agents; broad efficacy in different types of bipolar illness; valproate is relatively safe; clonazepam may be used as an adjunctive agent; antidepressants during manic or mixed phases can cause rapid cycling; addition of an antipsychotic may be necessary to control psychotic symptoms; antipsychotics such as quetiapine and aripiprazole are now used for bipolar disorder

NB: Catatonia may be seen in over 10% of inpatients in the psychiatric ward. It is more prevalent in mood disorders, especially bipolar, compared to schizophrenia. It may have a "retarded stuporous" form or an "excited delirious" form and is characterized by cataplexy, waxy flexibility, echophenomena, and negativism. Treatments include benzodiazepines, barbiturates, and ECT. DA antagonists and baclofen can worsen catatonia.

B. **Psychotic disorders**
 1. **Psychotic symptoms**
    a. Delusions: fixed, false beliefs (bizarre delusions are totally implausible)
    b. Thought disorganization: illogical progression of thoughts, association of unrelated ideas
    c. Disorganized behavior: behavior incongruous with surrounding stimuli and events
    d. Catatonia: motor immobility, motiveless hyperactivity or resistance to movement, or posturing
    e. Hallucinations (perception of nonexistent stimuli)
    f. Illusions (misinterpretation of real stimuli)
 2. **Psychosis due to physical illness**
    a. Neurologic: Wilson's, Huntington's, Parkinson's, encephalitis, epilepsy

NB: Forced normalization is a psychotic phenomenon occurring after achievement of good clinical seizure control or resolution of epileptiform discharges.

    b. General medical: hepatic encephalopathy, steroid use, acquired immunodeficiency syndrome, lupus, B_{12} deficiency, tertiary syphilis, porphyria
 3. **Schizophrenia**
    a. Epidemiology: approximately 1% of the population
    b. Genetics: approximately 50% concordance in twin studies; increased risk of schizophrenia in 1st-degree relatives of schizophrenics; increased risk of other psychotic disorders (schizotypal, schizoaffective, schizophreniform) in relatives of schizophrenics
    c. **Neuropsychiatric research findings**
       i. Anatomic: *increased size of lateral and 3rd ventricles; decreased size of temporal lobes,* caudate nucleus increases in size with treatment
       ii. Functional: altered metabolism in prefrontal cortex and striatum; saccadic breakdown of ocular tracking; poor working memory
       iii. Neurochemical: suggestions of *dopaminergic* hyperactivity in striatum come from hallucinations in parkinsonism and the efficacy of DA antagonists; studies of hallucinogens and antipsychotics suggest a role for *serotonin*; effects of phencyclidine (PCP; NMDA glutamate antagonist) and glutamate receptor agonists suggest a role for *glutamate* in pathogenesis of schizophrenia
    d. Diagnosis
       i. *At least 1 month of two of the following symptoms:* delusions, hallucinations, disorganized speech, disorganized behavior or catatonia
       ii. Social and/or occupational decline
    e. Differential diagnosis
       i. *Brief psychotic disorder: 1 month or less* of one psychotic symptom
       ii. *Schizophreniform disorder: 1–6 months* of schizophrenia
       iii. *Schizoaffective disorder:* schizophrenia with criteria simultaneously met for major depressive and/or manic episode
       iv. *Delusional disorder:* at least 1 month of *nonbizarre* delusions, without other symptoms of schizophrenia

     v. *Shared psychotic disorder (folie à deux):* a psychotic individual draws another into believing his/her delusions

  f. Course of illness

    i. Onset: 2nd decade in men; 3rd or 5th decade in women

    ii. Usually less severe in women

    iii. *Progressive decline in social, cognitive, and occupational function*

    iv. Prevention of exacerbations may slow deterioration

    v. *10% die of suicide; 50% attempt suicide*

    vi. *Most common cause of exacerbations is treatment noncompliance*

  g. Treatment

    i. Antipsychotic medication: *atypical agents are 1st-line treatment because of their reduced risk of EPS and TD;* patient must be informed about risk of TDs; intramuscular depot agents increase compliance

    ii. Augmenting agents include antimanic agents and benzodiazepines

    iii. Social support (housing, employment, group therapy)

C. **Anxiety disorders:** almost all can be treated with benzodiazepines and/or antidepressants

  1. Evidence for neurotransmitter involvement

    a. NE

      i. Ablation of locus ceruleus in primates abolishes fear.

      ii. β-Agonists and α_2 antagonists can induce panic in humans.

    b. Serotonin (5-HT)

      i. Serotonergic agents (SSRIs, tricyclics) are effective for treating anxiety.

      ii. Rapid titration of SSRI can cause acute anxiety.

    c. GABA

      i. GABA agonists can immediately relieve anxiety.

      ii. Flumazenil (GABA antagonist) can rapidly induce panic attacks.

      iii. Withdrawal from barbiturates or benzodiazepines causes anxiety.

  2. Anxiety caused by medical illness or medications

    a. Neurologic: Parkinson's, multiple sclerosis, neoplasm, stroke, migraine

    b. General medical: pheochromocytoma, allergic reactions, syphilis, carcinoid

    c. Medications: steroids, stimulants (xanthines), thyroid hormone

  3. Descriptions of the anxiety disorder diagnoses

    a. **Panic disorder:** recurrent unexpected panic attacks

      i. *Panic attack:* abrupt onset and peak (within 10 minutes) of four of the following: cardiac symptoms, sweating, tremor, dyspnea, choking, chest discomfort, GI distress, dizziness, derealization/depersonalization, fear of losing control, fear of dying, paresthesias, chills, or hot flushes

      ii. Can occur with or without *agoraphobia* (fear and avoidance of being in situations from which escape might be difficult or embarrassing)

      iii. May be an overreaction to internal fight-or-flight cues; breathing CO_2 can induce panic attacks in susceptible individuals; lactate infusion may cause panic attacks

      iv. Treatment: *antidepressants are the drugs of choice—start at low dose and titrate slowly, because they can induce panic attacks,* they take a few weeks to establish maximum effect; *benzodiazepines* work most rapidly—they are often started concurrently with an antidepressant and tapered after a few weeks; psychotherapy (cognitive therapy, relaxation, exposure/desensitization)

    b. **Phobias:** irrational fear of a subject or situation

      i. *Specific phobia:* a particular object or situation causes immediate and disabling anxiety. The anxiety or the patient's avoidance of the situation interferes significantly with his/her activities or daily functioning.

    ii. *Social phobia:* similar to specific phobia but cued by situations in which the patient feels he/she will be scrutinized or embarrassed.

    iii. Phobia is the most common psychiatric disorder in the United States.

    iv. Treatment: medications: antidepressants, benzodiazepines, → blockers; therapy: hypnosis, exposure/response-prevention, cognitive.

  c. **Obsessive-compulsive disorder (OCD)**

    i. *Obsession:* intrusive and recurrent sensation, fear, or idea that produces anxiety even though the patient recognizes that it is irrational (e.g., fear of contamination, irrational self-doubt, need for symmetry)

    ii. *Compulsion:* conscious, stereotyped behavior that often decreases anxiety when it is carried out (e.g., washing hands, counting ceiling tiles)

    iii. Prevalence: 2–3%

    iv. Treatment: serotonin reuptake inhibitors (clomipramine, SSRIs) are 1st-line treatment; benzodiazepines can be used as augmentation; DA blockade (risperidone, haloperidol); cognitive behavioral therapy may be as effective as medications

  d. **Post-traumatic stress disorder:** diagnostic features

    i. *Exposure* to an event involving a threat of serious injury to self or others. During the event, the person felt terrified, horrified, or helpless.

    ii. *Re-experiencing* of the event through: nightmares, flashbacks, dissociation, event-related hallucinations, or excessive reactivity when exposed to reminders.

    iii. *Avoidance* of stimuli associated with the event: patients may avoid any thoughts, activities, conversations, places, or people that recall the event; they may fail to recollect an important aspect of the trauma.

    iv. *General emotional numbing,* as exemplified by restricted affect, detachment from others, decreased participation in significant activities, and no expectations/hopes about the future.

    v. *Increased arousal,* exhibited as exaggerated startle, insomnia, irritability, poor concentration, and hypervigilance.

    vi. Treatment: there is no clearly established or overwhelmingly effective treatment; antidepressants: paroxetine, sertraline, venlafaxine, imipramine, amitriptyline; symptom-directed treatments: anxiety may be treated with benzodiazepines, insomnia can be addressed with sedatives and hypnotics, sedating antidepressants (e.g., trazodone, mirtazapine); flashbacks and hallucinations sometimes respond to antipsychotics; hyperarousal can be muted with clonidine (Catapres®), → blockers; aggression/agitation: antipsychotics, antimanic agents, antidepressants.

  e. **Generalized anxiety disorder**: diagnosis

    i. Persistent and excessive anxiety on most days, for at least 6 months

    ii. Lack of control over the anxiety

    iii. At least three of the following: restlessness, easy fatigability, poor concentration, irritability, muscle tension, insomnia

    iv. Treatment: antidepressants, buspirone, benzodiazepines (use on a limited basis)

D. **Substance-related disorders:** the board examination tends to focus on symptoms of withdrawal and intoxication and their treatment; however, you should also be familiar with persistent neurologic deficits that can be caused by substances of abuse and associated conditions (such as nutritional deficiency states)

  1. **EtOH**

    a. Epidemiology

      i. 10% of Americans who drink are alcoholic (they consume 50% of all alcohol).

      ii. Men 3× more likely to be affected with EtOH-related disorder.

      iii. EtOH is involved in 30% of suicides, 50% of homicides, 41% of highway crashes, and 86% of highway deaths.

      iv. EtOH accounts for 25% of hospitalizations in the United States (third, behind heart disease and cancer).

  b. Pharmacology

      i. Unknown neuronal effects. Some believe that EtOH causes *changes in cell membranes,* perhaps acutely increasing their fluidity, but chronically causing rigidity; *potentiation of GABA neurotransmission* is suspected, because of the similar effects of EtOH, benzodiazepines, and barbiturates. *GABA agonists are the only reliable treatment for EtOH withdrawal.*

      ii. Metabolism:

        (A) EtOH—[*EtOH dehydrogenase*] → acetaldehyde—[*aldehyde dehydrogenase*] → acetic acid

        (B) Average metabolism is 15 mg/dL/hour (faster in men and in chronic drinkers)

        (C) 90% metabolized by the liver; 10% excreted unchanged in breath and urine

        (D) Lower amount of serum EtOH dehydrogenase in women and some Asian populations causes easier intoxication

        (E) Aldehyde dehydrogenase deficiency (Asian populations) may cause quicker toxicity

        (F) Chronic alcohol users upregulate EtOH-metabolizing enzymes

  c. Intoxication

      i. *Legal limit for driving is 0.08% in most states*

      ii. General symptoms (blood alcohol concentration >0.05%): dysarthria, disinhibition, facial flushing, aggression, mood lability, posture/gait instability, impaired attention and judgment

      iii. "Blackouts" (conscious amnestic periods)

      iv. Severe symptoms: hypotension, hypothermia, loss of gag reflex

      v. Treatment

        (A) Supportive: *airway protection, fluid resuscitation, electrolyte replacement, nutrition,* warming

        (B) Protective: *thiamine* (to prevent Wernicke's encephalopathy), antipsychotics for agitation/aggression

        (C) Evaluate for presence of other substances

  d. EtOH withdrawal (can last for 14 days)

      i. Typical progression

        (A) Tremor (4–8 hours after last drink) is the earliest, most common symptom.

        (B) Autonomic arousal (6–8 hours): anxiety, agitation; tachycardia, mild hypertension; facial flushing, diaphoresis, mydriasis; *may be treated with clonidine or β blockers.*

        (C) Agitation, perceptual disturbances (8–12 hours).

        (D) Seizures (12–36 hours): EtOH withdrawal seizures are generalized. A *partial seizure should raise suspicion for an underlying CNS lesion or seizure disorder;* treat with parenteral benzodiazepines. Other antiepileptics are unnecessary and sometimes ineffective; *failure of benzodiazepines should initiate a search for other causes for the seizures.*

      ii. **Treatment of uncomplicated EtOH withdrawal**

        (A) Benzodiazepines: lorazepam (Ativan®), 2–4 mg q2–4h; chlordiazepoxide (Librium®), 25–50 mg q2–4h; diazepam (Valium®), 15–30 mg tid

(B) Antipsychotics: for severe agitation or hallucinations if benzodiazepines are ineffective; haloperidol, 1–2 mg q4h

iii. **Delirium tremens** (*72 hours to 1 week*)

(A) Occurs in 5% of hospitalized alcoholics

(B) *Mortality 20%;* death usually caused by intercurrent illness: cardiovascular collapse, pneumonia, renal or hepatic insufficiency

(C) Can appear without prior signs of withdrawal

(D) Rarely occurs in otherwise healthy individuals

(E) Hallmark symptoms: fluctuating arousal, from excitability to lethargy; autonomic instability; severe perceptual disturbances, paranoia, anxiety; dehydration, electrolyte imbalances

(F) Treatment: aggressive pharmacologic treatment for withdrawal; reduce stimulation (private room, lights low, reassurance); supportive care (hydration, correction of electrolyte and autonomic abnormalities)

e. **Other EtOH-related syndromes**

i. **Thiamine (B$_1$) deficiency syndromes**

(A) *Wernicke's encephalopathy:* develops over hours to days; pathology: petechial hemorrhages of periventricular structures; extrinsic oculomotor nuclei (III, VI); vestibular nuclei, cerebellar vermis; *clinical triad:* confusion, ophthalmoparesis (usually cranial nerve VI palsy), and gait disturbance (wide-based, lurching); treatment: *large doses (100–200 mg intravenously/intramuscularly qd) of thiamine for 3 days, glucose should not be given without thiamine*

NB: There may also be damage to the mamillary nucleus.

(B) *Korsakoff's amnesia:* the chronic stage of Wernicke-Korsakoff syndrome; pathology: lesions of Wernicke's, damage to inferomedial temporal lobes, thalamus, mamillary bodies; clinical features: anterograde and retrograde amnesia; disorientation, *other cognitive functions relatively preserved, confabulation* sometimes prominent, sometimes absent; treatment: *abstinence* from alcohol for life, *supplemental thiamine,* long-term nutritional support; improvement possible, but patients do not usually return to baseline

(C) *Beriberi:* develops over weeks to months; length-dependent *axonal* polyneuropathy (wallerian degeneration): frequent clinical features: paresthesias and/or pain of lower extremities, distal muscle weakness, decreased distal reflexes; other clinical features: cardiac dysfunction (tachycardia, palpitations, dyspnea), wet beriberi: pedal edema due to cardiac failure, blindness (optic neuropathy), hoarseness (laryngeal nerve dysfunction)

ii. **Niacin (B$_3$) deficiency—pellagra**

(A) Mnemonic: five Ds—dermatitis, *d*iarrhea, *d*elirium, *d*ementia, *d*eath

(B) Psychiatric: irritability, insomnia, depression, delirium

(C) Medical/neurologic: dermatitis, peripheral neuropathy, diarrhea

iii. **Fetal alcohol syndrome**

(A) Caused by fetal exposure to EtOH: usually occurs when mother drinks >80 g EtOH/day; milder forms are possible in social- or binge-drinking mothers

(B) **NB:** *Leading known cause of mental retardation in United States*

(C) Second most common cause of agenesis of corpus callosum

(D) Clinical features: growth retardation (height and weight <10th percentile); craniofacial anomalies: short palpebral fissures, smooth and/or long philtrum, thin upper lip; any of a number of cerebral abnormalities: developmental delay, hyperactivity, seizures

      (E) Prognosis: facial features become less prominent over time; small size and developmental delay persist

  iv. **Cerebellar degeneration**

      (A) EtOH is the most common cause of cerebellar degeneration

      (B) Progresses subacutely, over weeks to months

      (C) Pathology: atrophy of cerebellum, most prominent in vermis; cell loss, particularly among Purkinje cells

      (D) Clinical features: marked truncal ataxia; other signs of cerebellar dysfunction are usually absent; if limb ataxia is present, legs are worse than arms

      (E) Treatment: *abstinence* from EtOH and adequate nutrition

  v. **Marchiafava-Bignami disease**

      (A) *Demyelination of the middle portion of corpus callosum*

      (B) Variable presentations: bilateral frontal lobe dysfunction; sexual disinhibition

  vi. **Alcohol-induced persistent dementia:** it is unclear whether the dementia results specifically from exposure of the brain to EtOH, or from the accumulation of known effects of EtOH on all organ systems, combined with chronic nutritional deficiencies, CNS trauma (e.g., from falls, fights, or automobile accidents), and other maladies that affect alcoholics; cause notwithstanding, patients with chronic EtOH use often develop early and severe dementia

  vii. **Neuropathy:** clinically indistinguishable from neuropathy of beriberi

NB: Chronic alcoholic hallucinosis consists of auditory hallucinations that may persist during sobriety.

  2. **Amphetamine and related stimulants**

    a. Types

      i. "Classic" stimulants: dextroamphetamine (Dexedrine®), methamphetamine (Desoxyn®), methylphenidate (Ritalin®)

      ii. "Designer" stimulants: *3,4-methylenedioxy methamphetamine (Ecstasy),* N-ethyl-3,4-methylenedioxyamphetamine (MDEA), 5-methyoxy-3,4-methylenedioxyamphetimine (MMDA), 2,5-dimethoxy-4-methylamphetamine (DOM)

    b. Epidemiology

      i. Experimental use in 2% of general population

      ii. Young adults particularly affected (9% of 18–25 y/o report use)

    c. Pharmacology

      i. **NB:** *Classic drugs increase presynaptic release of catecholamines (DA > NE).*

      ii. Designer drugs cause catecholamine release, but additional 5-HT release probably makes them more hallucinogenic.

    d. Intoxication

      i. Behavioral symptoms: euphoria or affective blunting, hypervigilance, anxiety/tension/anger, stereotypies, poor judgment, *psychotic paranoia*

      ii. Physiologic symptoms (*autonomic arousal*): tachycardia/bradycardia, mydriasis, altered blood pressure, weight loss, diaphoresis, chills, dyskinesia, dystonia

      iii. Severe symptoms: seizures, respiratory depression, cardiac dysrhythmias, myocardial infarction

      iv. Symptoms typically resolve within 48 hours

    e. Withdrawal

      i. Progresses to peak in 72 hours, resolves in approximately 1 week

ii. Depression, suicidality, anxiety, tremulousness, lethargy, fatigue, nightmares, GI cramping, severe hunger

iii. The best-documented cases of substance-induced *cerebral vasculitis* have occurred in amphetamine users

3. **Caffeine**
    a. Epidemiology
        i. An average American adult consumes 200 mg caffeine per day.
        ii. 20–30% of adults consume >500 mg/day.
    b. Pharmacology: belongs to the methylxanthine family; acts as an antagonist at inhibitory G-coupled adenosine receptor, thus increasing intraneuronal cyclic adenosine monophosphate formation; probably hyperactivates DA and NE neurons
    c. Intoxication: restlessness, nervousness, insomnia, facial flushing, diuresis, GI disturbance, muscle twitching, tachycardia, agitation
    d. Withdrawal: headache, fatigue, depression, impaired motor performance, caffeine craving

4. **Marijuana (cannabis)**
    a. Epidemiology
        i. Probably the world's most-used illicit substance
        ii. 4.7% of the population >11 y/o have used in the past month
        iii. 2.5% of the population use >50 days per year
    b. Pharmacology
        i. Tetrahydrocannabinol binds to inhibitory G-protein–linked *cannabinoid receptors (hippocampus, basal ganglia, cerebellum)*
        ii. Affects monoamine and GABA neurons
    c. Intoxication
        i. Variable effects
        ii. Behavioral: ataxia, *euphoria, silliness,* temporal distortion, *poor judgment,* perceptual distortions
        iii. Physiologic: *conjunctival injection, hunger, dry mouth,* tachycardia
        iv. Euphoria from acute dose lasts up to 4 hours; psychomotor symptoms may last for 12 hours
    d. No well-recognized withdrawal syndrome, although chronic users can have psychologic dependence
    e. Other marijuana-related syndromes
        i. May cause a depression-like state with chronic use (*apathy,* decreased energy, sleep disturbance, poor attention/concentration, weight gain)
        ii. Can cause psychosis or anxiety
        iii. Causes acute and chronic pulmonary effects similar to tobacco smoking

5. **Cocaine**
    a. Epidemiology
        i. Used by approximately 0.7% of population >11 y/o
        ii. Frequent use by 0.3% of users (thus, almost one-half of all users are addicted)
        iii. Highest use in 18–25 y/o age group (1.3% reported use)
    b. Pharmacology
        i. Can be injected, smoked ("freebasing" or smoking "crack rocks"), inhaled (by "snorting" or "tooting" the fine powder), ingested (rarely)
        ii. **NB:** *Blocks presynaptic DA reuptake,* causing hyperactivation of mesolimbic dopaminergic system

   c. Intoxication
      i. Behavioral: euphoria, *hypervigilance, tension/anger,* poor judgment, hallucinations and paranoia, impulsivity, hypersexuality
      ii. Physiologic: *tachycardia, mydriasis, hypertension, weight loss, psychomotor agitation*
      iii. Severe: seizures, delirium, movement disorders, coma
      iv. Treatment: antipsychotics for paranoia, agitation, and hallucinations
   d. Withdrawal: depression and suicidality, fatigue, nightmares, altered sleep, increased appetite, psychomotor changes
   e. Other cocaine-related syndromes
      i. Cocaine is the most important cause of drug-related cerebrovascular accident: most often causes ischemic lesions; infarction can occur hours to days after use; spinal ischemia can be a complication of cocaine use
      ii. *Seizures* account for approximately 5% of cocaine-related emergency department visits
      iii. Users are at risk for *myocardial infarction,* dysrhythmias, cardiomyopathy
      iv. May cause cerebral vasculitis

6. **Hallucinogens**
   a. Synthetic: *lysergic acid diethylamide*
   b. Natural: *mescaline* (peyote cactus), *psilocybin* (mushrooms)
   c. Epidemiology: most commonly used by young adults (~1% report recent use)
   d. *Pharmacology*
      i. Data based on findings from lysergic acid diethylamide in animals
      ii. **NB:** Postsynaptic *5-HT receptor agonist*
      iii. Acute effects last 8–12 hours
   e. No recognized dependence or withdrawal syndrome; tolerance develops rapidly with continual use
   f. Intoxication
      i. Behavioral: anxiety/depression, paranoia, poor judgment, fear of losing one's mind
      ii. Perceptual: derealization, intensification of sensory experiences, hallucinations, illusions, synesthesia
      iii. Physiologic: diaphoresis, tachycardia, mydriasis, tremor, ataxia
      iv. Treatment: gentle reassurance ("talking down"), antipsychotics

7. **PCP**
   a. Pharmacology
      i. May be smoked (usually with marijuana) or injected
      ii. Effects peak in 30 minutes, can last for weeks
      iii. **NB:** Acts as *antagonist at NMDA glutamate receptor*
      iv. Also activates dopaminergic neurons in ventral tegmentum
   b. Intoxication
      i. Behavioral: *assaultiveness, belligerence, paranoia,* impulsivity, poor judgment, hypersexuality, inappropriate laughter, amnesia
      ii. *Physiologic:* **NB:** *vertical or horizontal nystagmus, hypertension, tachycardia, decreased pain response,* ataxia, dysarthria, seizures, hyperacusis, muscle rigidity, excess salivation
      iii. Patients can be extremely dangerous and often exhibit seemingly superhuman strength
      iv. Treatment

(A) Supportive: observe for rhabdomyolysis (from rigidity and hyperactivity), hydrate, decrease stimulation, attempt "talking down," protect airway

(B) Pharmacologic

    (1) Benzodiazepines: preferred for muscle spasms and seizures

    (2) DA blockade (antipsychotic): may be necessary to treat aggression

8. **Inhalants:** volatile substances (glue, solvents, aerosol propellants, thinners, fuel) and nitrous oxide

a. Epidemiology

    i. More common in whites, the poor, and adolescents

    ii. Account for 1% of all substance-related deaths (respiratory depression, cardiac dysrhythmias, aspiration)

b. Pharmacology

    i. May be sniffed or "huffed" (inhaled orally) from a tube, soaked rag, or plastic bag

    ii. Effects peak in minutes, may last for hours with repeated inhalations

    iii. Mechanism of action unknown: may enhance GABA activity or alter cell membranes

c. Intoxication

    i. Behavioral: belligerence, assaultiveness, apathy, poor judgment, euphoria, psychosis, sensory distortions

    ii. Physiologic: dizziness, nystagmus, dysarthria, tremor, lethargy, ataxia, coma

d. Other inhalant-related syndromes

    i. **NB:** *Neurologic*

        (A) **NB:** Subacute combined degeneration (nitrous oxide)

        (B) Lead intoxication (gasoline)

        (C) **NB:** Peripheral neuropathy (n-hexane)

        (D) Dementia, epilepsy, brain atrophy

    ii. General medical: renal failure, hepatic failure, fetal effects

9. **Nicotine**

a. Epidemiology

    i. 25% of Americans smoke

    ii. 1 billion smokers worldwide

    iii. Accounts for 60% of health care costs in the United States

    iv. Associated with 400,000 U.S. deaths per year

        (A) 25% of all deaths

        (B) 30% of cancer deaths (most lethal carcinogen)

    v. Demographics

        (A) Rate of smoking in women now almost equals rate in men

        (B) No race difference

        (C) Inverse correlation with education (17% of college grads vs. 37% of individuals who did not finish high school)

        (D) 50% in psychiatric patients (70% and 90% in bipolar I and schizophrenia, respectively)

b. **Pharmacology**

    i. Acts as an *agonist at nicotinic ACh* receptors

    ii. Increases concentration of circulating catecholamines

    iii. Increases mesolimbic dopaminergic activity

    iv. Most commonly used form is tobacco, which can be smoked or chewed

   c. Intoxication (no specific criteria defined by the 4th edition of the *Diagnostic and Statistical Manual of Mental Disorders*)
- i. Behavioral: improved concentration and attention, decreased reaction time, elevation of mood
- ii. Physiologic: increased heart rate, increased cerebral blood flow, relaxation of skeletal muscle
- iii. Toxicity: sialorrhea, diaphoresis, increased peristalsis, tachycardia, confusion

   d. Withdrawal
- i. Occurs within 24 hours of cessation
- ii. Depressed mood, insomnia, irritability, restlessness, poor concentration, decreased heart rate, hunger, or weight gain

   e. Other nicotine-related syndromes
- i. Direct
  - (A) Lung cancer (8× risk; 106,000 deaths per year)
  - (B) Emphysema, chronic bronchitis (51,000 deaths per year)
  - (C) Oropharyngeal cancer (from chewing tobacco)
- ii. Indirect
  - (A) *Increases risk of ischemic stroke 2–3×*
  - (B) 35% of myocardial infarctions are partially attributed to smoking
  - (C) Increases risk of bladder, esophageal, pancreatic, stomach, kidney, liver cancer

   f. Treatment of dependence
- i. Nicotine replacement, with gum or patch
- ii. Encouragement from nonsmoking physician is correlated with abstinence
- iii. Decrease nicotine withdrawal symptoms
  - (A) Bupropion (Zyban®) approved by U.S. Food and Drug Administration (FDA)
  - (B) Clonidine, fluoxetine, buspirone may be helpful

10. **Opioids**

   a. Epidemiology
- i. Heroin is the most commonly abused opioid (1.3% of population have used).
- ii. 90% of opioid abusers have another psychiatric diagnosis.
- iii. Tolerance and dependence can develop rapidly, even in individuals who are using prescription opioids appropriately.
- iv. Opioid use disorders are 3× more common in males.

   b. Pharmacology
- i. Opioids: available in injectable, smokeable, and ingestible forms
- ii. Opioid receptors
  - (A) μ Receptor: analgesia, respiratory depression, constipation, dependence
  - (B) κ Receptor: analgesia, diuresis, sedation
  - (C) δ Receptor: analgesia (?)
  - (D) Also inhibit locus ceruleus (noradrenergic) activity
- iii. Addiction probably mediated through enhanced mesolimbic dopaminergic transmission
- iv. *Endogenous opioids* (endorphins and enkephalins): related to euphoria, pain suppression, and neural transmission; released on injury

   c. *Intoxication*
- i. Behavioral: euphoria followed by apathy, poor judgment, psychomotor changes (usually retardation)
- ii. Physiologic: *miosis, constipation,* dysarthria, drowsiness, impaired cognition

d. *Withdrawal*
  i. *Physiologic withdrawal: an expected phenomenon, regardless of the reason (recreational or therapeutic) for opioid use*
  ii. Withdrawal may develop within minutes of cessation, usually peaks in 2 days; with meperidine (Demerol®), withdrawal symptoms can peak in 12 hours
  iii. Symptoms: dysphoria, *nausea/vomiting*, diarrhea, *lacrimation/rhinorrhea, yawning, mydriasis*, piloerection ("cold turkey"), diaphoresis, *myalgia*, headache, autonomic instability, *severe opioid craving*
  iv. Opioid withdrawal, although intensely uncomfortable, is *not life threatening*
e. **NB:** *Toxicity*
  i. *Symptoms: pinpoint pupils, respiratory depression, coma, vascular shock*
  ii. *Treatment*
    (A) Supportive: airway protection, telemetry, cardiovascular support
    (B) *Opioid antagonist—naloxone (Narcan®), 0.4 mg intravenously*
      (1) Doses may be repeated to total dose of 2 mg in 45 minutes
      (2) Can induce instant and severe withdrawal syndrome
      (3) *Short $t_{1/2}$—patient on long-acting opioid may suddenly relapse into coma*
f. Other opioid-related syndromes
  i. **NB:** Meperidine can induce seizures
  ii. *Needle-related complications*
    (A) *Most common and most dangerous complication of opioid use*
    (B) *Transmission of human immunodeficiency virus and hepatitis*
    (C) *Infective endocarditis* (20% progress to have stroke)
    (D) Abscesses at injection points
    (E) Injection and embolism of crushed pills
  iii. May cause CNS vasculitis
  iv. Anoxia and ischemia from respiratory/cardiovascular collapse
  v. The best-documented cases of substance-induced *myelopathy* have occurred in heroin users; resembles anterior spinal artery syndrome
  vi. *1-Methyl-4-phenyl-1,2,3,6-tetrahydropyridine (MPTP)*
    (A) Synthetic opioid manufactured in the 1970s
    (B) Converted in vivo to MPP+, a toxin taken up by dopaminergic neurons
    (C) *Induces parkinsonism*
g. Treatment of dependence
  i. Gradual decrease of opioid dosage
    (A) Clonidine to control withdrawal symptoms
    (B) Usually unsuccessful if not monitored closely
  ii. Replacement opioid
    (A) Methadone most frequently used
      (1) Eliminates needle-related complications
      (2) Easier to detoxify than heroin or morphine
      (3) Produces minimal euphoria or drowsiness but prevents withdrawal
      (4) Problems
        (a) Patient remains narcotic dependent.
        (b) In some programs, the patient must obtain the daily dose at clinic.
    (B) Buprenorphine (Subutex®) recently approved for detoxification
    (C) Levo-α-acetylmethadol is longer-acting than methadone and can be taken every other day
  iii. Opioid antagonist

(A) Attempt to decrease opiate use by blocking pleasant effects
(B) Naltrexone (ReVia®) has $t_{1/2}$ 72 hours
(C) Requires strong motivation and compliance from patient

Quick Reference Chart: Substances of Abuse

Substance	Receptor or neurotransmitter	Urine detection	Neurologic acute	Toxicity chronic
Alcohol	Cell membrane, GABA receptor	N/A	Wernicke	Korsakoff, beriberi, cerebellar atrophy, dementia, neuropathy
Amphet-amine	Catecholamine release	48 hrs	Seizures	Vasculitis
Caffeine	Adenosine antagonist	N/A	None	None
Marijuana	Cannabinoid receptor, GABA, catecholamines	4–5 days	None	None
Cocaine	Inhibits DA reuptake	48 hrs	Cerebrovas-cular accident, spinal ischemia	Vasculitis
Hallucino-gens	5-HT receptor agonist	N/A	None	None
PCP	NMDA antagonist	14 days	Rhabdomyolysis	None
Inhalants	Cell membrane, GABA receptor (?)	N/A	None (?)	Neuropathy, sub-acute combined degeneration, lead poisoning, dementia, epilepsy
Nicotine	Nicotinic ACh agonist	N/A	None	Cerebrovascular accident
Opioids	Opioid receptors	2–5 days[a]	Coma	Human immunode-ficiency virus, myelopathy, embolic stroke
Benzodiaz-epines[b]	GABA inducer	5–7 days[a]	None	Psychomotor slowing
Barbiturates[b]	GABA inducer	1–7 days[a]	None	None

N/A, not applicable.
[a]Depends on $t_{1/2}$ of specific compound.
[b]For more information on benzodiazepines and barbiturates, refer to the section on anxiolytics.

E. **Somatoform disorders:** these illnesses present with *physical complaints for which there is no adequate physiologic or anatomic explanation;* they are presumed to *allow patients to express their psychological discomfort in a culturally acceptable fashion* (i.e., physical illness); they may be present in up to *15% of patients in primary care settings;* in somatoform disorders, the *symptoms are not feigned or consciously produced;* the patients are subconsciously seeking *primary gain,* the resolution of internal conflict

1. **Somatization disorder** (preoccupation with *multiple, diffuse symptoms*)
   a. Demographics: young; female (20:1)
   b. Description: 2 years of more than five physical symptoms that are not fully explained by any detectable abnormality; the review of systems (particularly GI, genitourinary, cardiovascular, neurologic) is extremely positive; the patient is unable to accept medical reassurances of good health for more than a few weeks
   c. **NB:** *Treatment:* regular appointments, regardless of symptoms, will reduce the patient's need for "crisis" appointments
2. **Hypochondriacal disorder** (preoccupation with having *a particular defined disease*)
   a. Demographics: middle aged or elderly; history of physical illness; no gender specificity
   b. Description: at least 5 months of persistent preoccupation about having no more than two serious medical illnesses; worry about the illness impairs function or causes distress and *cannot be alleviated by medical reassurance*
   c. Treatment: avoid tests and treatment for nonobjective signs; regular appointments to reassure the patient he/she is not being abandoned
3. **Body dysmorphic disorder** (preoccupation with an *imagined flaw*)
   a. Demographics: usually begins in 2nd or 3rd decade of life
   b. Most frequent body parts are hair, nose, skin, and eyes
   c. Treatment: antidepressants, stress management techniques
4. **Conversion disorder** (presentation with a *pseudoneurologic symptom*)
   a. Demographics: more prevalent in rural, poorly educated, and low socioeconomic classes; female predominant; psychologically immature
   b. Description: patient presents with sudden onset of blindness, paralysis, numbness, etc., that does not follow a known physiologic pattern; the onset is often preceded by a psychologically conflicting event or situation; patients sometimes seem strangely unconcerned *(la belle indifférence)*
   c. Treatment: reassurance, symptom-directed therapy (e.g., physical therapy for paralysis), psychotherapy; *do not tell patients their symptoms are imaginary;* prognosis excellent with prompt therapy
F. **Factitious disorder**
   1. Symptoms are consciously feigned, but for primary gain (assuming the sick role)
   2. May also be *by proxy* (Münchhausen syndrome), in which the mentally ill person causes signs and symptoms in another (usually mother inflicts illness on child)
G. **Malingering:** symptoms are consciously feigned for a conscious *secondary gain*, such as financial gain, avoiding work, or escaping legal consequences.

Quick Reference Chart: Patients with Pseudosymptoms

	Conversion	Factitious	Malingering
Feigned symptoms	−	+	+
Conscious gain	−	−	+

+, present; −, absent.

H. **Dissociative disorders:**
   1. **Dissociative fugue**: patient goes on an unexpected journey away from familiar surroundings; behavior is organized, and self-care is maintained; he/she often experiences

amnesia for his/her prior identity during the trip, and amnesia about the journey once he/she returns home

2. **Dissociative identity disorder**: *"multiple personality disorder,"* the presence of multiple personality states that recurrently take control of the patient's behavior; each personality has its own distinct preferences and memories that may be inaccessible to the other personalities

I. **Eating disorders:**

1. *Anorexia nervosa*

   a. Diagnosis

      i. Refusal to maintain body weight *>85% of expected*

      ii. Irrational fear of gaining weight

      iii. Self-image influenced by *distorted perception* of weight and/or shape

      iv. *Amenorrhea*

   b. Treatment

      i. Medical: restore nutritional status, rehydrate, correct electrolyte imbalances

      ii. Psychiatric: psychotherapy, behavioral management; *no reliable medication*

2. *Bulimia nervosa*

   a. Diagnosis

      i. Recurrent episodes of eating a larger-than-normal amount during a discrete period, with a feeling of distress and lack of control over the binges

      ii. Compensation for bingeing (vomiting, excessive exercise, laxative abuse, fasting)

      iii. Self-esteem unduly influenced by weight and shape (patients are often normal or slightly overweight)

   b. Treatment

      i. Medical: sequelae of vomiting (dental decay, esophageal erosions, gastritis, hypokalemia, metabolic alkalosis) and laxative overuse (hemorrhoids, fissures) should be evaluated and repaired

      ii. Psychiatric: psychotherapy, antidepressant medications (not bupropion)

J. **Personality disorders:** these disorders describe an individual's pattern of responding to people and events in his/her environment; usually formed early in life and tend to be predictable and durable; patients with personality disorders do not recognize the maladaptive nature of their behaviors; treatment consists mainly of psychotherapy; medications are used to treat symptoms or comorbidities.

1. **Cluster A:** odd, suspicious

   a. *Paranoid:* suspects deception in others; doubts loyalty of friends and partner; believes others intend malice; persistently bears grudges; perceives nonexistent attacks on character/reputation; reads threats or injuries into benign statements

   b. *Schizoid:* no desire for close interpersonal relationships; chooses solitary activities; little interest in sex; little pleasure; few nonfamilial friends; indifferent to others' opinions; emotionally cold

   c. *Schizotypal:* ideas of reference; magical thinking or odd beliefs; perceptual distortions; odd thinking and speech; paranoia; inappropriate affect; unusual behavior; few close friends; social anxiety

2. **Cluster B:** dramatic, impulsive

   a. *Histrionic:* strives to be center of attention; sexually provocative behavior; shifting, shallow emotions; uses physical appearance to draw attention; impressionistic speech; theatrical; suggestible; overvalues relationships

   b. *Narcissistic:* inflated self-importance; fantasizes about unlimited success, power, or ideal love; believes he/she is special and should only associate with other special people; requires admiration; entitled; treats others as objects to satisfy his/her needs; lacks empathy; envious or suspects others of envying him/her; arrogant attitude

  c. *Antisocial:* repeated unlawful acts; deceitfulness; impulsivity; aggressiveness; irresponsibility; disregard for safety of self or others; lack of remorse; *history of conduct disorder as a child*

  d. *Borderline:* frantic avoidance of perceived abandonment; unstable and intense relationships; unstable self-image; impulsivity; recurrent suicidal behavior or self-mutilation; affective instability; chronic feelings of emptiness; difficulty controlling anger; stress-related paranoia or dissociation

NB: Instability of mood is the most consistent finding in borderline personality disorder.

 3. **Cluster C:** anxious

  a. *Avoidant:* avoids activities involving interpersonal contact; unwilling to form friendship unless assured of being liked; fears shame/ridicule in intimate relationships; preoccupied with fears of criticism/rejection; feels inadequate in new situations; poor self-image; does not take risks that may cause embarrassment

  b. *Dependent:* requires reassurance/advice to make decisions; needs others to be responsible for his/her life; unable to express disagreement; unable to initiate projects him/herself; does anything for approval of others; uncomfortable when alone; must be involved in relationship; preoccupied with fears of having to take care of him/herself

  c. *Obsessive compulsive: not related to obsessive-compulsive disorder;* preoccupation with rules, details, order instead of the main point; perfectionism interferes with progress; excessively devoted to work; inflexible about morality, ethics, or values; unable to discard worthless objects; reluctant to delegate; miserly; rigid and stubborn

III. Medical Ethics in Psychiatry: for the most part, laws governing ethical conduct are state specific; we have included some general principles that guide appropriate behavior vis-à-vis psychiatric patients.

 A. Informed consent
  1. Issues of informed consent are usually taken more seriously in psychiatry than in other fields, because patients with mental illnesses are vulnerable to exploitation
  2. Definitions
   a. Capacity: the ability to make informed decisions
    i. Mental illness is only one factor that can affect a patient's capacity.
    ii. Any physician can submit an opinion about whether a patient has capacity; a psychiatrist is usually asked to decide whether mental illness limits the patient's capacity.
    iii. Patients may have capacity for directing some aspects of care and lack capacity for others.
   b. Competence: a *judicial determination* about whether a patient is authorized to make decisions; if the patient is judged incompetent, a guardian is assigned to make decisions *in the patient's best interest*
  3. Consent for hospitalization
   a. In most states, a person being admitted to a psychiatric ward must give written consent to his/her admission, general medical treatment, and, *specifically,* for psychiatric treatment.
   b. When a patient requires hospitalization but is unable to give informed consent, a legal mechanism allows for involuntary admission to the hospital. In general, this

requires evidence that the patient has a mental illness *and* presents an *imminent* risk of harm to him/herself or others.

    c. *A patient's acceptance of hospitalization or treatment does not qualify as informed consent for hospitalization or treatment.*

        i. The patient must understand the reason for his/her hospitalization and treatment.

        ii. The patient must understand the likely outcome of accepting or refusing treatment.

    4. The presence of a severe mental illness does not automatically indicate that a patient lacks capacity to make decisions concerning his/her psychiatric or medical care

B. **Privacy**

    1. As with all medical records, privacy should be preserved at all costs.

    2. Health Insurance Privacy and Portability Act (HIPPA) guidelines *do* allow exchange of information to improve patient care, for operational purposes, and for third-party payment.

    3. The requirement to inform a potential victim of a psychiatric patient's intent to harm him/her was established in California in the *Tarasoff* case; that ruling, however, did not establish the same requirement in other states.

C. **Restraints**

    1. The use of "chemical restraints" is no longer considered appropriate.

      a. Treatment of agitated or aggressive behavior should be directed at the root cause, when possible.

      b. The first priority of emergency pharmacotherapy should be to reduce the risk of harm to the patient, and those around him/her—*not* to sedate or mute the patient.

      c. The patient should be given the option of accepting the medication, *if conditions permit a safe conversation.*

      d. Address escalation early, not before it becomes unsafe.

        i. Try redirection, "talking down"; offer the patient an empty room to calm down.

        ii. Offer medication to help calm the patient. Listen to the patient's suggestions about what he/she thinks may help.

    2. Physical restraints.

      a. Should be used as a last resort, with safety always in mind.

      b. Re-evaluate the need for restraints frequently.

      c. If improperly applied (too loose or too tight), restraints can be very dangerous for the patient.

      d. Physical restraints should always be used in combination with behavioral and pharmacologic approaches.

D. **Absolutely unethical behavior**

    1. A romantic relationship with a patient

    2. Lying to a patient

    3. Altering the medical record

    4. Exploitation of patients (e.g., getting free goods or services, requesting gifts)

ADDITIONAL NOTES

CHAPTER 23

Child Psychiatry

Child Pharmacology

I. General Concepts
  A. **Pharmacokinetics:** different in children
    1. Drug distribution
      a. Less fatty tissue (less drug storage in fat)
      b. Protein binding may be unpredictable
      c. Weight changes more rapidly, and changes are greater percentage of total weight
    2. Elimination is generally faster than in adults
      a. Higher glomerular filtration rate
      b. Larger hepatic capacity
  B. **Pharmacodynamics**
    1. Central nervous system <CNS> is still developing; effects of medications may change with CNS maturation.
    2. Surprising or paradoxic side effects may occur.
    3. Therapeutic drug levels may not apply.
  C. **Diagnosis:** may be more difficult in children (e.g., attention deficit hyperactivity disorder [ADHD] or bipolar? schizophrenia or autism?)
    1. Sometimes the diagnosis is established only after a response to pharmacotherapy.
    2. Symptom-directed treatment is common.
    3. Many childhood disorders have no specific treatment (autism, retardation, etc.).
  D. **Most psychotropics:** not U.S. Food and Drug Administration (FDA) approved for use in children
  E. **Electroconvulsive therapy and psychosurgery:** generally not indicated
  F. **Children are minors:** *the child's parents or guardians are the ultimate decision-makers;* treatment of any kind requires their informed consent

II. Psychotropics Used Mostly in Children
  A. **Medications for ADHD**
    1. *Amphetamines*
      a. Effects
        i. Increased release of catecholamines (norepinephrine [NE] and dopamine [DA])
          (A) Increased attention and concentration
          (B) Increased motivation
        ii. Reduced hyperactivity, aggression
        iii. Similar behavioral responses occur in children without ADHD (i.e., improvement with amphetamine is not diagnostic of ADHD)
      b. Specific drugs
        i. Methylphenidate (Ritalin®, Metadate®, Concerta®): the most frequently used
        ii. Dextroamphetamine (Dexedrine®)

   iii. Mixed amphetamine salt (Adderall®)
  c. Adverse effects
   i. Can worsen tics (which are often comorbid)
   ii. Insomnia, anorexia, nervousness
   iii. Potentially habit forming
   iv. If stimulants suppress growth, the effect is minimal, and growth catches up eventually
   v. Toxicity: hallucinations and seizures
 2. Pemoline (Cylert®)
  a. Nonamphetamine stimulant
  b. Longer acting than most amphetamines
 3. Antidepressants
  a. Tricyclics
   i. Likely work through NE reuptake inhibition
   ii. Therapeutic effect may be evident within days (unlike in depression)
   iii. *Desipramine: effective but associated with sudden cardiac death*
  b. Bupropion (Wellbutrin®)
   i. Increased NE and DA transmission
   ii. *Decreases seizure threshold*
 4. Atomoxetine (Strattera®)
  a. Nonstimulant; selective NE reuptake inhibitor
  b. May cause drowsiness
 5. Presynaptic α_2-noradrenergic agonists (not FDA approved)
  a. Clonidine (Catapres®), also available as a patch
  b. Guanfacine (Tenex®) may be more frontal lobe specific than clonidine
  c. Can cause hypotension, dysrhythmias, sedation
  d. *Rebound hypertension can occur if discontinued suddenly*
B. **NB: Medications for Tourette's disorder**
 1. Antipsychotics are the most effective treatments—probably work through DA blockade
  a. **NB:** Pimozide (Orap®): not frequently used but is a test answer
  b. **NB:** Haloperidol (Haldol®)
  c. Risperidone (Risperdal®)
  d. Risks
   i. *Extrapyramidal side effects, tardive dyskinesia*
   ii. *QT prolongation*—monitor with serial electrocardiographies
 2. Clonidine (less effective, but no risk of tardive dyskinesia)
C. **Medications for enuresis**
 1. Tricyclics
  a. Effective in 60% of patients
  b. Low doses, given approximately 1 hour before bedtime
  c. Clomipramine (Anafranil®): most commonly used
 2. Desmopressin
  a. Analogue of antidiuretic hormone
  b. Effective in approximately 50% of cases
  c. Dosed intranasally
  d. Can cause water retention
D. **Medications for self-injury (in developmental disorders)**
 1. Antimanic agents, such as *lithium and anticonvulsants*

2. Antipsychotics—risperidone in autism spectrum
3. Nonspecific sedatives, such as benzodiazepines and antihistamines
4. β-Blockers sometimes have a calming effect
5. Opioid antagonists naloxone (Narcan®) and naltrexone (Revia®)

Childhood Psychiatric Illnesses

Childhood psychiatric illnesses differ from adult illnesses in two ways. First, children may present with unusual symptoms of adult illnesses. Second, as in neurology, children have their own unique diagnoses that rarely present in adulthood. This chapter is not intended to be a comprehensive review of these illnesses but to present those that are likely to come to the attention of a neurologist (in real life or on an examination).

I. Mental retardation
A. *Categorization*
  1. Mild
     a. Intelligence quotient (IQ): 50–70
     b. 6th grade educable
     c. May be able to hold simple job
  2. Moderate
     a. IQ: 35–50
     b. 2nd grade educable
     c. May be able to function in sheltered workplace
  3. Severe
     a. IQ: 20–35
     b. May be able to talk or otherwise communicate
     c. Unlikely to benefit from vocational training
     d. May be able to protect self and perform simple hygiene
  4. Profound
     a. IQ: <20
     b. May develop rudimentary speech in adulthood
     c. Will require nursing care
B. *Causes*
  1. **NB:** Down syndrome
     a. *Trisomy 21:* most common cause
     b. Incidence: 1/700 live births (1/100 if mother >32 y/o)
     c. Signs
        i. Physical examination: hypotonia, oblique palpebral fissures, extra neck skin, protruding tongue, single palmar crease (simian crease).
        ii. Mental development seems normal until 6 months; IQ decreases after age 1 year.
        iii. As children, they are usually quite pleasant and placid.
        iv. Various behavioral problems can develop in adolescence.
     d. Prognosis/complications
        i. Frequent childhood infections (depressed immune system).
        ii. Outcome can range from holding jobs to lifelong institutionalization (10%).
        iii. **NB:** *Early-age Alzheimer's symptoms and neuropathology (age 30–40 years).*
        iv. *Atlantoaxial instability may cause myelopathy.*
  2. **NB:** Fragile X syndrome
     a. Caused by *trinucleotide repeat* at chromosomal locus Xq27.3
     b. Incidence: 1/1,000 males, 1/2,000 females
     c. Diagnosis

     i. Long head, large ears, hyperflexible joints, *macroorchidism*, short stature.
     ii. Mild to severe mental retardation.
     iii. These patients are often gregarious and pleasant.
     iv. Females are usually less severely affected.
     v. High frequency of ADHD and pervasive developmental disorders.

NB: Fragile X is the most common cause of inherited mental retardation (MR). Nearly all affected boys manifest attention deficit disorder (ADD) and have learning disabilities. The most common neurocognitive symptoms are abstract reasoning, complex problem solving, and expressive language. 33% meet criteria for autism. Female carriers can have a milder form of the disease.

3. **Prader-Willi syndrome**
   a. **NB:** *Paternal* chromosome 15q12 deletion
   b. Prevalence: 1/10,000
   c. Signs
      i. **NB:** *Compulsive eating (obesity)*
      ii. Can be oppositional, aggressive, and behaviorally labile
      iii. Hypogonadism
4. **Angelman's syndrome**
   a. **NB:** *Maternal* chromosome 15q12 deletion
   b. Diagnosis
      i. Developmental delay at 6–12 months
      ii. *Microcephaly* and seizures at early age
      iii. Speech impaired but often able to understand and communicate otherwise
      iv. **NB:** *Happy puppet*
         (A) Posture impairment and jerky gait
         (B) Flapping movements of hands
         (C) Excitable and tend to smile and laugh frequently
5. **Lesch-Nyhan syndrome**
   a. **NB:** *X-linked recessive (essentially affects only males)*
      i. Deficiency of hypoxanthine-guanine phosphoribosyl transferase
      ii. Causes accumulation of uric acid
   b. Incidence: 1/380,000
   c. Diagnostic features
      i. Patients typically present around 6 months old, with motor delay
      ii. *Medical:* uric acid tophi, nephrolithiasis, gout
      iii. *Neurologic:* microcephaly, seizures, movement disorders, pyramidal signs
      iv. *Psychiatric:* **NB:** *severe self-mutilation (biting lips, tongue, fingers)*, mental retardation
   d. Treatment
      i. Decrease uric acid
      ii. Allopurinol is used but fails to prevent progression
   e. Most patients die before 40 y/o

II. Learning Disorders
A. Diagnosed when one specific area of cognitive achievement is significantly below what would be expected for the child's age, schooling, and performance in other areas
B. **Types**
   1. Reading disorder
      a. 4% of children

b. Impaired word recognition and comprehension

c. If associated with right/left confusion, is called *dyslexia*

2. Mathematics

a. 5% of children

b. May present as simply as inability to count, or as complexly as failing geometry

3. Written expression

a. 3–10% of children

b. Possible genetic influence

4. Other types: spelling, mixed

III. Pervasive Developmental Disorders

A. **Characterized by:** severe, persistent impairment in developmental areas, particularly socialization

B. **Cognitive skill:** usually better than functional impairment would predict

C. **Autistic disorder**

1. Abnormal or failed development, before age 3 years, of language and communication, social attachment and interaction, or symbolic play

2. Incidence: 5/10,000 (males affected 3× more often than females)

3. Diagnosis: symptoms of dysfunction in three main areas

a. *Reciprocal social interaction:* poor eye contact; impaired use of body language; failure to develop peer relationships; lack of interest in sharing enjoyment; deviant responses to social cues

b. *Communication:* lack of language output, inability to maintain conversation; stereotyped or idiosyncratic use of language; lack of imitative play

c. *Repetitive or restricted patterns of behavior:* intense preoccupation with an unusual topic; compulsive adherence to rules or rituals; stereotyped motor mannerisms; preoccupations with object parts or nonfunctional elements of objects (color, texture, etc.)

4. Other symptoms

a. 10–30% have seizures

b. 60% are mentally retarded

c. Treatment

i. Behavioral therapy

ii. Symptomatic

(A) Antidepressants for compulsions, affective lability

(B) D2-blocking agents for tics

(C) Antimanics and antipsychotics for agitation and aggression

iii. Self-mutilation: data have shown efficacy of *risperidone*

D. **Asperger's syndrome:** autism without language disturbance

1. Incidence unclear because diagnostic criteria have changed frequently

2. Comparison to autism

a. Similar criteria for abnormal social interaction and repetitive patterns of behavior

b. **NB:** *No significant language delay*

c. Child maintains normal curiosity about environment and has normal nonsocial adaptive behavior

E. **Rett's disorder**

1. **NB:** *X-linked dominant*

2. **NB:** *Affects only females* (males die in utero or at birth)

3. Incidence: 1/20,000

4. Diagnosis

    a. **NB:** *Normal development until 5 months old*
    b. **NB:** *Deceleration of head growth between 5 and 48 months*
    c. **NB:** Characteristic wringing of hands (actually apraxic movements)
    d. Loss of social engagement
    e. Ataxia of trunk and gait
    f. Gait disturbance, scoliosis, seizures

IV. Attention Deficit and Disruptive Disorders
A. **ADHD**
    1. Incidence: 2–5% in American school-aged children
    2. Can persist into adulthood (15% of cases)
    3. Males affected 3× as frequently; females tend to have inattentive type
    4. Causes
      a. Some evidence for genetic cause (increased risk in twins and siblings)
      b. Hypofunction of NE?
      c. Hypofunction of DA?
      d. Impaired frontal lobe function?

NB: DA pathways have been recently implicated in the pathogenesis of ADHD, including the association between ADHD and polymorphisms in DRD4, DRD5, and SLC6A4, which encode D4 and D5 receptors and the DA transporter.

    5. Diagnosis
      a. *Inattention:* poor attention to detail; unable to sustain concentration; seems not to listen when spoken to; fails to follow through on instructions; poor organization; dislikes tasks that require attention; loses things; forgetful; easily distracted by extraneous stimuli/information
      b. *Hyperactivity/impulsivity:* fidgety; difficulty remaining seated; excessive running/climbing; difficulty playing quietly; talks excessively; on the go; has trouble waiting turn; intrusive
      c. Some evidence of symptoms before age 7 years
      d. Impairment in social, academic, or occupational function
      e. May be predominantly inattentive, predominantly hyperactive, or combined type
    6. Treatment
      a. Pharmacotherapy, as earlier
        i. Many clinicians give drug holidays on weekends and in the summer
        ii. Beware of rebound hyperactivity when medication is discontinued
      b. Therapy
        i. Family therapy
          (A) Instruct parents not to be overly permissive or punitive
          (B) Help parents develop useful behavioral interventions
        ii. Individual and group therapy
          (A) Build self-esteem
          (B) Refine interpersonal skills
      c. Associated illnesses
        i. Comorbidities: conduct disorder, depression, tics
        ii. Differential diagnosis: learning disorder, pervasive developmental disorder, bipolar disorder
B. **Oppositional defiant disorder**
    1. Diagnosis

    a. *Negative and hostile behavior:* loses temper; argues with adults; deliberately annoys people; defies adults' requests or rules; angry, resentful, and vindictive; irritable; blames others for his/her behavior

    b. Behaviors occur more frequently than would be expected for age and developmental level

    c. Behaviors last for at least 6 months

  2. Differential diagnosis: depression, conduct disorder, bipolar disorder, ADHD

  3. Treatment

    a. Family and behavioral therapy

    b. Symptom-directed pharmacotherapy, if necessary

C. **Conduct disorder**

  1. Diagnosis

    a. *Aggression:* bullies or threatens others; starts fights; has used a weapon; physically cruel to people or animals; has stolen while confronting the victim

    b. *Property destruction:* deliberate fire setting or other property destruction

    c. *Deceitfulness/theft:* has broken into a building or car; frequently lies; has stolen without confrontation

    d. *Rules violations:* stays out past curfew (before 13 y/o); has run away overnight at least twice; often truant (before 13 y/o)

    e. Must be <18 y/o

  2. 50% progress to antisocial personality disorder

  3. Treatment

    a. Poor prognosis

    b. Treat comorbidities (depression, ADHD, learning disorder)

    c. Individual therapy to improve problem-solving skills

    d. Family therapy

    e. Psychopharmacology directed at aggression (antimanics, antipsychotics, clonidine, antidepressants)

V. Tic Disorders

A. **NB: Tourette's disorder**

  1. Prevalence: 4/10,000

  2. Males are affected 3× more often than females

  3. Causes

    a. Genetic: higher coincidence in twins, autosomal dominant in some families

    b. Likely some degree of *DA hyperactivity* present

    c. May be *exacerbated by stimulants and cocaine* (both increase synaptic DA)

    d. Can be a tardive side effect of antipsychotic treatment

  4. **NB:** Diagnosis

    a. A *vocal tic* and *multiple motor tics* (not necessarily concurrent)

    b. Tics occur several times each day for at least 1 year, with no tic-free period >3 months

    c. Onset before age 18 years

    d. Differential: other movement disorders, Sydenham's chorea, Wilson's disease, obsessive-compulsive disorder, myoclonic disorders

  5. Comorbidities: depression, obsessive-compulsive disorder (OCD), ADHD, impulsivity/rage attacks

  6. **NB:** Treatment

    a. Low-dose, high-potency antipsychotics, or clonidine

  b. Psychotherapy generally ineffective
  c. Treatment of comorbidities can sometimes improve the tic
 B. *Motor or vocal tic disorder*
  1. Prevalence: 1/1,000
  2. Single or multiple vocal or motor tics
  3. *Treatment*
   a. As with Tourette's disorder
   b. Psychotherapy sometimes effective

VI. Miscellaneous Childhood Disorders

 A. *Separation anxiety*
  1. Epidemiology
   a. Most common anxiety disorder in children
   b. Prevalence: 3–4% of all school age children; 1% of adolescents
   c. No gender difference
  2. Diagnosis
   a. Excessive worry about becoming separated from loved ones; distress when separated; fear/refusal to go to school or elsewhere; separation nightmares; fear of being alone
   b. Occurs for a minimum of 4 weeks
   c. Onset before age 18 years
 B. *Selective mutism*
  1. Psychologically driven refusal or inability to speak in *some* situations
  2. 90% of affected children have some degree of social anxiety
  3. Treatment: family and behavioral therapy, fluoxetine (?)

VII. Differences from Adult Diagnostic Criteria

 A. **Depression**
  1. *Irritability* may replace depressed mood.
  2. *Failure to achieve appropriate weight gain* may replace loss of appetite or weight.
  3. Children often exhibit physical complaints.
  4. Children less frequently have trouble with sleep or appetite.
  5. Withdrawal from social and family activities may be more prominent.
 B. **Dysthymia and cyclothymia**
  1. Irritability can replace depressed mood.
  2. Symptoms present for 1 year (instead of 2).
 C. **Schizophrenia**
  1. Very rare in children <5 y/o
  2. Must be distinguished from pervasive developmental disorder or fantasy play
 D. **Bipolar disorder**
  1. Rare before adolescence
  2. Manic episodes may be less discrete than in adults

ADDITIONAL NOTES

CHAPTER 24

Neurobehavior and Neuropsychology

I. **Functional-Anatomic Correlations:** Review Chapter 21: Clinical Neuroanatomy to identify vessels supplying these important regions of the brain.
   A. **Frontal lobes**
      1. Luria description of functions
         a. Identification of problems or objectives
         b. Formulation of strategies and selection of an appropriate plan
         c. Execution of the plan
         d. Evaluation of outcomes
      2. Specific behavioral signs and symptoms of frontal damage
         a. Lateralized signs/symptoms
            i. Either frontal lobe: release of primitive reflexes (grasp, root, palmomental, suck, glabellar, snout); witzelsucht (inappropriate jocularity); depression
            ii. *Dominant frontal lobe: left hand apraxia* (inability to perform learned patterned movements); poor verbal fluency, including *Broca's aphasia*
            iii. *Nondominant frontal lobe:* decreased attention; loss of prosody (emotional content of speech); nonspecific behavioral symptoms; mania
            iv. **NB:** Bilateral damage: abulia, mutism; poor attention; rigid thinking; gait and sphincter disturbances
         b. By specific region
            i. *Orbitofrontal*—the region of social and interpersonal function: disinhibition, lability, euphoria, lack of remorse or social propriety

NB: *Wizelsucht* (inappropriate jocularity) is seen in patients with orbitofrontal cortex lesions.

            ii. *Dorsolateral*—executive function: poor planning, decreased motivation and flexibility, unable to resist reaction to environmental stimuli
            iii. *Medial:* apathy, akinetic mutism
   B. **Parietal lobes:** carry out diverse functions that help us to interpret the environment and our place within it; perform massive amounts of higher-order and multimodal processing of incoming sensory information
      1. Damage to either side
         a. Sensory extinction of the contralateral side of the body
         b. **NB:** *Hemineglect* of the opposite side of space
            i. May include neglect of body parts (amorphosynthesis)
            ii. Sometimes accompanied by anosognosia (unawareness of deficits); **NB:** More common with right-sided lesions
      2. **Dominant parietal lobe damage**
         a. Alexia (impaired ability to read)

      b. *Bilateral astereognosis*

      c. *Bilateral ideomotor apraxia*

      d. **NB:** Gerstmann syndrome: tetrad—dysgraphia, dyscalculia, right-left disorientation, finger agnosia; the individual signs of the syndrome are not localizing

   3. **Nondominant parietal lobe damage**

      a. Constructional apraxia (impaired ability to draw or copy figures)

      b. Loss of visuospatial memory

      c. Confusion (especially with acute damage, such as cerebrovascular accident)

NB: *Reduplicative paramnesia* (reduplication of place) has been associated with combined lesions in the right parietal and bifrontal areas.

NB: *Anosodiaphoria* (indifference to the condition despite recognition of the deficit) is seen with right hemisphere lesions.

   4. **Bilateral parietal damage**

      a. **NB:** Balint's syndrome

         i. Caused by damage to posterior superior watershed areas (Brodmann's areas 19 and 7)

        ii. *Simultanagnosia*—inability to relate objects presented together (e.g., looking at an American flag, a patient might say, "I see a white star," then, "I see a stripe")

       iii. *Inability to direct oculomotor function:* paralysis of optic fixation—inability to look into peripheral field; optic ataxia—clumsiness in responding to visual stimuli, inability to point to visual targets

      b. Spatial disorientation

C. **Temporal lobes:** the major functions associated with the temporal lobes are auditory processing, language, and memory

   1. **Hemispheric dominance**

      a. "Dominant" is that containing language function

      b. *Left hemisphere dominance* in 96% of right-handers, 70% of left-handers

      c. *Right hemisphere dominance* in 4% of right-handers, 15% of left-handers

      d. *Bilateral dominance* in 0% of right-handers, 15% of left-handers

   2. **Damage to either temporal lobe**

      a. Hallucinations (any sensory modality)

      b. Delirium

      c. Distortions in time perception

   3. **Damage to dominant temporal lobe**

      a. Aphasias

      b. Verbal amnesia

NB: Aphasias

Type	Speech	Comprehension	Repetition	Paraphasia	Localization
Wernicke's (sensory)	Fluent	–	–	+	Superior temp gyrus (area 22)
NB: Transcortical sensory	Fluent	–	+	+	Watershed zone between MCA and PCA (areas 40, 41, 42)

Type	Speech	Comprehension	Repetition	Paraphasia	Localization
Broca's (motor)	Nonfluent	+	–	–	Frontal opercu-lum (area 44)
Transcortical motor	Nonfluent	+	+	–	Anterior water-shed (above areas 44 and 45); **NB:** Supplemen-tary motor area
Global	Nonfluent	–	–	+	Perisylvian
Transcortical mixed	Nonfluent	–	+	–	Both watershed zones
Anomic	Fluent	+	+	–	Angular gyrus (area 39)
Conduction	Fluent	+	–	+	Arcuate fasciculus

+, normal; –, abnormal.

NB: Naming is poor in all of these syndromes; note that the transcortical (also called *extrasylvian*) aphasias have spare repetition.

NB: In advancing Alzheimer's disease, speech remains intact as language deteriorates. The result is an aphasia where the patient is fluent and paraphasic, with poor comprehensive but good repetition, similar to transcortical sensory aphasia.

4. **Damage to nondominant temporal lobe**
   a. Impaired performance with visual testing
   b. Impaired visual memory
   c. Impaired recognition of harmony and melody

NB: Topographic disorientation (impaired orientation and navigation in the environment) occurs with a lesion in the right posterior parahippocampal region or the infracalcarine cortex, but a milder form may be seen with a lesion in the right parietal area.

5. **Bilateral temporal damage**
   a. Korsakoff's dementia
   b. **NB:** *Klüver-Bucy syndrome*
      i. Usually with anterior temporal damage
      ii. Hyperorality, hypersexuality, apathy, hypermetamorphosis (overly sensitive or acutely aware of minute stimuli in the environment, resulting in preoccupation with these stimuli), and visual agnosia.
      iii. Aggression is not a component of the syndrome!
   c. Inability to ignore visual stimuli
D. **Occipital lobes:** receive visual input and performing visual processing; information encoded with the identity of objects is routed ventrally ("what" stream) toward temporal lobes; data about the location and movement of environmental objects ("where" stream) are routed dorsally, to the parietal lobes
   1. Damage to either occipital lobe can cause simple visual hallucinations

2. **Damage to dominant occipital lobe**
   a. Visual object agnosia (inability to identify objects by sight)
      i. **NB:** Interhemispheric fibers (from/to splenium) may be involved; disconnects primary visual cortex from language areas; signs: often associated with *color anomia, alexia without agraphia* (pure word blindness)
      (A) Patient *unable to read words*
      (B) Patient *able to write, speak, and spell*
      (C) Patient may be able to read individual letters and numbers
3. **Damage to nondominant occipital lobe**
   a. May cause contralateral visual neglect
   b. Visuospatial disorientation
   c. Visual illusions and hallucinations
4. **Bilateral occipital damage**
   a. **NB:** *Cortical blindness:* patient is unable to see; no response to visual threat; pupils remain reactive; **Anton's syndrome**—anosognosia for cortical blindness
   b. Achromatopsia (loss of color perception)
   c. **NB:** Balint's syndrome (see section I.B.4.a)
   d. **NB:** *Prosopagnosia* (inability to recognize faces)
      i. Can occur in the absence of other visual deficits
      ii. Commonly associated with achromatopsia
      iii. **NB:** Requires ventral occipitotemporal lesion ("what" pathway)
E. **Disconnection syndromes**
   1. *Callosal disconnection*
      a. **NB:** *Left posterior cerebral artery territory and splenium*
         i. Right homonymous hemianopsia—all visual information enters right hemisphere
         ii. Damaged posterior corpus callosum prevents right occipital lobe from communicating with language centers on the left; alexia (inability to read), color anomia (inability to name colors); the ability to copy words is spared—motor information crosses in anterior corpus callosum
      b. Anterior corpus callosum: disconnects right hemisphere motor and sensory integration centers from left hemisphere language areas: signs: apraxia of left hand, agnosia for fingers of left hand

NB: Callosal apraxia results from a lesion in the genu of the corpus callosum, resulting in limb kinetic apraxia. Tactile and auditory input cross the corpus callosum posteriorly and are therefore unaffected by a genu lesion!

      c. Complete callosotomy
         i. Alien hand (nondominant hand performs apparently independent acts)
         ii. Disconnection of dominant-sided sensory input (going to the nondominant side of the brain) from the patient's ability to describe or name the phenomena
   2. **NB:** *Arcuate fasciculus*—conduction aphasia
   3. *Subcortical fibers in dominant temporal lobe*
      a. Damages Wernicke's area and interhemispheric fibers
      b. No access of auditory input to language area
      c. Causes *pure word deafness*—sounds are appreciated, but not speech

II. Medical Diseases Causing Psychiatric Symptoms

A. **Cerebrovascular disease**
   1. Most common sequela is *depression.*
      a. 30–40% of stroke victims have depression.
      b. Previously associated with *left frontal* infarction in particular.
   2. Poststroke *mania associated with right-sided lesions.*

B. **Epilepsy**
   1. 30–50% have psychiatric illness
   2. Increased risk of suicide
   3. Auras—hallucinations and affective changes
   4. Ictal—rarely, complex partial seizures cause violent behavior
   5. Postictal—psychosis, confusion
   6. Interictal
      a. Personality disturbances
         i. Hyper-religiosity
         ii. Viscous ("complex partial personality"); circumstantial, pedantic, ponderous speech; hypergraphia
         iii. Sexual behavior: hyposexuality is the most common; fetishism, transvestism, deviant interests
      b. Psychosis
         i. Usually develops after years of epilepsy
         ii. Often preceded by other personality changes
   7. Medications: all compounds that suppress cerebral activity can cause changes in energy, sleep, appetite, and concentration
      a. **NB:** Topiramate
         i. Psychosis
         ii. Cognitive slowing
         iii. Anomia
      b. Benzodiazepines and barbiturates
         i. Cognitive impairment
         ii. Depression

C. **Multiple sclerosis**
   1. Depression
      a. 25–50% of patients
      b. Carries a higher risk of suicide
   2. Witzelsucht
      a. Frontal subcortical dementia
      b. Subsyndromal mania
   3. Personality change—irritability or apathy

D. **Movement disorders**
   1. **NB:** *Parkinson's disease*
      a. Depression: may be difficult to distinguish from masked facies and generalized bradykinesias that are part of the motor manifestations of Parkinson's disease
         i. Present in 30–45% of patients.
         ii. It may be presenting symptom, and it may not be correlated with motor severity.
      b. Dementia in 30%
      c. Psychosis
         i. Associated with dopamimetics, but can occur without

      ii. Approach

        (A) Rule out concurrent medical illness causing delirium

        (B) Decrease anti-Parkinson's medications, if possible

        (C) **NB:** Treat with *low-dose atypical antipsychotics (quetiapine or clozapine)*

  2. **NB:** *Huntington's disease*

    a. Can be accompanied by severe depression and suicidality.

    b. Dementia, psychosis, or irritability may precede motor dysfunction.

  3. **NB:** Wilson's disease

    a. Irritability and excessive emotionality may be first symptoms.

    b. Delirium and dementia may present late or early.

  4. Essential tremor

    a. Associated with anxiety

    b. Because of beneficial effects of ethanol, abuse may result.

E. **NB: Acute intermittent porphyria**

  1. Affects females > males between ages 20 and 50 years

  2. **NB:** *Recurrent triad:* abdominal pain, motor polyneuropathy, psychosis

  3. Seizures in 15%

  4. **NB:** Barbiturates and antiepileptics can exacerbate or precipitate attacks

  5. Treatment

    a. Glucose and hematin infusions (to inhibit aminoleuolunic acid [ALA] synthetase)

    b. Gabapentin for seizures

F. **NB: B$_{12}$ deficiency (subacute combined degeneration)**

  1. Usually results from poor absorption

    a. Failure to secrete required intrinsic factor, or

    b. Dysfunction of terminal ileum (absorption site)

  2. Psychiatric: depression, dementia, delirium, psychosis

  3. Neurologic abnormalities (present in 80%)

    a. Length-dependent demyelinating polyneuropathy

    b. Myelopathy (demyelination of posterior columns and lateral corticospinal tracts)

  4. Hematologic abnormalities

    a. Megaloblastic ("pernicious") anemia

    b. Hypersegmented neutrophils

    c. *May follow neuropsychiatric symptoms*

G. **Human immunodeficiency virus**

  1. Depression very common

  2. Dementia

  3. Neuropsychiatric disturbances from secondary infections

Neuropsychological Assessment

III. Intelligence

A. **Wechsler Adult Intelligence Scale and Wechsler Intelligence Scale for Children**

  1. **NB:** Most common test used in clinical practice

  2. Six verbal subtests: Information, Comprehension, Arithmetic, Similarities, Digit Span, Vocabulary

  3. Four performance subtests: Block Design, Picture Arrangement, Object Assembly, Digit Symbol

  4. Scores

    a. Mean = 100

    b. Standard deviation = 10

     c. Average range: 90–110

     d. Intelligence quotient <70 defines mental retardation (2.2% of population)

  5. Advantages

     a. Extremely high reliability

     b. High validity for detecting mental retardation and predicting school performance

     c. Can be used to localize cerebral dysfunction

     d. Can compare function in different domains

  6. Disadvantages

     a. Performance subtest is age-sensitive

     b. Some false lateralization with subcortical or parietal lesions

B. **Stanford-Binet Test**

  1. Once the gold standard for children, but now less popular than Wechsler Intelligence Scale for Children

  2. Mostly used in psychiatry and education

IV. Frontal Lobes

A. **Executive functioning and reasoning**

  1. **NB:** Wisconsin Card Sorting Test

     a. Subject sorts cards with objects of different shape, color, form, and number

        i. Initially, the patient does not know the rule.

        ii. The examiner tells the patient whether the sorting is correct.

        iii. Scored by the number of trials required to obtain ten consecutive correct responses.

        iv. Once goal is achieved, the examiner changes the rule again.

     b. Tests *cognitive flexibility* (ability to avoid perseveration) and *abstract thought*

        i. Sensitive to *frontal lobe* dysfunction

        ii. Also abnormal in patients with schizophrenia and caudate lesions

  2. Tower of Hanoi, Tower of London

     a. Subject moves blocks from starting arrangement to goal arrangement.

     b. Scored by number of moves required (the fewer moves, the better).

  3. **Bedside maneuvers**

     a. *Ability to perform nonutile motor sequences (Luria tests):* with minimal or no practice, the intact brain can learn simple motor sequences simply by mimicry; the more complex or variable the rhythm or sequence, the more sensitive the test is for frontal lobe dysfunction.

        i. Two-step hand sequence (reciprocally alternating fists and prone hands)

        ii. Three-step hand sequence ("fist-edge-palm")

        iii. Rhythm tapping

        iv. Alternating pattern (drawing alternating peaks and blocks)

     b. *Suppression of motor impulses:* the intact frontal lobes should be able to suppress the instinctive tendency to direct activity toward novel stimuli.

        i. Crossed response inhibition ("raise the hand that I don't touch")

        ii. Antisaccades ("look away from the finger that moves")

        iii. "Go/no-go"

     c. *Creativity:* the normal frontal lobes are able to categorize and retrieve items in memory that have concrete or abstract relationships to each other.

        i. "Thurstone" Controlled Oral Word Association Test ("all the words that start with the letter __")

        ii. Category fluency ("name all the [farm animals, cities] you can in one minute")

    d. *Suppression of primitive reflexes:* glabellar (Myerson's), snout, rooting, suck, Babinski, grasp (palmar and plantar), and palmomental reflexes are present in early life but sequentially extinguish as the frontal lobes myelinate and organize their function.

B. **Attention**
1. Three types of attention
   a. Focused attention—seeking and finding an objective
   b. Sustained attention or vigilance—extended monitoring of an objective
   c. Divided attention—ability to perform two tasks simultaneously
2. Tests
   a. **Trail-making** (connect-the-dots)
      i. *Trails A*—connect dots in simple numerical order (focused attention)
      ii. *Trails B*—connect dots with alternating sequence of numerical and alphabetical order (i.e., 1-A-2-B-3-C. . . .) (divided attention)
      iii. Scored based on time to perform each test and difference in performance between A and B
   b. **Stroop test**
      i. Reading of words on cards with increasingly difficult-to-ignore distractors
      ii. Most difficult is reporting the color in which a word representing a different color is printed (e.g., for the word "black" printed in green, the correct response is "green")

V. Memory

A. **Temporal categorization**
1. Working memory: a temporary storehouse for recently acquired (within the past minute) information; managed by the frontal lobes; usually able to store about seven or eight "chunks" of information
   a. Digit span and reverse digit span
   b. Memory for designs
   c. "N-back" test
2. **Recent memory:** the collection of events over the past few minutes to hours
   a. Word lists (Hopkins Verbal Learning Test, Rey Auditory Verbal Learning Test)
   b. Diagrams (Rey-Osterrieth Complex Figure)
3. **Recent past memory**: extends over the past few months; asking about recent events in the patient's life or in the news is a useful test
4. **Remote memory**: concerns events in the distant past
   a. Although preserved (relative to more recent memories) in dementias and amnesias, usually not intact

B. **Categorization by type of data**
1. Episodic memory: the recall of specific events (e.g., what you ate for breakfast today)
2. Semantic memory: the storage of knowledge and facts (e.g., semantic memory is the storage of knowledge and facts)
3. Procedural or implicit memory: preservation of learned automatic skills (e.g., riding a bicycle)
4. *Semantic and implicit memories do not deteriorate with normal aging;* episodic memory may decline slightly because of age-related inefficiency of frontal processing

VI. Perceptual and Motor Performance

A. **Bender Visual Motor Gestalt**
1. Originally developed to test cognitive maturity of children

2. Normal 12-y/o children can complete the test well
3. Consists of nine simple diagrams, which are directly copied by the patient
4. Used to screen for cerebral dysfunction (*sensitive, but nonspecific*)
B. **Benton Facial Recognition Test**
1. Patient is shown a head-on photograph of an unfamiliar face
2. Patient is shown the same face photographed in different ways (changed lighting or angle) and scored on the number of previously presented faces he recognizes
3. Specific for *posterior right hemisphere* lesions
C. **Hooper Visual Organization Test**—subject names fragmented objects

VII. Language Function
A. **Lengthy, comprehensive tests**
1. Boston Diagnostic Aphasia Examination
2. Western Aphasia Battery
3. Porch Index of Communicative Ability
B. **Brief, but fairly complete: Reitan Aphasia Screening Test**
C. **Specific tests**
1. Token Test: verbal comprehension
2. Boston Naming Test: naming pictured objects
3. Peabody Picture Vocabulary Test: auditory comprehension

VIII. Comprehensive Tests of Brain Function
A. **Halstead-Reitan Battery**
1. Domains tested
a. Tactile perception (stereognosis, manual dexterity, finger localization, graphesthesia, simultaneous tactile stimulation)
b. Auditory perception (rhythm discrimination, speech-sounds test)
c. Abstraction (categorization test)
d. Aphasia screening (naming, speech-sounds, body part identification)
e. Attention (trail-making test, flickering light)
f. Visual perception (flickering light)
g. Dexterity and motor speed (finger oscillation)
2. Long, intense test procedure
3. Reliably identifies subjects with brain damage
B. **Luria-Nebraska Neuropsychological Battery**
1. Tests broad range of cerebral function
2. Can localize dysfunction and identify particular disorders (i.e., sensitive and specific)
3. Can define hemispheric dominance

ADDITIONAL NOTES

ARE YOU *REALLY* READY?

50 Practice Questions

Select the best answer to each question. Each question is a test of the depth of your fund of knowledge. You are expected to correctly answer at least 70% of the questions. The distribution of topics or the degree of difficulty of each question is not a representation of the actual Board Examination. This section is mainly designed to provide you with a gauge of your readiness to sit for the Boards. Good luck!

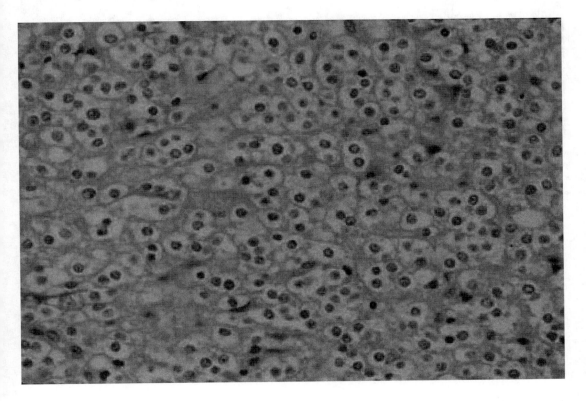

1. A 45-year-old man presents with his first episode of seizures. Brain biopsy reveals the above picture. The following statement(s) is/are NOT true:
   A. This tumor presents between the ages 30 and 50 years.
   B. It is calcified less than 50% of the time.
   C. The median survival is about 5 years.
   D. Treatment is surgical resection and chemotherapy, usually with good response to chemotherapy.
   E. None of the above.
   F. Two of the above.

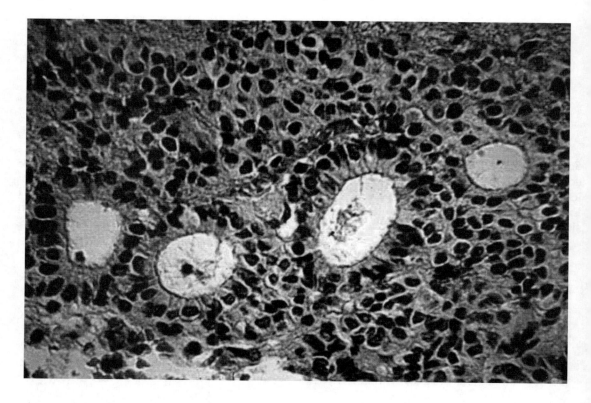

2. A 13-year-old girl presents with headache. The above picture shows the microscopic pathology. The following statement is NOT true:
A. Similar pathology can be seen with retinoblastoma and medulloblastoma.
B. The peak age incidence is between 10 and 15 years old.
C. Radiology often shows an intraventricular mass with contrast enhancement and frequent calcifications.
D. Treatment is surgical resection +/- radiation.
E. Five-year prognosis is less than 50% even after resection.
F. None of the above.

3. The following neurotransmitter is considered an "intermediate concentration neurotransmitter":
A. Aspartate
B. GABA
C. Glycine
D. Dopamine
E. Nitric oxide
F. Carbon monoxide
G. None of the above

4. The following compounds/conditions act by *blocking* the release of acetylcholine in the neuromuscular junction EXCEPT:
A. Botulinum toxin
B. Latrotoxin (black widow spider)
C. Eaton Lambert syndrome
D. Tick paralysis

E. Beta-neurotoxins of sea snakes
F. None of the above

5. The following agents are *reversible* cholinesterase inhibitors EXCEPT:
   A. Neostigmine
   B. Pyridostigmine
   C. Physostigmine
   D. Organophosphates
   E. None of the above

6. The *rate-limiting step* in dopamine synthesis is mediated by:
   A. Tyrosine hydroxylase
   B. DOPA decarboxylase
   C. Dopamine hydroxylase
   D. Vitamin B$_6$
   E. Phenylethanolamine-N-methyl transferase
   F. None of the above

7. Alzheimer's type 1 cells can be found in the following conditions EXCEPT:
   A. Alzheimer's disease
   B. Depakote toxicity
   C. Hepatitis
   D. Progressive multifocal leukoencephalopathy
   E. Wilson's disease
   F. B and C above

8. Neurofibrillary tangles can be seen in the following conditions EXCEPT:
   A. Down syndrome
   B. Lytico-Bodig disease
   C. Progressive supranuclear palsy
   D. von Economo disease
   E. Dementia pugilistica
   F. None of the above

9. The following disorders are due to excessive CAG repeats EXCEPT:
   A. Machado-Joseph disease
   B. Spinocerebellar ataxia type 6
   C. Spinobulbar atrophy
   D. Myotonic dystrophy
   E. Dentatopallidoluysian atrophy
   F. Huntington's disease

10. The following chromosomes are implicated in familial Alzheimer's disease EXCEPT:
    A. Chromosome 1
    B. Chromosome 14
    C. Chromosome 19
    D. Chromosome 21
    E. None of the above

11. The following chromosomes are implicated in autosomal dominant parkinsonism EXCEPT:
    A. Chromosome 2
    B. Chromosome 4
    C. Chromosome 6
    D. Chromosome 17
    E. None of the above

12. An upper extremity somatosensory evoked potential with an *absent* N18 response would suggest a lesion at the:
    A. Median nerve
    B. Erb's point
    C. Cervical cord
    D. Subcortical-thalamic area
    E. Thalamo-cortical area
    F. Hand region in the cortex

13. The following disorders are *X-linked dystrophies* EXCEPT:
    A. Emery-Dreifuss syndrome
    B. Duchene muscular dystrophy
    C. Beckers muscular dystrophy
    D. Limb-girdle muscular dystrophy
    E. None of the above

14. The following are true of Emery-Dreifuss muscular dystrophy EXCEPT:
    A. Predominantly humeroperoneal involvement
    B. Heart blocks are common
    C. Lots of contracture
    D. Absent emerin by immunochemistry
    E. X-linked dominant disorder
    F. None of the above

15. The following are clinical/laboratory features common in myotonic dystrophy EXCEPT:
    A. Hatchet-face appearance
    B. Frontal baldness
    C. Hypothyroidism
    D. Elevated CPK
    E. Pathology shows type 1 fiber hypertrophy and "ring fibers"
    F. None of the above

16. The following are characteristics of myopathy seen on muscle biopsy EXCEPT:
    A. Variable fiber size
    B. Small angulated fibers
    C. Fiber-type groupings
    D. Central nuclei
    E. Endomysial fibrosis
    F. Two of the above

17. The major *inhibitory* neurotransmitter in the spinal cord is:
    A. GABA
    B. Glycine
    C. Taurine
    D. Aspartic acid
    E. Glutamic acid
    F. None of the above

18. The following are NMDA *antagonists* EXCEPT:
    A. MK801
    B. Amantadine
    C. Felbamate
    D. Magnesium
    E. Zinc
    F. Glycine

19 The following are CAG repeats AND autosomal dominant EXCEPT:
  A. Huntington's disease
  B. Dentatopallidoluysian atrophy
  C. Machado-Joseph disease
  D. Kennedy's disease
  E. Spinocerebellar ataxia type 6
  F. None of the above

20. The following metabolic disorders have the *cherry-red spot* EXCEPT:
  A. Tay-Sach's disease
  B. Neimann-Pick disease
  C. GM1 gangliosidosis
  D. Sialidosis
  E. Mucolipidosis II
  F. None of the above

21. The following are X-linked *recessive* EXCEPT:
  A. Adrenoleukodystrophy
  B. Hunter's disease
  C. Ornithine transcarbamylase deficiency
  D. Lesch-Nyhan syndrome
  E. Duchene/Becker muscular dystrophy
  F. Menkes syndrome
  G. None of the above

22. The following are X-linked *dominant* EXCEPT:
  A. Incontinentia pigmenti
  B. Rett syndrome
  C. Aicardi syndrome
  D. Fragile X syndrome
  E. None of the above
  F. Two of the above

23. The following are autosomal recessive EXCEPT:
  A. Neurofibromatosis
  B. Tuberosclerosis
  C. von Hippel-Landau disease
  D. Huntington's disease
  E. Two of the above
  F. None of the above

24. The following disorders present with *facial dysmorphism* EXCEPT:
  A. GM1 gangliosidosis
  B. GM2 gangliosidosis
  C. Mucopolysaccharidosis
  D. Mucolipidosis
  E. Zellweger's syndrome
  F. None of the above

25. Which thalamic nucleus receives projections from the mamillary nucleus of the hypo-thalamus?
  A. Lateral geniculate
  B. Ventral anterior
  C. Dorsomedial
  D. Anterior

E. Pulvinar

F. None of the above

26. The following thalamic nuclei convey sensory information to the cortex EXCEPT:
    A. Ventral anterior
    B. Lateral geniculate
    C. Medial geniculate
    D. Ventral posterolateral
    E. Ventral posteromedial
    F. None of the above

27. Damage to the ventromedial nucleus of the hypothalamus leads to:
    A. Anorexia
    B. Obesity
    C. Shivering
    D. Sweating
    E. Polyuria

28. Damage to the suprachiasmatic nucleus leads to:
    A. Altered behavior
    B. Altered heat production
    C. Altered circadian rhythm
    D. Altered reproduction
    E. Polydipsia
    F. Weight loss

29. The following statement(s) about the autonomic nervous system is/are true:
    A. Acetylcholine is the neurotransmitter of the pre- and postganglionic parasympathetic and preganglionic sympathetic system.
    B. Norepinephrine is the neurotransmitter of the post-ganglionic sympathetic system.
    C. The preganglionic parasympathetic receptor is nicotinic while the post ganglionic parasympathetic receptor is muscarinic.
    D. Curare is a nicotinic receptor antagonist while yohimbine is an alpha2 receptor antagonist.
    E. All of the above.
    F. Three of the above.

30. The following are derived from the telencephalon EXCEPT:
    A. Cortex
    B. Amygdale
    C. Putamen
    D. Caudate
    E. Globus pallidus
    F. None of the above

31. The neural crest cells give rise to the following structures EXCEPT:
    A. Dorsal root ganglion
    B. Melanocytes
    C. Adrenal medulla
    D. Schwann cells
    E. Preganglionic sympathetic neurons
    F. None of the above

32. The following are true of Arnold-Chiari malformation type 2 EXCEPT:
    A. 100% have myelomeningocele
    B. Hydrocephalus

C. Skull base and upper cervical spine defects

D. Displacement of the medulla and 4th ventricle into the cervical canal

E. Occipital encephalocoele

F. None of the above

33. The following are true of Dandy-Walker malformation EXCEPT:

A. Due to failed or delayed development of the foramen of Magendie

B. Cystic dilatation of the 4th ventricle

C. Agenesis of the cerebellum and corpus callosum

D. Associated with cardiac and urinary tract abnormalities

E. Hydrocephalus

F. None of the above

34. The following are true of Miller-Dieker syndrome EXCEPT:

A. Associated with lissencephaly

B. Deletion of chromosome 17

C. Macrocephaly

D. Seizures

E. Cardiac defects

F. None of the above

35. The following statements are true of *caveolin-3* protein EXCEPT:

A. *Caveolin-3* protein is expressed exclusively in muscle cells.

B. A mutation in one *caveolin-3* allele produces an aberrant protein product capable of sequestering the normal *caveolin-3* protein in the Golgi apparatus of skeletal muscle cells.

C. Improper *caveolin-3* oligomerization and membrane localization result in skeletal muscle T-tubule system derangement, sarcolemmal membrane alterations, and large subsarcolemmal vesicle formation.

D. There are now over one dozen autosomal dominant *caveolin-3* mutations identified in the human population.

E. Mutations result in four distinct (sometimes overlapping) muscle disease phenotypes: limb-girdle muscular dystrophy, rippling muscle disease, distal myopathy, and hyperCKemia.

F. None of the above.

36. A 65-year-old woman with a known history of rheumatoid arthritis develops a constant headache, later followed by blurred vision. On examination, there is papilledema. ESR is slightly elevated, MRI shows an abnormal enhancement of the dura, including the sphenoid wing area. Biopsy of the dura reveals small mature lymphocytes, plasma cells, and epithelioid histiocytes, but no neoplasia, vasculitis, or infectious agents. The following statements are true EXCEPT:

A. This condition is commonly seen in rheumatoid arthritis, syphilis, Wegener's granulomatosis, tuberculosis, and cancer.

B. Headache, loss of vision, diplopia, ataxia, and seizures can be seen.

C. Corticosteroid therapy is the treatment of choice with minimal, if any, recurrence.

D. CSF cultures are almost always sterile.

E. None of the above.

37. The following statements are true of acute intermittent porphyria EXCEPT:

A. It is the most common of the disorders of pophyrin metabolism.

B. It results from an inherited partial deficiency of protopophyrin oxidase and is diagnosed by the excretion of excess ALA and porphobilinogen in the urine.

C. Its presentation is similar to hereditary coproporphyria and variegate porphyria.

D. Abdominal pain is the most common complaint.

E. None of the above.

38. The following statements are true about the genetics of epilepsy EXCEPT:

A. Both autosomal dominant and recessive modes of inheritance have been implicated in Juvenile Myoclonic Epilepsy (JME).

B. Five % of first-degree relatives of probands with JME develop epilepsy; over 30% of affected family members develop JME.

C. Susceptibility loci in JME have been reported in chromosomes 6q, 6p21.3, and 15q14.

D. Mutations in the CHRNA4 gene encoding the alpha-4 sub unit of the neuronal nicotinic acetylcholine receptor (nAChR) have been identified in idiopathic epilepsy autosomal dominant nocturnal frontal lobe epilepsy (ADN-FLE).

E. None of the above.

F. Two of the above.

39. The following statement(s) is/are true about Rett syndrome:

A. Rett syndrome is associated with mutations in the methyl-CpG binding protein 2 (MECP2) gene located on Xq28.

B. Typically, patients have a normal prenatal and perinatal period and a normal development in the first 6 months of life.

C. Both missense and nonsense mutations account for the majority of pathogenic mutations identified in Rett syndrome.

D. Patients with missense mutations carried a milder phenotype compared to those with truncating (nonsense) mutations.

E. All of the above.

F. Three of the above.

40. The following developmental milestone is NOT expected in a 12 month old child:

A. Waves good-bye

B. Stands alone

C. Seats self on the floor

D. Constantly responds with "no"

E. Prefers people over toys

F. None of the above

41. The following features can be found in a *dominant* parietal lobe lesion EXCEPT:

A. Alexia

B. Bilateral astereognosis

C. Bilateral ideomotor apraxia

D. Constructional apraxia

E. Dysgraphia, dyscalculia, right-left disorientation, and finger agnosia

F. None of the above

42. The following are true of Kluver-Bucy syndrome EXCEPT:

A. Usually affects posterior temporal lobe damage

B. Includes hyperorality and hypersexuality

C. They can be apathetic

D. None of the above

For items 43–45, match the following *callosal disconnection* features to their location:

A. Spleniun of the corpus callosum

B. Anterior corpus callosum

C. Complete callosotomy

43. Alien hand

44. Apraxia of the left hand

45. Alexia
46. The following statements are true regarding spinocerebellar ataxia (SCA) type 2 EXCEPT:
    A. It is an autosomal dominant condition discovered on chromosome 12q.
    B. Although the disease may have a variable phenotypic presentation, it is typically associated with slow saccades and/or ophthalmoplegia, ataxia, and peripheral neuropathy.
    C. Pathological studies show neuronal loss in the substantia nigra, striatum, and even neocortex, in addition to the degeneration of the olivopontocerebellar regions.
    D. It is responsible for an equal (minority) percentage of familial parkinsonism among whites and Asians.
    E. It can be associated with retinal degeneration and visual loss.
    F. Two of the above.

For questions 47–50, match the following neurocutaneous syndromes with their clinical characteristics/features:
    A. Neurofibromatosis type 1
    B. Neurofibromatosis type 2
    C. Tuberous sclerosis
    D. Ataxia telangiectasia
    E. Sturge-Webber syndrome
    F. von Hippel-Lindau disease
47. Axillary freckles
48. Pheochromocytoma, leukemia, and Wilms tumor
49. Adenoma sebacea
50. IgA and IgE immunodeficiency

ANSWERS TO THE PRACTICE QUESTIONS

1. B. *It is calcified less than 50% of the time.*
   The slide shows the "fried eggs" appearance typical of oligodendroglioma. This tumor commonly presents between ages 30 and 50 years. It is calcified in 50–90% of the time. Surgical resection and chemotherapy (usually with a good response) are the treatments.

2. E. *Five-year prognosis is less than 50% even after resection.*
   The slide shows "pseudorosettes" typical of ependymoma. Pseudorosettes can also be seen in retinoblastoma (Flexer-Wintersteiner rosettes) and medulloblastoma (Homer-Wright rosettes). Ependymomas occur most frequently in childhood and adolescence, with peak age between 10 and 15 years. Radiology often shows an intraventricular mass with contrast enhancement and calcifications. The treatment is surgical resection followed by radiation, which may include full spinal axis radiation. The 5-year survival rate is above 85% after resection.

3. D. *Dopamine.*
   Neurotransmitters such as dopamine, acetylcholine, norepinephrine, serotonin, and histamine are considered "intermediate concentration" neurotransmitters as they occur in the nanomole/gram concentration range. Glutamate, aspartate, GABA, and glycine occur in the micromole/gram ranges and are considered "high concentration" neurotransmitters. Nitric oxide and carbon monoxide are low concentration neurotransmitters.

4. B. *Latrotoxin.*
   The black widow spider acts by augmenting the release of acetylcholine (ACH) in the neuromuscular junction. While the rest act by blocking the release of ACH in the neuromuscular junction.

5. D. *Organophosphates.*
   Organophosphates (and Carbamates—a potent pesticide) are irreversible acetylcholinesterase inhibitors. Neostigmine, pyridostigmine, and physostigmine are reversible inhibitors.

6. A. *Tyrosine hydroxylase.*
   Tyrosine hydroxylase mediates the rate-limiting step in dopamine, epinephrine, and nor-epinephrine synthesis. DOPA decarboxylase requires Vitamin B_6 as a cofactor. NE is converted to epinephrine by phenylethanolamine-N-methyl transferase in the adrenal medulla only.

7. F. Alzheimer's type 1 and 2 astrocytes were described by Alois Alzheimer that indicates gliosis and astrocytosis. Alzheimer's type 1 astrocytes display abundant eosinophilic cytoplasm and can be seen in Alzheimer's disease (AD), Wilson's disease, and progressive multifocal leukoencephalopathy (PML). Alzheimer's type 2 cells are seen in hyperammonemic states and other hepatic disorders. The reaction consists exclusively of nuclear changes: swelling, contortion, central clearing of the chromatin, and the development of one or two prominent nucleoli.

8. F. *None of the above.*

   Neurofibrillary tangles are inclusions commonly seen in AD (along with granulovacuolar degeneration and Hirano bodies). It is also seen in other dementing conditions, Down syndrome, Lytico-Bodig disease, progressive supranuclear palsy, postencephalitic parkinsonism (von Economo disease), and dementia pugilistica. It can also be seen in tuberous sclerosis, meningioangiomatosis, and some ganglion cell tumors.

9. D. *Myotonic dystrophy.*

   Machado-Joseph disease, spinocerebellar ataxia type 6, spinobulbar atrophy, dentatopallidoluysian atrophy and Huntington's disease are due to excessive CAG repeats except for Myotonic dystrophy which is due to CTG repeats.

10. C. *Chromosome 19.*

    Chromosome 1 carries preseniline-2 protein, chromosome 14 carries preseniline-1, and chromosome 21 carries the amyloid precursor protein (APP) which have all been implicated in familial AD. Chromosome 19 carries APOE which is just a risk factor for AD and not implicated in familial AD.

11. C. *Chromosome 6.*

    Chromosome 2 carries park 3 that presents with autosomal dominant parkinsonism in the older population; chromosome 4 carries the alpha synuclein gene described in autosomal dominant early Parkinson's disease; chromosome 17 in autosomal dominant frontotemporal dementia with parkinsonism. Chromosome 6 carries the *parkin* gene in young-onset, usually autosomal recessive parkinsonism.

12. D. *Subcortical-thalamic area.*

    In a somatosensory evoked potential (SSEP), N9 represents the Erb's point; N13 represents the cervical cord; N18 represents the subcortical-thalamic area; N20 represents the thalamo-cortical area; and, P22 represents the hand region in the cortex.

13. D. *Limb-girdle muscular dystrophy.*

    Emery-Dreifuss syndrome, Duchene muscular dystrophy, and Beckers muscular dystrophy are X-linked dominant, except limb-girdle muscular dystrophy which is autosomal dominant (chromosome 5) or autosomal recessive (chromosome 15).

14. E. *X-linked dominant disorder.*

    Emery-Dreifuss is an X-linked recessive humeroperoneal muscular dystrophy presenting with biceps, triceps, and distal leg weakness, with contractures early in the course and cardiac conduction blocks. Pacemakers are often required.

15. D. *Elevated CPK.*

    Myotonic dystrophy is an autosomal dominant disorder (chromosome 19), usual onset is early childhood, and is characterized by premature frontal balding, protuberant lips, temporalis and masseter atrophy (giving the hatchet–face appearance), nasal voice, cardiac conduction abnormalities, testicular or ovarian atrophy, cataracts, retinal degeneration. CK is usually normal. EMG shows myotonia (spontaneous bursts of high-frequency and high-amplitude discharges) and pathology shows type 1 fiber hypertrophy and "ring fibers."

16. F. *Two of the above.*

    Muscle biopsy characteristics suggestive of myopathy include: fiber degeneration-regeneration (giving variable fiber size), myophagocytosis, fiber splitting, endomysial fibrosis, increased internal nuclei. Characteristics of neurogenic disease include: fiber-type groupings, group atrophy, and atrophic angular fibers of both type 1 and 2.

17. B. *Glycine.*

    Glycine, like GABA, stabilizes the membrane potential by increasing chloride conductance. Glycine is abundant in the spinal cord and brainstem while GABA is abundant in the higher centers. Strychnine non-competitively blocks glycine; tetanus toxin, in part, works by inhibiting release of glycine and GABA.

18. F. *Glycine.*
MK801 and Ketamine are non-competitive NMDA antagonists. Felbamate and lamotrigine both act on the NMDA receptor as well. Amantadine's anti-dyskinetic effect in PD has been attributed to its NMDA blocking effect. Mg and Zn are voltage blockers. Glycine, however, is obligate co-agonist acting at a different site on the receptor.

19. D. *Kennedy's disease.*
Although Kennedy's disease (adult bulbar muscular atrophy) is a trinucleotide repeat disease, it is X-linked recessive.

20. F. *None of the above.*
Tay-Sach's disease, Neimann-Pick disease, GM1 gangliosidosis, Sialidosis, and Mucolipidosis II can have a cherry-red spot.

21. G. *None of the above.*
In general, most of the metabolic disorders are autosomal recessive. Adrenoleukodystrophy, Hunter's disease, Ornithine transcarbamylase deficiency, and Lesch-Nyhan syndrome are a few of the exceptions. Duchene's and Becker's muscular dystrophy, Menkes syndrome are all X-linked recessive.

22. D. *Fragile X syndrome.*
Fragile X syndrome is an X-linked autosomal recessive disorder, while incontinentia pigmenti, Rett syndrome, and Aicardi syndrome are X-linked dominant; therefore only females can live to acquire the disorder.

23. F. *None of the above.*
Neurofibromatosis, tuberosclerosis, von Hippel-Landau disease, and Huntington's disease are all autosomal dominant disorders.

24. B. *GM2 gangliosidosis.*
GM1 gangliosidosis, Mucopolysaccharidosis, Mucolipidosis, and Zellweger's syndrome present with facial dysmorphism, gargoyle-like facial features, except GM2 gangliosidosis.

25. D. *Anterior.*
The anterior nuclei of the thalamus receives input from the mamillary nuclei of the hypothalamus, then projects to the cingulated gyrus.

26. A. *Ventral anterior.*
The ventral anterior nuclei project to the prefrontal, orbital, and premotor cortex. The ventral posterolateral and ventral posteromedial nuclei project to the sensory cortex, the lateral geniculate body project to the visual cortex, and the medial geniculate body project to the primary auditory cortex.

27. B. *Obesity.*
The feeding center is in the lateral hypothalamus and the satiety center is in the ventromedial nucleus. Damage to the feeding center leads to anorexia, while lesions in the satiety center lead to hyperphagia and obesity.

28. C. *Altered circadian rhythm.*
Many body changes are cyclically influenced by light-intensity changes that have a circadian rhythm. A retinosuprachiasmatic pathway reacts to changes in light intensity. Lesions in the suprachiasmatic nucleus cause loss of all circadian cycles.

29. E. *All of the above.*
All the statements are true regarding the autonomic nervous system. Curare and hexamethonium are nicotinic antagonists while atropine is a muscarinic antagonist. Yohimbine is an alpha2 antagonist while pheonxybenzamine, phenotolamine, and prazosin are

alpha1 antagonists. Alpha1 agonists are norepinephrine and phenylephrine, and an alpha2 agonist is clonidine.

30. E. *Globus pallidus.*

    The cortex, amygdale, putamen, and caudate are all derived from the telencephalon. The globus pallidus, including the thalamus and hypothalamus are derived from the diencephalon.

31. F. *None of the above.*

    The dorsal root ganglion, melanocytes, adrenal medulla, schwann cells, and preganglionic sympathetic neurons are all derived from the neural crest cells.

32. E. *Occipital encephalocoele.*

    Arnold-Chiari type 1 is characterized by displacement of the cerebellar tonsils into the cervical canal, causing a "kinked cord." In type 2, myelomeningocele, hydrocephalus, skull base and upper cervical spine defects, and displacement of the medulla and 4th ventricle into the cervical canal are present. Occipital encephalocoele is present in type 3.

33. F. *None of the above.*

    Dandy-Walker malformation is due to failed or delayed development of the foramen of Magendie. It is characterized by cystic dilatation of the 4th ventricle, cerebellar agenesis, hydrocephalus, agenesis of the corpus callosum, and is associated with cardiac and urinary tract abnormalities

34. C. *Macrocephaly.*

    Miller-Dieker syndrome is due to a deletion in chromosome 17. It is associated with lissencephaly and is characterized by microcephaly, hypotonia, craniofacial and genital defects, seizures, and cardiac defects.

35. D. *There are now over one dozen autosomal dominant caveolin-3 mutations identified in the human population.*

    Caveolin-3 protein is expressed exclusively in muscle cells. A mutation in one caveolin-3 allele produces an aberrant protein product capable of sequestering the normal *caveolin-3* protein in the Golgi apparatus of skeletal muscle cells. Improper *caveolin-3* oligomerization and membrane localization result in skeletal muscle T-tubule system derangement, sarcolemmal membrane alterations, and large subsarcolemmal vesicle formation. There are only 8 (not over a dozen) autosomal dominant *caveolin-3* mutations identified in the human population. Mutations result in 4 distinct (sometimes overlapping) muscle disease phenotypes: limb girdle muscular dystrophy, rippling muscle disease, distal myopathy, and hyperCKemia.

36. C. *Corticosteroid therapy is the treatment of choice with minimal, if any, recurrence.*

    This patient has idiopathic hypertrophic pachymeningitis, an uncommon disorder that causes a localized or diffuse thickening of the dura matter and has been associated with rheumatoid arthritis, syphilis, Wegener's granulomatosis, tuberculosis, and cancer. The main clinical features at presentation include headache, loss of vision, diplopia, papilledema, other cranial nerve involvement, ataxia, and seizures. MRI usually shows enhancement of the dura matter, ESR can be elevated, CSF may show lymphocytosis, but is always sterile. Biopsy of the dura shows infiltrates of small mature lymphocytes, plasma cells, and epitheliod histiocytes, but without neoplasia, vasculitis, or infectious agents. Corticosteroid therapy almost always improves vision and headache, but recurrence occurs in about half the cases, sometimes responsive to methotrexate or azathrioprine. (Neurology 2004; 62: 686–694).

37. B. *It results from an inherited partial deficiency of protopophyrin oxidase and is diagnosed by the excretion of excess ALA and porphobilinogen in the urine.*

Acute intermittent porphyria is an autosomal dominant condition resulting from the half-normal level of HMB synthease (also termed PBG deaminase), as a result, there is excess of ALA and porphobilinogen (PBG) in the urine. It is in variegate porphyria where the deficient enzyme is protopophyrin (PROTO) oxidase.

38. E. *None of the above.*
All of the above statements are correct. Both autosomal dominant and recessive modes of inheritance have been implicated in Juvenile Myoclonic Epilepsy (JME). Five % of first degree relatives of probands with JME develop epilepsy; over 30% of affected family members develop JME. Susceptibility loci in JME have been reported in chromosomes 6q, 6p21.3, and 15q14. Mutations in the CHRNA4 gene encoding the alpha-4 sub unit of the neuronal nicotinic acetylcholine receptor (nAChR) has been identified in idiopathic epilepsy autosomal dominant nocturnal frontal lobe epilepsy (ADN-FLE).

39. E. *All of the above.*
Rett syndrome is associated with mutations in the methyl-CpG binding protein 2 (MECP2) gene located on Xq28. Typically, patients have a normal prenatal, perinatal period and a normal development in the first 6 months of life. Both missense and nonsense mutations account for the majority of pathogenic mutations identified in Rett syndrome. Patients with missense mutations carried a milder phenotype compared to those with truncating (nonsense) mutations.

40. D. *Constantly responds with "no."*
Constantly responding with "no" is expected between 18 and 24 months. Waving good-bye, uttering first words, standing alone, opening cabinets, walking with some assistance, preferring people over toys, and seating self on the floor are all expected between 10 and 12 months.

41. D. *Constructional apraxia.*
Constructional apraxia is a feature of nondominant parietal lobe damage. Alexia, bilateral astereognosis, and bilateral ideomotor apraxia are features of dominant parietal lobe damage. The Gerstmann syndrome tetrad includes: dysgraphia, dyscalculia, right-left disorientation, and finger agnosia, which as a whole localizes to the dominant parietal lobe but individually are nonlocalizing.

42. A. *Usually affects posterior temporal lobe damage.*
Kluver-Bucy syndrome usually results from anterior temporal lobe damage. Hyperorality, hypersexuality, and apathy are common features.

43. C. *Complete callosotomy.*
Complete callosotomy can result in an alien hand syndrome.

44. B. *Anterior corpus callosum.*
Anterior corpus callosum lesions disconnect the right hemisphere motor and sensory integration centers from the left hemisphere language areas and result in apraxia of the left hand and agnosia of fingers on the left hand.

45. A. *Spleniun of the corpus callosum.*
Damage to the splenium prevents the right occipital lobe from communicating with language centers on the left, resulting in alexia, color anomia. However, the ability to copy words is spared as motor information crosses in the anterior corpus callosum.

46. F. *Two of the above.*
It is an autosomal dominant condition discovered on chromosome 12q. Although the disease may have a variable phenotypic presentation, it is typically associated with slow saccades and/or ophthalmoplegia, ataxia, and peripheral neuropathy. Pathological studies show neuronal loss in the substantia nigra, striatum, and even neocortex, in addition to

the degeneration of the olivopontocerebellar regions. It may be responsible for almost 10% of familial parkinsonism among Chinese, but rarely reported as a cause of parkinsonism among whites. SCA type 7 is commonly associated with retinal degeneration and visual loss. SCA type 2 and 17 is associated with cognitive impairment, and type 10 with seizures.

47. A. *NF Type 1.*

Neurofibromatosis type 1 is an autosomal dominant disorder, chromosome 17 characterized by café au lait spots, axillary freckles, Lisch nodules (white hamartomas in the iris), multiple cutaneous and subcutaneous tumors, acoustic neuromas, optic gliomas, spinal root tumors, pheochromocytoma, bone cysts, and pathologic bone fractures.

48. F. *von Hippel-Lindau disease.*

Also termed *hemangioblastoma of the cerebellum* is autosomal dominant in inheritance. Clinical features include ataxia and obstructive hydrocephalus. Cerebellar hemangioblastomas, retinal hemangioblastomas, hepatic and pancreatic cysts, renal tumors, polycythemia (because of increased erythropoietin), and pheochromocytoma are common.

49. C. *Tuberous sclerosis.*

Tuberous sclerosis is an autosomal dominant disease, chromosome 9. The classical triad of epilepsy, adenoma sebaceum, and mental deficiency is present in only one-third of patients. Primary criteria include: adenoma sebaceum, ungula fibroma, cerebral cortical tubers, subependymal nodules, and fibrous forehead plaques. Secondary criteria include: infantile spasms, ashleaf spots and shagreen patches, retinal hamartomas, phakomas, bilateral renal cysts, angiolipomas of the kidney, and rhabdomyosarcomas of the heart. Renal failure is the most common cause of death.

50. D. *Ataxia telangiectasia.*

Also called Louis-Bar syndrome is autosomal recessive in inheritance. The defect is in DNA repair. Clinical features include: ataxia, choreoathetosis, absent optokinetic nystagmus, apraxia of voluntary gaze, polyneuropathy, neoplasia especially lymphomas and gliomas, absent or decreased immunoglobulins.

INDEX

Note: Page references followed by *"f"* and *"t"* refer to figures and tables respectively.